PERONE dott. NICOLA
MEDICO CHIRURGO

NOVAK'S TEXTBOOK OF

Gynecology

EDMUND R. NOVAK, A.B., M.D. Assistant Professor in Gynecology, Johns Hopkins Medical School; Gynecologist, Johns Hopkins, Bon Secours, Hospital for the Women of Maryland, and Union Memorial Hospital, Baltimore

GEORGEANNA SEEGAR JONES, A.B., M.D. Associate Professor in Gynecology, Johns Hopkins Medical School, Baltimore

HOWARD W. JONES, JR., A.B., M.D. Associate Professor in Gynecology, Johns Hopkins Medical School, Baltimore

Seventh Edition

THE WILLIAMS & WILKINS COMPANY
Baltimore / 1965

First Edition, 1941

Second Edition, 1944

Third Edition, 1948
Reprinted February, 1950
Reprinted March, 1951

Fourth Edition, 1952
Reprinted June, 1953
Reprinted February, 1954
Reprinted July, 1955

Fifth Edition, 1956
Reprinted September, 1957

Sixth Edition, 1961
Reprinted May, 1962

Seventh Edition, 1965

Library of Congress Catalog Card Number 65–12648

Composed and Printed at the
Waverly Press, Inc.
Mount Royal and Guilford Avenues
Baltimore, Md.   21202   U.S.A.

TO OUR FAMILIES

Preface To The Seventh Edition

Our sixth edition of this textbook was the first in which the late Emil Novak did not participate. Although his guiding hand and dynamic style were sorely missed by us, most reviews were generally very complimentary towards our efforts. For this we are appreciative, and sincerely hope that this current edition will merit continued approval.

We have maintained the same general format that has been present since 1941. While several recent gynecological textbooks have utilized a panoramic approach with a progressive discussion of diseases in the female from birth through the postmenopausal era, we have always found this style inevitably led to considerable duplication and redundancy. This we hope to avoid.

Our aim is to provide the medical student with a thorough text, but one wherein the minutiae of our specialty are not overemphasized. For those who may, however, have a particular interest in any certain facet, we have attempted to provide an extensive and up to date bibliography for easy reference. Single case reports, however, unless dealing with an excessively rare problem, have generally been omitted.

Although certain critics have felt that our last edition's portrayal of vaginal and abdominal hysterectomy was "too much for the student, but not enough for the specialist," we have received overwhelming approval for continuance of this. Students and indeed graduates often welcome pictorial description of what amounts to approximately 90% of major operative gynecology. This has been repeated with appropriate revisions; indeed there have been few really major changes in this text. Yet the specialty of gynecology, especially endocrinology and cytogenetics, is so dynamic that a new edition of a book is almost archaic unless it is substantially revised every few years. This we have tried to accomplish along with new and improved pictures. The figures will be arranged in sequence for individual chapters rather than the whole; this allows late addition of any worthy pictures without completely disrupting the entire sequential order.

We are delighted to welcome Dr. Howard Jones as a co-author. In the last edition he was kind enough to make valuable contributions, and the reader familiar with his style will note fuller utilization of his considerable talents in this current text. We are most appreciative of Dr. John K. Frost for his diligent efforts in revising the rapidly changing and highly important cytopathological chapter. Dr. J. Donald Woodruff has continued to be generally helpful to us, especially in the chapters on the vulva and vagina, and to Don, as always, our thanks.

Lastly let us again acknowledge the excellent cooperation between the many nice people at The Williams and Wilkins Company and The W. B. Saunders Company for generously permitting interchange of many figures without specific acknowledgment. However, without Miss Helen Clayton in the office, and Miss Eva Hildebrandt in the laboratory, this textbook could never have gone into print, and these truly indispensable ladies are formally given our humble thanks.

THE AUTHORS

1

ANATOMY

The female reproductive organs are divisible into two groups, the external and internal. The former comprise the vulva and vagina; the latter the uterus, tubes, and ovaries.

THE VULVA

The vulva, representing the part of the genital apparatus visible externally, is a composite structure, its constituent parts being the following: (1) the labia majora, (2) mons pubis or mons veneris, (3) labia minora, (4) clitoris, (5) vestibule, (6) meatus urinarius, (7) vaginal orifice, (8) hymen (in virgins), and (9) vulvovaginal or Bartholin's glands.

Labia Majora. The labia majora are two longitudinal raised folds of adipose tissue covered by skin which, especially in brunettes, is rather heavily pigmented. They are markedly developed at puberty, as one of the secondary sex characters. Before puberty the vulva is rather flat, and the labia minora are much more conspicuous than the labia majora. In the postpuberal female, the latter extend posteriorly toward the perineum. On separating them posteriorly, a slightly raised connecting ridge, the *fourchette*, is seen. Just anterior to this, between it and the vaginal orifice, is a shallow, boat-shaped fossa, the *fossa navicularis*. The external surface of the labia shows a heavy growth of hair, usually curly, but the hair on the inner surface is much more sparse.

The substance of the labia majora is adipose tissue, although it contains also a light fascial layer which is the analogue of the dartos in the male. The labia themselves are to be looked upon as corresponding to the scrotum of the male. Mistakes in the diagnosis of the sex of pseudohermaphrodites have not infrequently been made because of the resemblance of the split scrotum to the labia majora of the vulva.

Mons Pubis. The mons pubis is a mound of fat covered by hair, situated just above the level of the symphysis pubis, at the lowest portion of the anterior abdominal wall.

Labia Minora. The labia minora are two firm pigmented folds which extend from the clitoris posteriorly to about two-thirds of the distance toward the perineum. Anteriorly they subdivide, one fold covering the glans clitoridis to form its prepuce (preputium clitoridis), the other passing beneath the glans to form, with its fellow of the opposite side, the frenulum clitoridis.

The skin covering the labia minora is devoid of hair follicles, but is very rich in sebaceous glands. Sudoriferous glands are exceedingly sparse, and, according to some, completely absent. The substance of the labia minora is described as being of the erectile type, though the degree of erectility is not comparable to that of the clitoris. It contains many venous spaces with much involuntary muscle tissue.

Clitoris. The clitoris is a small, cylin-

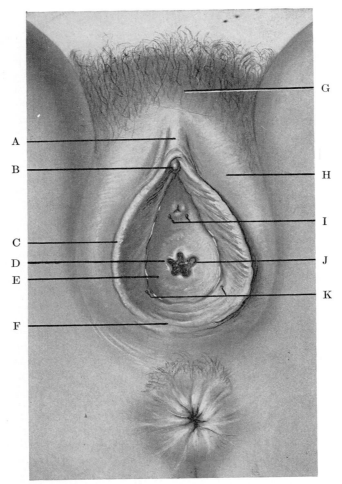

FIG. 1.1. The vulva. *A*, prepuce; *B*, clitoris; *C*, labia minora; *D*, hymen; *E*, vestibule; *F*, posterior commissure; *G*, mons pubis; *H*, labia majora; *I*, opening of Skene's ducts; *J*, vagina; and *K*, vulvovaginal (Bartholin's) glands.

drical, erectile organ corresponding to the male penis. Like the latter it consists of a glans, a corpus or body, and the crura. Only the *glans clitoridis*, about 6 to 8 mm. in diameter, is visible externally between the two folds into which the labia minora bifurcates anteriorly, the upper fold forming the *prepuce* and the lower the *frenulum* of the clitoris. The *body* extends upward toward the pubes beneath the skin dividing into two *crura* which are attached to the pubic bones. The clitoris is made up of erectile tissue, with many large and small venous channels surrounded by large amounts of involuntary

muscle tissue. The erectile tissue is arranged in two corpora cavernosa, and there is no corpus spongiosum as in the case of the male organ.

Vestibule. The vestibule is the boat-shaped fossa which becomes visible on separation of the labia. In it are seen the vaginal orifice and, anterior to this, the meatus urinarius. In the virgin the former is partly occluded by the *hymen*, a rather rigid membrane of firm connective tissue covered on both sides by stratified squamous epithelium. It is most frequently of annular or crescentic shape, but it may be cribiform or sievelike.

Under abnormal conditions it may be imperforate, occluding the vaginal orifice completely and leading to retention of the menstrual discharge.

Meatus Urinarius. The urethral meatus is the small slitlike or triangular external orifice of the urethra. It is visible in the vestibule, at about two-thirds of the distance from the glans clitoridis to the vaginal orifice. At each side of the meatus one usually sees a small pitlike depression in which there are a number of mucous glands, called the lesser glands of the vestibule, to distinguish them from the greater glands, which are the glands of Bartholin.

Just below the outer part of the meatus are the orifices of the *paraurethral or Skene's ducts*, which run in a tortuous fashion below and parallel to the urethra for a distance of about 1½ cm. Except near the orifice, where one finds stratified epithelium, the paraurethral ducts are lined by a transitional type of epithelium.

The *female urethra*, opening externally at the meatus, is lined proximally by a stratified transitional type of epithelium, while its distal portion is covered with stratified squamous epithelium which extends into the canal for a variable but considerable distance. The studies of Huffman have shown that the canal is surrounded by a labyrinth of *paraurethral glands* which he considers to be the homologues of the male prostate. Some of these paraurethral canals enter into the urethra and some into Skene's ducts which open just below the urethral meatus. Their chief clinical importance lies in the fact that they frequently harbor the Gonococcus, the infection often being intractable to any treatment except exci-

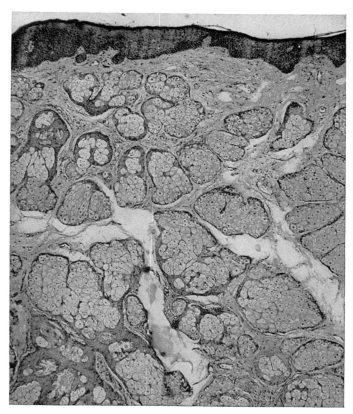

Fig. 1.2. Histological structure of labium minus, near clitoris, showing large number of sebaceous glands.

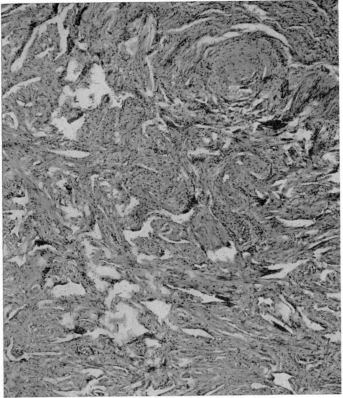

Fig. 1.3. Microscopic structure of clitoris

sion or destruction of the ducts. In addition, *suburethral diverticula* may occur as a sequel to infection and cystic enlargement of these glands.

Vulvovaginal or Bartholin's Glands. The vulvovaginal or Bartholin's glands are lobulated racemose glands situated one on each side of the vaginal orifice, at about its middle, and placed deeply in the perineal structures. They are frequently the seat of gonorrheal or other infections.

The main duct of the gland is lined by a stratified transitional type of epithelium, except for a very short distance within the orifice. As the ducts become smaller and smaller, the epithelium is flatter and flatter, so that in the finest branches it consists of a single layer of flat cells. The acini are lined by a layer of cuboidal cells with basal nuclei. The function of the gland is the secretion of mucus for lubri-

cation of the vaginal orifice and canal, especially during coitus.

THE VAGINA

The vagina is a musculomembranous canal which connects the vulva with the uterus. It is about 9 or 10 cm. in length, and, in the erect position of the woman, its direction is in general upward and backward from its vulvar to its uterine end. Its upper end expands into the cup-shaped *fornix*, into which the cervix uteri is fitted. The portions of the fornix in front of, behind, and at the sides of the cervix are designated as the anterior, posterior, and lateral fornices. The posterior fornix is of special surgical interest because it gives ready access to the peritoneal cavity, as the upper fourth or so of the posterior wall of the vagina is covered by peritoneum.

In the virgin, the *mucous membrane* of

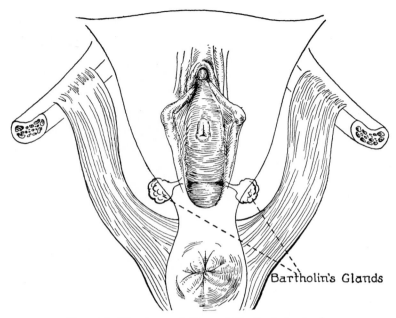

FIG. 1.4. The deep relations of Bartholin's glands

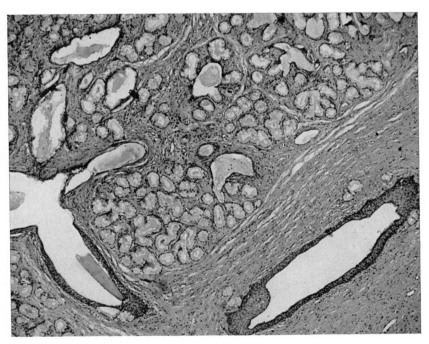

FIG. 1.5. Microscopic appearance of normal Bartholin's gland. Note the transitional epithelium in the large ducts, the flattened epithelium in the small ducts, and the cuboidal secretory epithelium in the gland acini.

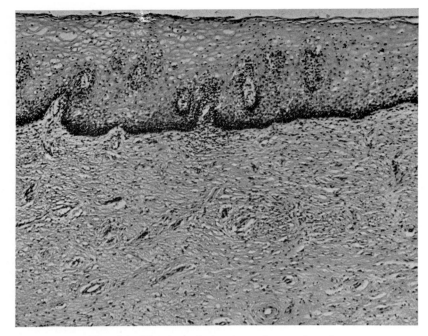

FIG. 1.6. Histological structure of normal vagina

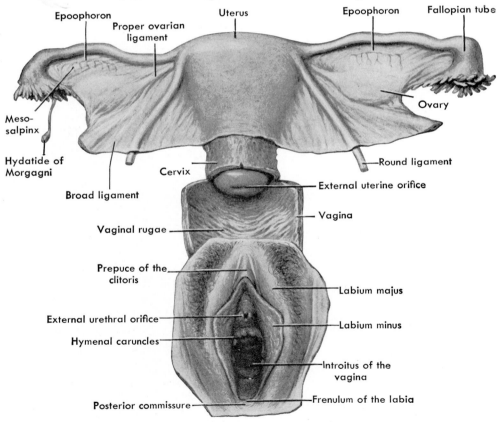

FIG. 1.7. The female reproductive organs. (From Rubin, I. C., and Novak, J.: *Integrated Gynecology, Principles and Practice*, Vol. 1. Blakiston Division, McGraw-Hill Book Company, Inc., New York, 1956.)

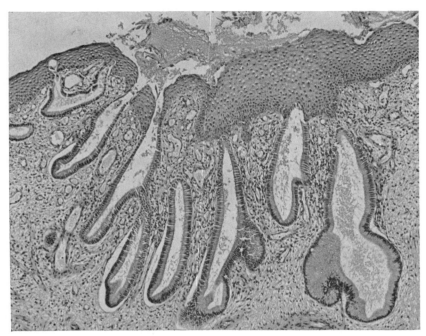

FIG. 1.8. Showing cervical glands opening on stratified squamous epithelium of cervix, as they often do in chronic inflammatory conditions (see Chapter 11).

the anterior vaginal wall is horizontally corrugated, with a central vertical ridge, thus producing the arbor vitae appearance. These ridges are absent in the widened canal of the woman who has borne children.

The mucous membrane of the vagina is reddish pink, and is lined by a stratified squamous epithelium into which project many tiny subepithelial papillae of the subjacent fibrous tissue. In the young child the epithelium shows only perhaps six or eight layers of cells, but in the postpuberal phase many more layers are present.

Beneath the mucous membrane is the muscular coat, made up of an inner circular and an outer layer. The outermost layer is the fibrous, derived from the pelvic connective tissue.

Cervix. The cervix is separated from the corpus externally by a slight constriction corresponding to the region of the internal os. The portion of the cervix above the level of the vagina is the supravaginal portion, that protruding into the vagina is the *pars or portio vaginalis*. The

cervical canal is somewhat spindle-shaped, terminating below at the *external os*, a small round or transversely slitlike opening averaging in the nulliparous woman about 5 mm. in diameter. At its upper end the cervical canal communicates with the uterine cavity through a constricted orifice called the *internal os*.

The *mucous membrane* covering the external or vaginal surface is of the stratified squamous variety, a continuation of that covering the adjacent vagina. From it arises the squamous cell or epidermoid carcinoma of the cervix, the most common of all gynecological forms of cancer. The cervical canal, on the other hand, is lined by an entirely different type of mucous membrane, the endocervix, which is distinguished by the following features.

(1) A tall, "picket" variety of columnar epithelium, with deeply stained nuclei placed close to the basement membrane, and a cytoplasm which is rich in mucin. There is a rather abrupt transition between this epithelium and the stratified squamous epithelium of the pars vaginalis

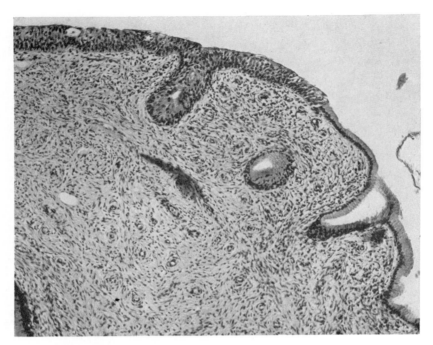

FIG. 1.9. Showing rather abrupt transition between columnar and stratified squamous epithelium of cervix in vicinity of external os.

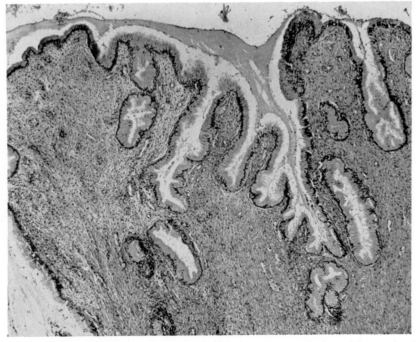

FIG. 1.10. Microscopic appearance of cervix, showing characteristic "picket" gland epithelium, racemose glands, and spindle-celled fibrous stroma.

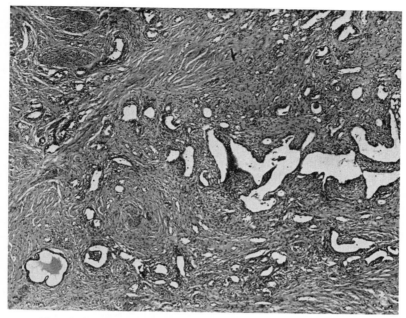

Fig. 1.11. Mesonephric tubules deep in the cervical substance

at or near the external os, and it is at this transition area that cancer is most apt to develop. *[handwritten annotation]*

(2) Glands of the racemose variety, lined by epithelium like that found on the surface.

(3) Stroma of fibrous tissue type, rich in spindle cell elements. *[handwritten annotation]*

The muscular coat of the cervix is well developed in the region of the internal os, but becomes increasingly sparse at a lower level, so that only a thin outer layer is present in the lower portion of the cervix, with a corresponding increase in the proportion of connective tissue. Glandlike vestiges of the mesonephric duct are occasionally observed deep in the cervical musculature.

THE UTERUS

The uterus is a hollow, thick-walled muscular organ which is situated in the pelvis, between the bladder anteriorly and the rectum posteriorly. It is placed almost at right angles to the vagina, with the bladder below and in front of it. It is somewhat pear-shaped, and measures in the nulliparous woman about 8 to 9 cm. in length, 6 cm. in its widest portion, and about 4 cm. in thickness. It is divisible into a *corpus* or body, and a *cervix* or neck. The upper domelike portion of the corpus is called the *fundus*, while the angle marking the attachment of the tube at each side is the *cornu*. The *uterine cavity* is rather conical, with the base above at the fundus and the apex, corresponding to the narrow internal os, leading into the cervical canal. Externally the corpus is covered with peritoneum.

The mucous membrane of the uterine body is the *endometrium*. This varies in thickness not only in individual women, but even more at different phases of the menstrual cycle. In general it is thinnest just after the periods, gradually increasing in thickness until just before the beginning of the next menstrual period, as will be described subsequently.

The *stroma* is a characteristic immature type of connective tissue, made up of a homogeneous mass of small cells with round or slightly oval nuclei and, in the early stages of the cycle, almost no cytoplasm. They are supported by an almost invisible light fibrillary supporting structure. The vascular supply of the endometrium is through two sets of vessels,

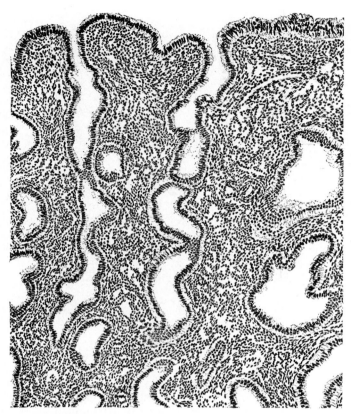

FIG. 1.12. Histology of endometrium. This, however, undergoes striking cyclical changes, which are described and illustrated in Chapter 4.

the spiral or coiled arterioles and the basal arterioles. The latter are the chief nutritional vessels, supplying especially the basal layers. The spiral arterioles, on the other hand, play an important part in the mechanism of the menstrual cycle and especially in menstrual bleeding.

The *muscular* coat of the uterus is made up of involuntary muscle fibers arranged in an interlacing fashion which, at least in the nonpregnant woman, is not disposed in any definite layer pattern. The serous coat consists of the peritoneum, which covers the entire corpus uteri.

The Ligaments of the Uterus. These are three in number on each side, as follows.

Broad Ligaments. Each of these consists of a broad double sheet of peritoneum which extends from the lateral surface of the uterus outward to the pelvic wall. At its upper border the broad ligament encircles the fallopian tube, and beyond the tube continues on to the pelvic wall as the *infundibulopelvic ligament,* through which the ovarian vessels make their way toward the tube and ovary. From the lower edge of the tube the broad ligament extends downward to surround the round ligament, this portion constituting a sort of tubal mesentery, or *mesosalpinx.* In this portion is found the parovarium (epoophoron or organ of Rosenmüller), which represents the lateral portions of the vestigial remains of the mesonephric tubules. To its medial side lies the paroophoron, likewise made up of vestigial mesonephric tubules, which, like those of the epoophoron, empty into the main mesonephric, or Wolffian, duct. It is the latter which in the male develops into the vas deferens. At its lower border the

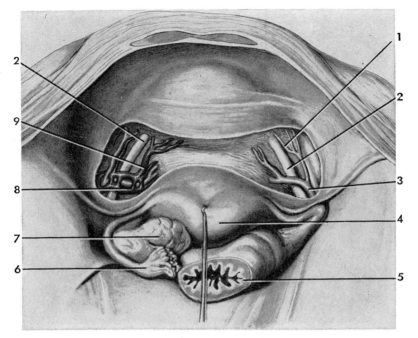

Fig. 1.13. The topic relationship between ureter and uterine vessels. *On the left side* both the arteries and veins are drawn; *on the right side*, only the arteries. *1*, Cervical branch of uterine artery; *2*, ureter; *3*, uterine artery; *4*, uterus; *5*, rectum; *6*, fallopian tube; *7*, ovary; *8*, uterine veins; and *9*, vesical vein. (From Rubin, I. C., and Novak, J.: *Integrated Gynecology, Principles and Practice*, Vol. 1. Blakiston Division, McGraw-Hill Book Company, Inc., New York, 1956; as redrawn from Tandler, J.: In *Handbuch der Gynäkologie*, Ed. 3, edited by W. Stoeckel, Vol. 1. J. F. Bergmann, Munich, 1930.)

broad ligament is thickened, with a condensation of connective tissue and some muscle fibers, forming the thonglike *cardinal ligament or ligamentum colli of Mackenrodt*. This structure is of prime importance in the support of the uterus, and its elongation is the chief cause of uterine prolapse.

Between the two layers of peritoneum which make up the broad ligament there is to be found, in addition to the structures already mentioned, a considerable amount of connective tissue, a small amount of involuntary muscle tissue, blood vessels, and nerves.

The Round Ligaments. These are two round, muscular bands which arise from the lateral aspect of the fundus on each side, a short distance below and anterior to the insertion of the tube. They course outward between the broad ligament layers in a curved fashion to the internal

inguinal ring, passing then through the inguinal canal, and spreading out in a fan-like fashion to fuse with the connective tissue of the groin. The thickness of these ligaments is very variable, but averages about 5 o 6 mm. They are made up of involuntary muscle continuous with that of the uterus itself, and their function seems to prevent retrodisplacement. They are probably more important during pregnancy, when they undergo marked hypertrophy.

Uterosacral Ligaments. The uterosacral ligaments are peritoneal folds containing, in addition to connective tissue, a considerable amount of involuntary muscle. They arise on each side from the posterior wall of the uterus at about the level of the internal os, and pass backward toward the rectum, around which they extend to their insertion on the sacral wall at about the junction of the second and third sacral

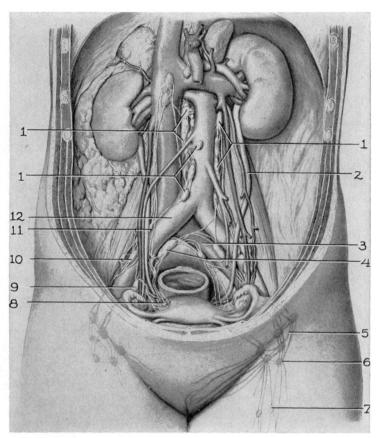

F<small>IG</small>. 1.14. The lymphatic system of the abdomen and pelvis. *1*, Lumbar or aortic nodes; *2*, ureter; *3*, common iliac vein; *4*, sacral lymph nodes; *5*, inguinal lymph nodes; *6*, subinguinal or inguinofemoral lymph nodes; *7*, femoral lymph nodes; *8*, parametric gland of Championière; *9*, hypogastric lymph node; *10*, external iliac lymph nodes; *11*, common iliac lymph nodes; and *12*, common iliac artery. (From Rubin, I. C., and Novak, J.: *Integrated Gynecology, Principles and Practice*, Vol. 1, Blakiston Division, McGraw-Hill Book Company, Inc., New York, 1956.)

vertebrae. In their course backward they describe an arclike curve, the concavity being directed toward the midline. They play an important part in the support of the uterus and cervix, so that when they are elongated the cervix sags abnormally downward and forward. In addition, they probably contain sensory nerve fibers which play a part in the production of dysmenorrhea.

Blood Supply. The blood supply of the uterus is derived from the ovarian and uterine arteries. The former, which correspond to the spermatic arteries of the male, arises from the abdominal aorta,

(the ovarian a.)

passing down behind the peritoneum to the infundibulopelvic ligament, through which it enters the mesosalpinx to supply the tube and ovary, finally anastomosing with the uterine artery to complete the utero-ovarian vascular arch.

The uterine artery arises from the anterior branch of the hypogastric artery, passing toward the uterus through the parametrium. It turns upward about $1\frac{1}{2}$ or 2 cm. lateral to the cervix, coursing upward in an extremely tortuous fashion to anastomose with the ovarian and giving off many branches to the uterine wall as it courses upward. As it turns upward at

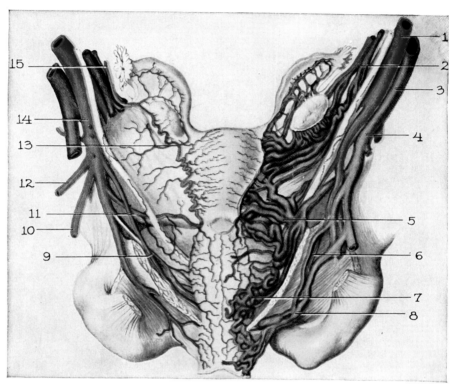

PLATE I.I. Arteries and veins of the female genital organs as seen from the dorsal side. *1*, Common iliac artery; *2*, ovarian plexus; *3*, common iliac vein; *4*, internal or hypogastric iliac vein; *5*, uterine venous plexus; *6*, internal pudendal artery; *7*, vaginal venous plexus; *8*, internal pudendal vein; *9*, vaginal arteries; *10*, caudal or inferior gluteal artery; *11*, uterine artery; *12*, cranial or superior gluteal artery; *13*, anastomosis between uterine and ovarian arteries; *14*, internal iliac or hypogastric artery; and *15*, ovarian artery. (From Rubin, I. C., and Novak, J.: *Integrated Gynecology, Principles and Practice*, Vol. 1. Blakiston Division, McGraw-Hill Book Company, Inc., New York, 1956.)

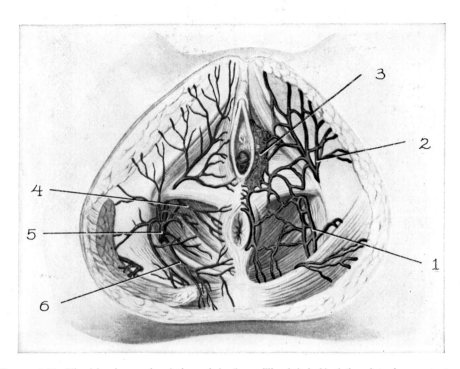

PLATE I.II. The blood vessels of the pelvic floor. The *left half of the plate* demonstrates the ramification of the internal pudendal artery; *the right side* shows the tributaries of the internal pudendal vein. *1*, Internal pudendal vein; *2*, anastomoses between pudendal and cutaneous veins; *3*, bulbus vestibuli; *4*, transverse perineal artery; *5*, internal pudendal artery; and *6*, inferior hemorrhoidal artery. (From Rubin, I. C., and Novak, J.: *Integrated Gynecology, Principles and Practice*, Vol. 1. Blakiston Division, McGraw-Hill Book Company, Inc., New York, 1956; as redrawn from Tandler, J.: In *Handbuch der Gynäkologie*, Ed. 3, edited by W. Stoeckel, Vol. 1. J. F. Bergmann, Munich, 1930.)

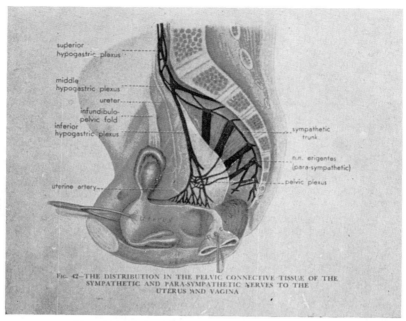

FIG. 42—THE DISTRIBUTION IN THE PELVIC CONNECTIVE TISSUE OF THE
SYMPATHETIC AND PARA-SYMPATHETIC NERVES TO THE
UTERUS AND VAGINA

FIG. 1.15. Sympathetic nerve pathways to pelvis

the level of the cervicovaginal juncture it is in close relation to the ureter, which passes *downward and inward*, behind the artery, on its course to the bladder. This is an exceedingly important relationship for the surgeon to bear in mind, as injury to the ureter is the chief bugbear in the operation of panhysterectomy.

The veins correspond in a general way with the arteries. The ovarian veins, on their way from the hilum of the ovary toward the vena cava, form, between the layers of the broad ligament, a rich network called the *pampiniform plexus*. On the right side the ovarian vein empties into the inferior cava itself, on the left into the left renal vein. The uterine veins follow the arteries and empty into the internal iliac veins.

Nerve Supply of the Female Genitalia. The genital tract is supplied by branches of both the autonomic and spinal nerve pathways. In the human certain higher centers as well as the *tuber cinereum* are of importance in regulating various sexual and menstrual functions, and one must always be cognizant of the highly important hypothalamic-

hypophyseal domination of ovarian function.

Various sympathetic and parasympathetic fibers of the *autonomic* system below the bifurcation of the aorta form the superior hypogastric plexus or presacral nerve, which is the chief supply of the uterus. As they pass caudal, they form the ganglion of Frankenhäuser or uterovaginal plexus located near the base of the uterosacral ligaments.

The clinician should be aware that the presacral nerve as it crosses the sacral promontory has fibers immediately adherent under the posterior peritoneum as well as others which directly overlie the bony protuberance. Both of these must be divided in the surgical procedure of presacral neurectomy, which is utilized in treating difficult cases of dysmenorrhea. The ovary is supplied not by the sacral fibers, but rather by branches of the renal and aortic plexuses which are located in the suspensory ligaments of the ovary.

The pudendal nerve of the *spinal* nervous system is the primary source of motor and sensory activation of the lower genital tract. This is derived from roots of

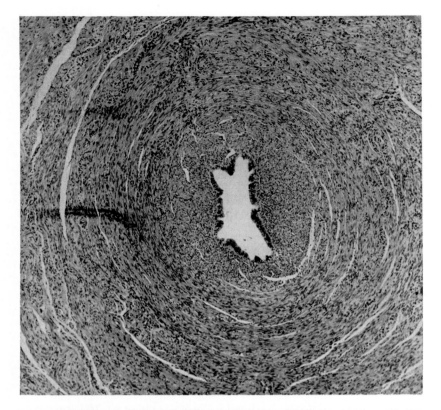

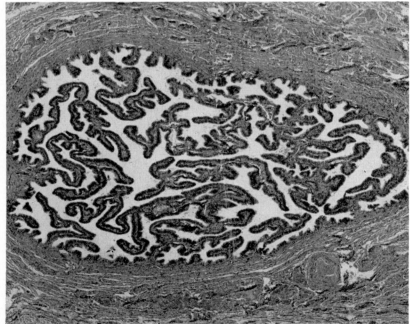

FIG. 1.16. Tube. *Top*, isthmic; *bottom*, ampullary portion

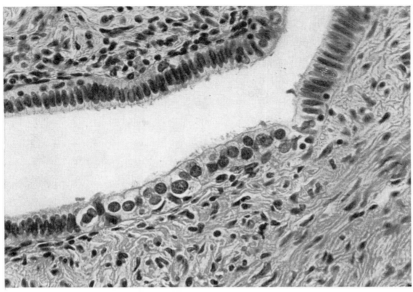

Fig. 1.17. The tubal epithelium, showing both ciliated and nonciliated cells. This epithelium exhibits definite cyclical changes in height and other characteristics.

the second, third, and fourth sacral nerves. It passes out of the pelvis via the greater and lesser *sciatic foramina*, and enters the pudendal canal of the *obturator fascia*. Various branches supply vulva, vagina, and perineum. Other nerves such as the ilioinguinal, genitofemoral, and cutaneous femoral nerve also contribute to the lower genital tract and perineum, but for details one is urged to consult appropriate neuroanatomical texts.

THE FALLOPIAN TUBES

The tubes are two musculomembranous canals which transport the ova from the ovaries to the uterus. They are about 11 or 12 cm. in length, and are divisible, for purposes of description, into four parts. (1) The *interstitial portion* is the narrow portion contained in the muscular wall of the uterus, which the tube penetrates to reach the uterine cavity. The uterine os of the tube is extremely minute, being about the diameter of a hairbrush bristle. (2) The *isthmus* is the narrow portion of the tube close to its insertion into the uterine cornu. (3) The *ampulla* is the wider, baggier middle portion of the tube. (4) The distal third or so is the *fimbriated extremity*, which is rather funnel-shaped,

the small orifice being surrounded by a number of peaked fringes or fimbriae.

Histologically, the tube consists of three coats, as follows: (1) the *serous coat*, which is formed by the encircling peritoneum of the upper margin of the broad ligament; (2) the *muscular coat*, arranged for the most part in an inner circular and an outer longitudinal layer; and (3) the *mucosa*, or endosalpinx, which is disposed in longitudinal folds or rugae, usually only three or four in number at the isthmus, but branching and subbranching longitudinally toward the fimbriated extremity, so that a cross section of the latter presents a very arborescent appearance as compared with the few folds at the isthmus. The lining *epithelium* is composed of a single layer of cells, superimposed on a rather cellular tunica propria. Like the uterine epithelium, the epithelium of the tube undergoes definite cyclical changes, although these are much less conspicuous than in the uterus.

THE OVARIES

The ovaries are two ovoid bodies which constitute the genital glands of the female. They are placed, one in each side of the pelvis, just below the tubes, the

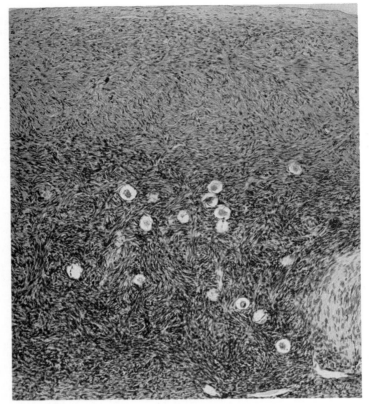

FIG. 1.18. Section of ovary showing primordial follicles and typical spindle-celled stroma

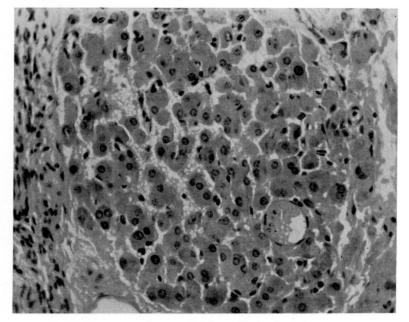

FIG. 1.19. Cluster of hilus cells in the ovary

Dorfman, R. I.: Determination of plasma estrone and estradiol-17B. Anal. Biochem., 5: 1963.

Ito, Y., and Higashi, K.: Studies on the prolactin-like substance in human placenta. II. Endocr. Japn., 8: 279, 1961.

Ittrich, G. von: Eine Methode zur chemischen Bestimmung von östrogenen Hormonen in Blut, Milch and Colostrum. Hoppe Seyler. Z. Physiol. Chem., 320: 103, 1960.

Johnson, S. G.: A clinical routine method for the quantitative determination of gonadotrophins in 24-hour urine samples. II. Normal values for men and women and all age groups from puberty to senscence. Acta Endocr. (Kobenhavn), 31: 209, 1959.

Jones, G. E. S., Delfs, E., and Stran, H. M.: Chorionic gonadotrophin and pregnanediol values in normal pregnancy. Bull. Johns Hopkins Hosp., 75: 359, 1944.

Jones, G. E. S., Gey, G. O., and Gey, M. K.: Hormone production by placental cells maintained in continuous culture. Bull Hopkins Hosp., 72: 26, 1946.

Josimovich, J. B., and Atwood, B. L.: Human placental lactogen (HPL), a trophoblastic hormone synergizing with chorionic gonadotropin and potentiating the anabolic effects of pituitary growth hormone. Amer. J. Obstet. Gynec., 88: 7, 1964.

Kaiser, I. H.: Histologic appearance of coiled arterioles in the endometrium of rhesus monkey, baboon, chimpanzee, and gibbon. Amer. J. Obstet. Gynec., 55: 699, 1948.

Kanematsu, S., Hilliard, J., and Sawyer, C. H.: The effect of reserpine on pituitary prolactin content and its hypothalamic site of action in the rabbit. Acta Endocr. (Kobenhavn), 44: 467, 1963.

Klooper, A., Strong, J. A., and Cook, L. R.: The excretion of pregnanediol and adrenocortical activity. J. Endocr., 15: 180, 1957.

Knauer, E.: Die Ovarientransplantation. Experimentelle Studie. Arch. Gynaek., 60: 322, 1900.

Kobayashi, T., Kigawa, T., Mizuno, M., and Amenomani, Y.: Influence of rat hypothalamic extracts and rat pituitary cells in tissue culture. Endocr. Jap., 10: 1, 1963.

Kumar, D., Azoury, R. S., and Barnes, A. C.: Studies on human premature births. I. Placental progesterone concentrations. Amer. J. Obstet. Gynec., 87: 126, 1963.

Lazo-Wasem, E. A., Neher, G. M., Shoger, R. L., and Zarrow, M. V.: Gelbkörperhormon in Blute männlicher Wirbeltiere. Endokrinologie, 31: 166, 1954.

Levan, A. B., and Szanto, P. B.: Frequency of anovulatory menstruation as determined by endometrial biopsy. Amer. J. Obstet. Gynec., 48: 75, 1944.

Li, C. H., Simpson, M. E., and Evans, H. M.: Physio-chemical characteristics of the interstitial cell stimulating hormone from sheep pituitary glands. J. Amer. Chem. Soc., 64: 367, 1942.

Loewe, S., and Lange, F.: Der Gehalt des Frauenharnes an brunsterzeugenden Stoffen in Abhängigkeit vom ovariellen Zyklus. Klin. Wschr., 5: 1038, 1926.

Longchampt, J. E., Gual, C. Ehrenstein, M., and Dorfman, R. I.: 19-Hydroxy-Δ⁴-androstene-3,17-dione an intermediate in estrogen biosynthesis. Endocrinology, 66: 3, 1960.

Loraine, J. A.: The renal clearance of chorionic gonadotrophin in normal pathological pregnancy. Quart. J. Exp. Physiol., 36: 11, 1950.

Lyons, W. R.: Preparation and assay of mammotropin. In Cold Spring Harbor Symposia on Quantitative Biology, Vol. 5, p. 198. Long Island Biological Association, Cold Spring Harbor, Long Island, New York, 1937.

MacCorquodale, D. W., Thayer, S. A., and Doisy, E. A.: The isolation of the principal estrogenic substance of liquor folliculi. J. Biol. Chem., 115: 435, 1936.

Macht, D. I.: Further historical and experimental studies on menstrual toxin. Amer. J. Med. Sci., 206: 281, 1943.

Marcotty, A.: Uber das Corpus Luteum menstruationis und das Corpus luteum graviditatis. Arch. Gynaek., 103: 63, 1914.

Markee, J. E.: Menstruation in intraocular endometrial transplants in the rhesus monkey. Contrib. Embryol., 28: 219, 1940.

Markee, J. E.: Morphological basis for menstrual bleeding. Antat. Rec., 94: 481, 1946.

Markee, J. E., Sayer, C. H., and Hollinsdead, W. H.: Adrenergic control of release of luteinizing hormone from hypophysis of rabbit. Recent Progr. Hormone Res., 2: 117, 1948.

Marrian, G. F.: The chemistry of oestrin. I. Preparation from urine and the separation from an unidentified solid alcohol. Biochem. J., 23: 1090, 1929.

Marrian, G. F.: Newly discovered urinary oestrogen metabolites. Acta Endocr. (Kobenhavn), 31: 27, 1957.

Marrian, G. F.: The urinary estrogens and their quantitative determination. Cancer, 10: 704, 1957.

Marsh, J. M., and Savard, K.: The activation of luteal phosphorylase by luteinizing hormone. J. Biol. Chem., 239: 1, 1964.

Mason, N. R., and Savard, K.: Conversion of cholesterol to progesterone by corpus luteum slices. Endocr. 75: 215, 1964.

McCann, S. M.: A hypothalamic luteinizing-hormone-releasing factor. Amer. J. Physiol., 202: 395, 1962.

McCann, S. M.: Effect of progesterone on plasma luteinizing hormone activity. Amer. J. Physiol., 202: 601, 1962.

McCann, S. M., Taleisnik, S., and Friedman,

H. M.: LH-Releasing activity in hypothalamic extracts. Proc. Soc. Exp. Biol. Med., *104:* 432, 1960.

Meites, J., Kahn, R. H., and Nicoll, C. S.: Prolactin production by rat pituitary "in vitro." Proc. Soc. Exp. Biol. Med., *108:* 440, 1961.

Myer, R.: Anovulatory cycle and menstruation. Amer. J. Obstet. Gynec., *51:* 39, 1946.

Noall, M. W., Alexander, F., and Allen, W. M.: Dehydroisandrosterone synthesis by the human ovary. Biochim. Biophys. Acta, *59:* 520, 1962.

Novak, E.: Superstition and folklore of menstruation. Bull. Hopkins Hosp., *29:* 270, 1916.

Noyes, R. W., Hertig, A. T., and Rock, J.: Dating the endometrial biopsy. Fertil. Steril. *1:* 3, 1950.

Odell, W. D., Swain, R. W., and Nydick, M.: The molecular weight of HPG as determined by radiation inactivation of biological activity. J. Clin. Endocr., *24:* 1266, 1964.

Odevlad, E., and Bostrom, H.: A Time-picture relation study with autoradiography on the uptake of labelled sulphate in the graafian follicles of the rabbit. Acta Radiol., *39:* 137, 1953.

Oertel, G. W.: Konzentration von oestrogenen in plasma nicht-schwangerer frauen. Klin. Wschr., *39:* 492, 1961.

Oertel, G. W., Weiss, S. P., and Eik-Nes, K. B.: Determination of progesterone in human blood plasma. J. Clin. Endocr., *19:* 213, 1959.

Palmer, A.: Basal body temperature determination in the management of menstrual disorders. Clin. Obstet. Gynec., *2:* 153, 1959.

Parker, F., Jr., and Tenney, B., Jr.: Further studies of hormone content of human tissues in pregnancy. Endocrinology, *26:* 527, 1940.

Parkes, A. S., and Bruce, H. M.: Pregnancy block in female mice placed in boxes soiled by males. J. Reprod. Fertil., *4:* 303, 1962.

Pearlman, W. H., and Thomas, M.: The progesterone content of human placental blood. Endocr., *52:* 590, 1953.

Peters, J. P., Man, E. B., and Heinemann, M.: Pregnancy and the thyroid gland. Yale J. Biol. Med., *20:* 499, 1948.

Pflüger, E.: *Uber die Bedentung und Ursuche der menstruation.* Berlin, 1865.

Preedy, J. R. K., and Aitken, E. H.: Plasma-oestrogen levels in late pregnancy, in the normal menstruating female, and in the male. Lancet, *1:* 191, 1957.

Purves, H. D., and Griesbach, W. E.: The site of thyrotropin and gonadotrophin production in the rat pituitary studies by McManus-Hotchkiss staining for glycoprotein. Endocrinology, *49:* 244, 1951.

Riddle, O., and Bates, R. W.: Concerning anterior pituitary hormones. Endocrinology, *17:* 689, 1933.

Riddle, O., and Braucher, P. F.: Control of the special secretion of the crop-gland in pigeons by an anterior pituitary hormone. Amer. J. Physiol., *97:* 617, 1931.

Robbins, E., and Marcus, P. I.: Blindness. Its relation to the age of menarche. Science, *144:* 1154, 1964.

Rossamn, I., and Bartelmez, G. W.: Delayed ovulation in the macaque monkey. Anat. Rec., *94:* 411, 1946.

Rothchild, J., and Rapport, R. S.: The themogenic effort of progesterone and its relation to thyroid function. Endocrinology, *50:* 580, 1952.

Rowlands, I. W., and Parkes, A. S.: Inhibition of the gonadotropic activity of the human pituitary by anti-serum. Lancet, *1:* 924, 1937.

Ryan, K. J.: The conversion of pregnenolone-7-³H and progesterone-4-¹⁴C to oestradiol by a corpus luteum of pregnancy. Acta Endocr. (Kobenhavn), *44:* 1, 1963.

Schroder, R.: Der mensuelle Gentialzyklus des Weibes und seine Storungen. In *Handbuch der Gynakologie,* edited by W. Stoecket, Vol. 1, Part 2. J. F. Bergmann, Munich, 1930.

Selye, H.: *Textbook of Endocrinology.* University of Montreal Press, Montreal, 1947.

Severinghaus, A. E.: The effect of castration in the guinea pig upon sex-maturing potency of the anterior pituitary. Amer. J. Physiol., *101:* 309, 1932.

Shedlovsky, T., Rothen, A., Greep, R. O., van Dyke, H. B., Chow, B. F.: The isolation in pure form of the interstitial cell stimulating (luteinizing) hormone of the anterior lobe of the pituitary gland. Science, *92:* 178, 1940.

Short, R. V., and Eaton, B.: Progesterone in blood. J. Endocr., *18:* 418, 1959.

Siebke, H., and Schuschania, P.: Ergebnisse von Mengenbestimmungen des Sexualhormons; Sexualhormon in Harn und Kot bei regelmassigem mensuellem zyklus zyklusstorungen und bei Hormontherapie. Zbl. Gynaek., *54:* 1734, 1930.

Smith, O. W.: Estrogens in the ovarian fluids of normally menstruating women. Endocrinology, *67:* 698, 1960.

Smith, O. W., and Arai, K.: Blood estrogens in late pregnancy and evaluation of method with improved recovery. J. Clin. Endocr., *25:* 1141, 1963.

Smith, O. W., and Ryan, K. J.: Estrogen in the human ovary. Amer. J. Obstet. Gynec., *84:* 2, 1962.

Smith, P. E., and Engle, E. T.: Experimental evidence regarding role of anterior pituitary in development and regulation of the genital system. Amer. J. Anat., *40:* 159, 159, 1927.

Soffer, L. J., and Fogel, M.: Effect of urinary "gonadotrophin - inhibiting substance" upon the action of human chorionic gonadotrophic (APL) and on human postmenopausal urinary gonadotrophin (Pergonal). J. Clin. Endocr., *23:* 9, 1963.

Stockard, C. R., and Papanicolaou, G. N.: The existence of a typical oestrous cycle in the guinea-pig with a study of its histological and physiological changes. Amer. J. Anat., *22:* 225, 1917.

Stricker, P., and Grueter, F.: Action du lobe anterieur de l'hypophyse sur la montee laiteuse. Compt. rend. Soc. Biol., *99:* 1978, 1928.

Svendsen, R.: A double isotopic derivative method for the quantitative determination of oestrone and 17β-estradiol in plasma. Acta Endocr. (Kobenhavn), *35:* 161, 1960.

Svendsen, R., and Sørensen, B.: The plasma concentration of unconjugated oestrone and 17β-oestradiol during the normal menstrual cycle. Acta Endocr. *45:* 245, 1964.

Taleisnik, S., and McCann, S. M.: Effects of hypothalamic lesions on the secretion and storage of hypophyseal luteinizing hormone. Endocrinology, *68:* 263, 1961.

Talwalker, P. K., Ratner, A., and Meites, J.: In vitro inhibition of pituitary prolactin synthesis and release by hypothalamic extract. Amer. J. Physiol., *205:* 213, 1963.

Tenny, B., Jr., and Parker, R., Jr.: Estrogenic content of cirrhotic livers. J. Clin. Endocr., *2:* 293, 1942.

Trenkle, A., Li, C. H., and Moudal, N. R.: Studies of pituitary lactogenic hormone. Arch. Biochem., *100:* 255, 1963.

Venning, E. H., and Browne, J. S. L.: Urinary excretion of sodium pregnandiol glucuronidate in the menstrual cycle (an excretion form of progesterone). Amer. J. Physiol., *119:* 417, 1937.

Villee, C. A.: In *Modern Trends in Human Reproductive Physiology*, Ch. 6, edited by H. M. Carey, Butterworths, Washington, 1963.

Wade, R., and Jones, H. W.: Effect of progesterone on oxidative phosphorylation. J. Biol. Chem., *220:* 553, 1956.

Westman, A.: Investigations into transit of ova in man. J. Obstet. Gynaec. Brit. Comm., *44:* 821, 1937.

Wilson, J. G.: Reproductive capacity of adult female rats treated prepubertally with estrogenic hormones. Anat. Rec., *86:* 341, 1943.

Witten, C. L., and Bradbury, J. T.: Hemodilution as a result of estrogen therapy. Estrogenic effects in the human female. Proc Soc. Exp. Biol. Med., *78:* 626, 1951.

Wolfe, J. M.: The action of a synthetic estrogenic agent on the anterior pituitary of the castrated female rat. Amer. J. Physiol., *115:* 665, 1936.

Wong, A. S. H., Engle, E. T., and Buxton, C. L.: Anovulatory menstruation in women. Amer. J. Obstet. Gynec., *60:* 790, 1950.

Zander, J.: Steroids in the human ovary. J. Biol. Chem., *232:* 1, 1958.

Zander, J., Brendle, E., von Munstermann, A. M., Diczfalusy, E., Martinsen, B., and Tillinger, K. G.: Identification and estimation of oestradiol-17β and oestrone in human ovaries. Acta Obstet. Gynec. Scand., *38:* 724, 1959.

Zander, J., Forbes, T. R., von Munstermann, A. M., and Neher, R.: Δ⁴-3-Ketopregnane-20α-ol and Δ⁴-3-ketopregnane-20β-ol, two naturally occurring metabolites of progesterone. J. Clin. Endocr., *18:* 337, 1958.

Zondek, B., and Aschheim, S.: Das Hormon des Hypophysenvorderlappens Testobjekt zum Nachweis des Hormones. Klin. Wshr., *6:* 248, 1927.

Zondek, B., and Goldberg, S.: Placental function and foetal death. J. Obstet. Gynaec. Brit. Comm., *64:* 1, 1957.

3

CYCLICAL HISTOLOGY OF THE GENITAL TRACT

Thorough familiarity with the appearance of the endometrium at different stages of the cycle will permit the experienced pathologist to express an accurate opinion as to the approximate time of the menstrual cycle. It is our own feeling that there is so much variation among different women as to make it impossible to date the endometrium to the day, although certain pathologists make this claim (Noyes and coworkers). Indeed we doubt if the endometrium of the same woman would necessarily show the same pattern in successive months.

The endometrium, under the immediate influence of the two ovarian hormones, estrogen and progesterone, exhibits certain characteristic cyclical changes, which may be most conveniently divided into four phases.

Postmenstrual Phase. The endometrium is thin, measuring ordinarily only 1 or 2 mm. in thickness. The surface epithelium, as well as that lining the glands, is of cuboidal type. The glands are straight, narrow, and collapsed, while the stroma is dense and compact. This phase may arbitrarily be put as including the 4 or 5 days immediately following cessation of a period. There is some evidence to indicate that a period of *rest* may at times occur just after

menstruation, but this applies chiefly to women with abnormally long cycles, with marked prolongation of the preovulatory phase.

Proliferative Phase. By a gradual transition the postmenstrual phase is followed by the interval stage, during which the continued action of estrogen brings about increased thickness of the uterine mucosa. The surface epithelium becomes taller and columnar, as does that of the glands, while mitotic figures are quite numerous, more so than in the immediately postmenstrual phase. The *early interval* phase antedates ovulation, and during this period no evidence of secretory activity is to be seen in the gland epithelium, as the secretion of progesterone has not yet begun. This non-secretory portion of the cycle is usually spoken of as "proliferative" and is characterized primarily by growth.

Whereas the proliferative phase of the cycle involves primarily growth activity, the action of progesterone after ovulation causes a profound secretion of glycogen. Thus it is obvious that every cycle is dedicated to preparing the endometrium as the best possible site to nourish an implanted pregnancy in case fertilization has occurred this particular month.

Secretory or Progestational Phase.

48

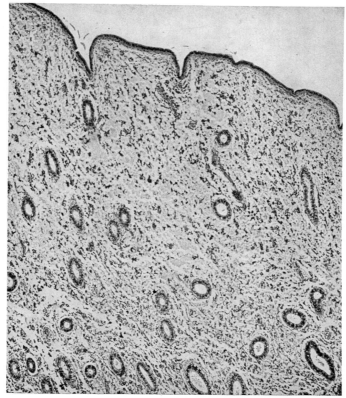

FIG. 3.1. Postmenstrual endometrium

After ovulation, however, in what may be called the *late interval* or *secretory* phase, the evidence of secretory activity in the gland epithelium becomes more and more marked. If, for example, differential staining for glycogen is carried out, granules of glycogen are demonstrable, at first only few in number and within the cytoplasm of the cells, but later more abundant in the cells and present also in increasing amount in the gland lumina. Subnuclear vacuoles, which are believed to represent a prosecretion phase, begin to crowd the nuclei from the base of the cells toward the lumen. Despite some uncertainty, it is generally assumed that these prosecretion vacuoles represent the earliest stages of progesterone activity. The stroma is more abundant and more vascular than in the postmenstrual phase, particularly in the later stage of the interval, which extends to within a week of the next menstrual phase.

Premenstrual Phase. During this stage the secretory function of the now fully mature corpus luteum brings about a full-blown secretory response in the endometrium, which now is soft, velvety, and edematous, measuring from 4 or 5 mm. to as much as 6 or 7 mm. in thickness. While the surface epithelium is still tall and cylindrical, that of the glands is now low, the nuclei having receded toward the base of the cells, and the cytoplasm appearing to melt into the lumen, so that the edge is apt to appear frayed.

The glands are wide and assume a characteristic corkscrew pattern, the convolutions producing tuftlike accumulations of epithelium on either longitudinal or cross section. The necks of the glands often remain rather narrow and straight, the tortuosity involving chiefly the middle or spongy zone of the endometrium. The growing tips of the glands in the basalis, in immediate contact with the muscula-

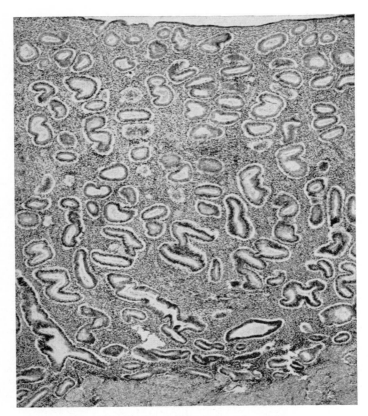

FIG. 3.2. Early proliferative endometrium

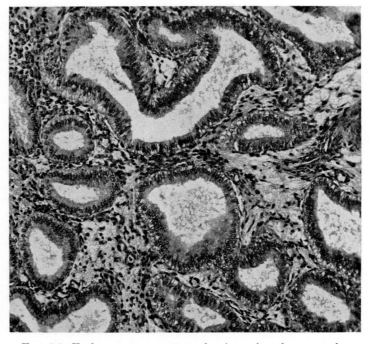

FIG. 3.3. Early secretory pattern showing subnuclear vacuoles

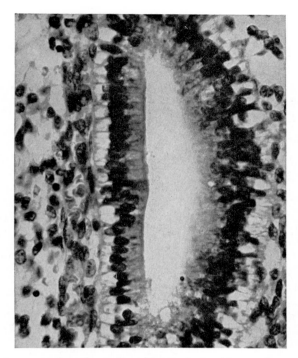

FIG. 3.4. Subnuclear vacuoles, the earliest histological evidence of secretory activity (high power).

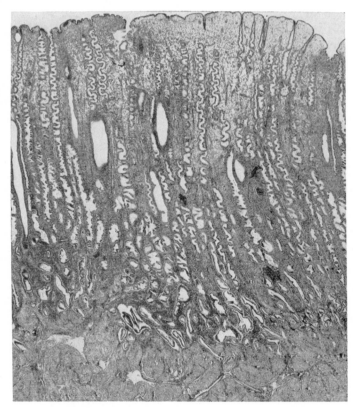

FIG. 3.5. Late interval endometrium showing definite secretory activity

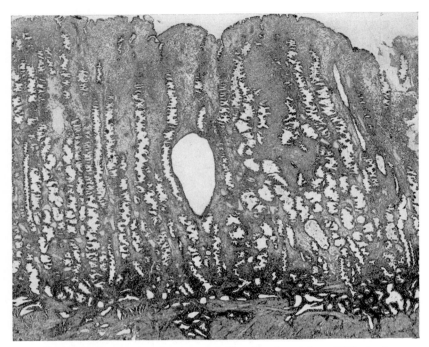

Fig. 3.6. Premenstrual or progestational endometrium (25th day)

ture, are lined by an immature type of epithelium which is apparently unresponsive to progesterone, so that secretory reaction is lacking.

The stroma becomes edematous and loose textured, especially in its superficial layer or *stratum compactum*, and its constituent cells undergo hypertrophy, with an increased amount of cytoplasm. This gives them an appearance suggesting decidual cells, and in many cases the resemblance is so striking that one might well suspect the existence of early gestation. In others, however, the hypertrophic stromal changes are much less marked.

In this phase one can distinguish the same three layers which one sees even more sharply delimited in the young decidua. The uppermost layer is compact in appearance, consisting of broad fields of hypertrophied stroma cells between the rather narrow necks of the glands. It is called the *stratum compactum*. The middle zone presents a lacy, labyrinthine appearance because of the preponderance of dilated and tortuous glands, with very little intervening stroma. It is therefore spoken of as the *stratum spongiosum*. Finally, the deepest layer (*basalis*) in contact with and often penetrating for short distances the muscularis, is made up of the growing tips of the glands, with a dense, compact stroma surrounding them.

The compacta and spongiosa together make up the portion of the endometrium chiefly participating in the cyclical phenomena of menstruation, so that together they comprise the so-called *functional* zone. The basalis, on the other hand, is the layer responsible for growth and regeneration of the endometrium.

It is not uncommon to find even large areas of unripe endometrium, often showing the Swiss cheese pattern of hyperplasia (see Chapter 14) in endometria which otherwise are typically secretory or progestational in character. It is easy to see, therefore, why curettings from such a uterus would show a mixture of secretory and unripe endometrium, constituting the so-called *mixed endometrium*. Such localized areas of unripe or hyperplastic endometrium appear to produce

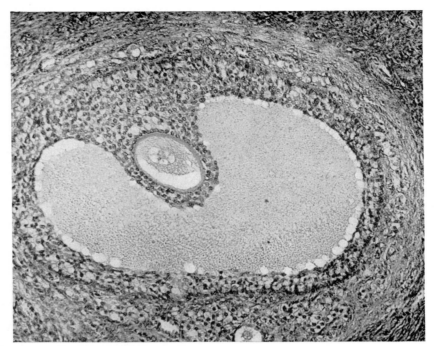

FIG. 3.24. Maturing Graafian follicle showing ovum embedded in cumulus oophorus

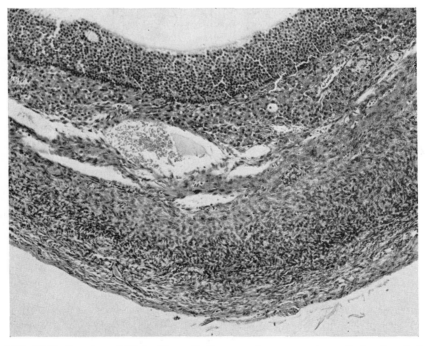

FIG. 3.25. Wall of mature follicle. Beneath the granulosa, note the well developed theca interna.

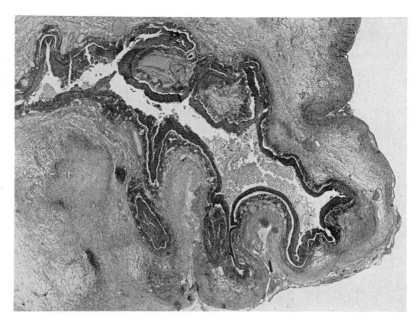

FIG. 3.26. Freshly ruptured follicle showing crumbling of wall

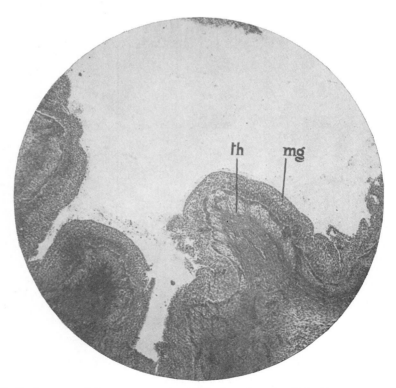

FIG. 3.27. Early corpus luteum, removed on 10th day of cycle. Note the vascular line of demacation between the two layers; *mg*, membrana granulosa; *th*, theca interna.

(c) The *membrana granulosa*.

(d) The central cavity or *antrum*, filled with the liquor folliculi.

(e) The *cumulus oophorus* or *discus proligerus*.

(f) The *corona radiata*, the layer of cells of the discus immediately surrounding the egg, and arranged in radial fashion.

(g) The *zona pellucida*, a thin, refractile, amorphous zone just within the corona radiata.

The rupture of the follicle is attended by extrusion of the egg and, with it, of the zona pellucida, corona radiata, and a considerable number of the cells of the cumulus. No one but a pathologist will understand the extreme difficulty in distinguishing between a mature follicle and an early corpus luteum, because the luteim changes in granulosa and theca cells are not abrupt but very gradual in their evolution. The collapse of the follicle with the subsequent crumbled festooned pattern is probably the most reliable index of ovulation.

Metabolic studies suggest that the granulosa cells which convert to true lutein cells lack 17α-hydroxylase, so that the biosynthetic pathway cannot progress beyond progesterone. Theca cells, currently presumed to be estrogenic, apparently contain this enzyme allowing further metabolism to estrogen production. The absence of blood vessels in the preovulatory granulosa layer of the follicle suggests that progesterone manufactured by these, passes through the theca zone to be excreted as estrogen; when there is a direct (postovulation) vascular supply the luteinized granulosa

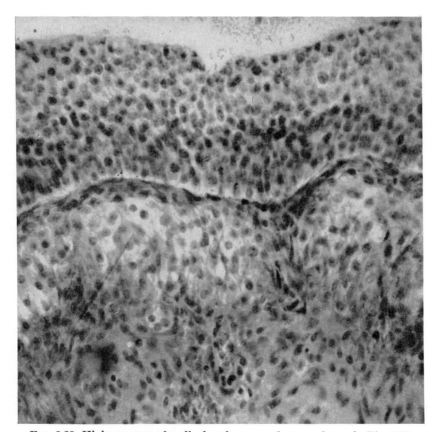

Fig. 3.28. Higher power of wall of early corpus luteum shown in Fig. 3.23

cells secrete progesterone into the circulation unchanged.

Strassman has shown that the theca interna forms a wedgelike cone directed toward the surface of the ovary and thus playing an important mechanical role in ovulation. The cavity collapses with the escape of the follicular fluid, and the second or corpus luteum phase of development now begins, reaching its maximum several days before the onset of the next menstrual period. It should be stressed, however, that the corpus luteum is only a modified follicle, and an exact line of demarcation is histologically impossible. For purposes of description, its life cycle can be divided into the following stages, according to the plan originally suggested by Meyer.

(a) The stage of proliferation or hyperemia, immediately following rupture of the follicle. As might be expected, therefore, the wall of the corpus luteum in its earliest stage is identical with that of the fully mature follicle. The granulosal layer, however, soon shows evidence of beginning transformation into the large, polyhedral, often vacuolated cells known as lutein cells. Between the granulosa and theca there is a zone of blood vessels known as the perigranulosal vascular wreath.

Grossly the corpus luteum in this early stage is a very inconspicuous structure, its thin wall being crenated and folded on itself because of shrinkage of the cavity. There is no such festooning of the wall as is seen in later stages, and its color is a grayish yellow instead of the bright carroty yellow of late stages.

(b) The stage of vascularization. This phase is so designated because its chief characteristic is an invasion of the layer of now definite lutein cells by blood vessels from the theca. These channels extend to the very lumen, and hemorrhage into the latter is a normal feature of this phase. Characteristically it is of limited amount, the blood forming a zone along the lumen edge of the lutein zone. At times, however, the cavity may be distended with blood. The theca interna has

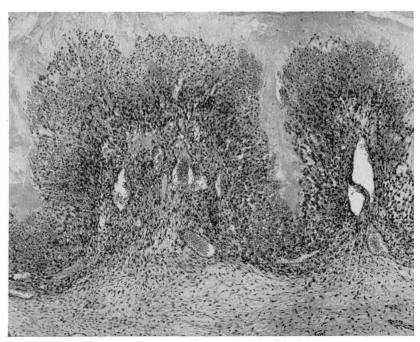

FIG. 3.29. Corpus lutem in stage of vascularization

undergone retrogressive changes, its cells having shrunken through disappearance of the rich lipoid content of the earlier phase.

Grossly, the corpus luteum is now a rather large structure of hemorrhagic appearance. It may measure 10 or 12 mm. in diameter, and is usually recognizable on the surface of the ovary, where it often forms a slight mound. On section the bright yellow lutein zone is seen to be fairly wide and moderately festooned, its color contrasting sharply with the blood which is present in the lumen.

(c) The stage of maturity, which parallels the progestational phase in the endometrium. The broad yellow lutein zone is thrown into festoons like bunting, the color being due to the presence of the pigment carotene. The theca pushes down into the lutein zone in wedgelike septa which divide the lutein into broad folds and alveoli. The cells of the theca themselves often show luteinization, constituting the theca lutein or paralutein cells, although these are always much smaller than the granulosa lutein cells. Along the inner edge of the lutein zone a layer of fibroblastic tissue appears to shut off the lutein cells from the cavity. The latter contains a varying amount of fluid, including usually unresorbed blood elements from the preceding stage.

The gross appearance of a mature corpus luteum is not always the same, nor is its size, which varies from 10 to 20 mm. in diameter. Its yellowish color can often be seen shimmering through the surface of the ovary, above which it may project as a more or less conspicuous mound, at times actually polypoid. In other cases the corpus may seem to lie

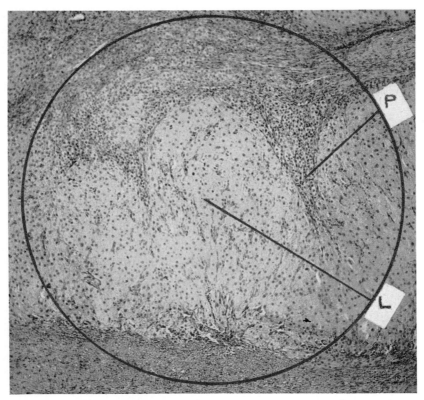

Fig. 3.30. Wall of mature corpus luteum (27th day). Showing lutein (L) and theca-lutein or paralutein (P) cells. The latter are not always so well marked.

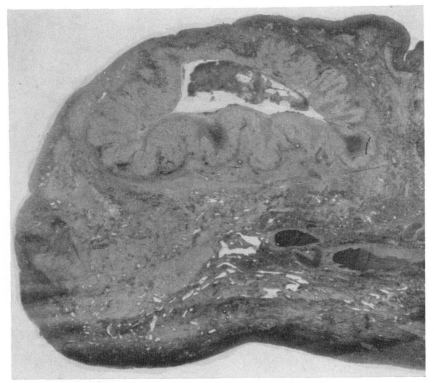

FIG. 3.31. Mature corpus luteum near surface of ovary

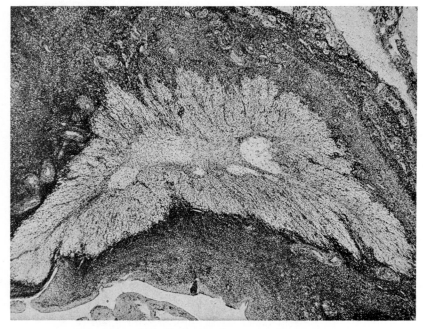

FIG. 3.32. Retrogressive corpus luteum

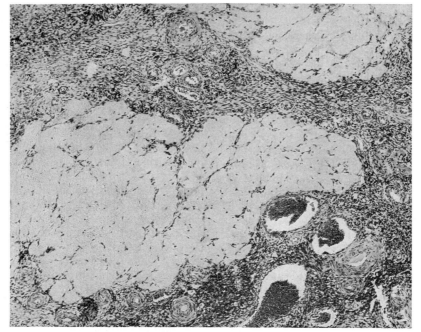

FIG. 3.33. Corpus albicans

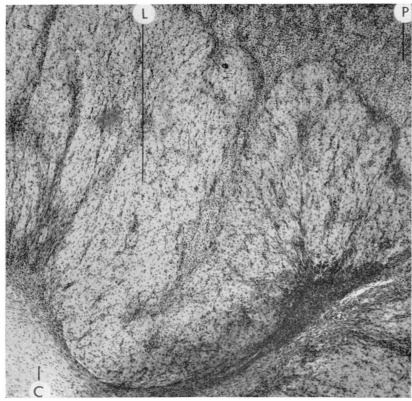

FIG. 3.34. Corpus luteum of early pregnancy. Showing lutein cells (L), paralutein cells (P), and organization along inner wall to lutein layer (C).

beneath the surface, being revealed only by cutting into the ovary. The cavity may be small, with only a small amount of fluid, or it may be very large and distended with a yellowish fluid.

(d) The stage of retrogression. The maximum development of the corpus luteum is attained, not a day or two before the onset of menstruation, as was formerly believed, but probably as early as the 4th to the 6th day before the appearance of menstrual bleeding. This has been well established by the study of Brewer on this subject. The retrogression of the corpus is marked by fatty degeneration, fibrosis, and later by hyalinization of the lutein zone, with increase of the cicatricial tissue within the cavity. The yellowish color may persist for a long time, even several months, but ultimately it disappears.

The end product is the *corpus albicans* or corpus candicans, appearing as a whitish, hyalinized, convoluted structure which slowly decreases in size. Its mor-

phology has recently been discussed by Joel and Foraker.

While as a rule only one follicle each month reaches full maturation, many others advance to various stages of incomplete maturation and then are blighted (*atresia folliculi*). The ovum dies, and this is followed by degeneration and later disappearance of the granulosa, with not infrequently distention of the cavity with fluid. Such small follicular cysts are found in all normal ovaries during reproductive life, but under some conditions, such as chronic pelvic inflammatory disease, they may be so numerous that they produce the so-called "cystic ovary." The process of atresia is also exaggerated during pregnancy.

The cystic stage is followed by cicatricial obliteration proceeding slowly from the periphery toward the center (obliterative phase). The end result is the *corpus fibrosum*, a convoluted zone of hyalinized tissue surrounding a small central cicatrix. Its much smaller size and the narrow and

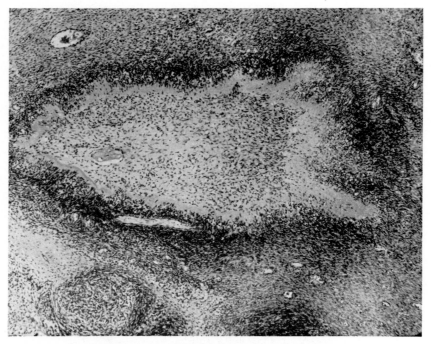

Fig. 3.35. Atretic follicle in obliterative stage

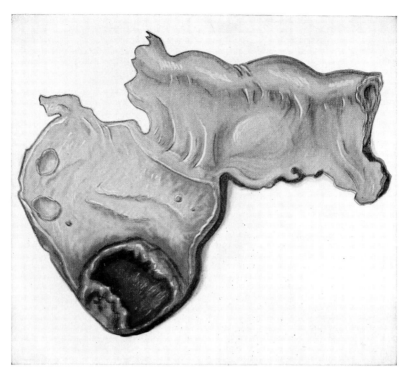

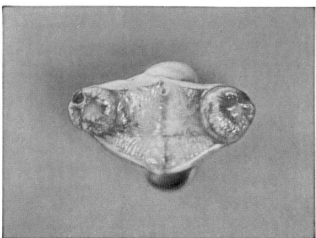

PLATE III.I. *A* (*top*), corpus luteum in stage approaching maturity; *B* (*bottom*), mature corpus luteum.

have found a typical progestational endometrium 6 years after the menopause in one case, and in another fully 10 years after x-ray induction of the menopause which had been done at the age of 46 because of functional bleeding. Such instances, however, are exceedingly rare. It is well to advise the menopausal woman to continue her precautions for 1 year after her last menstrual period.

Vasomotor Symptoms. The most characteristic symptoms of the climacterium are the so-called *vasomotor group:* hot flushes, which involve chiefly the head, neck, and upper part of the thorax and the sweats, often profuse, which frequently immediately follow the flushes.

The frequency and severity of these vasomotor symptoms are exceedingly variable, being almost absent in some women, very moderate in most, and severe in a minority of patients. In the latter case, organotherapeutic treatment is often called for, and usually is successful in ameliorating the symptoms, as is discussed in the chapter on treatment of menopausal symptoms.

The *cause* of the vasomotor symptoms is the cessation of ovarian function with estrogen withdrawal. The characteristic flush certainly involves a vasomotor mechanism, perhaps not unlike that concerned in the phenomenon of blushing. Just what pathways are involved in the production of the vasomotor phenomena is not known.

Other Symptoms. Aside from the vasomotor phenomena such a legion of other symptoms has been ascribed to the menopause, that the public is apt to attribute almost any symptom that happens to occur in the middle-aged woman to the "change of life." In this connection we wonder whether many of our colleagues are not at times to blame in suggesting to the woman, or in acquiescing in her own ready suggestion, that the menopause is responsible for all sorts of indefinite symptoms, especially when a more likely cause for the latter is not patently clear.

A distinction should be made between (1) those symptoms which are clearly menopausal in origin, in the sense that they are the physiological results of the cessation of ovarian activity, and (2) those frequently seen in women passing through the menopause but which are only indirectly or secondarily of menopausal origin and therefore not characteristic. To illustrate what is meant, let us take the example of an average uninformed woman who approaches the menopause with a considerable degree of apprehensiveness. The occurrence of frequent hot flushes and sweats, often disturbing her rest at night and awakening her with a panicky feeling, increases her nervous instability and makes her irritable. Why should not such a woman have headaches, vertigo, depression, a tendency to insomnia, loss of appetite, other digestive-symptoms, or any of many other subjective manifestations? These are certainly not the direct result of any endocrine disturbance, but a part of this particular woman's menopausal disturbance.

Postmenopausal Ovarian Function. There is growing evidence that the postmenopausal ovary is not necessarily the atrophic, functionless organ it has been presumed to be. Randall and Harkins have indicated a persistence of estrogen effect in a considerable percentage of women who have had no vaginal bleeding for years. Although the adrenal can on occasion manufacture estrogen, it is difficult to deny that the ovary is also of some importance, perhaps by virtue of certain hyperplastic stromal cells (ovarian stromal hyperplasia).

Certainly Masters, also Griffith, are adamant in their contention that the ovary has a continued role in body metabolism and general hormone balance. A more complete discussion is found in Chapter 33.

Treatment. See Chapter 33.

REFERENCES

Albright, F.: Studies on ovarian dysfunction; menopause. Endocrinology, *20:* 24, 1936.
Arey, L. B.: Degree of normal menstrual irregularity. Amer. J. Obstet. Gynec., *37:* 12, 1939.

Corner, G. W.: *Attaining Manhood*. Harper & Brothers, New York, 1939.

Corner, G. W.: *Attaining Womanhood*. Harper & Brothers, New York, 1939.

Engle, E. T.: Relation of anterior pituitary gland to problems of puberty and of menstruation. Res. Publ. Ass. Res. Nerv. Ment. Dis., *17:* 298, 1936.

Engle, E. T., and Shelesnyack, M. S.: First menstruation and subsequent menstrual cycles of pubertal girls. Hum. Biol., *6:* 431, 1934.

Fluhmann, C. F.: Period of puberty and inception of menstruation. Amer. J. Obstet. Gynec., *31:* 573, 1936.

Fluhmann, C. F.: *Menstrual Disorders*. W. B. Saunders Company, Philadelphia, 1939.

Glueck, H. I., and Mirsky, I. A.: Clotting mechanism of menstrual blood. Amer. J. Obstet. Gynec., *42:* 267, 1941.

Griffith, G. C.: Oophorectomy and cardiovascular tissues. Obstet. Gynec., *7:* 749, 1956.

Hervey, G. W., McIntire, R. T., and Watson, V.: Low hemoglobin levels in women as revealed by blood donor records. J. A. M. A., *149:* 1127, 1952.

Huggins, C., Vail, V. C., and Davis, M. E.: Fluidity of menstrual blood; a proteolytic effect. Amer. J. Obstet. Gynec., *78:* 46, 1943.

Kennedy, W. P.: Menarche and menstrual type; notes on 10,000 case records. J. Obstet. Gynaec. Brit. Comm., *49:* 792, 1933.

Lozner, E. L., Taylor, J. E., and Taylor, F. H. L.: So-called coagulation defect in menstrual blood. New Eng. J. Med., *226:* 481, 1942.

Masters, W. H.: Sex steroid influence in the aging pattern. Amer. J. Obstet. Gynec., *74:* 733, 1957.

Novak, E. R.: The menoapuse. J. A. M. A., *156:* 575, 1954.

Price, D. C., Forsyth, E. M., Cohn, S. H., and Cronkite, E. P.: The study of menstrual and other blood loss, and consequent iron deficiency by Fe[59] whole body counting. Canad. Med. Ass. J., *90:* 51, 1964.

Randall, C. L.: Ovarian function and women after the menopause. Amer. J. Obstet. Gynec., *73:* 1000, 1957.

Randall, C. L., and Harkins, J. L.: Ovarian function after the menopause. Amer. J. Obstet. Gynec., *74:* 719, 1957.

Simmons, K., and Graulich, W. W.: Menarchal age and height, weight and skeletal age of girls age 7 to 17 years. J. Pediat., *22:* 518, 1945.

Stevenson, R. A., Stinson, J. C., Jr., and Keuhne, B. A.: Quantity of menstrual flow. Texas Rep. Biol. Med., *3:* 371, 1945.

Thoma, A.: Age at menarche, acceleration and heritability. Acta Biol. Acad. Sci. Hung., *11:* 241, 1960.

Wuest, J. H., Dry, T. J., and Edwards, J. E.: Coronary atherosclerosis in bilaterally oophorectomized women. Circulation, *7:* 801, 1953. (See also references to Chapter 33).

5

GYNECOLOGICAL HISTORY, EXAMINA-
TION, AND OPERATIONS

This chapter will be directed to the more strictly professional aspects of the gynecological consultation, although it may be stressed that the female patient, because of the often intimate nature of her problems, will be doubly grateful for sympathy, tact, and understanding on the part of the physician whom she has chosen to consult. It likewise seems unnecessary to go into any detail as to the equipment of the gynecologist's consulting room, with reference to such items as examining table, instruments, etc. In this day and age of frequent medicolegal problems it is imperative that a full and accurate history be maintained if only for the physicians' defense in case of a lawsuit.

GYNECOLOGICAL HISTORY

The aim of each history should be to obtain as complete a picture as possible of the patient and her illness at the time of her examination. Indeed, a strongly presumptive diagnosis can, not infrequently, be made from the history alone, before examination. The value of such records for statistical and literary purposes, and many other advantages need hardly be stressed. In taking a gynecological history, the first emphasis should be put on the fact that the patient is not merely another gynecological case, but

that she is a woman who happens to be suffering from a gynecological complaint. Various methods of taking histories are employed, but should always include the patient's full name along with her husband's, age, social condition (single, married, divorced, or separated), occupation, religion, referring physician. Index files by name and history number are desirable.

Patient's Complaint. The general nature of the patient's complaint should be ascertained at the beginning of the consultation, and should be stated as nearly as possible in the patient's own language. This may not always be very precise, or even literate, but it will at least be authentic, and will often point the way to later questioning.

Family History. Special attention should be directed to familial diabetes, tuberculosis, or cancer. It should be emphasized that cancer is not directly hereditary. However, the woman in whom there is a strong family background of this disease stands a better than average chance of contracting it. The actual risk of gynecological malignancy in the aging female has been computed accurately by Randall in a recent review. It would appear that the incidence of clinical cervical cancer is decreasing, endometrial carcinoma seems more common, but ovarian malignancy is markedly increased. At least one cause for this changing ratio in genital cancer is an increased longevity of today's woman.

Past History. A record of the patient's previous illnesses, and especially of any operations which she has undergone, is of obvious importance. It is remarkable how little many women know as to the nature of operations to which they have submitted. Such information is often of such significance in the diagnosis and treatment of later gynecological disease that it is often wise to secure more accurate information from the surgeon who officiated at the previous operation, or from the hospital at which the operation was performed.

Menstrual History. Since menstrual symptoms, with the possible exception of pain, are of more significance than any other group in gynecological patients, a complete menstrual history should be obtained in every case. This should include the following data.

Age at Onset. An unusually early menarche, especially when accompanied by general developmental changes, may be indicative of certain endocrinopathies, and an occasional case of this sort may be seen in association with certain tumors of the ovary, adrenal, or pituitary. On the other hand, certain other endocrinopathies are characterized by the very late appearance of puberty.

Intervals. While the traditional menstrual interval is 28 days, there are wide individual variations even in normal women, as will be discussed in a later chapter. Departures from the woman's norm, however, are frequently produced by either functional or anatomical abnormalities, so that marked irregularities of rhythm constitute important symptoms of gynecological disease, and should always be noted in the history.

Duration. The same general statement may be made concerning the duration of the flow. Most frequently this parallels the quantity, a prolonged flow being usually an excessive one, and a very short period being usually scanty, but a 2- to 6-day flow represents normal variation. There are, however, numerous exceptions to this general rule.

Amount. While variations in the amount of blood lost at menstruation by different women are wide, a marked diminution is significant, usually of an endocrine or constitutional abnormality of some sort, while menstrual excess is produced by either functional or structural lesions, very often the latter. A very rough idea as to the amount of menstrual flow may be obtained by inquiry as to the number of napkins used.

Character of Menstrual Discharge. The menstrual blood is characteristically of dark venous appearance, and normally is unclotted. When menstruation is excessive, however, the blood may be bright red and under such circumstances clotting is common. As a matter of fact, it is not unusual to find some clotting even when menstruation is of normal amount, and this is without any very great pathological significance. When clots are numerous and large, however, dysmenorrhea is usually a complaint.

Menstrual Pain. Pain in association with menstruation is one of the most common of gynecological symptoms, and any one or more of many factors may be responsible. These need not necessarily be of anatomical or structural character, for often constitutional, psychogenic, and other general factors may be concerned. In questioning patients, it is wise to inquire as to the character of the pain, which is usually of either a bearing down or colicky character, and also as to the time of its onset and its duration. For example, in the common type of primary dysmenorrhea, it most characteristically begins a day or two before the onset of the period, and disappears after menstruation has been well established. In other cases, it may persist throughout the flow or even beyond. Any increased dysmenorrhea should require further elucidation.

Intermenstrual Bleeding. It is important to ascertain whether or not there is bleeding between the menstrual periods, and whether this is apt to occur after coitus or other contact. The mere fact that bleeding of this type is the most characteristic symptom of early cervical cancer is evidence enough of its importance, although it is common also with such lesions as cervical polyp or erosion.

The Date of the Last Menstrual Period. When this is inquired for, the physician will in a large proportion of cases find the patient's memory very hazy, and this item in the history is sure to be inaccurate in many cases. Yet it is often of great importance, as in cases of possible early gestation, intra- or extrauterine. When possible, it is desirable also to secure the menstrual date preceding the last period, as well as information as to the normalcy of the period, subsequent spotting, etc.

Vaginal Discharge. Leukorrhea is such a common gynecological symptom that it merits a special heading. The duration of the leukorrhea, the character, color, possible odor, and possible irritativeness of the discharge are among the items of inquiry.

Obstetrical History. Whether the patient is single or married, and, if the latter, how long, is of obvious significance. Even more so is the history of the pregnancies and labors, with especial reference to their number, character, and possible complications. Other important items concern miscarriages or abortions, either spontaneous or induced. On the other hand, a history of sterility, when there has been no contraception, may be of great significance, although necessarily in a qualified sense because of the possible responsibility of the husband.

Urinary Symptoms. The great frequency of urinary symptoms among women, not only in association with urinary tract disease but also with various gynecological disorders, makes it important to inquire as to such items as increased frequency, pain, incontinence, nocturia, and hematuria. A history of previous urinary tract disease, such as cystitis or pyelitis, may likewise be of much value in the interpretation of existing urinary symptoms.

Gastrointestinal Symptoms. Loss of appetite is frequently observed with gynecological disease, especially when the latter is accompanied by marked debility, hemorrhage, or marked nervousness and anxiety. Other digestive symptoms, such as bloating, belching, and discomfort after eating, may be secondary to gynecological disease, or they may rather suggest functional or organic abnormalities of some of the abdominal viscera. The same statement may be made concerning nausea and vomiting. The latter symptoms, when associated with amenorrhea, would naturally make the physician think of the possibility of pregnancy, to give only one illustration of their possible significance. Constipation, so frequent among women in general, is especially common in gynecological patients but may be a rather direct result of certain pelvic lesions associated with pressure or rectal pain. Bleeding on defecation is often due to hemorrhoids, but the frequent responsibility of other pelvic or rectal lesions should always be borne in mind.

Present Illness. Last and perhaps most important comes the most comprehensive heading, that of the history of the present illness, which constitutes a summation of those previously mentioned. The physician's queries should take cognizance of all the body systems, so that all other factors bearing on the case may be brought out. The questions will often be inspired by the general nature of the patient's complaint or by her very appearance (see "Sample Case History").

GYNECOLOGICAL EXAMINATION

While the gynecologist's examination will naturally be directed chiefly toward the pelvic and abdominal organs, it must include a general survey of the entire physical make-up. This can be elaborate or comparatively simple, depending upon the requirements of the individual case.

General. Among the general items which should rarely be omitted are the

Sample Case History

No.: 21875
Name: Smith, Mary A. (John C.)
    36 N. Main Boulevard
    Johnston, S. C.

Date: March 18, 1965
Referred by: Dr. Paul A. Brown
    262 N. Centre St.
    Jonesville, S. C.

Age: 64

C. C.: "Bleeding after the change of life."

F. H.: Mother died of cancer of the cervix; father of gastric cancer; otherwise negative.

P. H.: D. & C. 1950, "Bleeding," Johns Hopkins Hospital. Appendectomy approximately 1918. Possible rheumatic fever without cardiac involvement as child. Otherwise only c.c.d.

G. U.: History of apparent cystitis 30 years ago with only pregnancy. No present hematuria, dysuria, urgency, etc.

G. I.: Chronic constipation; otherwise negative.

M. H.: LMP 1952 after uneventful menstrual life. (1 D. & C. as noted above.)

Ob. H.: Para 1-1-0.0.1. One uncomplicated pregnancy at age 32 after 8 years involuntary sterility; no other pregnancies; never contraception.

P. I.: LMP 16 years ago. No further bleeding until 1 month ago when noticed bright red spotting, at first intermittent, but now more or less constant, so requires pad. Never excessive flow and no pain of any kind. No known estrogen therapy although is taking butazolidine for arthritis.

Menses generally normal though D. & C. in premenopausal area for flooding. No sequelae and LMP about 1 year later. Para 1 after 8 years sterility and no other pregnancies. G. U.-G. I. essentially negative as above.

P. E.: Shows an obese rather flushed W. F. 64. (Wt. 220; B.P. 210/120.) *Thyroid* not enlarged. *Breasts* pendulous without masses. *Abdomen*—marked panniculus. No masses or tenderness. C-V angles nontender. *Pelvic*—external genitalia normal. Outlet parous with no relaxation anterior or posterior. Cervix small and smooth, almost flush with the vault. Fundus normal postmenopausal size, midposition, regular, and free. Adnexa not palpable. *Speculum*—no present bleeding. Cervix clean. Vaginal mucosa well supported.

Rectal—small hemorrhoids at 3, 6, and 10 o'clock. Otherwise essentially negative and confirmatory.

Impression: (1) Postmenopausal bleeding.
    (2) Adenocarcinoma fundus (?).

Rx: Papanicolaou smear and cervical biopsy taken.
Urine (cath.) for microscopic and culture taken.
Old D. &. C. specimen to be reviewed.
To be admitted 3/28/65 for glucose tolerance, cholesterol, and routine laboratory studies. Medical consultation (EKG, chest x-ray, etc.) 3/29/65. For D. & C. and possible radium application, 11:30 a.m. See letter to Dr. Brown.

height, weight, and general build of the patient, and, in the case of obese patients, the regional distribution of the adipose tissue, as well as any abnormalities of hair distribution. The thyroid should be examined, and at least a superficial examination of the heart and lungs made. The blood pressure should be taken, and the urine examined for albumin and sugar, with, usually, a microscopic examination.

Examination of the Breast. Certain gynecological textbooks have attempted to include sections on the diagnosis and treatment of breast cancer, and indeed one of our own texts formerly featured such a chapter. Unfortunately this was predestined to be incomplete and unsatisfactory, for breast disease is so complex and so highly specialized that it warrants not a chapter but a textbook of its own. In our own locale, breast surgery is the domain of the general surgeon; in many areas it falls within the realm of the gynecologist and, indeed, operative surgery on the breast is fully sanctioned by the American Board of Obstetrics and Gynecology. Whether he performs mammary surgery himself, or refers it to a fellow surgeon, palpation of the breast by the gynecologist is mandatory as part of a gynecological "check-up," for breast cancer is nearly twice as common as any other form of carcinoma which the female may acquire.

Although we feel that a gynecological textbook should not include a short and incomplete chapter on breast disease, we should like simply to list *verbatim* a certain set of rules, advocated by Montgomery, Bowers, and Taylor which exemplify our own feelings in regards to palpation of the breast. Incidently, evaluation of the breast, particularly in the obese woman, is one of the greatest problems with which the gynecologist comes in contact.

1. There is some safety in numbers: to wit, bilateral diffuse induration of the breast is rarely cancerous and offers no site of selection for biopsy. Such cases should be observed periodically.

2. Cancer may appear in an area of chronic mastitis by coincidence, or possibly as a result of cause and effect. Any local change of texture or development of a 'dominant' lesion should therefore be biopsied promptly.

3. Unilateral persistent fibrocystic disease, such as appears frequently in the upper and outer quadrant of the breast, should be freely excised and studied in multiple section.

4. Enlarged glands of the axilla adjacent to such areas of induration should also be excised for study, even though the breast area itself is benign.

5. In the case of patients appearing with a well defined mass in the breast, arrangements should be made for prompt biopsy and mastectomy at the same sitting if the tissue is positive.

6. In a slender undernourished woman, the whole fabric of the breast may be revealed to a degree suggesting fibrocystic disease or even small neoplasms.

7. Lipoma-like masses in the breast of aged women often harbor scirrhous carcinoma. *Be strongly suspicious of any lesion of the breast after the menopause* (italics ours).

8. Questionable areas of nodulation in the breasts of pregnant women should be biopsied under local anesthesia, the biopsy examined in paraffin section, and the definitive therapy carefully planned.

9. Small apparent lesions of the breast ← discovered at examination just before menstruation should be rechecked after the period is over; they may disappear.

10. Minute and doubtful lesions which seem scarcely deserving of biopsy even though they persist after the period should be rechecked every 6 to 8 weeks until the problem is resolved.

11. The patient with serous discharge from the nipple should be biopsied whenever the secretion can be traced or whenever induration is palpable at any point around the areola or adjacent breast tissue.

12. A patient with fibrocystic disease may have to be biopsied several times in the course of years to satisfy the physician that cancer is not developing. In some such cases, simple mastectomy becomes the ultimate solution.

13. The patient who complains most of pain is least likely to have carcinoma, unless she has an enormous lesion.

14. The patient with extensive fibrocystic disease or adenosis of the breast, and a strong family history of cancer, had better have a simple mastectomy.

15. Postmenopausal patients should be discouraged in the prolonged use of estrogens because of the untoward effect on the breasts."

With all of the dicta so specified, we are in full accord. Like Montgomery, Bowers, and Taylor, we are inclined to wonder how deleterious to the patient simple biopsy may be, and why immediate mastectomy must be carried out if frozen section, frequently of poor quality and not always representative, should suggest carcinoma. We are able, however, in this community to permit the surgeon to shoulder this burden. An equally important and equivocal question that is frequently related is whether the young menstruating woman should be castrated, and this poses an enigma that can hardly be resolved by anyone in our present ignorance of certain endocrinological functions; today's opinion is in the affirmative.

The Relation of the Ovary to Breast Cancer. Like the uterus, the breast is an end organ insofar as stimulation by the ovarian hormone is concerned. It has recently been pointed out by Randall and Harkins that a significant number of women continue to show evidence of estrogen effect on the vaginal mucosa for many years after the cessation of their menses, and there is general agreement that certain postmenopausal women possess this capability. It has been well documented that in certain animals, even of the male sex, breast cancer can be produced by treatment with large, protracted doses of estrogen. It has likewise been noted that women with breast cancer who are subjected to oophorectomy reveal a considerable degree of so-called "ovarian stromal hyperplasia," and thus such gonads seem to harbor cells morphologically akin to the theca cells which normally secrete estrogen. It would therefore seem highly rational, as noted by Rosenberg and Uhlmann, to advocate routine castration in the menstruating woman to avoid further stimulation of an already proved malignant end organ. Patterson and Russell suggest irradiation as an effective and simple method of ablating ovarian functions.

Unfortunately, the problem is not nearly so simple, for it is well established that the adrenal gland is quite capable of estrogen secretion. A recent review by Brown, Falconer, and Strong indicates that *castrated* patients treated with adrenocorticotrophin (ACTH) have a large measurable amount of urinary estrogen, almost certainly of adrenal origin. For this reason, certain gynecologists, surgeons, and endocrinologists have adopted a policy of oophorectomy for the young menstruating patient and adrenalectomy for the older patient, especially when there has been evidence of metastatic disease. That this approach is not entirely satisfactory is suggested by a series of recent articles by Bulbrook and Greenwood. In a limited number of patients with advanced breast cancer, who had been subject not only to oophorectomy and adrenalectomy but also to hypophysectomy, the level of urinary estrogen was nearly equivalent to that found at certain stages of the cycle in normally menstruating women. We can merely speculate as to what is the source of this estrogenic substance; but is it too far-fetched to wonder if it may be ingested by female and male alike as part of the daily diet, perhaps as cholesterol which can be synthesized to the steroidal hormones. Probably only a few convert to estrogen.

Castration with Breast Cancer. At this writing there is no positive set of regulations that can be postulated for the management of breast cancer, but a recent collective review of the effect of castration deserves the utmost consideration. Lewison, one of the very real students of mammary disease, has made an exhaustive study of the literature to which he has compounded an outstanding clinical experience. His current thoughts may be summarized as follows.

Twenty-two per cent of all female cancers (over 50,000 annually) will originate in the breast, and about 20,000 of these women will be in the *premenopausal age group* although women of any age are susceptible. Although a minority of these females will have a cancer that is hormone dependent, approximately 25% of youthful women seemingly exhibit a beneficial response if immediate therapeutic surgical castration is carried out. Results with irradiation are more variable, slower to appear, and less convincing than comparable patients treated surgically.

Lewison points out the current difficulties in ascertaining which lesion will respond to castration, and indicates that it may in no way be equated with estrogen assay or cytologic maturation index. In any case, the possibility of exacerbation of the disease by castration may be discounted, but the relative frequency (25% noted by Kasilag and Rutledge) with which metastatic breast cancer spreads to the ovary would likewise warrant consideration. It might seem, therefore, preferable to attempt an optimal salvage by means of prophylactic castration rather than carry out mere therapeutic palliation especially where there is axillary or other metastatic tumor.

Although it would appear that over-all salvage is increased by prophylactic oophorectomy, there is still some uncertainty. If this question could be verified, however, it would seem that castration should be regarded as mandatory, and part of the initial planned treatment. Hormone therapy, adrenalectomy and hypophysectomy, all on less well substantiated data, might be reserved for palliation of recurrent or metastatic disease. It should also be emphasized that oophorectomy or ablation of other endocrine glands in the usual postmenopausal woman is probably not worth the effort.

In a very recent conversation with Lewison we have been informed that there is a controlled study by a number of surgical clinics to systematically study mammary cancer, its extent with metastasis, the effect of pregnancy, along with the time and degree of initial surgery. These will be equated with the pre- or postmenopausal status with particular emphasis on castration, subsequent hormone or chemotherapy, and ablation of adrenal or hypophysis. Irradiation will likewise be evaluated, but currently it seems appropriate primarily for advanced disease. It would appear that this joint study by many clinics, all utilizing rigid criteria and patient-treatment selection will produce some clarification in the confusion attendant to proper treatment of breast cancer in the different age groups. It is hoped that the ever constant salvage of approximately 50% will show some improvement, but this figure remains about the same irrespective of the type of therapy. An early report by Goldenberg would suggest a 20% remission by usage of testosterone

proprionate, especially where there is vast skin-node involvement.

As a consequence of the above opinions, we have formulated certain generalizations for women with breast cancer, none of which, however, are absolute. (1) Conservation of ovaries in the young where there is no evidence of metastatic disease, but castration if there is proved evidence of axillary or other spread. (2) Castration, even in the young woman who has had recurrence after radical mastectomy. (3) Castration in the older woman with metastatic or recurrent cancer *only* if the vaginal smear shows evidence of sustained high estrogen effect. (4) Pregnancy is to be avoided, and if other than simple curettage is indicated for therapeutic abortion, probably hysterectomy with castration is preferable to hysterotomy. Indeed, if hysterectomy by any approach or for any reason is contemplated, probably it is well to practice simultaneous oophorectomy, except in the very youthful woman.

Although these tenets must not be regarded as absolute, and although there are unquestionably certain exceptions, they have at least provided us with a general working rule in regard to the management of a highly controversial subject. Obviously certain religious and individual indications on occasion influence our expressed intentions, and we would be the first to admit that our opinions are by no means based on firmly established facts.

Steroid therapy of advanced breast cancer is likewise highly unpredictable. Brilliant results have sometimes been obtained by usage of large dosage of testosterone proprionate (100 mg. daily) where there is local or soft tissue involvement. Similar large dosage of estrogenic substances for bony metastasis may be utilized. Landau, Ehrlich, and Huggins feel that benefits are obtained by daily injections of progesterone and estradiol, especially where previous oophorectomy or adrenalectomy had induced tumor regression. Since breast cancer like endometrial adenocarcinoma is on occasion presumed to be estrogen-dependent, it would seem that mammary cancer might show the striking remission often exhibited by fundal disease. Opinion, however, is far from uniform.

That there are occasional dramatic remissions of the disease following drug therapy no one will deny. Certainly cure is infrequent, and in any case, the critical physician will recall that on occasion there may be dramatic spontaneous remission of malignancies. Where there is no overt evidence of continued estrogenic function, however, we are in full accord with a trial of large dosage steroid therapy where there is advanced or recurrent cancer. The place of corticoids, as well as such procedures as adrenalectomy and hypophysectomy, seems less certain.

Abdominal Examination. Simple inspection will reveal such abnormalities as undue prominence or asymmetrical contour, as well as the abnormalities of abdominal and pubic hair distribution so common in women. Previous pregnancies will be indicated by the characteristic abdominal striae. Palpation will yield further information as to the thickness of the adipose layer and the tone or lack of tone of the muscle. Tenderness at any point should be carefully noted. Particular attention should be directed toward certain cardinal areas, especially the adnexal regions, McBurney's point, the gall bladder region, the epigastrium, and the kidney areas. Scars of previous operations should be noted.

Abnormal masses are carefully searched for, and here again, gentle palpation will usually be far more productive than rough handling, which makes the patient apprehensive, causes pain, and brings about involuntary tightening of the abdominal muscles. If an abnormal mass of any kind is felt, its position and its relation to any abdominal or pelvic organ or region should be noted, together with its size, shape, contour, consistency, movability, and tenderness or lack of tenderness. Percussion will yield still further information along the same line, and is of special value in the case of cer-

tain large tumors, such as ovarian cysts, which must be distinguished from ascites.

Pelvic Examination. It is in the examination of the pelvic organs proper that the special training of the gynecologist comes into play. The more experienced, thorough, and methodical he is, the more he will learn from the examination.

Preparation and Position of the Patient. The clothing having been removed below the abdomen, the patient lies in the dorsal recumbent position, with flexed thighs and knees, the feet resting on the stirrups of the examining table, and the limbs and lower abdomen being draped with a sheet. The presence of a nurse, or of a female relative or friend, should be looked upon as essential for obvious reasons. It is of great importance that the patient's bladder be emptied just before the examination.

The examining hand is covered with a rubber or "throw-away" plastic glove, for the protection of the physician perhaps even more than of the patient, and the index finger is well lubricated with tincture of green soap or one of the proprietary lubricating jellies. The traditional examining hand of the gynecologist is the left, and the expert gynecologist soon learns to feel both sides of the pelvis equally well with the left hand; indeed, the use of the left hand has apparently become a mark of the guild, and most gynecologists would feel awkward using the right routinely. A reason for use of the left hand is that the stronger and more useful right hand is left free to handle the instruments which are at times called for during the examination. The importance of a good light for the examination, usually from a lamp of the goose-neck variety, over the examiner's left shoulder, cannot be too strongly emphasized.

Careful inspection of the external genitalia is the first step of the pelvic examination. This will take cognizance of the presence of any anatomical or pathological abnormalities, the presence of any skin lesions or of any inflammation or

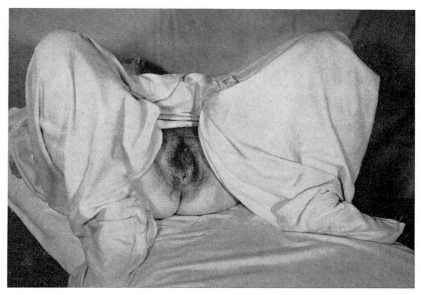

Fig. 5.1. Position of patient for ordinary pelvic examination

irritation of the vulvovaginal mucosa and urethra, the presence or absence of the hymen, the size of the clitoris or whether there is any outlet relaxation or vaginal protrusion, uterine prolapse, cystocele, or rectocele. The presence or absence of hemorrhoids, fissure, or fistula is likewise noted.

Before proceeding with the vaginal examination, the presence of urethral or Bartholin's gland disease should be excluded. Urethral caruncle or erosion will usually be evident on inspection, but the distal portion of the urethra should be gently stripped to ascertain whether a purulent exudate can be milked from either the urethra, the subjacent Skene's ducts, or a suburethral diverticulum infection.

One or more fingers well lubricated, are then introduced into the vagina, and as the fingers pass into the vagina one can note the degree of relaxation if any is present. Ordinarily the patient is asked to bear down for a moment, as this will give one a good idea of the degree of any cystocele, rectocele, or uterine descensus which may be present.

In the case of unmarried patients in whom an intact hymen would render digital examination of the vagina undesirable and often impossible or very painful, the examination of the pelvic organs should be made *per rectum*. While this may seem to the beginner a rather unsatisfactory makeshift, it will be found with practice to yield almost as satisfactory information concerning the uterus and adnexa as does vaginal examination. Occasionally examination under anesthesia is desirable, especially in the case of young girls.

The examination of the internal genitalia begins with careful *palpation of the cervix*, making note of such data as its size and shape, the size of the external os, the direction in which the cervix points, whether or not there is any laceration or hypertrophy, the possible presence of polyps or any unusually hard, raised, or roughened areas, and whether or not such digital contact with the cervix causes bleeding, as it so commonly does with certain lesions (polyp, cancer). Just as important as palpation is careful inspection, but this is best deferred until the completion of the palpatory examination.

The examining fingers now seek to determine the size, shape, and position of the uterus, and now for the first time the external hand is called into play, and the real *bimanual procedure* begins. The purpose is to map out the organs between the internal fingers and the hand externally, and the cooperation of the patient is indispensable for good results. A few explanatory and reassuring remarks to her, with often the suggestion that she breathe through the mouth and untighten the abdominal muscles, will help a great deal, especially if the examiner is very gentle in his manipulations. It is rarely necessary to cause any great amount of pain, even in the presence of very painful and tender pelvic lesions. When the abdominal wall is very thick and obese, one can scarcely expect to be able to outline the organs as clearly and sharply as in the case of women with thin and flabby abdominal walls.

A common complaint of beginners is that the fingers are too short to permit satisfactory outlining of the internal genital organs. During the examination the fingers should hug the posterior rather than the anterior wall, for pressure against the urethra may cause much discomfort. On the other hand, the perineum can be pressed backward toward the rectum quite freely and painlessly. By passing the finger along the front of the cervix one comes to the anterior surface of the uterine body, which can be felt through the anterior vaginal fornix, especially if the external hand gently presses the uterus down toward the internal. Between the two the fundus can then be clearly felt, and one can determine its size, contour, and movability

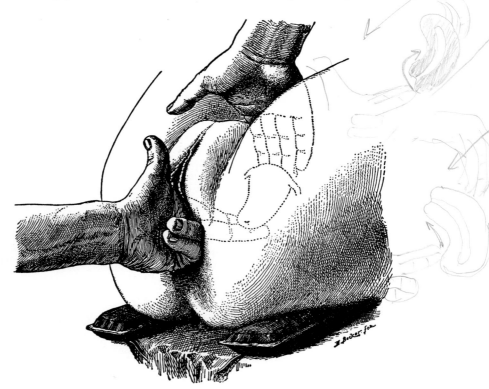

Fig. 5.2. Bimanual palpation of pelvic viscera. (From Kelly, H. A.: *Operative Gynecology*. D. Appleton-Century Company, Inc., New York, 1898.)

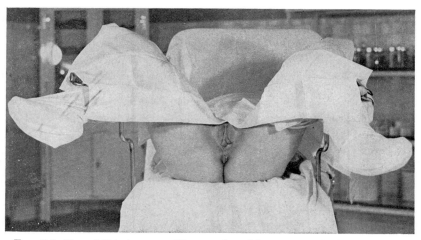

Fig. 5.3. Dorsal lithotomy position employed for most vaginal operations

quite accurately. An irregular, knobby outline, combined with enlargement of the uterus, for example, makes it quite certain that the uterus contains myomatous tumors. The posterior wall can likewise be readily palpated in most cases.

When, on the other hand, the fundus cannot be felt anteriorly, the finger passed upward along the posterior surface of the uterus encounters the firm uterine body posteriorly, so that retroversion or retroflexion can be easily diagnosed; or the uterus may not be felt either anteriorly or posteriorly, in which case it will be about vertical in position as a result of slight retroversion. The idea, in other words, is simply to play one hand against the other, groping gently about to outline the various normal or abnormal pelvic contents. In palpating behind the cervix one incidentally notes any tenderness or thickening in the uterosacral region, sometimes due to inflammatory thickening of the ligaments themselves but often to the presence of prolapsed, inflamed, and adherent adnexa. Or one may feel large or small tumor masses in this region.

The sides of the pelvis are then carefully and gently explored by groping about in a stroking fashion with the external hand in an effort to feel the lateral organs between the two hands. In most cases the normal ovaries are readily palpable and are tender to palpation. Any enlargement is noted, as well as the movability or fixation of the organ. Although the normal tube cannot be felt, any noteworthy enlargement, as with pyosalpinx, makes it easily felt as a definite, usually fixed and adherent mass of varying size, and not under these circumstances separable from the ovary, which cannot be outlined in most such cases.

The bimanual examination over, one may now proceed with the *speculum examination of the cervix*, for without this no gynecological examination is complete. Any one of the "duckbill" or bivalve types of speculum may be used, with proper lubrication. A good light is absolutely essential, the usual source being a strong spotlight or goose-neck lamp behind the left shoulder of the examiner. The presence of polyps, erosion, eversion, or retention cysts must be looked for, and the character, amount, and probable source of any discharge noted. The vaginal mucosa should likewise be inspected. The Gonococcus may be sought for in the secretion from the cervical canal or urethra, whereas the Trichomonas can be found in the exudate exposed by the speculum in the posterior fornix. The technique for these various tests is described in the appropriate chapters.

Perhaps the most important field for very careful and painstaking speculum inspection of the cervix is in cases of suspected malignancy of the cervix. Although the later stages of cancer are ordinarily unmistakable, the early lesions are not so characteristic and present no specific appearance. One must suspect any cervical lesion and settle the question definitely, as it can practically always be settled, by *biopsy*. Cytological studies should be routine, especially for parous women over 30 years of age. These and other special diganostic methods are discussed in Chapter 12, "Carcinoma of the Cervix."

Examination of the Rectum. Finally, examination of the rectum is of importance, especially in those cases in which rectal symptoms, especially bleeding or pain, have been complained of. External hemorrhoids, fissures, and fistulous openings are readily seen, but other abnormalities require digital or proctoscopic examination. Certainly digital examination should be a routine part of the gynecological examination in all such cases. Frequently, combined examination, with one finger in the vagina and one in the rectum, will be most informative.

GYNECOLOGICAL OPERATIONS

We have always felt (and still do) that a textbook on clinical gynecology cannot satisfactorily include adequate coverage of operative gynecology. Attempts to achieve this have invariably resulted in rather obvious shortcomings in discussion of the surgical methods or of such aspects as pathology or endocrinology—which are even more important to the student or general practitioner than is operative technique. However, we have also speculated as to whether it might not be advisable to describe only a few gynecological operations which, with certain

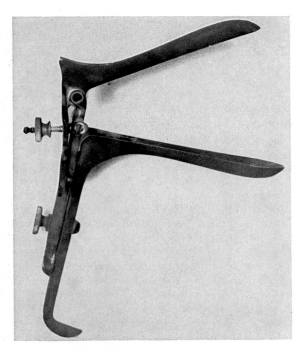
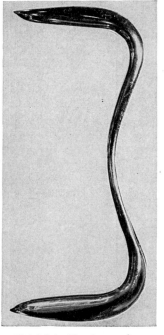

Fig. 5.4. Vaginal speculums. *A* (*left*), Graves' bivalve; *B* (*right*), Sims' speculum

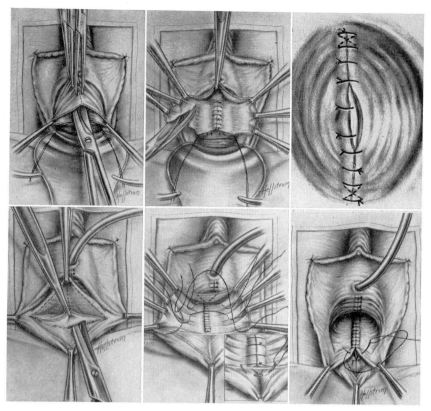

FIG. 5.6B. Vaginal hysterectomy (*continued*). *Top left*, if cystocele repair is desired, it is performed after suspension of the vagina; note separation of mucosa from bladder and fascia. *Top middle*, excision of redundant mucosa after approximation of pubocervical fascia (plication of sphincter where necessary). *Top right*, closure of vault with excision of redundant vaginal mucosa. *Bottom left*, posterior repair begun by elevating mucosa. *Bottom middle*, approximation of levator ani (repair of perirectal fascia is often desirable). *Bottom right*, running lock suture of posterior vaginal wall. From Gray, L. A.: *Vaginal Hysterectomy*, Charles C Thomas, Springfield, Ill., 1955.)

dures as ventrofixation and other types of suspension can make subsequent vaginal hysterectomy of considerable difficulty. One of the nicest features of the vaginal approach to hysterectomy is that it spares the surgeon the decision as to how to handle the ovaries. These are rarely removed during the course of the average vaginal operation, although this would often technically be easy. Vaginal hysterectomy (with or without adnexectomy) is occasionally expedient in treating endometrial adenocarcinoma as noted by Pratt, Symmonds, and Welch.

We cannot justify morcellation of large, myomatous uteri so that hysterectomy may be achieved vaginally, nor can we advocate ovarian or tubal surgery as a routine by the vaginal approach. There are certain individual patients with large fibroids whose problems may include the desirability of vaginal surgery. When there is any doubt as to whether all of the operation can be accomplished from below, we generally post the patient for a combined procedure.

Combined Procedure. This generally implies the necessary repair of anterior or posterior relaxation with urethral plication if there is incontinence followed by laparotomy. If, however, hysterectomy is deemed desirable and can be accomplished easily from below, well and good. If the uterus is too bulky or fixed for satisfactory removal from below, we complete the vaginal repair and then redrape the patient for laparotomy. Because of the posting of a "combined procedure" a laparotomy table is available, and we are able to carry out the abdominal procedure with little delay.

Urinary Complications of Vaginal Surgery. A rather frequent complication of any vaginal procedure, especially cystocele repair, is urinary retention, which is always transient but frequently of considerable nuisance value with associated mental trauma. Repeated catheterization is the rule, with infection of the urinary bladder a common sequel; therefore some discussion of bladder inflammation in general seems in order. Tidal drainage is an excellent prophylaxis against, as well as treatment for, urinary retention (Fig. 5.7). For details the reader is referred to a recent review by Kass and Sossen.

Acute Cystitis. This condition may occur as an apparently specific entity, although it has been postulated that the short length of the female urethra facilitates upward extension from such primary vectors as the heavily coliform rectum. On the other hand, there is no question that acute infection of the lower genitourinary tract may ensue as a sequel to activation of a quiescent upper tract infection; in most cases, however, the actual etiology is obscure.

Specific agents may lead to an acute cystitis. An indwelling catheter, the mechanical trauma known as "honeymoon cystitis," or irradiation or surgical trauma can induce acute bladder infection, which is manifested by frequency, urgency, dysuria, and occasional hematuria. Pyuria and hematuria should be searched for by catheterized specimen, and it should be emphasized that *valid urinalysis of any woman cannot be made on the basis of a voided specimen*, as pus cells caused by vaginitis are common in voided urine.

Catheterization for microscopic study should frequently include culture, with concomitant tests for sensitivity to penicillin, erythromycin, tetracycline, Chloromycetin, Furadantin, and other appropriate drugs. Different strains of *coli-aerogenes,* α- and β-*streptococci, Staphylococcus albus* and *Staphylococcus aureus,* and Proteus are the usual organisms. Occasional resistance is found, in which case mere empirical therapy must be evoked; however, when there is adequate suggested response the resultant antibiotic should be instituted. Before the culture-sensitivity report is obtained simpler measures, such as treatment with Gantrisin, Kynex, Mandelamine, or Pyridium, may be instituted. Such palliative alkalinizing and antispasmodic agents as the following should be utilized:

Bladder Mixture

Tincture of hyoscyamus.......	30 cc.	(1 oz.)
Potassium citrate.............	30 cc.	(1 oz.)
Water, *ad*....................	180 cc.	(6 oz.)

Sig. 2 tbs. b.d.

Chronic Cystitis. On occasion a persistent low grade infection may be present, characterized only by minor symptomatology. It may be a residuum of an incompletely cured acute cystitis or an aftermath of an indwelling catheter, repeated catheterization, or urinary retention. Other causes include upper tract disease, cystocele with a residual urine, or idiopathic or unknown causes.

The appropriate forms of chemotherapy or antibiotic treatment should be instituted after culture-sensitivity reports are obtained. Irrigation of the bladder with 1/1000 silver nitrate or 2% boric solution (30 cc.) is helpful. When prompt relief of symptoms is not obtained, more thorough study of the urinary tract is advisable. Intravenous pyelography should be supplemented by retrograde study *via* water or air cystoscopy. The latter is particularly useful in allowing visualization of a discrete Hunner (elusive) ulcer, which is frequently amenable to topical application of Argyrol, use of fulguration, or, more recently, cortisone instillations. Such unusual entities as

mesenchyme and referred to as medullary cords; and (4) germ cells which have wandered in from the outside as previously described and which seem to accumulate beneath the germinal epithelium.

The derivation and subsequent development of the structures referred to above has been the subject of considerable difficulty and controversy. For purposes of simplicity the views of Witschi will be followed. According to this authority the cellular cords referred to above constitute the *medulla* of the gonads. Further condensation of cells in the upper portions of the gonad establishes solid connection between these cords and mesonephric tubules, the primordial efferent ductules (Fig. 6.4).

According to Witschi, when the migrating germ cells enter the primitive gonad they selectively accumulate under the celomic epithelium but the cords, which may now be referred to as medullary cords, do not contain many germ cells in embryos of 8-mm. length (5 weeks). Suddenly the behavior of the germ cells changes and at this time many of them pass from the cortex to the medulla along the medullary sex cords. During this transit they seem to carry with them some somatic cells from the cortex which, according to Witschi's view, later become Sertoli cells. The significance of this observation lies in the attempt to explain the estrogenic production of the Sertoli cells in the adult testis, which is primarily the development of the medulla of the primitive gonad. This explanation assumes that estrogenic production must be of cortical origin. Finally, by the 14-mm. stage (slightly older than 6 weeks) the indifferent gonad is composed of an outer cortex containing many germ cells and an internal medulla comprising sex cords also provided with germ cells.

Differentiation of the Testis. According to Gillman the differentiation of the testis first becomes recognizable in an embryo with a crown rump length of 14 to 16 mm. (6 to 7 weeks). The medullary cords which become the seminiferous tubules of the testis acquire a prominence. During this same time the cortex de-

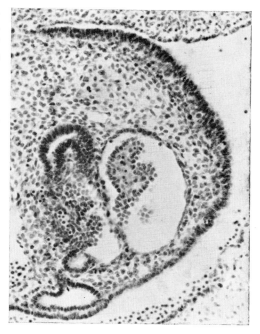

FIG. 6.3. Human embryo 7.4 mm. Cross section through left urogenital fold at indifferent gonad stage. The cortex consists of the much thickened celomic epithelium and contains several germ cells. The medulla is composed of a nucleus of blastema cells, more or less distinctly organized as cords radiating from the mesonephros toward the cortex. A narrow albuginea with a few mesenchyme cells separates cortex and medulla. (Reprinted by permission from Jones, H. W., Jr., and Scott, W. W.: *Hermaphroditism, Genital Anomalies and Related Endocrine Disorders.* The Williams & Wilkins Company, Baltimore, 1958.)

generates, the germ cells disappear from the cortex, the cells of the outer epithelium flatten, and a connective tissue layer develops between the sex cords and the covering epithelium. In a male fetus the sex gland of a 27-mm. embryo (about 8 weeks) is a typical testis (Fig. 6.4).

According to Gillman's studies the interstitial cells show their first signs of specialization in a fetus of about 31-mm. crown rump length (about 10 weeks). By the time the fetus reaches 50 mm. (about 11 weeks), they begin to increase enormously and the medullary tubules now properly called seminiferous tubules, are

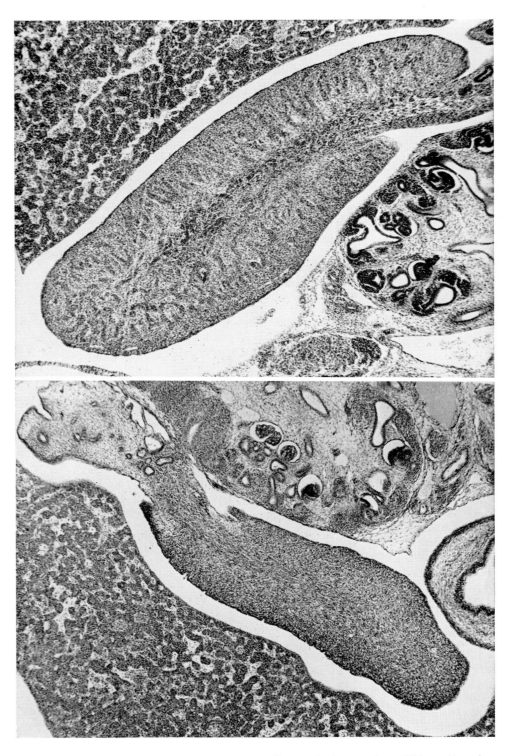

FIG. 6.4. Sections of gonads of human fetuses. *Top*, male 27 mm. long. This section shows short, straight testicular tubules connected with the rete testis which are darker in the center. *Bottom*, female embryo 25 mm. long. Note the cellular cortex with the poorly developed rete and the inconspicuous medulla. (Reprinted by permission from Jones, H. W., Jr., and Scott, W. W.; *Hermaphroditism, Genital Anomalies and Related Endocrine Disorders*. The Williams & Wilkins Company, Baltimore, 1958.)

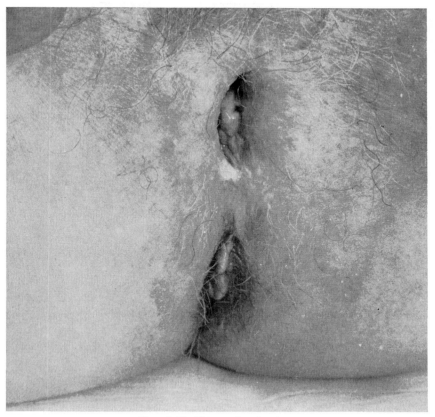

FIG. 9.17. Kraurosis of vulva

The many terms that have been applied to these primary hyperkeratoses need some interpretation.

Leukoplakia has been used to describe a variety of whitish lesions since the term could be applied to any "white patch." More accurately, it should designate that hyperkeratotic, elevated, pruritic lesion which often demonstrates linear excoriations. As noted above, microscopically the problem is similarly confused in that the characteristic features of leukoplakia, namely hyperkeratosis, acanthosis and inflammatory infiltrate, are also those of chronic forms of neurodermatitis, eczematoid dermatitis, and lichen planus. It would seem wiser to eliminate such descriptive terms as applied to specific disease for a designation which would relay information as to the malignant potential such as "hyperplastic

vulvitis" with the modifying degrees, mild, moderate, or marked to explain the degree of anaplastic activity to the clinician.

Lichen sclerosus et atrophicus applies to a skin lesion which begins as a small bluish white papule. Frequently coalescence of these papules produces a picture of diffuse whitish change over the entire vulva and perianal region (Fig. 9.18). In its terminal stage this disease simulates *atrophic leukoplakia* and *kraurosis* in that there is loss of the subcutaneous tissue with flattening of the labial folds and constriction of the outlet. Actually *kraurosis* is simply a descriptive term meaning "shrinkage." The microscopic pictures of atrophic leukoplakia, lichen sclerosus et atrophicus, and kraurosis are similar.

These lesions commonly appear in the early postmenopausal years. Nevertheless, atrophy of a primary type may be seen

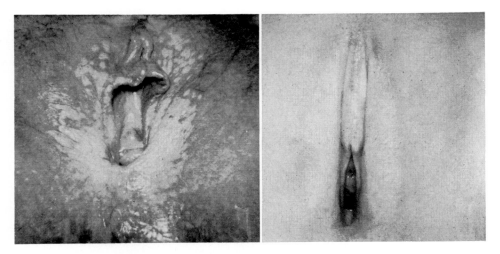

FIG. 9.18 (*left*). Lichen sclerosus et atrophicus in 56-year-old female showing isolated lesions with confluence at fourchette.

FIG. 9.19 (*right*). Lichen sclerosus in 6-year-old-child.

prepubertal (Fig. 9.19), and patchy lichen sclerosus et atrophicus is not infrequently seen in the fourth decade of life.

Although *atrophy* has been applied to these lesions, certain studies have indicated that the thinned epithelium is not metabolically inactive. Clark *et al.*, noted that the uptake of radioactive phosphorus is as great in these *atrophic* lesions as in carcinoma-in-situ. Similar findings have been recognized in our laboratory using other methodologies. Although, metabolic activity cannot be correlated directly with anaplasia, the changes do not justify the designation of atrophy. Furthermore, these lesions must be followed carefully as carcinoma can develop in this context (Fig. 9.20). It is important to remember that any irritative lesion may become malignant although the thickened, elevated, hyperkeratotic type seems to be more prone to anaplastic alteration. Of major importance in the study and therapy of the lesions are the use of the biopsy and the elimination of scratching with the use of antipruritics, particularly hydrocortisones and antihistamines, intravaginal estrogens postmenopause, the treatment of specific vaginitis, the removal of local irritating medications, etc., and if necessary some

variety of nerve block. Plastic procedures to increase the caliber of outlet are often necessary to eliminate the dyspareunia and allow for satisfactory coitus. Vulvectomy is of importance if anaplastic changes are noted in the tissue study.

Finally it must be recognized that *carcinoma-in-situ* (Fig. 9.21) and *invasive cancer* can and frequently do appear as whitish lesions. As a consequence any hyperkeratotic area must be biopsied and followed carefully. Again therapy for the common symptomatology is imperative.

PRURITUS VULVAE

Pruritis, or itching, of the vulva is one of the most distressing and often one of the most baffling and intractable of gynecological symptoms. Although it is only a symptom and not a disease entity, it is often difficult to ferret out the underlying cause. It is believed that itching represents a subpain response, and that it has its origin in the epidermis rather than in the subcutaneous nerves. When the vulva is the seat of a definite dermatological lesion, such as eczema, dermatitis, or leukoplakia, it is easy to understand how itching would probably be a symptom, just as with a similar lesion elsewhere. In other cases

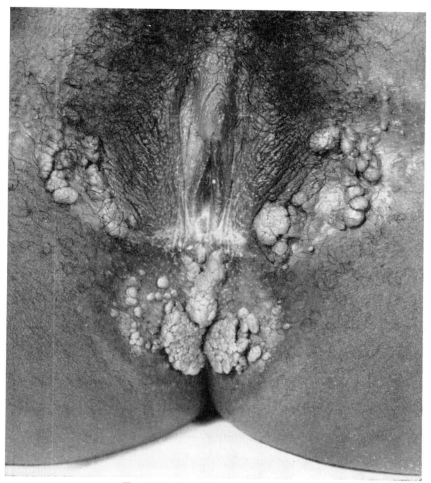

FIG. 9.25. Condylomata acuminata

rarely in the upper vagina and even on the cervix.

When numerous they tend to become confluent, forming large clusters. They undergo pronounced hypertrophy during pregnancy, sometimes forming huge cauliflower masses which may even offer obstacles to delivery (per vaginam). Actually, many may regress spontaneously postpartum if removal is not necessary during the pregnancy. Malignant degeneration may occur, but is rare, and only a few such cases have been seen in this country.

Formerly, the preferred treatment of condyloma was by excision, although fulguration or use of the high frequency current has been employed by some Topical application of 25% podophyllin in tincture of benzoin or mineral oil is quite effective in the treatment of the smaller lesions, and this is the customary method of therapy. To avoid a chemical burn, care must be taken to wash off the treated area within a few hours after application. Topical sulfonamides have been used effectively by some observers.

4. Angioma. Although angiomata are rare, the congenital type cause problems due to irritations of diapers, urine, and feces. However, it is important to take no action if possible, since most of these congenital types regress as the child grows (Fig. 9.26).

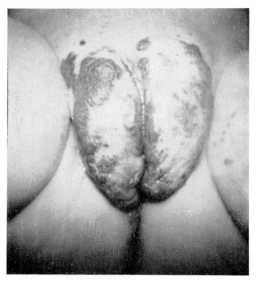

FIG. 9.26. Congenital hemangiomata on both labia, appearing at 2 months of age and at year much reduced without treatment.

5. Hidradenoma of Vulva. While this is a rare lesion, it is of some importance because it is so frequently mistaken for adenocarcinoma, not clinically but microscopically (Fig. 9.27). The lesion arises from the vulvar sweat glands, and with rare exceptions it is benign. Clinically it appears as a small nodule usually raised above the surrounding surface, and having a fibroma-like appearance and consistency (Fig. 9.28). In some cases the overlying skin may be reddened, granular, or ulcerated. In such cases there may be slight bleeding. Most frequently there are no symptoms, although occasionally itching is present. The usual location of the lesion is on the inner surface of the labia majora, but it may be on the labia minora or the adjacent perineum. The treatment consists of simple excision. Only a rare malignancy

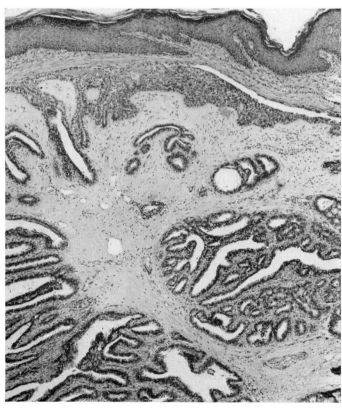

FIG. 9.27. Hidradenoma of vulva. A rare lesion which may be mistaken for adenocarcinoma

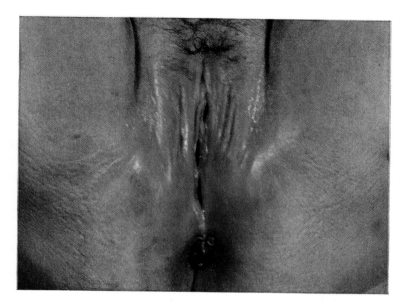

PLATE IX.I. Diabetic vulvitis often associated with mycotic infection

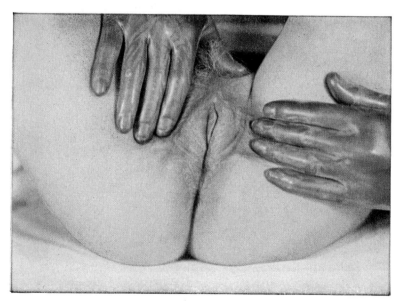

PLATE IX.II. Mycotic vulvitis

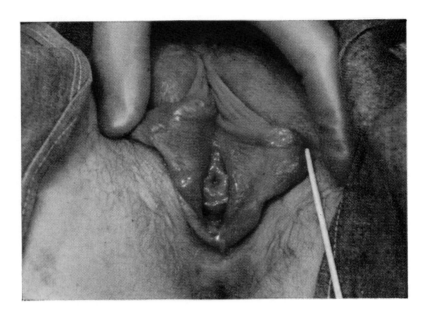

PLATE IX.III. Chancroid of vulva

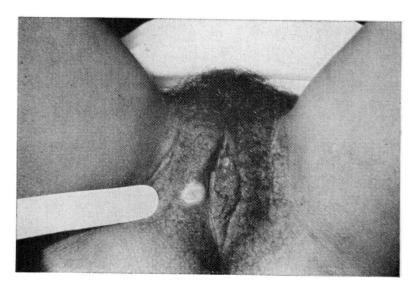

PLATE IX.IV. Chancre of vulva

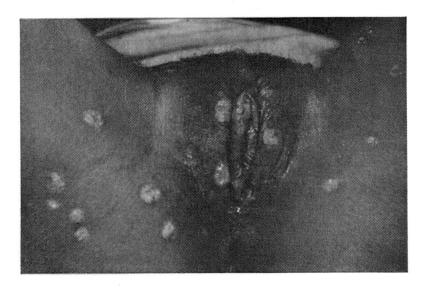

PLATE IX.V. Condylomata lata of vulva and perineum

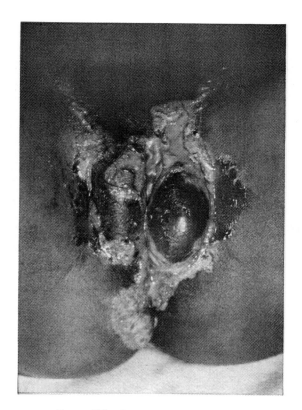

PLATE IX.VI. Granuloma inguinale

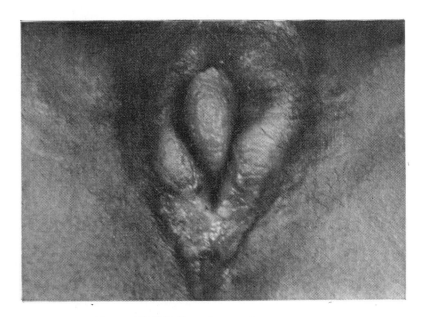

Plate IX.VII. Lymphogranuloma venereum

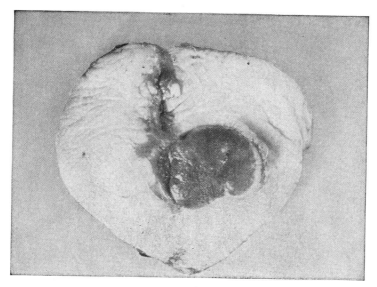

PLATE IX.VIII. Carcinoma of vulva after excision by vulvectomy

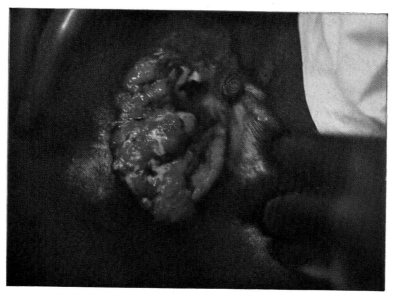

PLATE IX.IX. Carcinoma of vulva in colored woman 45 years of age

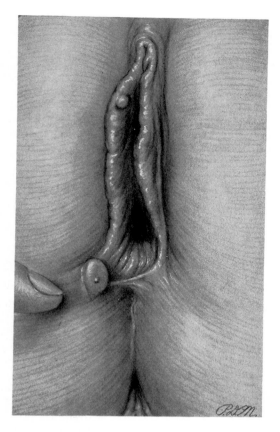

FIG. 9.28. Gross appearance of hidradenoma of vulva

is noted in the recent comprehensive review of Chung and Greene.

Supernumerary breast tissue may be found on the vulva and microscopically simulates the apocrine adenoma since the breast is a modified apocrine gland.

6. Granular Cell Myoblastoma of Vulva. This rather uncommon tumor, composed of irregular clumps of large pale staining cells with eosinophilic cytoplasmic granules, is most commonly found in the tongue, but has been found at many sites. Although called myoblastoma, the tumor is felt to arise from the myelin sheath of the nerve. Of interest is the pseudo-epitheliomatous change in the overlying epithelium suggesting epidermoid cancer. Rubin brings up to 23 the total number of such vulvar myoblastomas and, although these are included under benign tumors, he points

out that incomplete removal may lead to recurrence.

7. Nevus. The nevus is an important lesion on the vulva since although the vulvar skin makes up only 1% of the entire body surface, 7 to 10% of malignant melanoma in the female occur on the external genitalia. This may be due to the many irritants which affect this area as well as the fact that junction activity is common in the vulvar nevus.

CARCINOMA OF THE VULVA

The most important of vulvar tumors is carcinoma, the third most common of all primary pelvic cancers, being exceeded in frequency only by uterine (Cervix and corpus) and ovarian cancer. Vulvar cancer accounts for 3 to 4% of all primary malignancies of the genital canal.

Carcinoma-in-situ of the vulva is a definite entity, although far less common than intraepithelial cancer of the cervix. Intraepithelial cancer of the vulva has the same relation as the comparable cervical disease in its tendency to exist at the periphery of invasive cancer or to precede true infiltrative cancer. Indeed, some of the patterns of the so-called hypertrophic leukoplakia bear the same relation to early cancer that atypical cervical epithelium does to cervical intraepithelial cancer. By definition intraepithelial cervical cancer connotes full thickness replacement of the lining epithelium by undifferentiated abnormal cells, often of basal type; and similarly, intraepithelial cancer of the vulva shows abnormality of the lining epithelium with abnormal mitotic activity. However, vulvar cancer is characteristically spinal in type, and some degree of differentiation of the component cells is often found despite undeniable intraepithelial anaplasia. It is important, however, to recognize that a pure cytologic type of in situ cancer of vulva is as rare as a similar pure lesion in the cervix. A variety of terms such as Bowen's disease, erythroplasia of Queyrat, etc., have been used to describe types of in situ cancer, but basically the microscopic pictures are not sufficiently distinctive to be specific. Grossly the anaplasias may appear as granulomatous, leukoplakic, or variegated pigmented, whitish (Fig. 9.29), slightly elevated lesions and are commonly multicentric in origin (Fig. 9.30).

Paget's disease of the vulva is a specific form of in situ cancer characterized grossly by a reddish lesion interspersed with white epithelial islands (Fig. 9.31) and microscopically by the large pale "Paget" cells. While the similar lesion of the breast is usually associated with an underlying carcinoma, such is rare on the vulva.

Invasive carcinoma is preeminently a disease of elderly women, the great majority of cases occurring after the age of 50. The average age in Taussig's large series was 59, and the decade between 60 and 70 shows the highest incidence. The exception occurs in those cases preceded by granulomatous disease where the average age is about 40 years as noted by Salzstein, Collins, and Alexander. The disease begins on any part of the vulva, most frequently the labia, the region of the clitoris, the vestibule, or the vulvovaginal gland. In all of these locations the cancer is of squamous cell or epidermoid variety (Fig. 9.32), except that primary carcinoma in Bartholin's gland which may be either adenocarcinoma, transitional or epidermoid in character. In such instances a hard stony mass can be felt in the region of the gland.

The gross appearance may be whitish, ulcerated, or granulomatous depending on the primary lesion (Fig. 9.33 and Plates IX.VIII and IX.IX). As noted previously several authors have reported the premalignant nature of the granulomata and leukoplakic diseases.

Basal cell carcinoma is rare and appears as on the skin elsewhere as a superficial ulcer with "rolled" edges.

In the usual forms of vulvar cancer,

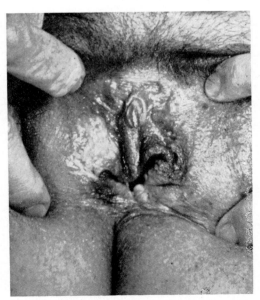

Fig. 9.29. In situ cancer of the vulva with major area on right labium majus, but multiple sites on both labia.

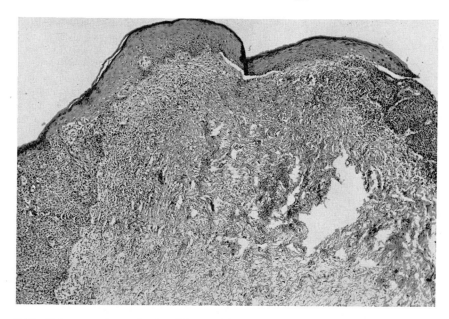

FIG. 9.30. Vulvar carcinoma in situ. Note multicentric origin with intervening normal tissue

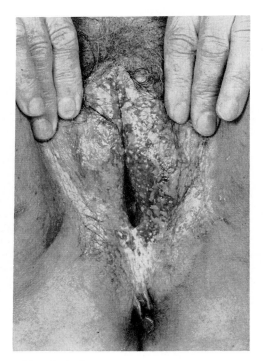

FIG. 9.31. Paget's disease of the vulva. (Dark areas are red in color, and white "leukoplakoid" area are as seen).

the initial lesion becomes steadily larger, with increasing induration, ulceration, and surrounding edema. If neglected, the destruction of the disease may involve most of the vulvar structure. Metastatic involvement of the superficial and deep inguinal glands, as well as the lymph glands at the femoral ring, soon develops, while the richness of the lymphatic communications with the pelvis leads to extension in that direction.

The *symptoms* in the early stage are apt to be very slight, consisting only of slight soreness and itching, although the latter is not invariably present. In many instances, however, there is a history of long standing pruritus antedating the appearance of carcinoma. As the ulceration and infiltration extend, the pain increases, and in the advanced cases it may be persistent and intolerable unless controlled by narcotics.

Not uncommonly there is an unfortunate delay of $1\frac{1}{2}$ to 2 years between the appearance of symptoms and diagnosis of the disease. Much of this delay is due to reluctance of the older patient to seek medical consultation, however, in about

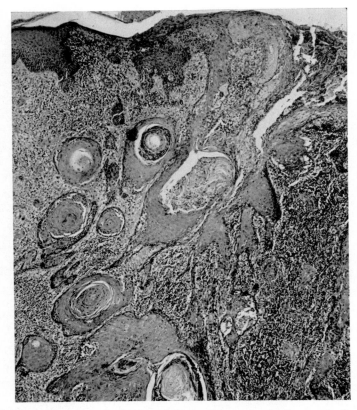

FIG. 9.32. Epidermoid carcinoma of vulva. Spinal cell type developing in a leukoplakia base

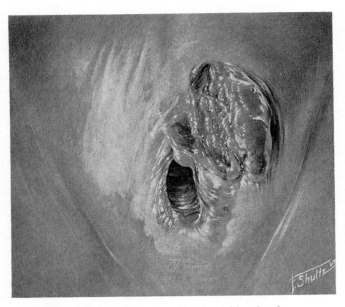

FIG. 9.33. Carcinoma and leukoplakia of vulva

one-third of the cases the physician is at fault as noted by Howson and Montgomery. In the early stage the patient suffers very little discomfort, and the lesion may seem even to the physician a rather unimpressive one unless he is familiar with its potentialities. *Biopsy and microscopic examination* are of decisive importance, and they should *never* be omitted when an ulcerative vulvar lesion is observed in elderly women. Upon this diagnostic procedure one must depend for the differentiation from other ulcerative lesions, such as syphilitic ulcers, or lymphogranuloma venereum.

Prophylaxis is of considerable importance, for it has been noted that both leukoplakia and various granulomatous or other irritative lesions are frequent precursors of cancer. Fortunately these generally cause such intense pruritus and discomfort as to lead to medical attention, but haphazard use of various ointments, lotions, and sprays can only be condemned if biopsy of any suspicious lesion is not performed.

Treatment of Vulvar Cancer. There can be no doubt that the main treatment for carcinoma of the vulva is surgery. Vulvectomy is sufficient in those instances of in situ disease, however, thorough study of the removed tissue must be carried out to eliminate invasion. Radical vulvectomy is mandatory for invasive cancer. Lymphadenectomy is the rule, but there is considerable difference of opinion as to how extensive this should be. The presence of palpable nodes should not be the criterion; since in one-third of the cases in which nodes are enlarged the enlargement is not due to cancer but to infection. Likewise, in one-third of the cases in which there is metastatic disease to the nodes, the nodes are not clinically enlarged.

Way emphasizes that vulvectomy must be so extensive as to disallow primary closure; and although we do not necessarily concur, we agree that *radical* removal of the vulva is the *essential part* of a surgical approach to this disease. The value of lymphadenectomy is less

certain, for if the removed nodes show cancer, the salvage is markedly impaired. Nevertheless, Taussig's publications on the Bassett operation, *i.e.*, radical vulvectomy with extensive lymphadenectomy, did result in a remarkably increased 5-year salvage. Perhaps this was by virtue of merely a more radical vulvar excision, for there is no doubt that if removed nodes contain cancer, recurrence may be delayed, but salvage approximates only 10%.

Green, Ulfelder, and Meigs perform a one-stage "crescent incision" to carry out simultaneous vulvectomy and bilateral lymphadenectomy (Fig. 9.34). The New Orleans approach (Collins *et al.*) is more radical with an extended lymphadenectomy and freely utilizing exenteration if adjacent organs (vagina, urethra, or rectum) are involved without extrapelvic metastases. McKelvey, believing that complete excision of the local disease is paramount to salvage, feels that vulvectomy with superficial node dissection (one-stage under local anesthesia) is adequate treatment.

Collins has also pointed out that curability roughly parallels the extent of the lesion when seen, and he notes 3 cm. as the critical size below which cure is usual and above which, unlikely. A 5-year salvage of all patients should approximate 50% if adequate surgery is carried out. X-ray therapy is felt to be rarely indicated by most authors; however, some Scandanavian schools have suggested extensive fulguration of the local growth and x-ray therapy to the nodes.

Although ultraradical surgery may be an unjustifiably extensive approach for the age group usually affected and results in a rare salvage if the high nodes are involved, nevertheless operative therapy is generally accepted as the therapeutic approach of choice. The lesion is slow to metastasize and often does so in a superficial fashion. Wide local invasion and extension often precedes lymphatic or hematogenous dissemination. Such a disease process obviously deserves a wide local radical excision with some form of bilateral lymphadenectomy. The frequent crossover of lymphatics from one to the other side demands bilateral operation.

Other Vulvar Malignancies. *Sarcoma* of the vulva is exceedingly rare, only about 30 cases having been reported. *Malignant melanoma* is also rare; however,

it is the second most common malignancy in the vulvar area. As in other parts of the body, its origin is usually in pigmented moles. Its tendency to widespread dissemination is well known, and a fatal termination is common. Symmonds has reported improved results with early and

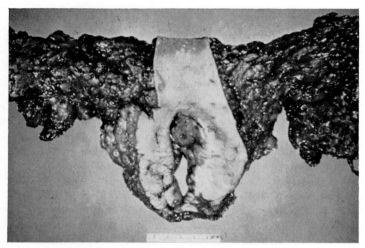

Fig. 9.34. Specimen from one stage radical vulvectomy and node dissection. (Cancer noted at clitoris.)

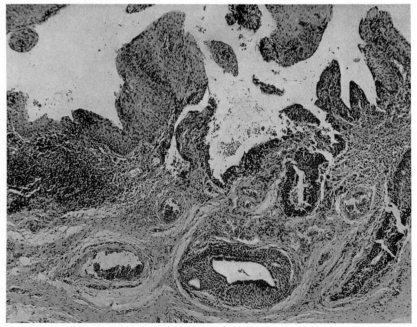

Fig. 9.35. Chronic urethritis. Resection of marked urethral eversion

radical surgery. A recent publication by Woodruff and Brack describes these and other unusual types of vulvourethal lesions.

URETHRA

Although the urethra is technically not part of the genital canal, the diseases that affect the area commonly involve the genitalia. Urethral infection is often gonoccocal, the vulvovaginal glands and cervix being also frequent sites of involvement. Actually the urethra may be the primary organ invaded by the gonococcus, however, the symptoms are usually very transient. Residuae may remain in the urethral glands or Skene's ducts (Fig. 9.35).

Many other organisms also involve the posterior portion of the urethra, as well as of the trigone. The clinician must be mindful of the possibility that the sub-urethral gland infection may result in the formation of a diverticulum. This may be the cause of a recurrent cystitis. Palpation of the urethra may reveal a saclike outpouching from which pus can be "milked out," through the urethral meatus. Occasionally endoscopic examinations with urethrographic studies, as suggested by Davis and Cian, are necessary.

Although surgical excision of a diverticulum is the preferred treatment, simple urethritis, either acute or chronic, is frequently amenable to alkalinization of the urine and to the administration of sulfonamides or antibiotics. More helpful, particularly in the low grade, chronic infections, is the topical application of 2 to 5% silver nitrate. If the immediately adjacent Skene's glands are involved, as indicated by expression of pus on palpation, they may be easily fulgurated.

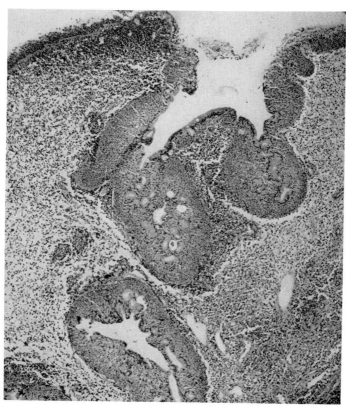

Fig. 9.36. Microscopic appearance of urethral caruncle of papillomatous type

A real but frequently overlooked entity is the postmenopausal senile or atrophic urethritis. This frequently occurs in conjunction with a similar type of vaginitis as a sequel to estrogen deprivation. There is a reddening of the meatus as edema and exfoliation of the urethral mucosa lining occur, and the resultant appearance is much like a urethral caruncle. Local pain, terminal burning on urination, strangury, and even hematuria may occur, but prompt remission and relief are achieved by estrogen therapy. Stilbestrol intravaginal suppositories, 0.5 mg., applied nightly for 2 to 3 weeks, are perhaps preferable to systemic steroid therapy. Fulguration, the preferred treatment for a caruncle, is not necessary in this form of urethral disease.

Benign tumors are uncommon, the most frequent being the caruncle (Fig. 9.36). This small, reddish pedunculated lesion is occasionally tender and may bleed. Fulguration after biopsy is the treatment of choice.

The urethra may be the site of other pathological entities, such as stricture or fistula (frequently postirradiation or postoperative), granulomatous infection by lymphopathia or granuloma inguinale, prolapsed mucosa, and even carcinoma. The latter is rare and carries a poor prognosis, less than 50%. Treatment is generally radiation, as indicated by Brack and Farber, but occasionally radical surgical procedures are performed particularly in the radio resistant lesion.

REFERENCES

Alexander, L. J., and Shields, T. L.: Squamous cell carcinoma of vulva secondary to granuloma inguinale. Arch. Derm., 67: 395, 1953.

Anderson, N. P.: Hidradenoma of vulva. Arch. Derm. Syph., 62: 873, 1950.

Barclay, D. L., and Collins, C. G.: Intraepithelial cancer of vulva. Amer. J. Obstet. Gynec., 86: 95, 1963.

Brack, C. B., and Dickson, R. J.: Carcinoma of the female urethra. Amer. J. Roentgen., 79: 472, 1958.

Brack, C. B., and Guild, H. G.: Urethral obstruction in the female child. Amer. J. Obstet. Gynec., 76: 1105, 1958.

Buckingham, J. C., and McClure, J. H.: Reticulum cell sarcoma of vulva. Obstet. Gynec., 6: 121, 1955.

Chung, J. T., and Greene, R. R.: Hidradenoma of vulva. Amer. J. Obstet. Gynec., 75: 310, 1958.

Clark, D. G., Zumoff, B., Brunschwig, A., and Hellman, L.: Preferential uptake of phosphate by premalignant and malignant lesions of the vulva. Cancer, 13: 775, 1960.

Cockerell, E. G., Knox, J. M., and Rogers, S. F.: Lichen sclerosus et atrophicus. Obstet. Gynec., 15: 554, 1960.

Collins, C. G., Borman, R. G., McMahon, B., and Avent, J. C.: Vulvectomy for benign diasease. Amer. J. Obstet. Gynec., 76: 363, 1958.

Collins, C. G., Collins, J. H., Nelson, E. W., Smith, R. C., and MacCallum, E. A.: Vulval cancer. Amer. J. Obstet. Gynec., 62: 1198, 1951.

Collins, C. G., Kushner, J., Lewis, G. N., and LaPointe, R.: Noninvasive malignancy of the vulva. Obstet. Gynec., 6: 339, 1955.

Cosbie, W. G.: Treatment of carcinoma of the vulva. Amer. J. Obstet. Gynec., 63: 251, 1952.

Davis, H. J., and Cian, L. G.: Positive pressure urethrography; a new diagnostic study. J. Urol., 75: 753, 1956.

Dennis, E. J., Hester, L. H., Jr., and Wilson, L. A.: Primary carcinoma of Bartholin's glands. Obstet. Gynec., 6: 291, 1955.

Douglas, C. P.: Lymphangioma venereum and granuloma inguinale of the vulva. J. Obstet. Gynaec. Brit. Comm., 69: 871, 1962.

Falk, H. C., and Hyman, A. B.: Diagnosis and treatment of pruritus vulvae. Clin. Obstet. Gynec., 2: 461, 1959.

Gardiner, S. H., Stout, F. E., Arbogast, J. L., and Huber, C. D.: Intraepithelial carcinoma of the vulva. Amer. J. Obstet. Gynec., 65: 515, 1953.

Green, T. H., Ulfelder, H., and Meigs, J. V.: Epidermoid carcinoma of the vulva. Amer. J. Obstet. Gynec., 75: 834, 1958.

Greenblatt, R. B., Baldwin, K. R., and Dienst, R. B.: Minor venereal diseases. Clin. Obstet. Gynec., 2: 549, 1959.

Hawson, J. V., and Montgomery, T. L.: Delay period in diagnosis of genital cancer. Amer. J. Obstet. Gynec., 57: 1098, 1949.

Herndon, E. G.: Leukoplakic vulvitis and its relationship to the development of carcinoma of vulva. J. Bowman Gray Sch. Med., 4: 35, 1946.

Hester, L. J.: Granuloma venereum of cervix and vulva. Amer. J. Obstet. Gynec., 62: 312, 1951.

Huber, C. P., Gardiner, S. H., and Michael, A.:

Paget's disease of vulva. Amer. J. Obstet. Gynec., *62:* 778, 1951.

Huffman, J. W.: Detailed anatomy of paraurethral ducts in adult human female. Amer. J. Obstet. Gynec., *55:* 86, 1948.

Hyman, A. B., and Falk, H. C.: White lesions of the vulva. Obstet. Gynec., *12:* 407, 1958.

Isaacs, J. H., and Topek, N. H.: Carcinoma of the vulva. Amer. J. Obstet. Gynec., *73:* 1277, 1957.

Jeffcoate, T. N. A.: Dermatology of vulva. J. Obstet. Gynaec. Brit. Comm., *69:* 888, 1962.

Kanter, A. E., and Strean, B. J.: Melanoma of the vulva. Obstet. Gynec., *12:* 516, 1958.

Knight, R. V.: Bowen's disease. Amer. J. Obstet. Gynec., *6:* 514, 1943.

Lacy, G. R.: Hydradenoma and hydradenoid carcinoma of vulva. Amer. J. Obstet. Gynec., *51:* 268, 1945.

Lang, W. R.: Genital infections in female children. Clin. Obstet. Gynec., *2:* 428, 1959.

Langley, I. I., Hertig, A. T., and Smith, G. van S.: Relation of leucoplakic vulvitis to squamous carcinoma of vulva. Amer. J. Obstet. Gynec., *62:* 167, 1951.

Lipschütz, B.: Ulcus Vulvae acutum. In *Jadassohn's Handbuch der Haut- und Geschlechtskrankheiten.* Julius Springer, Berlin, 1927.

Marcus, S. L.: Basal cell and basal-squamous cell carcinomas of the vulva. Amer. J. Obstet. Gynec., *79:* 461, 1960.

Marcus, S. L.: Multiple squamous cell carcinomas involving the cervix, vagina, and vulva. Amer. J. Obstet. Gynec., *80:* 802, **1960.**

Masterson, J. G., and Goss, A. S.: Carcinoma of Bartholin gland. Amer. J. Obstet. Gynec., *69:* 1323, 1955.

McKelvey, J. L.: Carcinoma of vulva. Obstet. Gynec., *5:* 452, 1955.

Mering, J. H.: A surgical approach to intractable pruritus vulvae. Amer. J. Obstet. Gynec., *64:* 619, 1952.

Miller, N. F., Riley, G. M., and Stanley, M.: Leukoplakia vulvae. Amer. J. Obstet. Gynec., *64:* 768, 1952.

Newman, B., and Cromen, J. K.: Multicentric origin of carcinomas of the female anogenital tract. Surg. Gynec. Obstet., *108:* 273, 1959.

Nolan, J. F.: Carcinoma of the vulva. Amer. J. Obstet. Gynec., *78:* 833, 1959.

Novak, E., and Novak, E. R.: *Gynecologic and Obstetric Pathology,* Ed. 4. W. B. Saunders Company, Philadelphia, 1958.

Novak, E., and Stevenson, R. R.: Sweat gland tumors of vulva, benign (hidradenoma) and malignant (adenocarcinoma). Amer. J. Obstet. Gynec., *50:* 641, 1945.

Plachta, A., and Speer, F. D.: Apocrine gland adenocarcinoma and extra-mammary Paget's disease of the vulva. Cancer, *7:* 910, 1954.

Rainey, R.: Association of lymphogranuloma inguinale and cancer. Surgery, *34:* 221, 1954.

Rubin, A.: Granular cell myoblastoma of the vulva. Amer. J. Obstet. Gynec., *77:* 292, 1959.

Saltzstein, S. L., Woodruff, J. D., and Novak, E. R.: Postgranulomatous carcinoma of the vulva. Obstet. Gynec., *7:* 80, 1956.

Siegler, A. M., and Greene, H. J.: Basal-cell carcinoma of vulva. Amer. J. Obstet. Gynec., *62:* 1219, 1951.

Stening, M., and Elliott, P.: Primary carcinoma of the vulva, with special reference to leukoplakia. J. Obstet. Gynaec. Brit. Comm., *66:* 897, 1959.

Symmonds, R. E., Pratt, J. H., and Dockerty, M. B.: Melanoma of the vulva. Obstet. Gynec., *15:* 543, 1960.

Taussig, F.: *Diseases of Vulva.* D. Appleton-Century Company, New York, 1921.

Taussig, F.: Leukoplakic vulvitis and cencer of the vulva. Amer. J. Obstet. Gynec., *18:* 472, 1929.

Taussig, F.: Cancer of vulva. Amer. J. Obstet. Gynec., *40:* 764, 1940.

Taylor, C. W.: Dermatology of the vulva. J. Obstet. Gynaec. Brit. Comm., *69:* 881, 1962.

Thomas, W. A.: Clinical study of granuloma inguinale with a routine for the diagnosis of lesions of the vulva. Amer. J. Obstet. Gynec., *61:* 790, 1951.

Tomskey, G. C., Vickery, G. W., and Getzoff, P. L.: Successful treatment of granuloma inguinale, with special reference to use of podophyllin. J. Urol., *48:* 401, 1942.

Ulfelder, H.: Radical vulvectomy with bilateral inguinal, femoral and iliac node resection. Amer. J. Obstet. Gynec., *78:* 1074, 1959.

Wallace, H. J.: Vulva leukoplakia. J. Obstet. Gynaec. Brit. Comm., *69:* 865, 1962.

Way, S.: *Malignant Disease of the Female Genital Tract.* Blakiston Company, Division of McGraw-Hill Book Company, Inc., New York, 1951.

Way, S.: Carcinoma of the vulva. Amer. J. Obstet. Gynec., *79:* 692, 1960.

Wharton, L. R., and Everett, H. S.: Primary malignant Bartholin gland tumors. Obstet. Gynec. Survey, *6:* 1, 1951.

Woodruff, J. D.: Paget's disease of the vulva. Obstet. Gynec., *5:* 175, 1955.

Woodruff, J. D.: Premalignant lesions of the vulva. In *Treatment of Cancer and Allied Diseases,* edited by G. Pack and I. Ariel. Paul B. Hoeber, Inc., New York, 1962.

Woodruff, J. D., and Brack, C. B.: Unusual

malignancies of vulvourethral region. Obstet. Gynec., *12:* 677, 1958.

Woodruff, J. D., and Hildebrandt, E. E.: Carcinoma in situ of the vulva. Obstet. Gynec., *12:* 414, 1958.

Woodruff, J. D., and Richardson, E. H., Jr.:

Malignant vulvar Paget's disease. Obstet. Gynec., *10:* 10, 1957.

Woodruff, J. D., and Williams, T. J.: Multiple sites of anaplastic change in the lower genital system. Amer. J. Obstet. Gynec., *85:* 724, 1963.

10

DISEASES OF THE VAGINA

VAGINITIS

Vaginitis (of bacterial or parasitic origin) comprises a sizable percentage of most gynecological practice. It is difficult for the clinician to be enthusiastic about such patients, whose complaints are truly valid, but the infection is never of serious import and is often difficult to eradicate. Since the histology of the vagina varies at different age periods, it is not strange that certain types of inflammatory involvement are characteristic of certain age periods. During reproductive life, for example, the vaginal epithelium is many layers thick. This fact, together with the absence of glands, makes gonorrheal infection very rare as compared to its incidence in the young child. In the latter, only a few layers of vaginal epithelial cells are seen, and the Gonococcus gains an easy foothold, so that gonorrheal vaginitis is most common in children. Again, in the senile phase of life, there is marked atrophy of the vaginal wall, so that infection by various organisms, including not infrequently the Gonococcus, occurs quite readily.

The *normal flora* of the vagina may include many types of organisms (Streptococcus, Staphylococcus, Döderlein's bacillus, diphtheroid organisms, etc.) including some of pathogenic type, and not infrequently fungi of various sorts. The bacteriology of the vagina, however, is still very confusing. It seems clear, however, that the so-called bacillus of Döderlein, a normal inhabitant, plays an important role in maintaining the acidity which characterizes the normal vaginal secretion. This acidity is due to the presence of lactic acid formed from the splitting up of the glycogen present in the vaginal epithelial cells. The pH of the normal vaginal secretion averages from 4.5 to 5.

Causes. The *bacteria* most often responsible for vaginitis are the Gonococcus (more particularly in the infantile vagina, but not during reproductive life) and various strains of Streptococcus, the *Staphylococcus aureus*, colon bacillus, diphtheroid, and other organisms.

Other frequent causes are the *Trichomonas vaginalis*, *Hemophilus vaginalis*, and certain *yeast fungi*, especially the *Monilia* or *Candida albicans*, the same parasite which produces thrush in the oral cavity of the infant. These receive special consideration later in this chapter. Certain *general diseases* may, by the lowering of general vitality, predispose to the disease. Especially important in this connection is diabetes, which through the presence of large amounts of sugar in the blood and urine, may also predispose to the invasion and growth of yeast fungi. In the occasional case the presence of *foreign bodies*, especially neglected pessaries, may be followed by vaginitis, and a transient form of the latter may follow the use of *douches* which are too hot or which are chemically irritating. Another possible cause is infection by *discharges from the uterine* cavity or cervix. Finally, the acute *exanthematous diseases* may in rare cases cause vaginal inflammation.

Symptoms and Signs. The outstanding symptom of vaginitis, the one which as a rule leads the patient to seek advice, is *vaginal discharge*, which is commonly milky but in other cases thinner in consistency, and the addition of mucus from the cervix may make it mucopurulent. There is often much *local irritation* from the discharge, with vulvar and perineal *itching* and *burning*, especially on urination. The vulvovaginal mucosa is reddened and congested, and on speculum examination the entire vaginal mucous membrane likewise shows intense *redness* and *hyperemia*. In certain types the surface shows small reddish granular patches (follicular vaginitis).

Special types of vaginitis, especially those due to the Gonococcus in children, and the Trichomonas and yeast fungi in adults, present special characteristics, as will be described below.

Diagnosis of Nonspecific Form. While the diagnosis of vaginitis is made easily enough by simple *inspection* of the vagina, the assumption of its nonspecific nature is not permissible except by *exclusion of a more specific etiology*. In the adult this means especially exclusion of the Trichomonas, Hemophilus, and yeast fungus infections, which produce a clinical picture often not distinguishable from nonspecific vaginitis, except through demonstration of the causative organism.

In the frequent cases of nonspecific vaginitis in children and virgins, speculum examination is not possible or desirable, but in these it is possible to inspect the vaginal surface by means of a vesical speculum of the Kelly type, the patient being placed in the knee-chest position.

Treatment The nonspecific forms of vaginitis respond readily to simple measures of treatment. *Mild antiseptic douches*

are useful, and frequently triple sulfa or Gantrisin cream is helpful.

Trichomonas Vaginitis

Although the organism known as the *Trichomonas vaginalis* was described by Donné as far back as 1836, its importance as the etiological factor in a frequent and troublesome form of vaginitis was not appreciated until recent years. As a matter of fact, there are still some who believe that it alone, without the presence of certain pathogenic bacteria, especially various strains of streptococci, cannot produce the vaginal inflammation with which it is often associated.

Incidence. The infection is an extremely common one, many looking upon the trichomonas variety as being the most frequent form of vaginitis. In a report of 5712 obstetrical and gynecological patients examined routinely for the Trichomonas, Peterson states that 24.6% of the smears were positive for this parasite. Bland and Goldstein, as well as others, have shown that the infection is exceedingly common in pregnant women.

Symptoms. The chief manifestation of trichomonas vaginitis is *leukorrhea*, almost invariably associated with *vaginal soreness, burning*, and often *itching*. The discharge may be rather thin and milky, but often it is very thick and whitish or yellowish white. When the patient is examined with a speculum, one often sees a pool of pus in the vaginal fornix, and characteristically this has a rather foamy or bubbly appearance. As might be expected, *dyspareunia* is a not infrequent complaint. The infection shows little tendency to involve the urethra or vulvovaginal glands, as does the gonococcal, although such infection may occur.

The appearance of the vagina is usually quite characteristic. The mucous membrane is reddened and inflamed, and the posterior fornix often presents a granular or *strawberry-like appearance* which is almost pathognomonic. Small petechial erosions may be seen on the cervix.

Diagnosis. The diagnosis is made by demonstration of the Trichomonas, and this is usually very easy if one uses the proper technique. The patient is cautioned to take no douche on the day of examination. A bivalve speculum is introduced without the use of a lubricant, as this destroys the activity of the parasite. A drop of pus is taken and a smear is then made on a warm slide, using a considerable amount of normal saline solution to dilute the pus and to avoid too rapid drying out of the smear. A cover glass may be used, but is not essential.

The slide is examined under a moderately high power, part of the illumination being cut off. The organisms, when present, are readily recognizable as motile, pear-shaped parasites, with long flagellae at the narrow end, and with an undulating cell membrane. They are intermediate in size between the ordinary pus cells and the pavement epithelial cells which are found in practically all vaginal smears. The active movements of the flagellae are readily seen, but must be distinguished from sperm cells.

Methods of Infection. There is still much uncertainty as to the source of vaginal infection with the Trichomonas. Infection from the rectum suggests itself as a possible source, and this view is held by many, although the recent studies of Allen and Butler do not support it. Contamination from bath water, or from towels, hands, and instruments must all be considered, although in the individual case the explanation is rarely clear. The evidence that the organisms are not infrequently transmitted through coitus seems uncertain.

Treatment. An extensive literature has developed on the subject of the treatment of vaginal trichomoniasis, and a great variety of methods have been proposed. This in itself would indicate that none of these plans has been found altogether satisfactory, and such, in fact, is the view of those who have had the greatest experience in this field. There is general agreement that almost any of the many methods which have been employed will give good immediate results, the difficulty being in avoiding frequent re-

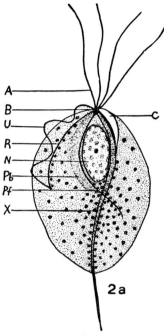

FIG. 10.1. Trichomonas vaginalis. *A*, four anterior flagella; *B*, blepharoplast; *U*, undulating membrane; *R*, chromatic basal rod; *N*, nucleus; *Pb*, parabasal body; *Pf*, parabasal fibril; *X*, cytostome. (From Davis, C. H. (Editor): *Gynecology and Obstetrics*. W. F. Prior Company, Inc., Hagerstown, Maryland, 1933.)

currences of the condition, which are not uncommon.

Silver Picrate. One of the most popular, and apparently one of the most effective forms of treatment, is with silver picrate. About 5 gm. of the silver picrate powder preparation, readily available commercially and consisting of 1 % silver picrate dispersed in kaolin, is blown into the vagina by some form of insufflator, after preliminary cleansing and drying. Following this the patient is instructed to insert a 2-grain suppository of silver picrate every night for 2 weeks, and then to return. Good results are reported.

β-Lactose Treatment. There has been some popularity of methods designed to promote the growth of the normal vaginal flora, especially the bacillus of Döderlein, which are looked upon as constituting the normal defense against the growth of pathogenic organisms. This they do by maintenance of vaginal acidity. For example, while the pH of the vagina averages about 4.5, it is often as high as 7 or more in cases of trichomonas infection. In such cases there is depletion of the normal glycogen content of the vaginal epithelium, and this may be prevented by the use of such carbohydrate substances as β-lactose, which has the further virtue of absorbing moisture very effectively. Frequent insufflation is probably no more satisfactory than self-application of lactose powder in gelatin capsules (Butabs).

Floraquin Method. Diodoquin (Floraquin) is inserted into the posterior fornix. The patient is instructed to insert 1 moistened tablet into the posterior fornix night and morning thereafter for 7 days, then 1 at night only for 7 days, and finally 1 every other night for a week to 10 days.

Daily morning douches of 3 tablespoonfuls of vinegar to 2 quarts of warm water may be used, followed in the active stage by the insertion of 1 tablet into the fornix. After 3 weeks of intensive treatment, a tablet should be inserted two or three times a week for about 3 months. A cure can be assumed if the parasites cannot be demonstrated after the third menstrual period.

Antibiotics. Although various types of systems and local antibiotic therapy have been suggested, we question whether they ever should be used. Although they may be effectively bactericidal, this very effectiveness may disrupt the synergistic relationship of vaginal fungi and bacteria. Thus, the patient may end up with a much more severe and intractable yeast infection and be even more symptomatic than she was before.

Other Methods of Treatment. Among other popular methods of treatment have been those employing arsenical compounds of one sort or another, chief among which have been such commercial preparations as carbarsone, acetarsone, Devegan, and Milibis. Although good results have been reported, it would seem

that these substances are less widely used than formerly. Numerous other commercial trichomonacides have been introduced, especially to be mentioned is tricofuron.

Flagyl. In recent years, flagyl has been introduced and although there was a long delay in its acceptance by the F. D. A., it has been approved. The medication, given in doses of 250 mgm. three times a day by mouth for 10 days, offers an effective therapy especially for the stubborn cases resistant to local treatment. It has been extremely effective, nontoxic, and useful in the recurrent or recalcitrant cases which comprise a major nuisance in every day gynecological practice. The cure rate has exceeded 90% in most reported series (Searle).

Treatment in Pregnancy. As already mentioned, trichomonas infection is extremely common in pregnant women. The methods of treatment are essentially the same as in the nonpregnant condition, and they can be carried out with safety until the last month of pregnancy, when they should be discontinued. The discontinuance of douches as early as possible seems advisable.

Mycotic Vaginitis (Fungous or Monial Vaginitis)

As with trichomonas infection, the frequency and importance of the mycotic form has been recognized only in recent years. Hesseltine states that about 10% of nonpregnant women who complain of vaginal discharge harbor fungi of the yeast group, and that in about one-third of pregnant women such fungi are to be found in the vagina, although only a small proportion have symptoms sufficiently troublesome to seek medical relief. The vulvovaginal inflammation so often seen in diabetes is almost always due to the presence of fungi which thrive in the presence of the carbohydrate-rich environment characterizing that disase. It is most common in postmenopausal women.

The organisms responsible for this type of infection are fungi of the yeast group, similar to those which so often produce thrush in the oral cavity of the infant. There is still some confusion as to nomenclature, and various names are applied to the causative organism, *viz.*, *Monilia albicans, Saccharomyces albicans, Oidium albicans*, but it is usually believed that the *Candida albicans* is the one most commonly involved.

Symptoms. The disease is characterized by a *discharge* which varies between a thin watery to a thick purulent character, *pruritus* which may be intense, *local irritation*, and marked *reddening* of the entire vaginal or vulvovaginal mucous membrane. In addition, there are often *thrushlike patches* on the vagina, vulva, or both. When the vulva is extensively involved, its surface may show large whitish or grayish areas of the aphthous deposit, and itching may be exceedingly distressing, so that scratch marks are often present.

Diagnosis. While the above described clinical picture should at once suggest the probability of the mycotic etiology, the diagnosis is made positive by microscopic demonstration of the fungi. A smear is made from the exudate, and this is stained with the Gram stain. The fungi appear in the form of long threadlike fibers or *mycelia*, to which are attached the tiny buds or *conidia*. For confirmation, the organism may be cultured on Sabouraud's or Nickerson's medium.

Methods of Infection. As with Trichomonas, the mode of contamination is rarely clearly explainable, although it seems certain that dissemination is by means of the hands, towels, coitus, clothing, bath water, or instruments.

Treatment. Although gentian violet used to be almost the specific treatment for yeast infection, it is so "messy" that it has been pretty well discarded. During the past few years the intravaginal use of Propion gel or Aci-gel has become very popular, and it is usually promptly effective in the relief of symptoms from monilial vaginitis. This jelly is introduced by the patient herself by means of a syringe applicator, usually twice a day for a

period of several weeks. More recently even this has been more or less supplanted by the use of nystatin (Mycostatin) suppositories nightly for several weeks.

Hemophilus vaginalis Vaginitis

This agent as a sole or contributory cause to vaginitis has been noted by Gardner and Dukes (1955), Brewer, Halpern, and Thomas (1957), and others. Culture is taken with the use of Casman's blood agar medium as well as thioglycolate broth. The organism may be grown and identified, and although its importance as the sole agent in producing vaginitis is uncertain, it is frequently present.

The usual symptoms of leukorrhea, pruritus, and dyspareunia are produced, and it would seem that the Hemophilus must be considered a possible pathogenic cause in certain types of vaginitis that are recalcitrant to the usual treatment. Terramycin-polymyxin B was abandoned by Brewer despite success in eradicating the Hemophilus organisms, because of the frequent occurrence of *Candida albicans*. In its place he recommends the use of hexetidine, available commercially as Sterisil vaginal gel. Most methods of treatment lay be helpful at one time or another.

Gonorrheal Vulvovaginitis in Children

While the histological structure of the adult vagina, with its many layers of squamous eipithelium and its lack of glands, protects it from the attacks of the Gonococcus, this is not true of the immature vagina of the young child, with its thin mucous membrane covered with only a few layers of epithelial cells. Gonorrheal vaginitis, involving usually also the vulvar mucosa (vulvovaginitis) is not an uncommon disease. It is far less frequently encountered in private practice than in the dispensary type of patient.

Mode of Infection. The disease is spread through contact with infected persons, often other infected children, but the dissemination is usually an indirect one, through the medium of the fingers,

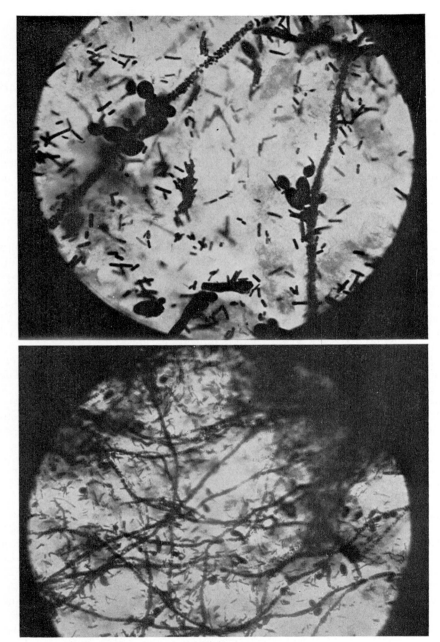

Fig. 10.2. Monilia in a vaginal smear. *Above*, high-dry power; *below*, mycelial forms with budding elements as well as other organisms (oil immersion). (From Plass, E. D.: In *Gynecology and Obstetrics*, edited by C. H. Davis. W. F. Prior Company, Inc., Hagerstown, Maryland, 1933.)

towels, toilet seats, or bathtubs. While the method of spread can by proper investigation be explained in some cases, in many others this may be altogether im-

possible. In institutions like school, hospitals, or children's homes, the disease used to assume epidemic proportions. In a certain proportion of cases the infection is caused by rape, often incited by the superstition still prevalent among ignorant men that coitus with a child will cure gonorrhea.

Symptoms. The chief and often the only symptom is persistent vaginal discharge, often very slight, at times rather profuse, so that the child's clothing is soiled with the whitish or yellowish discharge. There is apt to be considerable local irritation, which may at times lead to masturbation. The course of the disease if untreated is extremely chronic, with alternation of periods of remission and exacerbation, but the tendency is to disappearance of the vaginal inflammation and discharge with the onset of puberty.

Diagnosis. There is no question that many errors of diagnosis occur through failure to recognize the fact that other causes than the Gonococcus may be re-

sponsible for vaginal discharges in children. Among these may be mentioned pinworms, foreign bodies, and infection with such organisms as the *Micrococcus catarrhalis*, Streptococcus, or colon bacillus. The only criterion of diagnosis is the microscopic demonstration of the Gonococcus, but even better is to obtain a positive culture; and here also there are pitfalls to be encountered and errors are not infrequent. The finding of the typical coffee bean, Gram-negative organisms within the cells (intracellular) is essential for diagnosis. Greenhill states that "there must be more than 10 typical Gram-negative diplococci intracellularly in the same slide and two or more within the same cell" in order to permit of positive diagnosis.

Treatment. Up to recent years there were few diseases so unsatisfactory to

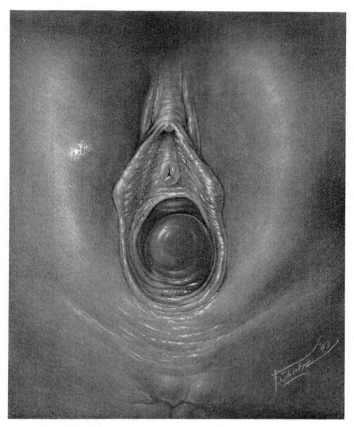

FIG. 10.3. Unusually large vaginal inclusion cyst

treat as the gonorrheal vulvovaginitis of children. Protracted treatment with all sorts of local antiseptics, such as silver nitrate, Argyrol, or Mercurochrome, was commonly employed, with notoriously unsatisfactory results. The introduction of the *estrogenic plan of treatment* in 1933 has now been largely replaced by intramuscular or even oral penicillin for 3 to 4 days. Results are uniformly good.

Senile Vaginitis

The atrophy of the vaginal mucosa which takes place normally at the time of the menopause makes it thin and pasty, and renders it very prone to infection. Frequently tiny superficial areas of granulation or ulceration develop, giving rise to slight vaginal staining. In seeking for the cause of slight postmenopausal bleeding, senile vaginitis, like the corresponding condition in the cervix and corpus uteri, must be borne in mind as a not infrequent one. The most characteristic symptoms, however, are discharge, itching, burning, and soreness in the vaginal region. The discharge is usually rather thin, and it may, as already mentioned, be blood-tinged. In later stages there may be contraction of the vaginal lumen, with dyspareunia or complete inability to carry on marital relations.

Treatment. Here again *estrogenic therapy* is often invoked with benefit, and this should always be local unless there is some other reason for oral administration. We usually prescribe nightly *vaginal suppositories of stilbestrol* (0.5 mg.) for 3 to 4 weeks or some form of estrogenic vaginal cream combined with daily vinegar douches. It must be remembered that too vigorous estrogenic therapy may produce uterine bleeding, an undesirable occurrence because of the suspicion it may excite of adenocarcinoma of the uterus.

For the local pruritus and irritation, one may resort to any of the measures described in the section on pruritus vulvae (Chapter 9).

Emphysematous Vaginitis

A rare variety of vaginitis is the so-called vaginitis emphysematosa. This condition has been found to be associated with pregnancy and also with cases of heart failure. It is characterized by the

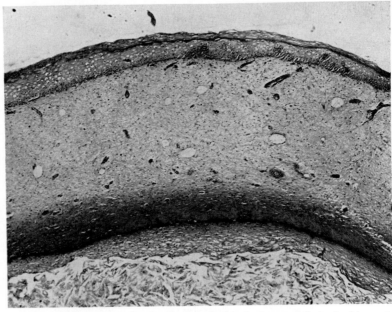

Fig. 10.4. Microscopic appearance of wall of vaginal inclusion cyst (*below*); skin surface *above*

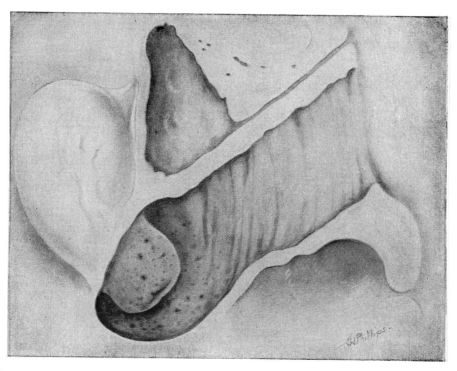

PLATE X.I. *Trichomonas vaginalis* vaginitis. (From Davis, C. H. (Editor): *Gynecology and Obstetrics*. W. F. Prior Company, Inc., Hagerstown, Maryland, 1933.)

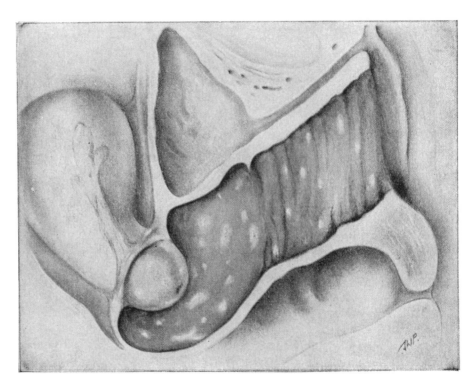

PLATE X.II. Thrush vaginitis during pregnancy. (From Davis, C. H. (Editor): *Gynecology and Obstetrics*. W. F. Prior Company, Inc., Hagerstown, Maryland, 1933.)

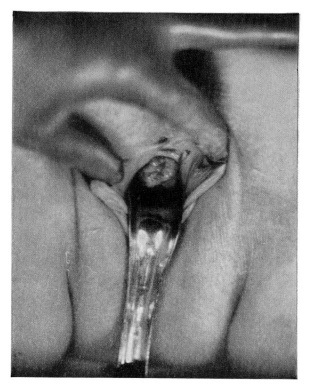

PLATE X.III. A rather extensive carcinoma of posterior wall of vagina

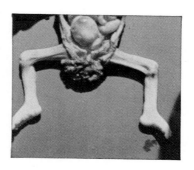

PLATE X.IV. Autopsy specium of sarcoma
botryoides in a 2-year-old child.

vaginalis and *Trichomonas intestinalis.* Amer. J. Obstet. Gynec., *39:* 1005, 1940.

Lang, W. R.: Premenarchal vaginitis. Obstet. Gynec., *13:* 723, 1959.

Livingston, R.: *Primary Carcinoma of the Vagina.* Charles C Thomas, Springfield, Ill., 1950.

Marcus, S. L.: Müllerian mixed sarcoma (sarcoma botryoides) of the cervix. Obstet. Gynec., *15:* 47, 1960.

Marcus, S. L.: Primary carcinoma of the vagina. Obstet. Gynec., *15:* 673, 1960.

McGoogan, L. S.: The treatment of vaginitis. Clin. Obstet. Gynec., *2:* 450, 1959.

McVay, L. V., Evans, L., and Sprunt, D. H.: New method of treatment of *Trichomonas vaginalis.* Surg. Gynec. Obstet., *99:* 177, 1954.

Merrill, J. A., and Bender, W. T.: Primary carcinoma of the vagina. Obstet. Gynec. *11:* 3, 1958.

Novak, E., Woodruff, J. D., and Novak, E. R.: Probable mesonephric origin of certain genital tumors. Amer. J. Obstet. Gynec., *68:* 1222, 1954.

Ober, W. B., and Edgcomb, J. H.: Sarcoma botryoides in the female urogenital tract. Cancer, *7:* 75, 1954.

Pace, H. R., and Schantz, S. I.: Nystatin (Mycostatin) in treatment of monilial and nonmonilial vaginitis. J. A. M. A., *162:* 268, 1956.

Palumbo, L.: Primary carcinoma of vagina. Southern Med. J., *47:* 356, 1954.

Reich, W. J., Nechtow, M. J., Zaworsky, B., and Adams, A. P.: Investigation and management of the patient with vaginal discharge. Clin. Obstet. Gynec., *2:* 441, 1959.

Russ, J. D., and Collins, C. G.: Treatment of prepuberal vulvovaginitis, with new synthetic estrogen (diethylstilbestrol); preliminary report. J. A. M. A., *114:* 2446, 1940.

Searle, G. D.: Symposium on flagyl. Research, *56:* 26, 1964.

Sheets, J. L., Dockerty, M. B., Decker, D. G., and Welch, J. S.: Primary epithelial malignancy in the vagina. Amer. J. Obstet. Gynec., *89:* 121, 1964.

Singh, B. P.: Primary carcinoma of vagina. Cancer, *4:* 1073, 1951.

Smith, F. R.: Primary carcinoma of vagina. Amer. J. Obstet. Gynec., *69:* 525, 1955.

Smouth, F. R.: Primary carcinoma of vagina. Amer. J. Obstet. Gynec., *69:* 525, 1955.

Studdiford, W. E.: Vaginal lesions of adenomatous origin. Amer. J. Obstet. Gynec., *73:* 641, 1957.

Thomas, H. H.: Candidal vulvovagnitis. Obstet. Gynec., *9:* 163, 1957.

Westerhout, F. C., Hodgman, J. E., Anderson, G. V., and Sack, R. A.: Congenital hydrocolpos. Amer. J. Obstet. Gynec., *89:* 957, 1964.

11

CERVICITIS AND CERVICAL POLYP

Inflammation of the cervix uteri, or cervicitis, may be either acute or chronic, and may involve the portio, the endocervix, or, more frequently, both. The etiology of cervicitis is usually bacterial, the organisms concerned being the Gonococcus, or any one of a number of other bacteria which are normal inhabitants of the genital canal or which are introduced from the outside. In this latter group the various strains of streptococci are most important. Viral and fungal infestation is likely, although uncertain. The Gonococcus is almost always introduced through coitus, but the nongonorrheal variety of infection is not always easy to explain except on the general basis of an *increased pathogenicity of the genital flora*, especially in the presence of recent or previous *trauma* of some sort.

Most important in the nongonorrheal group is *childbirth*, with commonly associated trauma and minute lacerations of the cervix which become secondarily infected. In certain serious forms of infection, especially in the case of criminal abortion, the portal of entry is the cervix, whence it spreads to other pelvic structures by way of the lymphatics (lymphangitis and perilymphangitis) and veins (phlebitis and periphlebitis) of the broad ligaments. More frequently the infection is of a milder form, and entrenches itself in chronic form in the cervix, which has frequently suffered some degree of laceration. Here it may persist for many years, its only symptom usually being a persistent leukorrhea.

ACUTE CERVICITIS

Pathology. In the acute stage, which clinically is seen in most typical form in acute gonorrheal infection, the cervix is reddened, congested, and somewhat swollen, while from the canal there escapes a profuse, purulent exudate, sometimes white and sometimes yellowish. *Microscopically*, this phase is characterized by intense polymorphonuclear infiltration of the mucosa and immediately underlying tissue, hyperemia, and more or less edema. The gland lumina may be distended with an exudate consisting of large numbers of dead leukocytes, desquamated epithelial cells, and mucus.

Clinical Symptoms. By far the most constant and usually the only symptom of cervicitis is *leukorrhea*. In the acute stage this is purulent, and in the gonorrheal type, especially where there is associated urethritis, there may be much vaginal and urinary irritability, suggesting cystitis. During this stage the infection is very active, and in the gonorrheal cases, the causative organisms can be readily found in large numbers in the purulent discharge. There

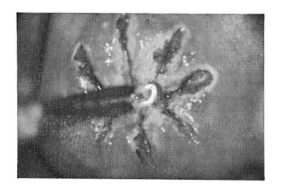

PLATE XI.III. Appearance of cervix just after radial electrocauterization. Complete healing usually requires 6 to 8 weeks.

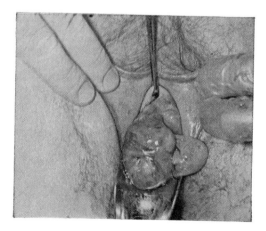

PLATE XI.IV. Huge bilobed benign cervical polyp presenting at introitus.

12

CARCINOMA OF THE CERVIX

Carcinoma of the cervix uteri is probably the most important of all diseases with which the gynecologist must contend, because of its great frequency and its extreme gravity to the individual patient. Although breast cancer is more frequent, cervical cancer is more lethal; more than 10,000 women in the U.S.A. succumb annually to this form of genital malignancy.

More is known about the natural history of epidermoid carcinoma of the cervix than about any other cancer. Invasive symptomatic cancer may develop from the normal epithelium by a slow process which consumes many years. From the time of appearance of intraepithelial carcinoma, which is now generally considered as carcinoma in the true sense of the word, until invasion of surrounding connective tissue by the malignant tissue, 10 or more years may elapse. Even prior to full blown intraepithelial carcinoma certain microscopic changes in the epithelium have been considered by some authors as precancerous in nature. If these atypical findings be considered as the first step to malignancy, 15 or more years may elapse from initiation of the first changes to death from untreated epidermoid cancer of the cervix.

INCIDENCE

The death rate from cancer of the cervix is impossible to state with great accuracy as it is only in recent years that cancer of the cervix has been separated from cancer of the uterus (entire) in the list of official causes of death. However, the National Office of Vital Statistics annually gives a rate of about 10 per 100,000.

Of much greater accuracy are the various incidence studies which have been carried out on population groups under the auspices of the United States Public Health Service. For example, Haenszel and Hillhouse report an age-adjusted incidence rate for invasive cancer of 14.9 per 100,000 for the total female population in New York City. The rates varied for the different social and ethnic groups from a low of 3.6 per 100,000 for Jewish women to a high of 97.6 per 100,000 for Porto Rican women. Negro women had a rate of 47.8 per 100,000, and other white women of 13.5 per 100,000. The rates naturally vary with the age of the population and with the stage of the cancer.

Several screening studies of asymptomatic women have given *prevalence* rates very much higher than the *incidence* rates just quoted. For example, Davis and many others have found rates in excess of 1,000 per 100,000 for intraepithelial cancer among women age 30 to 45. The extraordinarily high figures are understandable when it is realized that the *prevalence* (disease existing at any given time) rates include all those cases which will become invasive and, therefore, symptomatic in future years while the *incidence* figures given above by definition include only those cases which have become symptomatic in the year in question. Such comparative figures represent one line of evidence supporting the view that intraepithelial cancer exists for many years before invasion.

Many recent publications have stated a changing ratio of cervical to endometrial cancer which formerly was quoted in the ratio of 6 or 8 to 1. Webb, Margolis, and Traut note that in their own clinic (California) cervical carcinoma is only three times as common as the fundal variety, and Tweeddale finds that in Lincoln, Nebraska, there is an actual prepondernace of the corporeal disease. One must, while accepting the validity of their reports, consider how patient selection in a hospital may flavor the statistics. Novak and Villa Santa have found that at the Johns Hopkins Hospital the ratio of cervical to endometrial cancer is 6.7:1, or if intraepithelial carcinoma is excluded, 5.8:1. At another local hospital, a few miles away, the ratio is 1.2:1 or 1.1:1, respectively. This disparity is quite easily reconciled if one considers that the Hopkins patient load comprises a considerable proportion of colored ward women; at the other the patient load is almost exclusively white and private in nature.

ETIOLOGICAL FACTORS

In a biological sense the cause of carcinoma of the cervix, like the cause of all cancer, is unknown. However, certain circumstances are so closely associated with it that they may be regarded as etiological factors.

There have been many efforts devoted to studying the diverse economic and sociological factors that may contribute to the varied incidence of cervical cancer. All are agreed that cervical cancer is relatively rare in the Jewish woman, and Wynder *et al.* indicate that its occurrence is about one-eighth as common as in similar groups of gentiles. In a recent review, based on the large material of Mount Sinai Hospital in New York City, Rothman and his coworkers find that carcinoma of the cervix is nine times as frequent in non-Jewish women as in Jewish women. On the other hand, the two groups show no significant difference as regards the incidence of endometrial cancer. Similar notations have been made by others, most recently Tennis and Oalmann.

The low incidence of cervical cancer among Jewish women has led to the suspicion that coitus with an uncircumcised male might act in some way as a causal influence, with poor penile hygiene and resultant smegma being particularly suspected, as noted by Fischer. Indeed Heins, Dennis, and Pratt-Thomas have recently noted the development of cervical cancer in certain strains of mice subjected to stimulation by human smegma for at least 14 months. Wynder *et al.* have published an extensive review on the importance of varied extraneous factors, and are forced to conclude that carcinogenesis can be regarded only as a result of many exogenous and endogenous stimuli. Such factors as mixed sexual partners, incomplete circumcision, and lack of adherence to the mosaic doctrine which forbids intercourse for 1 full week after menstruation must always be considered. However, Jones and his coworkers have detected no significant difference in cervical cancer, irrespective of the state of circumcision of the male partner. In a comprehensive report from the University of Madras, Rewell has found the incidence of cervical cancer to be the same among Moslems (males circumcised) and Hindus (males uncircumcised). The supposed relationship between circumcision and cervical cancer was critically studied by Lilienfeld and Graham who showed there was a 34.4% disagreement between examination and statement among 213 male patients. All in all, there is little except supposition to support this supposed etiological relationship.

On the other hand, within the past decade some half dozen major studies have examined the relationship between

the histological zones, (2) the anatomical areas with reference to the histological zones, (3) the various normal histological findings in the area of the squamocolumnar junction, and (4) the sites of origin of carcinoma in situ proposed by various investigators.

There are three histological zones: the portio vaginalis (histological portio), the transitional zone, and the endocervix. The histological portio is defined as cervical stroma without glands covered by squamous epithelium (Fig. 12.4). Thus, portio epithelium indicates squamous epithelium of the histological portio. The transitional zone lies between the histological portio and the endocervix (Fig. 12.4, Drawings III and IV) and consists of endocervical stroma with glands covered with some form of squamous epithelium. Other authors arbitrarily designate a portion of the endocervix abutting the histological portio as the transitional zone (Fig. 12.4, Drawings I and II). The histological endocervix consists of endocervical stroma containing glands with surface and glandular epithelium of columnar cells (Fig. 12.4).

The anatomical areas are considered to be (1) the portio vaginalis and (2) the endocervix. The anatomic portio is that portion of the cervix lying external to the external os, the surface of which is visualized by the clinician with a bivalve speculum; this includes, not only the squamous-epithelium and subepithelial stroma, but also the columnar epithelium and glandular stroma within the area everted by laceration of the original external os and within a clinical erosion. The endocervix is that portion of the cervix that cannot be visualized by the clinician, lying above the external os and below the internal os.

The relationship between the histological zones and the anatomic areas varies; it depends on the position of the external os with reference to the histological zones. Thus, if the external os lies at *arrow 2* in Fig. 12.4, the anatomical portio consists of the histological portio in all four variations of the squamocolumnar junction and the anatomical endocervix consists of the histological endocervix (Fig. 12.4, Drawings I and II) and of the transitional zone and histological endocervix (Fig. 12.4, Drawings III and IV). If the external os lies at *arrow 3* in Fig. 12.4, the anatomical portio consists of the histological portio and histological endocervix (Fig. 12.4, Drawings I and II) and of the histological portio and histological transitional zone (Fig. 12.4, Drawings II and IV); if it is at *arrow 4*, the anatomical portio consists of the histological portio, histological transitional zone, and histological endocervix (Fig. 12.4, Drawings I to IV). If the external os lies at *arrow 1* (as it frequently does in postmenopausal women) the anatomical portio consists of the histological portio but the anatomic endocervix consists of the histological portio and histological endocervix (Fig. 12.4, Drawings I and II) or of the histological portio, histological transition zone, and histological endocervix (Fig. 12.14, Drawings III and IV). In the majority of cervices of women of the childbearing age the external os lies at *arrow 3* or *4* of Fig. 12.4. Thus, the cervical atypias frequently found in the transitional zone are wholly or partially on the anatomical portio. Once these relationships are understood, it is seen that the cellular origin of precancerous lesions is unrelated to the anatomical area in which the lesion is found.

The normal squamocolumnar junction, in which the normal histological portio abuts the normal histological endocervix, is illustrated in Fig. 12.4, Drawing I. In women of the childbearing age, this rarely occurs.

A pathological erosion of the histological portio and adjacent endocervix is shown in Fig. 12.4, Drawing II. A pathological erosion is an area in which the surface epithelium has been lost and the denuded stroma is inflamed. The pathological or true erosion must be distinguished from the clinical erosion in which there is a reddened area about the external os. The clinical erosion may be caused by eversion of the endocervix, metaplastic or anaplastic squamous epithelium, squamous epithelium in the process of healing a pathological erosion, or an unhealed pathological erosion.

Figure 12.4, Drawing III depicts squamous epithelium within the transitional zone that is morphologically indistinguishable from the squamous epithelium of the histological portio and that is not only contiguous to, but continuous with, the portio epithelium. The origin of this type of epithelium is controversial.

The four cellular sites of origin of carcinoma in situ that have been proposed are indicated by A, B, C, and D in Fig. 12.4. A indicates the basal cells of the histological portio epithelium; B, the basal cells of the histological portio epithelium at the margin of an old pathological erosion; C, the basal cells of the portio epithelial component involved in erosion healing; and D, the subcylindrical cells of the endocervix adjacent to the histological portio.

It has been proposed that carcinoma in situ may sometimes arise in the subcylindrical cells of the endocervix adjacent to the histological portio (Fig. 12.4 D). This supposition is based on several pieces of evidence: (1) the resemblance of the cytological features and the morphologic pattern of growth of some forms of carcinoma in situ to subcylindrical cell metaplasia; (2) atypical and anaplastic subcylindrical cells in areas contiguous to the carcinoma in situ; (3) the most frequent occurrence of carcinoma in situ in the transitional zone over endocervical portio exclusively; and (4) the sharp vertical line of demarcation between carcinoma in situ and the normal squamous epithelium.

The high association of carcinoma in situ with anaplasia and subcylindrical cell anaplasia suggests that carcinoma in situ may be preceded by one or both of these lesions. The site of the carcinoma in situ, often surrounded by anaplasia, suggests that the carcinoma in situ arose within the field of anaplasia. Furthermore the position of the anaplasia and carcinoma in situ with subcylindrical cell

anaplasia at the periphery further suggests that either or both of these lesions may be preceded by subcylindrical cell anaplasia.

It was proposed by Johnson *et al.* that the histogenesis of invasive cancer occurs most frequently as shown schematically in Figure 12.5. This scheme is an extension of Fluhmann's drawing of the evolution of cervical cancer. A covert potential cancerous field is in the subcylindrical cells of the endocervix, in the transitional zone (Fig. 12.5, Part 1). These cells, with unknown stimuli, proliferate in an abnormal way to form anaplastic subcylindrical cells (Fig. 12.5, Part 2). Perhaps the most common evolution occurs from anaplasia (Fig. 12.5, Part 3) which gradually develops into carcinoma in situ (Fig. 12.5, Part 4), which in turn minimally invades the stroma (Fig. 12.5, Part 5) and ultimately develops into clinically invasive cancer (Fig. 12.5, Part 6). Alternatively, however, there may be a faster evolution (perhaps with an increased dose of carcinogen or an increased response from the host) whereby subcylindrical cell anaplasia is converted directly into carcinoma in situ (Fig. 12.5, Part 2a) or even converted in a relatively short period of time into early stromal invasion (Fig. 12.5, Part 2b).

As was indicated above, not all observers agree with the subcylindrical cell concept. There are at least two problems, (1) the general difficulty of establishing the origin of cell lines by microscopic technique, and (2) the necessity of calling upon an indifferent cell in the adult to provide a cell of origin for a tumor.

The difficulty of establishing the cell or tissue by microscopic technique is well known and has plagued descriptive embryology to this day. While the technique has been extraordinarily helpful and is the basis for most of our embryological understanding, we need only to recall the difficulties in establishing the origin of the vagina, or the origin of the primary and secondary sex cords of the ovary, or, indeed, the origin of the primitive germ cell, which was argued for years, to realize

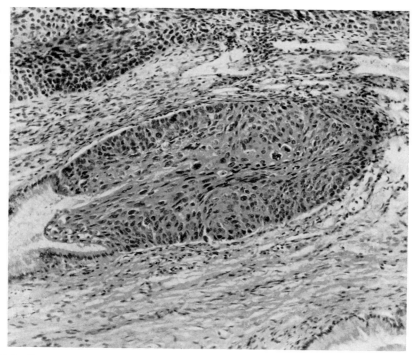

Fig. 12.8. Carcinoma in situ with gland extension, although this in itself is not considered indicative of histological invasiveness.

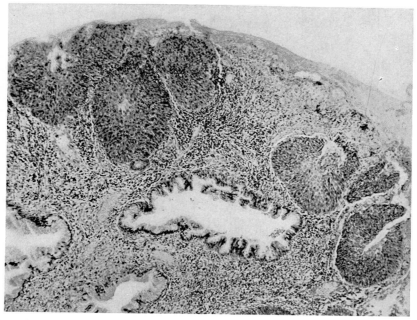

Fig. 12.9. A characteristic pattern in early epidermoid carcinoma. Whether there is only glandular extension or early stromal invasion is a difficult diagnosis.

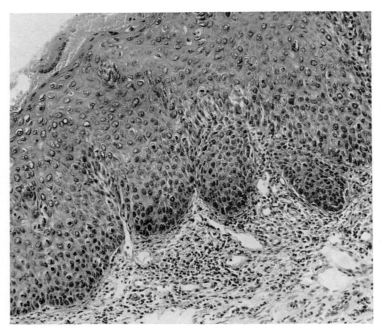

FIG. 12.10. Rather marked· basal cell hyperactivity but not suggesting carcinoma in situ

covering epithelium by immature undifferentiated basal cells does not warrant a diagnosis of in situ cancer *unless* there is *complete* absence of stratification and lack of mature cells.

These incomplete degrees of aberration of the lining epithelium are variously designated as *atypical cervical epithelium*, *basal cell hyperplasia*, *dysplasia*, or *hyperactivity*, and many other terms. Their significance is not completely understood, but it would appear that major degrees may either antedate or exist at the periphery of invasive cancer, thereby exhibiting the same relationship to intraepithelial cancer that this lesion does to invasive cancer. On the other hand, minor degrees of these cervical changes appear to be of little significance, for they are frequently transient and likely to be associated with cervical infection or irritation. A term formerly often applied to abnormal cervical architecture, the leukoplakia of Hinselmann, with his four-grade rubric pattern, has been rather generally discarded. Actually leukoplakia is a clinical term denoting various types of whitish plaquelike areas, but neither this

nor any other clinical picture is characteristic of intraepithelial cancer or basal cell hyperactivity, which may exist in an innocuous appearing cervix (Figs. 12.10 and 12.11).

To lend confusion to an already confused subject, increasing numbers of cases of marked degrees of basal cell hyperactivity, and even of intraepithelial cancer, have been reported as undergoing complete regression (Wespi and others). A certain number of these lesions have been noted in pregnant women and some still believe that pregnancy can produce changes in the cervix that may be histologically indistinguishable from cancer but which may regress with termination of pregnancy. At this writing, however, most of us agree with Greene and his associates, who emphasize that, irrespective of a concomitant pregnancy, the microscopic pattern of true intraepithelial cancer is indicative of a real preinvasive cancer. In other words, the pregnancy is merely incidental; however, there is rarely need for haste, and the pregnancy is allowed to progress to term under careful observation with final evaluation of the problem

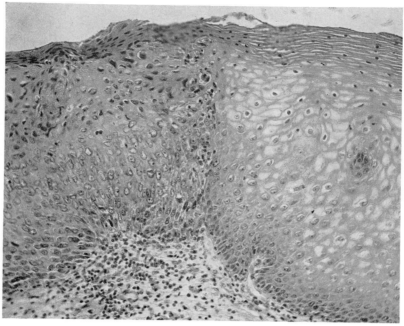

FIG. 12.11. Definite line of demarcation between normal squamous epithelium on *right* and moderate basal cell hyperactivity on *left*.

postpartum. Occasionally conization is necessary to exclude invasion (Fig. 12.12).

Invasive Carcinoma. As with carcinoma elsewhere, the microscopic diagnosis of invasive carcinoma of the cervix is based on two chief characteristics: (1) an abnormal pattern or architecture, and (2) abnormalities in the constituent cells.

(1) Whereas in the normal epithelial surface the epithelial cells are sharply demarcated from the stroma by the basement membrane, in cancer the latter is broken through, so that the epithelium pushes into the stroma, at first in small buds, but later in the form of long columns which grow deep into the stroma, much as the roots of a tree grow down into the soil. In all but the earliest phases, therefore, a reasonably certain diagnosis can usually be made with the low power alone, as this suffices to reveal the disorderly and illegitimate invasion of the stroma by the epithelium. It is this invasiveness, with the dissemination of cells by the lymphatics, which is responsible for the characteristics traditionally asso-

ciated with malignancy, such as local infiltration, metastasis, and recurrence after incomplete removal.

(2) While the normal epithelium is made up of cells of adult, differentiated type, that of cancer shows varying degrees of immaturity and unripeness. Histologically this is indicated by such features as disparity in the size of cells and nuclei, hyperchromatosis, mitoses, either normal or abnormal, and karyorrhexis.

Our own laboratory utilizes the histological classification proposed by Martzloff. According to this, growths made up dominantly of highly differentiated cells resembling those of the prickle cell layer are designated as the *spinal cell* group, making up approximately 15% of the total; at the other extreme, the type in which the constituent cells resemble the basal layers of the epithelium, or even more the spindle cells of fat tissue, is spoken of as the *basal or spindle cell* variety, seen in only about 10% of the cases. The large intermediate group, with

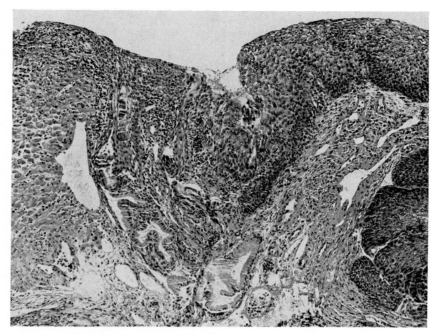

FIG. 12.12. "Pregnant" cervix; decidual reaction to *left* and markedly atypical epithelium to *right*.

transitional cell characteristics, makes up the largest proportion, about 75% of all (Figs. 12.13–12.15).

Perhaps even more popular is the plan of designating various numerical groups or grades, as suggested by Broders. In Grade I the dedifferentiation is least, in Grade IV most extreme, with Grades II and III between.

The significance of such plans of classification lies in the accepted fact that, generally speaking, the clinical malignancy of a tumor parallels the degree of unripeness of its cells. On the other hand, it must be remembered that the greater the degree of unripeness of the cells, the more favorable their response to radiotherapy. There are exceptions to both these rules, however, while from the standpoint of prognosis *the stage of the disease is much more important than is the cell type.*

Again, it must be recalled that the great majority of cases do not exhibit a pure cell type, that biopsy does not always give an accurate picture, and that individual pathologists will differ about the grouping of certain cases. For this reason the determination of the cell type is not as important as it might at first thought appear, although spinal cell malignancies of the cervix were at one time regarded as being notoriously radioresistant.

The elapsed time from cervical atypia to invasive cancer is of considerable importance and has been studied by a number of workers. From an historical point of view one of the first reasons for suspecting the prolonged duration of intraepithelial carcinoma was the great difference in the average age of women with intraepithelial cancer as contrasted with invasive cancer. For example, McKay, Hertig, and Younge noted a mean age of 48 years for invasive cancer, 38 years for intraepithelial cancer, and 34.9 years for atypical hyperplasia. Many other workers have similar statistics. Dunn, in a study of data from the population screening of 53,585 women, concluded that intraepithelial carcinoma lasted about 5 years but that 3 or 4 additional years elapsed

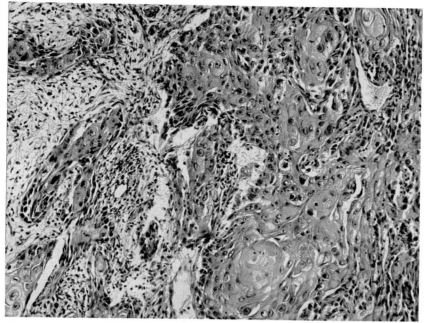

FIG. 12.13. Spinal cell type of epidermoid carcinoma showing pearl formation by highly differentiated cells, but many anaplastic forms are obvious.

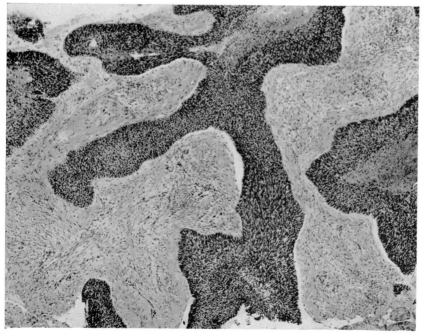

FIG. 12.14. Epidermoid carcinoma of basal cell type

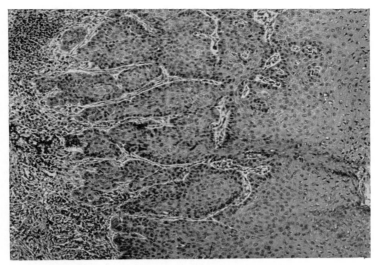

Fig. 12.15. A very early and small epidermoid carcinoma measuring only a few millimeters in diameter, but showing the same characteristics of cell change and invasive pattern found in much ater lesions. This is a transitional cell lesion.

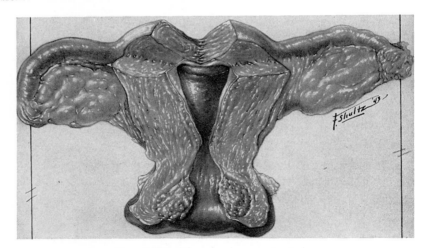

Fig. 12.16. Adenocarcinoma of cervix

after pathological invasion before the onset of symptoms. The practical and fortunate point is that there is an opportunity of several years duration during which the diagnosis of the disease may be made in its very curable stage.

ADENOCARCINOMA OF CERVIX

As has already been said, cervical adenocarcinoma is much the least common of the three forms of uterine carcinoma, being only from one-fifteenth to one-twentieth as common as the epidermoid cervical variety. While it usually begins within the cervical canal, the initial lesion may appear at or near the external os, and in the later stages it may form a large vegetative growth presenting on the vaginal surface of the cervix. More characteristically, however, the growth produces increasing involvement of the cervix and adjoining tissues without extensive external lesions on the vaginal surface (Figs. 12.16 and 12.17).

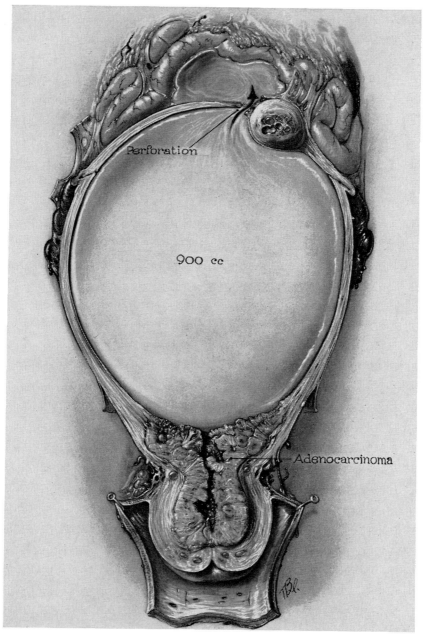

Perforation

900 cc

Adenocarcinoma

FIG. 12.17. Adenocarcinoma of cervix with associated pyometra and perforation. (Courtesy of Dr. Erle Henricksen, Los Angeles, California.)

Microscopically it is characterized by the atypical gland pattern so distinctive of adenocarcinoma, in striking contrast with the orderly distribution and appearance of the normal cervical glands. In some cases the departure from normal is moderate, in others the abnormal gland pattern is intricate and highly atypical.

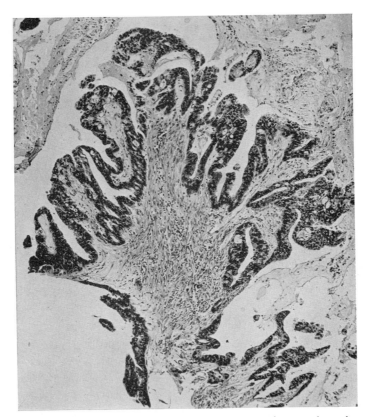

FIG. 12.18. Microscopic appearance of adenocarcinoma of cervix

The same variations in degree apply to the cell changes. In some adenocarcinomas the gland epithelium may be for the most part of one cell thickness, and many of the cells may still retain the mature columnar shape of normal cervical epithelium. In others the gland epithelium may be many layers thick, and may even fill the lumina so completely that in individual areas the carcinoma may appear to be of the solid epidermoid variety (Figs. 12.18 and 12.19).

On the basis of such variations in the same family of tumors, systems of *histological gradation* have become popular, the one most commonly employed being that suggested by Broders. The least undifferentiated variety is Grade I (often mucinous); the most undifferentiated type is Grade IV, with Grades II and III as intervening varieties.

Adenoacanthoma of the cervix may oc-
cur as a primary disease or, more frequently, by direct extension from the corpus (see "Carcinoma of the Endometrium," in Chapter 15). We prefer to confine the term "adenoacanthoma" only to *malignant* adenomatous disease with associated *benign* squamous metaplasia which may confuse the picture but in no way alters the prognosis. It is unfortunate that various European writers use this term to signify a mixed epidermoid-adenocarcinoma. With this dual malignancy, a very different process than our interpretation of adenoacanthoma is present. The term *adenoepithelioma*, as proposed by Way, seems more appropriate and much less confusing.

When adenocarcinoma or adenoacanthoma is found in the cervix it is important to know if it is primary or secondary to endometrial tumor. Differential curettage of the endocervix and uterine

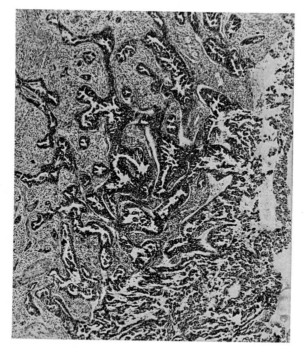

FIG. 12.19. Another pattern of adenocarcinoma of cervix

cavity is frequently helpful. If it appears likely that the cervix is the primary site of the adenocarcinoma, our policy is to irradiate only as with epidermoid cancer. Should the cervical adenocarcinoma be secondary to fundal disease, we irradiate both cervix and endometrium and later perform a hysterectomy.

A rare variety of cervical adenocarcinoma has its *origin from the tubular or glandlike mesonephric vestiges* which may at times be noted deep in the cervical structure, as described in Chapter 1. The adenocarcinoma arising from these elements may show no connection with the endocervix, and microscopically it may be characterized by a rather tubular pattern. Carcinomas of the cervix which occur in children are exclusively of this variety.

CARCINOMA OF CERVICAL STUMP

With the increasing employment of total hysterectomy, this is becoming an increasingly less common gynecological problem, although it is by no means rare

to see such cases today. In close to 50 % of patients with malignancy of the cervical stump the disease is detected less than a year after subtotal hysterectomy, making it appear probable that the cancer was present at the time of the incomplete and inadequately studied hysterectomy. Routine preoperative biopsy or smear of all cases where only a subtotal operation seems possible (as in severe cases of endometriosis or pelvic inflammatory disease) or similar routine study of a preserved cervix might lead to detection of this "coincidental cancer."

Cancer of the stump has acquired a reputation for being unusually difficult to treat and attended by a poor prognosis. In our experience this stigma is not deserved if treatment is modified to fit the individual (see "Treatment"). Salvage is just as good, and complications no more frequent. Actually it seems that the woman who has had a subtotal operation with a resultant surgical menopause is much more apt to seek medical advice if bleeding occurs than the complacent woman of 45 who interprets any menstrual irregularity as being due to change of life. Cervical stump cancer may be epidermoid or adenocarcinoma in type, and obviously the prognosis will vary as to the histological pattern and degree of disease.

CLINICAL CHARACTERISTICS OF CERVICAL CARCINOMA

As was mentioned previously, the mean age of patients with symptomatic cancer of the cervix is about 48 years. In contrast, patients with intraepithelial carcinoma average 38 years of age. Intraepithelial carcinoma is basically asymptomatic. However, clinical studies of patients with this condition usually result in the listing of a series of symptoms, most of which are coincidental. For example, Younge, Hertig, and Armstrong reported that 46% of 135 patients had absolutely no symptoms, 24% complained of leukorrhea and 30% had abnormal bleeding of some kind.

Pain is not a symptom of cervical carcinoma until the late stages of the disease, and even then it is not always very severe. Ignorance of this fact is one of the most important obstacles in the campaign for the early recognition of cancer. In the majority of cases the first symptom is *bleeding*, although this is usually slight. Characteristically it is of intermenstrual type if the patient is still within the reproductive years. It is apt to be noted after coitus, severe exertion, or the straining of defecation. The "contact" bleeding following coitus or simple pelvic examination is especially characteristic. Unfortunately in some cases bleeding does not occur until the disease has obtained a fairly good foothold and extended into the lymphatics, so that even an alert and intelligent patient may be doomed before the appearance of symptoms. In the intracervical forms of cancer, moreover, bleeding is apt to be later in appearance, because of the more protected position of the lesion.

Abnormal discharge, usually rather watery, may at times be noted even before the appearance of the bleeding, especially with adenocarcinoma. As the disease advances, both *bleeding and discharge* become more persistent and profuse, and the increasing ulceration and secondary infection make the discharge increasingly offensive. Other symptoms, such as *bladder irritability*, may arise from involvement of the vesicovaginal septum with corresponding *rectal discomfort* from posterior extension. Heavy, aching *pain* is now usually a prominent symptom and may become severe as the disease advances. Fistulas into the bladder or rectum may develop, adding tremendously to the patient's misery. Increasing lateral infiltration obstructs the ureters, and *uremia is the terminal cause of death* in perhaps the largest proportion of cases.

DIAGNOSIS OF CERVICAL CANCER

Recent years have witnessed a complete revision in our methods of evaluating office patients as regards the diagnosis of uterine cancer, especially cervical. Indeed previous editions of this text stressed the importance of a careful questioning for contact bleeding, the gross appearance of the cervix, the value of palpation, and certain other methods which must now be regarded as of purely secondary status.

Exfoliative Cytology. The development of an *accurate cytological method* for assessing asymptomatic women with a completely normal appearing cervix has led to the diagnosis of many cases of early cancer long before symptomatology or overt pathological abnormalities are apparent. If routine smear cannot be carried out on all patients, certainly every parous woman over 30 is entitled to a cancer smear, which is inexpensive (in our community currently $5.00) and which we sincerely tell patients is the best investment they can make.

Nevertheless, a thorough history as regards intermenstrual bleeding should be taken, and careful palpation of the cervix and speculum examination should be carried out. Where there is a typical cancer present or even a definite but merely suspicious lesion, biopsy should be per-

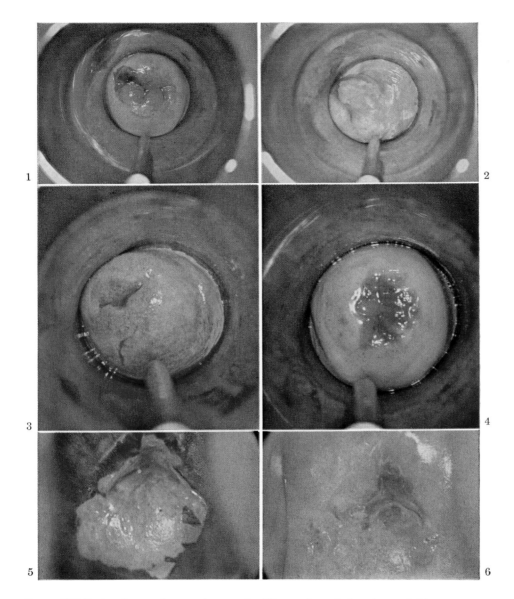

PLATE XII.I. An abnormal appearing cervix. Biopsy showed chronic cervicitis.

PLATE XII.II. This cervix may be described as showing leukoplakia, which is a clinical term. Biopsy showed only chronic cervicitis.

PLATE XII.III. A rather normal appearing cervix. Biopsy showed intraepithelial carcinoma.

PLATE XII.IV. A grossly abnormal cervix, but a diagnosis on appearance alone is not possible. Biopsy showed intraepithelial carcinoma.

PLATE XII.V. A low power colposcopic view of a cervix showing a positive Schiller's test. The unstained area is to be considered suspicious of malignancy. Biopsy proved this area to be intraepithelial cancer. The Schiller test may be used without the colposcope. (Courtesy of Dr. Hugh Davis.)

PLATE XII.VI. A low power colposcopic view of the same cervix shown in Plate XII.V before the application of the iodine solution. The prominent capillary network and the ground glass mosaic appearance are suspicious features. Biopsy proved to be intraepithelial cancer. (Courtesy of Dr. Hugh Davis.)

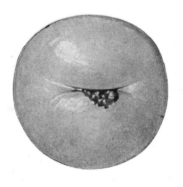

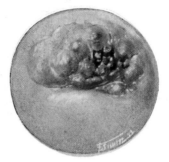

PLATE XII.VII. Clinical appearance of epidermoid carcinoma of cervix in early (*top*) and moderately advanced (*bottom*) stages.

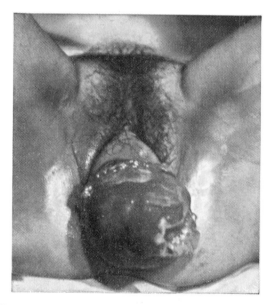

PLATE XII.VIII. Carcinoma (at 3 o'clock) developing with prolapse, a rather rare occurrence. (Case of Dr. Diaz-Bazan, from Novak, E., and Novak, E. R.: *Gynecologic and Obstetric Pathology.* W. B. Saunders, Company, Philadelphia, 1958.)

the desirability of primary surgery in favorable Stage I and Stage II cases with the argument that irradiation has little effect on the intrapelvic lymph nodes—a statement that they have already modified. Certainly many studies would seem to indicate that irradiated patients show considerably less nodal involvement than control patients if routine lymphadenectomy be carried out. Since, however, the question of surgery *versus* irradiation is a current issue, it seems only fair to present both sides of the discussion.

Irradiation. This can be utilized for any stage of disease and is applicable for the very obese, the elderly, or the poor medical risk. Although irradiation complications may occur, there is not the mortality or morbidity associated with radical surgery.

The end results from radiation vary considerably from clinic to clinic depending upon clinical material, technique, and intangible factors. Perhaps the best idea of what can be accomplished by this modality is obtained from the combined figures from over 100 clinics published in the *"Annual Report."* Thus, for the 5-year period 1953 to 1957 as reported in the 13th edition, the end results from 61,776 patients are available. The recovery rates for Stages I, II, III, and IV were 74.9, 53.0, 30.2, and 8.1%, respectively. The over-all recovery rate for these stages combined was 48.5%.

Over the years the recovery rates as reported in the *"Annual Report"* have gradually improved. For example in 1941 the over-all rate was 30.9% and this has gradually improved to the most recent 48.5%. The improvement has resulted partly from a shift of clinical material into earlier stages and partly from improved results by stage.

The technique of irradiation varies in different clinics and the details are beyond the scope of this text. Different combinations of x-ray, radium, and radioactive materials are utilized, all seeking to apply an adequate cancerocidal dosage to the cervix, parametrium, and pelvic lymph nodes. At the same time the effect on such vital structures as bladder, and bowel must be kept at a minimum.

The radiological treatment usually consists of the local application of radium to the cervix by any one of a number of applicators. This is followed by external radiation by x-rays or cobalt. The treatment must be planned as a unit, especially with respect to dose of radium, dose of external therapy, and elapsed time. In order to express dose in the cervix, Tod and Meredith a number of years ago proposed that dosage be related to two theoretic points, *viz.* A, defined as 2 cm. lateral to the axis of the external canal and 2 cm. above the vaginal fornix, and B, 3 cm. lateral to A (Fig. 12.21). It is considered desirable to deliver a minimum of 5,000 to 6,000 rads to A and B within 6 weeks. The average radium application can achieve this at A but the dose at B seldom exceeds 2,000 rads from radium alone. For this reason external roentgen or cobalt therapy is necessary. The average radium treatment delivers about 20,000 rads to the cervix. Normally the radium is given in divided doses at an interval of 2 weeks followed by the external therapy. The entire therapy is completed in about 6 weeks.

Special mention may be made of the effect of radiation on lymph node metastasis, since this has been widely discussed. Information on this point must be deduced from the average lymph node involvement in various stages of the disease as compared with involvement after radiation. Morton *et al.* have recently compiled the reported incidence of lymph node involvement by stage as follows: Stage I, 16.5%; Stage II, 31.9%; and Stage III, 46.7%. Figures for involvement after radiation vary considerably but most reported series show a figure considerably below this so that it may be considered that radiotherapy is effective in destroying cancer metastasis in at least some patients.

Morton *et al.* found that the average incidence of lymph node involvement postradiation was about 10% in Stage I and about 20% in Stage II. It may be estimated, therefore, that about one-third

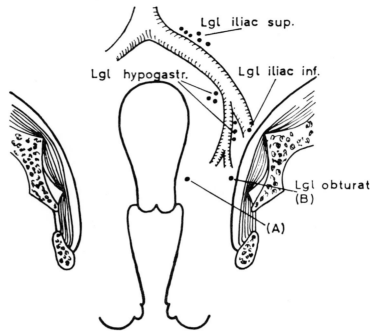

Fig. 12.21. Diagram showing irradiation targets, Points *A* and *B*

of the patients with positive lymph nodes have them sterilized by radiation.

Lymphangiography has been used to acertain the presence of metastases in lymph nodes (Fig. 12.22).

Indeed, the Sloane Hospital group (Gray, Gusberg, and Guttman) feel that supervoltage irradiation is so effective that lymphadenectomy should never be employed as an adjunct to radical surgery. Not only is this form of x-ray destructive to cancerous lymph nodes, but in addition it is not attended by the high morbidity rate associated with lymph node dissection. Above all complications the authors specify postoperative pelvic lymphocyst, in which there may be sufficient retroperitoneal collection of lymphatic fluid to seriously compromise the function of the urinary tract, the large vessels, etc. Rutledge and Fletcher, from the M. D. Anderson Hospital, also question routine lymphadenectomy, while pointing out the cancerocidal nature of deep x-ray therapy to the pelvis.

Despite all precautions, it is inevitable that irradiation should have some complications. Many women notice varying degrees of bladder irritability, diarrhea, and rectal bleeding during and after therapy, but in most cases these are transitory and short-lived. Far more distressing and troublesome are the bowel or bladder fistulas that may occur at any stage after treatment, even in the complete absence of cancer. It must be borne in mind that the initial ulcerative and destructive effect of irradiation is replaced by a later stage of marked scarification and fibrosis. An endarteritis may occur with gradual obliteration of the blood supply, with rectal or vesical fistula the result. Since the fistula is a direct result of tissue ischemia and impaired circulation, surgical repair is sometimes extremely difficult because the devitalized necrotic tissue simply will not heal. In the absence of cancer, however, even these patients may be helped to lead a comfortable if not ideal existence by such procedures as colpocleisis, colostomy, or ureteral transplantation, as noted by Dean and Taylor. Every clinic must expect a certain percentage of fistulas (as high as 10%) or else the sal-

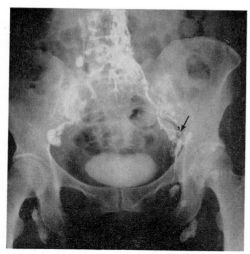

FIG. 12.22. External lymphangiogram obtained by intralymphatic injection. This shows malignant invasion of left external iliac lymph nodes verified at laparotomy. (From Pattillo, R. A., Foley, D. V., and Mattingly, R. F.: Internal pelvic lymphography. Amer. J. Obstet. & Gynec., *88:* 110, 1964.)

vage will be poor. It is just not technically possible to deliver effectively cancerocidal doses to cervix and parametrium without occasionally damaging adjacent structures. In addition it seems probable that certain individuals are unduly sensitive to irradiation and, where this seems likely after the first application, further dosage should be decreased. In cancer of the cervical stump it is likewise important to diminish the radium dosage; the fundus usually acts as a type of screen and, if this is absent, severe irradiation damage may occur.

Surgery. The recent resurgence of surgery as the primary treatment is directly attributable to such medical advances as improved anesthesia, well equipped blood banks, antibiotic drugs, etc., which have made it possible to perform extensive, radical surgery with minimal operative mortality. Surgical proponents feel that irradiation has no effect on the pelvic lymph nodes, which can, however, be removed by surgery. Certain types of cervical cancer are resistant to irradiation and show no response

to therapy. The surgeons also argue that removal of the uterus prevents local recurrence and that operation avoids irradiation complications.

Meigs and others have suggested the routine use of an improved radical Wertheim hysterectomy and pelvic lymphadenectomy in medically fit women with Stage I and early Stage II lesions. There is no question but that a skilled operator can perform this procedure with negligible mortality, but even in expert hands there is a sizable number of postoperative fistulas (especially ureteral) plus other morbidity.

Unfortunately there are few clinics where all patients with Stage I and Stage II disease are treated by surgery. Thus, surgical series are selected and end results must be interpreted with this in mind. Just as with radiation, surgical results vary greatly from institution to institution probably due to the degree of patient selection. Nevertheless, the 5-year figures quoted below for abdominal radical hysterectomy and lymphadenectomy (Wertheim) may be considered representative. Liu and Meigs reported that for Stage I, they obtained a 74% recovery rate in 116 patients and for Stage II 57% for 49 patients. Parsons, Cesare, and Friedell reported 78% recovery rate for Stage I, 85% for Stage IIa, and 45% for Stage IIb in a relatively small selected series. Welch, Pratt, and Symmonds reported 85.7% for Stage I and 80% for Stage II, again with a selected series. It is regrettable that there is no compilation of very large numbers of patients or a true alternate treatment series so that a comparison with the end results from radiation may be made.

Some clinics, primarily European, have advocated the radical vaginal hysterectomy (Schauta) for cancer of the cervix. Navratil reported an 83.3% survival rate for 294 patients with Stage I and 51.7% for 203 patients with Stage II. With this operation, no lymphadenectomy is routinely done and postoperative radiation to the lymph nodes is ordinarily carried out.

The curability of lymph node metastasis by surgery has received special attention just as it has with radiation. There is no doubt that lymph node involvement is of ominous prognostic significance. Nevertheless all authors are able to report some curability with lymph node involvement. For example, Liu and Meigs with a 74% over-all survival rate for Stage I, cured but 5 of 14 patients who had lymph node involvement. Other authors report similar figures.

On the other hand, Rauscher and Spurny reported the relative cure rates for 315 patients, 158 of whom had hysterectomy without lymphadenectomy and 157 of whom had hysterectomy with lymphadenectomy. The cure rates for Stages I and II combined were 75.04 and 75.79%, respectively.

Surgical therapy, like radiation, is associated with complications principally to the urinary tract. Ureteral or vesical fistulas may occur in up to 10% of patients.

Combined Irradiation and Surgery. It is our feeling that this should not be a routine form of treatment, and for two different reasons. First, there is no doubt that irradiation, by virtue of its tendency to cause increased vascularity, edema, and scarring, makes subsequent surgery more difficult—with a resultant increase in complicating fistula. Of even more importance, however, is the tendency of surgery to undo one of the most important and vital irradiation effects. In addition to an immediately destructive and lethal effect on cancer, both radium and x-ray lead to later fibrosis and scarring that may entrap and hold in check microscopically viable appearing tumor cells. Surgery tends to cut across and break down these fibrotic barriers with dissemination of malignant cells into lymphatic and vascular channels, and we have observed this apparent sequence in more than one instance. However, Stevenson, Carter *et al.*, and others have reported excellent results by utilizing combined irradiation and surgery. Although patient selection is confined to certain favorable Stage I and early Stage II lesions, their resultant 85% 5-year salvage rate seems impressive.

TREATMENT OF RADIORESISTANT CANCER

A certain small percentage (probably less than 5%) of cervical cancer is completely resistant to any amount of irradiation, and the clinician will be alerted to this by a consistently positive biopsy. Actually biopsies may remain positive for several weeks following completion of therapy, but experience suggests that persistence of tumor more than 8 to 10 weeks posttherapy indicates failure of response.

Evaluation of postirradiation biopsies is an exceedingly difficult and sometimes impossible task. Novak has indicated that degenerative changes closely mimic neoplastic ones, and at certain times it is impossible to distinguish viable from nonviable tumor cells. Yet this is of paramount importance, and where biopsies are equivocal it is sometimes desirable to perform conization to establish failure of response to irradiation. Although the British feel that sequential biopsies during and after therapy are helpful in formulating a prognosis, we are frequently dissatisfied with them as a means of early detection of radioresistance. In any case, biopsy of the cervix is unfortunately not an index of lymphatic spread.

Infinitely more promising but still unproved is the work of the Grahams, who feel that they can accurately forecast the behavior of the tumor by cytological methods. Cells obtained in vaginal smears can be identified as being responsive to irradiation and, if there is a good sensitization response (SR), a favorable result will be had by irradiation. Cytology is also utilized during the course of treatment and the radiation response (RR) can also be assessed. A poor SR or RR indicates surgery. Jones and his associates have suggested the use of the buccal smear as indicative of host resistance.

There are usually only two indications for surgery in the average conservative clinic that utilizes irradiation as standard therapy. The first of these is the detection of *radioresistance* and, if this can be detected early, while the disease is localized, the prognosis is that much better.

The second is *recurrence after complete adequate irradiation*. Experience has shown that once a postirradiation recurrence has appeared, no further amounts of radiotherapy will be effective.

We would emphasize the extreme difficulty as well as importance of making a diagnosis of resistant or recurrent lesion. Where cervical biopsy or smear is unequivocally positive this is simple, but where this clue is absent the problem is formidable. A high index of suspicion should be reserved for increasing radiating backache, pelvic pain with induration, dilatation of the urinary tract, leg or vulvar edema, etc. However, even earlier diagnosis should be striven for if there is to be any hope for successful surgery in the face of radioresistance. Although premature unfounded suspicion should not mandate radical complicated surgery, nevertheless the patient who does poorly following radiation generally will show a recurrent or resistant tumor even though proof may be difficult to obtain. We favor hospital admission, with examination under anesthesia, conization, and curettage as well as cytological studies, pyelography, and other x-ray study. If there should be positive or even suggestive evidence of radioresistance or recurrence, some operative procedure may be considered, but Burns and Brack point out that this is generally performed too late.

The surgery will of necessity depend on the extent of the disease when resistance or recurrence is noted. If early, a *radical hysterectomy with pelvic lymphadenectomy may be utilized*, but this is insufficient for advanced degrees of disease. Recent years have seen experimental programs in which ultraradical surgery was carried out, as proposed by Brunschwig. The procedure of *complete pelvic exenterations* involves removal of all pelvic organs, bladder and rectum, and transplantation of the ureters into an exteriorized colon or ilial segment. A handful of 5-year survivors can be reported, but we feel very strongly that use of this heroic procedure for purely palliative purposes is not indicated. The surgeon must decide for himself whether the rare survivor is compensation for the extensive suffering, financial sacrifices, prolonged hospitalization, and ultimate death for the vast majority.

Less radical procedures can be utilized where the rectum is free of disease, so that only the bladder and pelvic organs need be removed along with ureteral transplantation. These so-called *anterior exenterations* are apt to develop severe kidney difficulties at a later date, particularly if the urinary tracts are already damaged when the ureter is implanted.

Where the rectum is involved but the bladder is free of disease, a *posterior exenteration* can be utilized which, of course, leaves the patient with a colostomy. Either one of these partial exenterations is utilized by most clinics on occasional selected and qualified patients with less distaste than for the complete operation. All of these show a not inconsiderable mortality and morbidity even if done by trained gynecologists, and unfortunately many poorly qualified surgeons attempt these procedures. With recurrent or resistant irradiated cancer, one must admit that there is no other chance for cure than surgery.

Where partial exenteration or a radical Wertheim operation is feasible, the results are worthwhile, as indicated by the reports of Thompson and Brack from our own clinic, Brunschwig, Douglas, Schmitz, and others. We utilize such surgery for those women who have a *proven* radioresistance or recurrence. Results with Wertheim hysterectomy approach 50% salvage of operable patients and, with partial exenteration, 20%, *if no lymph node involvement is encountered*. Should there be evidence of lymphatic cancer, salvage is minimal, and it should be apparent to all of us that even meticulous lymphadenectomy is not the answer to cure of cancer after radiation. If the nodes *are* involved, are they an absolute barrier to malignant cells, and is it not likely that tumor has spread beyond the nodal borders so that no form of lymphadenectomy will be beneficial? Because of our belief in this tenet, plus the increased morbidity as opposed to the beneficial results of therapy, we cannot help but feel that routine lymphadenectomy in radical surgery after radiation is merely a gesture.

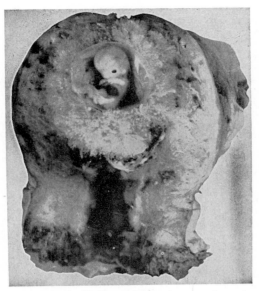

FIG. 12.23. Epidermoid carcinoma of cervix associated with pregnancy of 6 to 8 weeks.

TREATMENT OF CERVICAL CANCER IN PREGNANCY

This must of necessity vary in different cases, depending chiefly on the stage of the disease and the stage of pregnancy at which the cancer is recognized, although there are often other factors to be considered, such as the religious beliefs of the patient and her family. Fortunately, cancer of the cervix in the pregnant woman is relatively rare.

If careful study of the cervix, by conization if necessary, indicates that the disease is intraepithelial, the pregnancy may be allowed to go to term with the treatment of the cervix deferred until after delivery. For more advanced cancer the disease should be treated without regard to the pregnancy.

In general, if the cancer is recognized in the early stages of pregnancy, irradiation is the best plan, in the hope of inducing abortion. Others prefer to do therapeutic abortion or hysterotomy, followed by either irradiation or radical operation,

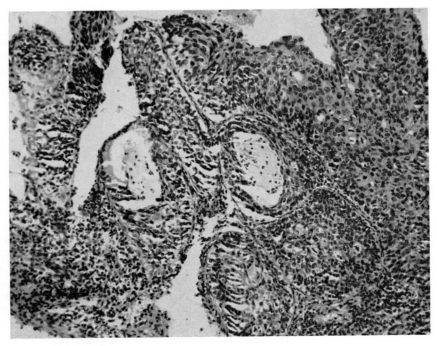

FIG. 12.24. Intraepithelial carcinoma found during pregnancy; same pattern postpartum and in hysterectomy specimen.

depending upon the stage of the disease and the personal predilection of the clinician. In later stages, one can wait a short time for viability, or, if this has been reached, deliver the baby by the abdominal route, followed usually by irradiation. There are various modifications of this general plan which may be indicated in individual cases, but the prime motive is to treat the cancer with disregard of the pregnancy, although occasional individualization is practiced. The results by stage are somewhat inferior to those obtained in the nonpregnant (Figs. 12.23 and 12.24).

REFERENCES

Annual Report on the Results of Treatment in Carcinoma of the Uterus, Vol. 13. Stockholm, 1963.

Boyd, J. R., Royle, D., Fidler, H. K., and Boyes, D. A.: Conservative management of in situ carcinoma of the cervix. Amer. J. Obstet. Gynec., 85: 322, 1963.

Brack, C. B., Everett, H. S., and Dickson, R.: Irradiation therapy for carcinoma of the cervix; its effect upon the urinary tract. Obstet. Gynec., 7: 196, 1956.

Broders, A. C.: Grading of carcinoma. Minnesota Med., 8: 726, 1925.

Brunschwig, A.: Complete excision of pelvic viscera for advanced carcinoma; a one-stage abdominoperineal operation with end colostomy and bilateral ureteral implantation into the colon above the colostomy. Cancer, 1: 177, 1948.

Brunschwig, A.: Surgical treatment of stage I cancer of the cervix. Cancer, 13: 34, 1960.

Burns, B. C., and Brack, C. B.: Prognostic factors in radioresistant cervical cancer. Obstet. Gynec., 16: 1, 1960.

Carter, B., Parker, R. T., Thomas, W. L., Creadick, R. N., Peete, C., Cherny, W. B., and Williams, J. B.: Follow-up of patients with cancer of cervix treated by radical hysterectomy and radical pelvic lymphadenectomy. Amer. J. Obstet. Gynec., 76: 1099, 1958.

de Alvarez, R. R.: The sites of metastasis in carcinoma of the cervix. Western J. Surg., 61: 623, 1953.

Dean, R. E., and Taylor, E. S.: Surgical treatment of complications resulting from irradiation therapy of cervical cancer. Amer. J. Obstet. Gynec., 19: 34, 1960.

Diaz-Bazan, N.: Prolapso uterino y cancer del Cuello. Arch. Col. Med. El Salvador, 5: 15, 1952.

Douglas, R. G., and Sweeney, J. H.: Exenteration operations in advanced pelvic cancer. Amer. J. Obstet. Gynec., 73: 1169, 1957.

Dunn, J. E., Jr.: Preliminary findings of the Memphis-Shelby County uterine cancer study and their interpretations. Amer. J. Public Health, 48: 861, 1958.

Enterline, E. T., Arvan, D. A., and Davis, R. E.: The predictability of residual carcinoma in situ from study of cervical cones. Amer. J. Obstet. Gynec., 85: 940, 1963.

Epperson, J. W. W., Hellman, L. M., Galvin, G. A., and Busby, T.: Morphologic changes in cervix during pregnancy, including intraepithelial carcinoma. Amer. J. Obstet. Gynec., 61: 50, 1951.

Fidler, H. K., Boyes, D. A., Aversperg, N., and Lock, D. R.: The cytology program in British Columbia. Canad. Med. Ass. J., 86: 779, 1962.

Fischer, R.: Possible role of smegma in etiology of squamous cell carcinoma of cervix. Obstet. Gynec. Survey, 8: 232, 1953.

Fluhmann, C. F.: Carcinoma in situ and the transitional zone of the cervix uteri. Obstet. Gynec., 16: 424, 1960.

Gagnon, F.: Contribution to study of etiology and prevention of cancer of cervix of uterus. Amer. J. Obstet. Gynec., 60: 516, 1950.

Galvin, G. A., Jones, H. W., and Te Linde, R. W.: Clinical relationship of carcinoma in situ and invasive carcinoma of the cervix. J. A. M. A., 149: 744, 1952.

Galvin, G. A., Jones, H. W., and Te Linde, R. W.: Significance of basal cell hyperactivity in cervical biopsies. Amer. J. Obstet. Gynec., 70: 808, 1955.

Graham, R. M., and Graham, J. B.: Cytological prognosis in cancer of the uterine cervix treated radiologically. Cancer, 8: 59, 1955.

Gray, M. J., Gusberg, S. B., and Guttman, R.: Pelvic lymph node dissection following radiotherapy. Amer. J. Obstet. Gynec., 76: 629, 1958.

Greene, R. R., and Peckham, B. M.: Preinvasive cancer of the cervix, and pregnancy. Amer. J. Obstet. Gynec., 75: 551, 1958.

Greene, R. R., Peckham, B. M., Chung, J. T., Bayly, M. A., Benaron, H. B. W., Carrow, L. A., and Gardner, G. H.: Preinvasive carcinoma of cervix during pregnancy. Surg. Gynec. Obstet., 96: 71, 1953.

Haenszel, W., and Hillhouse, M.: Uterine cancer morbidity in New York City and its relation to the pattern of regional variation within the United States. J. Nat. Cancer Inst., 22: 1157, 1959.

Heins, H. C., Jr., Dennis, E. J., and Pratt-Thomas, H. R.: Possible role of smegma in carcinoma of the cervix. Amer. J. Obstet. Gynec., 76: 726, 1958.

Henriksen, E.: The lymphatic spread of carcinoma of the cervix and body of the uterus. Amer. J. Obstet. Gynec., 58: 924, 1949.

Hertig, A. T., and Younge, P. A.: What is

cancer in situ of the cervix? Is it the preinvasive form of true carcinoma? Amer. J. Obstet. Gynec., *64:* 807, 1952.

Hinselmann, H.: Davis and Carter Gynec. and Obstet. *3:* Ch. 4. W. F. Pryor Co., Hagerstown, Md.

Johnson, L. D., Easterday, C. L., Gore, H., and Hertig, A. T.: The histogenesis of carcinoma in situ of the uterine cervix. Cancer, *17:* 213, 1964.

Jones, E. G., McDonald, I., and Brestlow, L.: Epidemiologic factors in carcinoma of the cervix. Amer. J. Obstet. Gynec., *76:* 1, 1958.

Jones, H. W., Jr., Galvin, G. A., and Te Linde, R. W.: Intraepithelial carcinoma of cervix and its clinical implications. Int. Abstr. Surg., *92:* 521, 1951.

Jones, H. W., Jr., Goldberg, B., Davis, H. J., and Burns, B. C., Jr.: Cellular changes in vaginal buccal smears after radiation. An index of the radiocurability of carcinoma of the cervix. Amer. J. Obstet. Gynec., *75:* 1083, 1959.

Kottmaier, H. L.: Current treatment of carcinoma of the cervix. Amer. J. Obstet. Gynec., *76:* 243, 1958.

Lilienfeld, A. M., and Graham, S.: Validity of determining circumcision status by questionnaires as related to epidemiological studies of cancer of the cervix. J. Nat. Cancer Inst., *21:* 713, 1958.

Liu, W., and Meigs, J. V.: Radical hysterectomy and pelvic lymphadenectomy. Amer. J. Obstet. Gynec., *69:* 1, 1955.

Martzloff, K. H.: Carcinoma of the cervix uteri. Bull. Hopkins Hosp., *40:* 960, 1927.

McKay, D. G., Hertig, A. T., and Younge, P. A.: Carcinoma in situ. J. Int. Coll. Surg., *21:* 212, 1954.

McKelvey, J. L., Stenstrom, K. W., and Gillam, J. S.: Results of experimental therapy of carcinoma of cervix. Amer. J. Obstet. Gynec., *58:* 896, 1949.

Meigs, J. V.: *Surgical Treatment of Cancer of the Cervix.* Grune & Stratton, Inc., New York, 1954.

Meigs, J. V.: Radical hysterectomy with bilateral pelvic-lymph-node dissection for cancer of the uterine cervix. Clin. Obstet. Gynec., *1:* 1029, 1958.

Meigs, J. V., and Brunschwig, A.: Proposed classification for cases of cancer of the cervix treated by surgery. Amer. J. Obstet. Gynec., *64:* 413, 1952.

Meyer, R.: Basis of histologic diagnosis of cervical carcinoma, and similar lesions. Surg. Gynec. Obstet., *73:* 14, 1941.

Morton, D. G., Lagasse, L. D., Moore, J. C., Jacobs, M., and Amromin, G.: Pelvic lymphnodectomy following radiation in cervical carcinoma. Amer. J. Obstet. Gynec., *88:* 932, 1964.

Navratil, E.: Indications and results of the Schauta-Amreich operation with and without postoperative roentgen treatment in epidermoid carcinoma of the cervix of the uterus. Amer. J. Obstet. Gynec., *86:* 141, 1963.

Novak, E. R.: Radioresistant cervical cancer. Obstet. Gynec., *4:* 251, 1954.

Novak, E. R., and Villa Santa, U.: Factors influencing the ratio of uterine cancer in a community. J. A. M. A., *174:* 1395, 1960.

Parsons, L., Cesare, F., and Friedell, G. H.: Primary surgical treatment of invasive cancer of the cervix. Surg. Gynec. Obstet., *109:* 279, 1959.

Pattillo, R. A., Foley, D. V., and Mattingly, R. F.: Internal pelvic lymphography. Amer. J. Obstet. Gynec., *88:* 110, 1964.

Petersen, O.: Spontaneous course of cervical precancerous conditions. Amer. J. Obstet. Gynec., *73:* 1063, 1957.

Rauscher, H., and Spurny, J.: Results with the radical Wertheim operation with and without obligatory lymphadenectomy. Geburtsh. Frauenheilk., *19:* 651, 1959.

Rewell, R. E.: Population structure and apparent incidence of cancer; a study of endometrial carcinoma in England and South India. J. Obstet. Gynaec. Brit. Comm., *65:* 590, 1958.

Rothman, A.: Carcinoma of cervix in Jewish women. Amer. J. Obstet. Gynec. *62:* 160, 1951.

Rotkin, I. D.: Relation of adolescent coitus to cervical cancer risk. J. A. M. A., *179:* 110, 1962.

Rutledge, F. N., and Fletcher, G. H.: Lymphadenectomy after supervoltage irradiation. Amer. J. Obstet. Gynec., *76:* 321, 1958.

Schiller, W.: Untersuchungen zur Entstehung der Geschivulste. I. Collumcarcinom des Uterus. Virchow. Arch. Path. Anat., *263:* 279, 1927.

Schmitz, H. E., Smith, C. J., Foley, D. V., and Schack, C. B.: Evaluation of surgical procedures employed following the failure of irradiation therapy in cancer of the cervix. Amer. J. Obstet. Gynec., *74:* 1165, 1957.

Schmitz, R. L., Schmitz, H. E., Smith, C. J., and Molitor, J. J.: Details of pelvic exenteration evolved during an experience with 75 cases. Amer. J. Obstet. Gynec., *80:* 43, 1960.

Stevenson, C. S.: Treatment of carcinoma of the cervix with full irradiation therapy followed by radical pelvic surgery. Amer. J. Obstet. Gynec., *75:* 888, 1958.

Tennis, M., and Oalmann, M. C.: Carcinoma of the cervix; an epidemiologic study. J. A. M. A., *174:* 155, 1960.

Thompson, J. D., and Brack, C. B.: Radical surgery for radioresistant cancer. Obstet. Gynec., *10:* 676, 1957.

Thornton, W. N., Fox, C. H., and Smith, D. E.: Relationship of the squamo-columnar junction and the endocervical glands to the site of origin of carcinoma of the cervix. Amer. J. Obstet. Gynec., *78:* 1060, 1959.

Tod, M. C., and Meredith, W. J.: The treatment of cancer of the uterine cervix. Brit. J. Radiol., *11:* 809, 1938.

Tod, M. C., and Meredith, W. J.: Treatment of cancer of the cervix uteri. A revised "Manchester Method." Brit. J. Radiol., *26:* 252, 1953.

Towne, J. E.: Carcinoma of cervix in nulliparous and celibate women. Amer. J. Obstet. Gynec., *69:* 606, 1955.

Tweeddale, D. N., Gorthey, R. L., Harvey, H. E., and Tanner, F. H.: Cervical *versus* endometrial carcinoma; relative incidence. Obstet. Gynec., *2:* 623, 1953.

Way, S.: *Malignant Disease of the Female Genital Tract.* Blakiston Company, Division of McGraw-Hill Book Company, Inc., New York, 1951.

Webb, G. A., Margolis, A. J., and Traut, H. F.: Adenocarcinoma of the endometrium; evaluation of factors influencing prognosis and outline of plan of therapy based on these factors. Western J. Surg., *63:* 407, 1955.

Welch, J. S., Pratt, J. H. and Symmonds, R. E.: The Wertheim hysterectomy for squamous cell carcinoma of the uterine cervix. Thirty years' experience at the Mayo Clinic. Amer. J. Obstet. Gynec., *51:* 978, 1961.

Wespi, H.: *Early Carcinoma of the Uterine Cervix.* Grune & Stratton, Inc., New York, 1949.

Woodruff, J. D., and Mattingly, R. F.: Epithelial changes preceding spinal cell carcinoma of cervix uteri. Amer. J. Obstet. Gynec., *77:* 977, 1959.

Wynder, E. L., Cornfield, J., Schroff, P. O., and Doralswami, K. P.: A study of environmental factors in carcinoma of the cervix. Amer. J. Obstet. Gynec., *68:* 1016, 1954.

Younge, P. A., Hertig, A. T., and Armstrong, D.: A study of 135 cases of carcinoma in situ of cervix at Free Hospital for Women. Amer. J. Obstet. Gynec., *58:* 867, 1949.

13

RELAXATIONS, FISTULAS, AND MALPOSITIONS

Structure of the Vaginal Outlet. The pelvic floor, closing the outlet of the pelvis, is made up of a number of muscular and fascial structures which are pierced by the rectum, vagina, and urethra as these canals pass to the exterior of the body. The most important of the muscles is the levator ani, which forms a broad muscular sheet, concave above and convex below, and which extends like a diaphragm from one side of the pelvis to the other. It consists of a pubic portion which arises from the pubic bone anteriorly, and passes backward to encircle the rectum, while the iliac portion arises from the so-called white line of the pelvis and passes downward to meet its fellow of the opposite side in the midline, extending to the tip of the coccyx behind. Most of its fibers pass behind the rectum and, according to the majority of anatomists, few or no fibers pass between the vagina and the rectum.

Even more important in the support of the pelvic organs is the pelvic fascia. The superior or pelvic fascia covers the upper surface of the muscular diaphragm, extending from the white line of the pelvis on one side to that of the other, and giving off fascial coverings to the vaginal and rectal canals as they pass through the pelvic floor.

The inferior or external pelvic fascia, found beneath the levator diaphragm, is divisible into two parts, one anterior and one posterior to a line between the tuberosities of the ischia. The posterior covers the under surface of the levator muscles, while the anterior constitutes the so-called urogenital diaphragm or inferior triangular ligament. This is a dense fascial sheet which fills in the triangle formed by the pubic arch, the rami, and a line drawn between the two tuberosities. It is composed of a superficial and a deep layer. The superficial perineal muscles are placed superficial to the urogenital diaphragm, but the deeper group, with other important structures, are situated in the space between the two layers (Figs. 13.1–13.3).

LACERATIONS OF THE PERINEUM

These are best subdivided into those of the *incomplete* and *complete* varieties. In the former, the laceration does not involve the sphincter ani, whereas in the latter this muscle is partly or completely torn. Incomplete tears are sometimes subdivided into those of *first* and *second degrees*, according to their extent, the complete variety being considered as of the *third degree*. In the overwhelming majority of cases *lacerations of the genital canal* are due to childbirth, but other forms of trauma, such as coitus, attempted rape, or external violence may at times be responsible. The cervix and

252

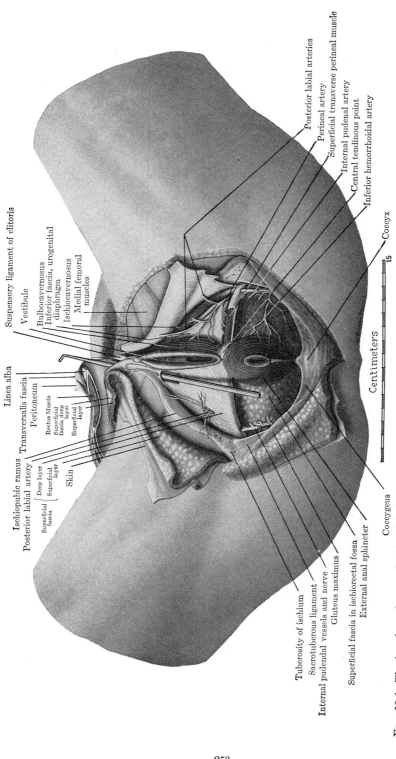

Linea alba

Suspensory ligament of clitoris

Ischiopubic ramus

Posterior labial artery

Vestibule

Bulbocavernosus
Inferior fascia, urogenital diaphragm
Ischiocavernosus
Medial femoral muscles

Transversalis fascia

Peritoneum

Rectus Muscle
Superficial fascia deep layer
Superficial layer

Superficial fascia { Deep layer / Superficial layer

Skin

Posterior labial arteries
Perineal artery
Superficial transverse perineal muscle
Internal pudenal artery
Central tendinous point
Inferior hemorrhoidal artery

Tuberosity of ischium

Sacrotuberous ligament

Internal pudendal vessels and nerve

Gluteus maximus

Superficial fascia in ischiorectal fossa

External anal sphincter

Coccygeus

Coccyx

Centimeters

15

FIG. 13.1. The female perineum. On the right half of the urogenital triangle the superficial fatty layer has been turned aside to display the deep layer of the superficial fascia; the latter, on the left half, has been reflected to show the contents of the superficial perineal compartment. (From Anson, B. J.: in *A Textbook of Gynecology*, Ed. 6, edited by A. H. Curtis and J. W. Huffman, W. B. Saunders Company, Philadelphia, 1950.)

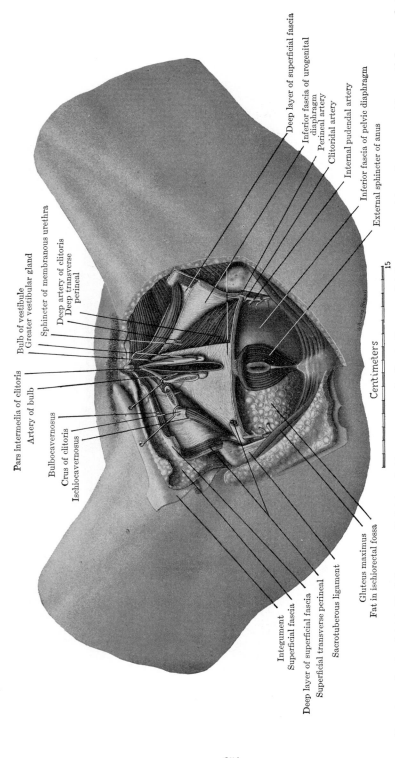

Pars intermedia of clitoris
Artery of bulb

Bulbocavernosus
Crus of clitoris
Ischiocavernosus

Bulb of vestibule
Greater vestibular gland
Sphincter of membranous urethra
Deep artery of clitoris
Deep transverse
perineal

Deep layer of superficial fascia

Inferior fascia of urogenital
diaphragm
Perineal artery
Clitoridal artery

Internal pudendal artery

Inferior fascia of pelvic diaphragm

External sphincter of anus

Integument
Superficial fascia
Deep layer of superficial fascia
Superficial transverse perineal
Sacrotuberous ligament

Gluteus maximus
Fat in ischiorectal fossa

Centimeters

15

Fig. 13.2. On the right half of the urogenital triangle the cavernous bodies in the superficial compartment have been exposed by partial removal of the superficial perineal muscles; on the left, the inferior fascia of the urogenital diaphragm has been reflected to show the musculature in the deep perineal compartment. In the anal triangle, on the left side, the superficial (fatty) tissue has been removed from the ischiorectal fossa. (From Anson, B. J.: in *A Text-book of Gynecology*, Ed. 6, edited by A. H. Curtis and J. W. Huffman, W. B. Saunders Company, Philadelphia, 1950.)

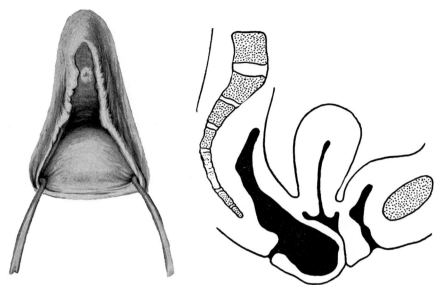

Fig 13.7. Sagittal view of rectocele and cystocele. (From Davis, C. H. (Editor): *Gynecology and Obstetrics.* W. F. Prior Company, Inc., Hagerstown, Md., 1933.)

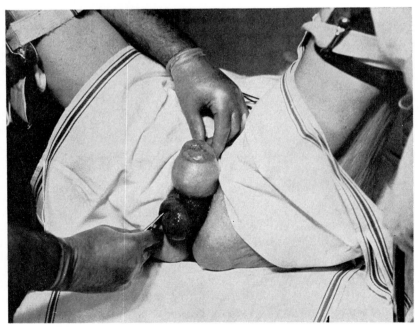

Fig. 13.8. Unusually extensive birth injury in which the rectum was avulsed from its posterior attachments. The patient had had complete incontinence of feces for 30 years. It was possible to repair this injury at a single operation, with resulting satisfactory bowel control.

Symptoms of Genital Relaxation. Even extensive relaxation of the outlet may be entirely symptomless, while in other cases there is a complaint of *loose-ness and heaviness in the vaginal region*, especially after prolonged standing. The patient not infrequently describes her symptoms as a sensation of "everything dropping out." There may be some *bearing-down discomfort in the lower abdomen*, and *backache* may be complained of. However, troublesome backache should always lead to a search for other far more frequent causes, such as abnormalities of the back itself, or the presence of marked backward displacements of the uterus.

Where relaxation is associated with *complete perineal laceration*, at least partial *fecal incontinence* is produced. In the latter, the patient may have fairly good control, but if the stools are rather loose, distressing incontinence develops.

While moderate *cystocele* often causes no symptoms, the more marked degrees bring about increasing *difficulty in emptying the bladder*. As a matter of fact, in extreme cases the patient may be unable to void unless the bladder is first pushed back in the vagina with the finger. In the more marked cases, the bladder may contain much residual urine, and *cystitis* is almost always the result, with the possibility of ascending infection. There is, therefore, a complaint of *increased frequency of urination*, with perhaps *tenesmus*, the symptoms being most troublesome during the day, and improved by night or when the patient is in the recumbent position. *Incontinence of urine* is frequent, especially where there is a definite urethrocele, and this *incontinence* is usually of the *stress* variety, with escape of urine on coughing, laughing, sneezing, or other muscular effort. Although stress incontinence may occur with cystocele or urethrocele, it may occur with no obvious relaxation and from many causes as indicated in the excellent text on urinary incontinence by Ullery.

Rectocele, like cystocele, may produce few symptoms, but where the protruding rectal pouch is large, there may be a deflection of feces into the pouch, with in creasing *difficulty of defecation* and *constipation*, because of the impaired overstretched rectal wall. *Hemorrhoids* frequently develop, adding to the patient's discomfort. Finally, in cases associated with *prolapse of the uterus*, there is added the strain of symptoms characterizing the latter, especially the discomfort produced by the *protrusion* of the prolapsed uterus, bladder, and rectum.

Diagnosis. The diagnosis of relaxation is usually simple, but a thorough diagnostic study should include an appraisal of its exact nature and of the structures involved. This is of obvious importance when operation is contemplated but the degree of relaxation may not parallel the symptoms.

The simpler *relaxations of the vagina* are usually evident, even on simple inspection, from the gaping appearance of the orifice and the separation of the anterior and posterior vaginal walls, normally in juxtaposition. Where there has been extensive laceration, scar tissue may be plainly visible, either in the midline or in one or both sulci. When the examining fingers are introduced, and the patient is asked to strain down, one can at once note the *absence of the resistance of the muscles* surrounding the lower vagina.

Cystocele and rectocele, when large, may be at once visible on inspection, but often they recede when the patient is lying flat. It is always important to ask the patient to strain, this bringing out the cystocele and rectocele so that their extent can be seen. The presence of *urethrocele* is indicated by marked bulging just below the urethral orifice. This condition should always be borne in mind, as its surgical correction involves certain specific features. The demonstration of a rectocele can be made more striking by introducing a finger into the rectum and pushing it upward and forward into the rectal pouch. By thrusting the finger forward, the anterior rectal wall can be hooked outward from the vagina, the rectovaginal septum being exceedingly thin and atrophic in such cases as this.

When *complete laceration* exists, there is often a deep midline cleft from the posterior vaginal margin through the perineum into the rectum, and sometimes extending upward into the anterior rectal wall. Under such circumstances, the rectal mucosa is commonly everted, presenting as a bright red spongy area. Even when the anus seems intact, the sphincter may have been injured. Here, as in the case of the vagina, a demonstration of the adequacy or inadequacy of the sphincter control may be made by asking the patient to "draw in" on the inserted finger.

Stress Incontinence

The diagnosis of *stress incontinence* is not always easy, for urgency due to infection, leakage from fistulas, and other modes of urinary loss are sometimes difficult to exclude. A good history is of course paramount. Various methods of elevating the vaginal wall by two fingers (Bonney test) or Allis clamps (Marchetti test) tend to prevent loss of urine on straining. Urinalysis, cystoscopy, cystometric studies, and urethrocystograms with or without a metallic bead chain as advised by Hodgkinson and Green are occasionally necessary. The uncertain mechanism of incontinence has resulted in many different types of treatment, and a recent symposium edited by Lund fully treats the complicated subject of urinary incontinence. The student, however, should be aware of the fact that many, if not most, women especially if they have borne children, will occasionally experience trivial degrees of urinary loss which needs no treatment.

When the patient is in the childbearing age, and when she is anxious for further pregnancies, the conservative plan is always advisable with the more moderate degrees of relaxation, and when symptoms are absent or slight, as they so often are, plastic correction can in a large proportion of cases be deferred until after the completion of childbearing. Occasionally the "perineometer" will encourage development of muscles of the bladder neck so that stress incontinence is markedly improved.

Treatment. Correction of any of these forms of genital relaxation is possible only by surgical procedures, but in a large proportion of cases operations may safely be deferred for long periods of time, and in the less pronounced cases they may be avoided altogether. Jeffcoate points out the frequency of dyspareunia if injudicious, too snug, posterior repair is utilized. Indeed, even if an adequate vagina is preserved in the menstrual era, postmenopausal atrophy superimposed on a vagina of borderline caliber may lead to distressing dyspareunia. Our own tendency is to avoid posterior repair in the younger woman unless there are really major degrees of relaxation.

Reparative Surgery. When any type of vaginal plastic procedure is contemplated, the rational gynecologist will at once consider the possibility of *vaginal hysterectomy* with appropriate repair. As to the age-old question, "Isn't she too young?" the thinking gynecologist will reply that only a rare woman is "too young" for hysterectomy if she has completed her family. Admittedly, one stroke of lightning could wipe out that family with the woman unable to have more children, but this is certainly a pessimistic approach to life in general. Nevertheless the conscientious gynecologist will discuss this possibility with the patient and her husband.

We see many 30-year-old women with a 50-year-old pelvis. If their doubts and superstitions regarding the "dire effects" incurred by hysterectomy can be resolved, then certainly they are better relieved of a symptomatic prolapsed uterus—an organ which annually is the site of 15,000 fatal cancers. We are not attempting to justify prophylactic hysterectomy; we simply state our preference for vaginal hysterectomy in the symptomatic woman with anatomical defects where conservative operation, if followed by subsequent pregnancy, might well undo the most proficient repair.

We likewise feel that tubal ligation (in conjunction with repair) is an archaic procedure, thus preserving a functionless uterus which may well become the seat of myoma, cancer, etc. Indeed tubal ligation, except in the immediate postpartum or poor risk patient hardly seems a justifiable operation, although admittedly morbidity is low. Hysterectomy, generally by the vaginal route, has just about superseded this procedure; similarly, uterine suspension is a rare procedure in our clinic. Where possible, judicious use of pessaries often (not always) obviates the necessity for any operative procedure until after the family has been completed, at which time, irrespective of age, definitive surgery can be accomplished. We do not, however, believe in vaginal hysterectomy merely as a sterilizing measure in the asymptomatic patient.

Above all, it should be emphasized that repair of the pelvic outlet is an elective procedure. There is nothing urgent about cystocele, rectocele, or prolapse, and only if those are symptomatic should surgery be contemplated. Where protrusion out the introitus is constant, however, chafing of the mucosa with ulceration and bleeding is inevitable, and this degree of relaxation, although otherwise asymptomatic, warrants treatment.

FISTULAS

Genital Fistulas

A genital fistula is an abnormal communication between some part of the genital canal, on the one hand, and either the urinary tract or intestinal canal, or both.

Etiology. By far the most common cause of genital fistulas in past years was *obstetrical trauma*, especially in cases of prolonged and difficult labor. In such cases the fistula is due to necrosis and sloughing of the genital canal, usually the vagina, and also of the wall of the subjacent viscus, generally the bladder. The *improper use of forceps* likewise added to the incidence of such fistulas. The great improvement in obstetrical management which has occurred in recent years has very greatly lessened the frequency of fistulas due to this group of causes.

On the other hand, the enormous development of major *surgery* and the widespread *employment of radium* for many gynecological indications have brought with them a not inconsiderable incidence of genital fistulas. As a matter of fact, the majority of fistulas seen nowadays are the result of injury to the bladder, ureter, or rectum in the course of operations, particularly radical hysterectomy, or they result from necrosis and sloughing produced by the application of radium. Other causes are the *destruction of tissue* by *malignant tumors, ulceration due to foreign bodies*, especially vaginal pessaries, and occasionally, cystocele repair.

Urinary Fistulas

Even the most accomplished gynecological surgeon will at one time or another inadvertently damage the urinary tract, and Graben, O'Rourke, and McElrath have indicated that serious injury (accidental laceration) of the bladder occurs in almost 2% of the hysterectomies. Complications are minimized if the damage is recognized, but serious problems may ensue (as fistula) if the injury is not noted. The causative factors and

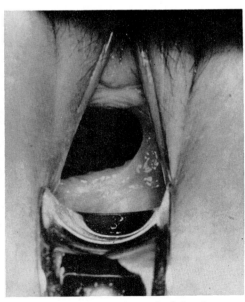

Fig. 13.9. Large vesicovaginal fistula cured surgically. (Courtesy of Dr. Albert Brown, Saskatoon, Canada.)

("sump") drainage will close a high fistula but will often minimize autodigestion of the adjacent tissues.

MALPOSITIONS

Displacements of the Uterus

Normal Position of Uterus. Normally the uterus occupies a position in the pelvic cavity between the bladder anteriorly and the rectum posteriorly. The long axis of the uterus is in the nearly horizontal plane, and forms an approximate right angle with the long axis of the vagina. The easy mobility of the uterus is an important characteristic, as can be noted in pelvic examinations of normal women. Under abnormal conditions it is greatly restricted, as when the uterus is fixed by surrounding inflammatory disease.

Normal Supports of the Uterus. The normal position of the uterus is maintained by three factors.

(1) THE PELVIC FLOOR. The fascial planes of the pelvic floor are inserted at about the level of the internal os, the strongest band being the fasciomuscular condensation in the base of the broad ligament, constituting the so-called ligament of Mackenrodt or cardinal ligament.

(2) THE UTERINE LIGAMENTS. Of these the most important in the support of the uterus are the broad and the uterosacral ligaments. This is true particularly because in the base of the former is the fascial condensation above alluded to as the cardinal ligament, while the uterosacral ligament likewise includes a strong fascial band stretching backward to the junction of the second and third sacral vertebrae. The round ligaments, formerly spoken of picturesquely as exerting a guy-rope function on the fundus, are now looked upon as having no supporting function except perhaps during pregnancy, when they become thick and hypertrophic, and may even, as some believe, help to direct the presenting part of the child downward toward the pelvic canal during labor. In the non-pregnant uterus, their laxity and their circuitous course make it difficult to believe that they can have a supporting function.

(3) INTRAABDOMINAL PRESSURE. Normally this not inconsiderable force is directed upon the posterior surface of the uterus, driving it downward and forward, and thus tending to accentuate the normal position of the organ. Intestinal loops are, so to speak, deflected into the posterior cul-de-sac, and are not normally found between the uterus and bladder. The same intraabdominal force can become a power for evil if the uterus is displaced backward, as it is then exerted on the anterior uterine surface, tending to crowd the uterus farther backward and downward.

Anterior Displacement of the Uterus

Anteflexion can be most simply defined as a bending forward of the uterus, which involves chiefly the body. The anteflexed uterus often shows some degree of hypoplasia, although most often of rather slight degree. *Anteversion* needs no treatment. Hypoplasia in the degree suggesting a really infantile uterus often responds to the stimulus of the estrogenic hormone.

Retrodisplacements of the Uterus

Of far greater importance to the gynecologist than the anterior displacements are the retrodisplacements. These may be either *congenital or acquired*, the latter being the more important, especially when complicated by other pelvic lesions, such as pelvic inflammatory disease or endometriosis.

Types and Degrees. *Retroversion* refers to the retrodisplacement in which the uterus is tilted backward on its transverse axis to a greater or lesser degree. When the tilting is comparatively slight, so that the fundus is about vertical or pointing no farther back than the sacral promontory, the retroversion is spoken of as of the *first degree*. When the fundus is within the hollow of the sacrum but not below the level of the cervix, the designation of *second degree* is commonly employed. Finally, when the uterus is so far back that the fundus is below the level of the cervix, the retroversion is of the *third degree*.

Retroflexion, simply defined, is a bending backward of the uterus, *i.e.*, of the body upon the cervix. The latter may still be directed normally downward and backward, but more frequently has tilted downward and forward (erect position of the woman) toward the symphysis as the fundus falls backward.

Retrocession of the uterus, much less frequent, refers to an abnormally posterior location of the organ, so that it occupies a position much closer to the sacrum than normal.

Causes. The causes of retrodisplacements of the uterus may be grouped as follows.

(1) CONGENITAL. Retrodisplacement of one type or another is frequently observed in the uteri of fetuses or very young children. This condition often persists into adult life, probably as a result of certain developmental deficiencies.

(2) ACQUIRED. Retrodisplacement of a previously normally placed uterus may occur from a number of causes, the most important of which may be grouped as follows.

(a) *Puerperal.* This group embraces a considerable number of possible factors which may develop following full term delivery, or, much less frequently, miscarriage. After parturition, the uterus is large and soft during the period of involution. Persisting overdistention of the bladder may tend to displace the uterus backward, as may chronic constipation, which crowds the cervix forward and thus tends to swing the fundus backward.

Much more important are injuries of the supporting structures, especially the fascial structures of the pelvic floor. When these are injured or when they are overstretched, the cervix drops forward and downward, tending to swing more and more into the long axis of the vagina. Once this process has started, it tends to continue, the fundus falling backward, after which the intraabdominal pressure

tends to further accentuation of the backward displacement, whether retroflexion or retroversion. It is easy to understand, therefore, why some degree of descensus of the uterus is seen in almost all cases of acquired retrodisplacement. While the above sequence of events may occur even after comparatively simple normal deliveries, it is far more likely to be the result of difficult and protracted labors, in which case other birth injuries of the maternal tissues are frequently associated.

(b) *Adnexal Disease.* The complicated form of retroflexion is as a rule associated with adnexal disease, either inflammatory or endometriotic The sequence may be in the order of retrodisplacement followed later by adnexitis or endometriosis, or *vice versa*. In either case the retrodisplaced fundus, instead of being free and movable, is adherent to other structures, especially the adnexa or the rectum, or both.

(c) *Neoplasms.* The effect of pelvic neoplasms of one sort or another in producing retrodisplacements is a mechanical one. For example, a large myoma developing in the anterior wall of the uterus will tend to push the uterus backward, while certain ovarian tumors impacted deep in the cul-de-sac may, by pushing the cervix far forward, cause backward displacement of the corpus.

(d) *Trauma.* The question of whether acute displacement can occur as a result of trauma is not infrequently of medicolegal importance. The protected position of the uterus, and the nature of its support, makes it difficult to believe that any but the most severe trauma could bring about displacement. The generally accepted opinion is that such acute traumatic displacement can occur, but that it is exceedingly rare.

Symptoms. Simple uncomplicated retrodisplacements of the uterus are often entirely symptomless. There are some authors who believe that this is practically always true, while others take the view that in a considerable proportion they give rise to various symptoms,

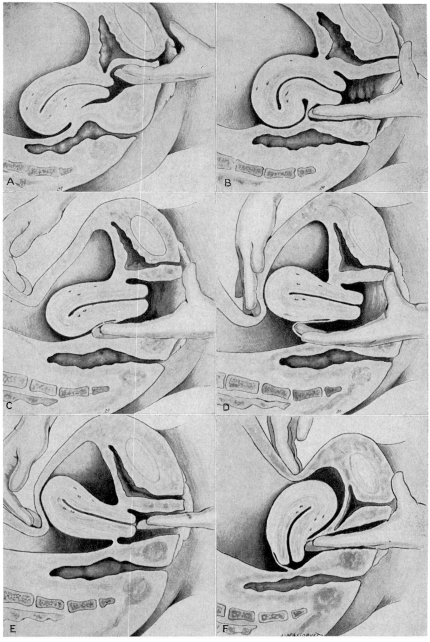

Fig. 13.13. The three degrees of retrodisplacement of the uterus and the touch signs of each. *A*, first degree, corpus out of reach of examining fingers, both above and below; *B*, second degree, vaginal fingers feel posterior surface of corpus uteri extending directly back; *C*, third degree, vaginal fingers impinge on corpus uteri turned down into the posterior cul-de-sac; *D*, grasping the fundus through the abdominal wall and pushing it upward with internal finger; *E*, further replacement by pushing backward and upward on cervix; *F*, continuing this maneuver to full replacement. (From Crossen, H. S., and Crossen, R. J.: *Diseases of Women*. C. V. Mosby Company, St. Louis, 1935.)

especially *backache*. The truth is probably somewhere between these two more extreme points of view. Certainly every gynecologist, in the course of routine examinations, encounters innumerable cases of even marked retrodisplacement in which not the slightest backache nor often any other symptom has been complained of which might be linked up with the displacement. Even when backache is a symptom, it is often due to other causes than the position of the uterus.

BACKACHE. One of the most frequent complaints found in any gynecological practice is backache, for the average woman with such a problem will immediately make the diagnosis that "her womb is out of place." Far more often, of course, the difficulties are due to musculoligamentous or osseous ailments of the back itself, and are in the realm of what most practicing gynecologists refer to as an "orthopedic backache," *i.e.*, they require orthopedic consultation.

Occasionally a probable "orthopedic backache" will coexist with minor degrees of prolapse or retroposition, and the astute clinician will obtain appropriate consultation before contemplating surgery. Unfortunately, the most adroitly performed vaginal plastic or abdominal suspension operation will not relieve backache unless uterine malposition is the cause. Minor degrees of gynecological pathology with major complaints are the hardest to evaluate, but, mindful of the old axiom, "Fools rush in . . . ," the wise clinician will not promise the moon without preoperative orthopedic advice.

The Causes of Backache, Other than Pelvic. These are legion and may merely be summarized.

(a) Postural: This may be found either in the obese woman whose body load is simply too much for her musculoligamentous skeleton, or in the "long, lean, lanky" woman who has acquired bad habits of posture. In either case it may be accentuated in middle age as muscular atony begins, and there is no doubt but that psychoneurosis may accentuate the problem. Weight loss in appropriate

cases, supportive garments, heat, rest, simple analgesics, etc. will be of considerable aid as indicated.

(b) Musculoligamentous injuries: Frequently there is a history of some vigorous form of exercise such as housecleaning, followed by low back pain, with tenderness over both sacroiliac regions, accentuated by assuming certain positions. With such history and physical findings, a trial of simple therapy as noted above seems worthwhile for a few weeks.

(c) Skeletal disease: Where symptoms are acute or are unresponsive to simple measures, orthopedic consultation should be arranged. Various congenital anomalies may be found or a history of trauma may suggest coccygodynia or a ruptured intervertebral disc. X-rays and myelography may be required to establish the existence of the latter. Arthritis, tuberculosis, spina bifida, tumors, etc., are among the other causes of backache which are all best handled by our medical or orthopedic confreres. Intravenous pyelograms as well as careful abdominal and pelvic examination should first be carried out to avoid any embarrassing omissions.

Backache Due to Pelvic Cause. Retrodisplacement may be associated with backache, especially when there is a marked retroflexion producing a boggy, edematous fundus. Frequently there is some degree of concomitant prolapse, and in either case the backache may be accentuated around the menses or when the patient has been on her feet a great deal. The mechanics of the forces of gravity tend to further aggravate the anatomical deformity, and we prefer this explanation to the so-called generalized "pelvic congestion" phenomenon. Endometriosis and pelvic inflammatory disease frequently are associated with a backache, in part as a result of a fixed retroversion, but in part because of turgor of the adherent pelvic structures. Large posterior tumors may be painful by virtue of pressure or impingement on the sacral plexus.

A very ominous type of backache may occur with certain pelvic malignancy,

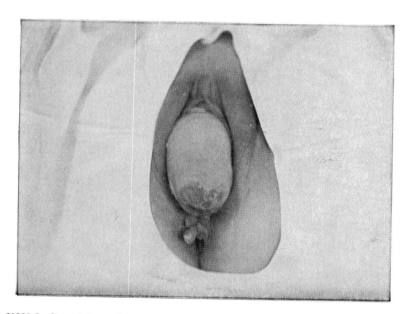

PLATE XIII.I. Complete prolapse of uterus with large cystocele. Note the superficial ulceration of the cervix, and also the rather large hemorrhoidal tags.

especially *carcinoma of the cervix*. It is not unlike the type of backache associated with a herniated disc, but in the cancer patient, treated or otherwise, it is generally the harbinger of involvement of the iliac nodes. Enlargement of these may ensue, even before obvious lymphedema, with irritation of the sciatic nerve trunks and severe pain radiating down the back of the leg. In the patient treated for carcinoma of the cervix this is often the first sign of recurrence before nodes are palpable. Pyelograms and x-rays of the spine should be obtained, but even if these appear normal, the gynecologist will keep his fingers crossed when this typically suggestive symptom appears. Unfortunately, he is not yet justified in making a diagnosis of recurrent malignancy; when he is able, the patient has generally passed beyond the stage of operability. In no other gynecological problem is the matter of clinical judgment so necessary, and this vital problem is discussed in Chapter 12, "Carcinoma of the Cervix."

Our own experience has been that the simple congenital retrodisplacement has little or no tendency to cause backache. In the acquired type, however, in which the uterus is often heavy, subinvoluted, and edematous, premenstrual backache is often produced and may occasionally be relieved by suspension of the uterus after trial by pessary.

Menstrual disorders may or may not be present. A prolonged flow with protracted, tarry staining of odoriferous nature is often noticed and seems quite in keeping with a retroflexion that opposes the forces of gravity. Should the cervix be pointing toward the symphysis, it is obvious that *infertility* might be incurred.

If pregnancy occurs in a retrodisplaced uterus, there seems to be general agreement that the hazard of miscarriage is slightly increased. This is not the usual occurrence, because even a markedly retroflexed pregnant uterus will ordinarily, before the end of the third month, lift itself above the pelvic brim into the abdomen. In some cases of marked retroflexion, especially if the uterus is adherent, the enlarging uterus is crowded more and more into the hollow of the sacrum, where it is incarcerated, with miscarriage as the usual result. It will be seen, therefore, that the management of retroflexion combined with pregnancy calls for special supervision and for occasional use of a pessary through the first trimester.

After the menopause, women with uncorrected retrodisplacements ordinarily experience marked mitigation in symptoms, as a result of the lessened congestion, the abolition of menstruation and the general shrinkage of the organs.

The effect of pregnancy upon retrodisplacements is variable. In the milder forms, especially of retroversion, the uterus, after the termination of pregnancy, may resume its normal position. Where the displacement is marked, and especially where there is a pronounced retroflexion, the displacement will usually persist or may be aggravated after the termination of gestation.

Diagnosis. The symptoms are of little value in diagnosis. Certainly the mere existence of backache is anything but characteristic, contrary to the lay view. Careful elimination of postural, spinal, and other causes is essential before one is justified in attributing backache to a retrodisplacement, as noted previously.

Pelvic examination is necessary for diagnosis, and this is usually easy. The cardinal points are as follows.

(1) The cervix usually points toward the symphysis, instead of downward and toward the sacrum.

(2) The fundus cannot be felt anteriorly, where it should be placed, but it can be palpated posteriorly. When bimanual examination is difficult because of obesity or extreme abdominal rigidity, the diagnosis is often possible from internal palpation alone. By the usual methods of bimanual palpation, one not only determines the position of the uterus, but also its size and its degree of movability. A part of such an examination is to determine the presence of complicating pelvic pathology, such as adnexitis or tumors.

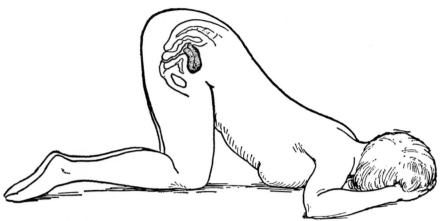

FIG. 13.14. Knee-chest posture showing the pelvic structures in outline and the tendency of the uterus to gravitate forward. (From Crossen, H. S., and Crossen, R. J.: *Disease of Women.* C. V. Mosby Company, St. Louis, 1935.)

In virgins the examination must be made *per* rectum, and even in married women vaginorectal examination may yield worthwhile information. Occasionally anesthesia may be required.

Differential Diagnosis. While the diagnosis is usually easy enough, there are certain cases in which it may be exceedingly difficult, even if the conditions for palpation are satisfactory. A myoma of the posterior wall may be difficult to distinguish from a retroflexed fundus, while on the other hand, a sharply retroflexed fundus may feel like a myoma. A firm inflammatory mass densely adherent to the posterior wall may likewise simulate a retroflexed uterus. A pregnant retroflexed fundus may even be mistaken for an ovarian cyst, and various other possibilities for error may be encountered. In the occasional case where differentiation is important, it may be necessary, under strict aseptic preparations, to insert a uterine sound in order to determine the position of the uterus. It need scarcely be said that this is not to be done when there is any suspicion of pregnancy.

Treatment. POSTURAL. The use of the knee-chest position is advocated by many both in prophylaxis and in the management of cases which respond to bimanual replacement, as well as in the uncomplicated cases in which satisfactory replace-

ment and vaginal pessaries are not possible. There is some difference of opinion as to its value, but we believe it to be useful in many cases, especially postpartum. As soon as a woman assumes the knee-chest posture, and air distends the vagina, a freely movable uterus falls toward the front. As a matter of fact, this procedure will often accomplish replacement of the uterus when bimanual manipulation fails. The maintenance of the normal position is often made more certain by instructing the patient to assume the knee-chest position three or four times a day for a period of 5 minutes at a time. The indications for a *pessary* will be discussed in a subsequent portion of this chapter.

Suspension Operations. Suspension operations should never be contemplated unless a preliminary trial by pessary has been carried out. If a pessary should anatomically replace a retroposed uterus with complete relief of symptoms, it is significant. If removal of the pessary is followed by a subsequent retrodisplacement, with a return of the previously alleviated symptoms, this might suggest that the patient is a suitable candidate for suspension. Failure to improve following *proper* application of a pessary should of course contraindicate uterine suspension, and it should be mandatory that *trial of a pessary should precede any operation for retroposition* unless, of course, the uterus is fixed posteriorly.

Although there is some difference of opinion, most gynecologists feel that an occasional suspension operation is indicated in the correction of *infertility.* As Tompkins has pointed out, this is justifiable only when the uterus cannot be maintained anteriorly by a pessary, when all the usual sterility tests have been performed and found normal, and when there has been a 2-year span of infertility after all minor defects have been corrected.

What type of operation is to be done must be determined according to the operative findings and the judgment and individual preferences of the surgeon. Some type of suspension (hysteropexy), frequently combined with plication of the uterosacral ligaments, is most often indicated in the noncomplicated cases, while in those complicated by other pelvic disease, various types of operation, sometimes including hysterectomy, may be called for.

Prolapse of the Uterus
(Descensus Uteri)

This is an extremely common condition, being far more frequent in elderly women than in young patients. This is explained by the increasing laxity and atony of the muscular and fascial structures in later life. The effects of childbirth injuries may thus make themselves evident, in the form of uterine prolapse, many years after the last pregnancy.

What has been said as to the causes of the acquired puerperal types of retrodisplacement will apply to the etiology of prolapse. As a matter of fact, many cases of the latter are preceded or accompanied by retrodisplacement of the uterus. The important factor in the mechanism of prolapse is undoubtedly injury or overstretching of the pelvic floor, and especially of the cardinal ligaments (ligaments of Mackenrodt) in the bases of the broad ligaments. Combined with this there is usually extensive injury to the perineal structures, producing marked vaginal relaxation, and also frequent injury to the fascia of the anterior or posterior vaginal walls, with the production of cystocele or rectocele. Usually various combinations of these conditions are seen, although at times little or no cystocele or rectocele is associated with the prolapse. Occasional cases are seen, for that matter, in women who have never borne children, and in these the prolapse apparently represents a hernia of the uterus through a defect in the pelvic fascial floor. When the cervix of the prolapsed uterus, usually pointing in the axis of the vagina because of the associated retrodisplacement, is well within the vaginal orifice, the prolapse is spoken of as of the *first degree.* In prolapse of the *second degree,* the cervix is at or near the introitus. Finally, when the cervix protrudes well beyond the vaginal orifice, the prolapse is of *third degree* (*procidentia uteri*). Complete prolapse of the posthysterectomy (abdominal or vaginal) vagina may occur and is often difficult to repair if a functioning vagina is desired.

Pathology. Aside from the prolapse of the uterus, and the frequently associated cystocele or rectocele, there are other possible pathological sequelae of this condition. Ulceration (decubitus ulcer) of the cervix not infrequently occurs, as a result of friction against the patient's thighs or the rubbing against clothing or the protective napkins which many of these patients wear. *Hypertrophy* of the cervix is another common concomitant, this portion of the uterus being often enormously elongated, even in the nulliparous woman, and this would seem to represent merely a congenital malformation.

When the relaxation is marked, there may be complete inversion of the vagina, the canal being literally turned inside out. The drying effect of the air produces a skinlike thickening of the vaginal mucosa, but ulceration and bleeding may occur. In addition, marked degrees of prolapse and cystocele may lead to angulation of the ureter at the urethrovesical junction,

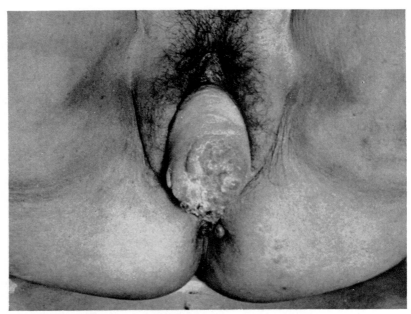

FIG. 13.15. Epidermoid carcinoma developing in cervix of completely prolapsed uterus. (Courtesy of Dr. Narcisco Diaz-Bazan, San Salvador.)

with significant degrees of upper tract dilatation.

Cervical Cancer with Prolapse

This combination is considered very rare so that relatively few cases are encountered in gynecological literature. Diaz-Bazan reports an astounding number of cases from El Salvador, which amount to almost 20% of all cases in the world literature, and since he has been good enough to send us pictures and microscopic sections, we can testify to the accuracy of his findings.

El Salvador certainly has relatively low standards of living, but they do not differ from other Central American countries where combined procidentia and cervical cancer are rare. Other factors must operate, and we would agree with Diaz-Bazan that the high incidence in El Salvador deserves investigation.

Symptoms of Prolapse

As with other forms of uterine displacement, there are marked individual differences in the symptomatology. Even the most complete prolapse may be associated with no symptoms except the discomfort produced by the mechanical protrusion of the uterus. In most cases, however, there is likely to be some degree of bearing down and heaviness in the lower abdomen and some backache, both of these being probably due to traction on the uterine ligaments and the venous congestion produced by the prolapse. Cystocele and rectocele are often associated and productive of their respective symptoms.

Diagnosis. The diagnosis is usually simple, and, as a matter of fact, the usual complaint of the patient when she presents herself is that she has "falling of the womb." She is generally, but not always, correct in her surmise. While the history of difficult or instrumental labors is suggestive, it is of no great value in diagnosis, which must be made from pelvic examination.

Inspection will, in many cases, at once reveal the prolapse, if this is of the complete type. In such cases the cervix, even with the patient lying down, protrudes beyond the outlet, often occupying a position between a soft boggy cystocele anteriorly and a pouchlike protrusion of the rectocele posteriorly, should these

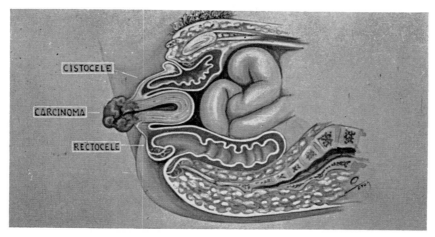

FIG. 13.16. Sagittal diagram of condition illustrated in Figure 13.15

coexist. Frequently, however, a markedly hypertrophic cervix may protrude without significant uterine prolapse.

Even in cases of complete prolapse, however, the protrusion usually recedes when the patient lies down, while in first or second degree prolapse no external protrusion exists. In such cases the patient is asked to strain, this bringing the cervix far down into the vagina and perhaps beyond the introitus. The same straining effort will ordinarily reveal the cystocele and rectocele, should they be present. In the complete variety, if straining does not restore the protrusion, gentle traction on the cervix with a light tenaculum will usually do so. Or, the patient is made to stand and strain, when the prolapsed uterus ordinarily promptly reappears.

The palpatory signs of first degree prolapse are like those of retrodisplacement except for the low position of the cervix. Occasionally, however, even a uterus in anterior position may prolapse.

Differential Diagnosis. The chief source of possible error is to mistake for prolapse the *simple hypertrophy of the cervix* which is seen at times, even with little or no vaginal relaxation. The cervix may become so elongated as to present at or beyond the introitus. Careful examination, however, will show that the cervical elongation is all below the cervicovaginal junction, and that the latter

is still high up in the vaginal canal. Cystocele and retocele are usually not present. Gainey has pointed out that remarkable degrees of *vaginal prolapse* or *inversion* may exist with only minor degrees of cystocele, rectocele, or uterine prolapse.

A large *cystocele or rectocele* is often mistaken by the patient for prolapse of the uterus, and the physician himself may make the same error if his examination is too superficial. Such a cystocele or rectocele may occur with no uterine prolapse whatsoever, and this can easily be determined by the examining finger, which reveals the cervix high in the vaginal vault. Finally, the larger cervical or uterine polyps, either glandular or myomatous, may develop long pedicles and present at the orifice of the vagina, and thus simulate a prolapsed cervix. Simple vaginal palpation is all that is necessary to make the differentiation.

Treatment. There are a number of factors which must necessarily influence the management of this condition. Chief among these are the patient's age, marital status, and general health, on the one hand, and on the other, the degree of the prolapse and the presence or absence of any associated pathologic conditions.

SURGICAL. This is best deferred until the family has been completed, for further pregnancy, even over an adequately repaired pelvic floor, will often undo the best surgical results. Although many operations have been devised for the correction of prolapse, 99% of such cases are satisfactorily handled by any one of the following procedures (along with appropriate repairs).

(1) *Vaginal Hysterectomy* (see Chapter 5). This is suitable for all but the most massive degrees of prolapse and, if combined with adequate anterior or posterior repair, gives excellent results. It furthermore removes the usual site of later cancers, tumors, or bleeding, and is obviously sterilizing. It should be stressed that abdominal hysterectomy and suspension of the vaginal vault from above is *not* the proper operation for prolapse; removal from below with adequate building up of the weakened and attenuated structures is the only feasible surgical approach. The composite operation which preserves the uterine isthmus while removing fundus and cervix has won no wide support.

While most vaginal procedures are uncomplicated, there may be problems such as massive intraperitoneal hemorrhage or severe vaginal bleeding. When this occurs, prompt reoperation is indicated, and if resuture of the bleeding area is difficult because of the proximity of the ureter, ligation of the hypogastric arteries is an alternate solution.

(2) *Manchester Operation.* Although this is the usual English manner of surgically correcting any degree of prolapse, American gynecologists seem to utilize this procedure primarily for the lesser degrees of prolapse, especially in association with a large cystocele. Curet-

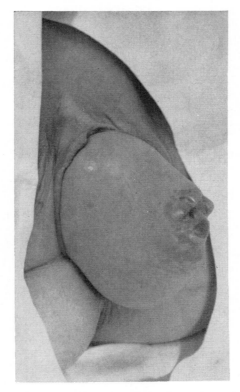

FIG. 13.17. Complete inversion of vagina with cystocele, rectocele, and entrerocele (lateral view). (Note ulceration of cervix.)

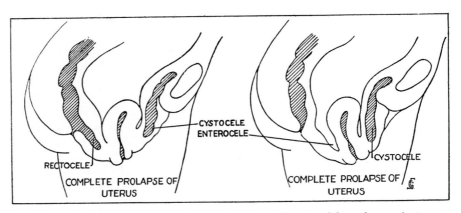

FIG. 13.18. Sagittal section to show anatomical relations with prolapse of uterus

tage to exclude malignancy should precede the operation, and it should rarely be done in the childbearing era, for cervical amputation (although not included in the original Manchester procedure) seems an integral part of the operation. A modified Watkins procedure affords excellent results where hysterectomy is not feasible or desired. Pregnancy after either of these procedures is apt to be complicated and to mandate cesarean section.

(3) *Colpocleisis (Le Fort Operation)*. Occasional cases of massive procidentia, often failures by other procedures, require closing the vagina. Obviously this operation is performed only in the elderly spinster or widow, although various modifications allow partial vaginal function. Colpocleisis is generally easily and quickly performed and may of course be preceded by vaginal hysterectomy. This type of surgery should be a last resort, but is almost infallible if properly performed.

NONSURGICAL. There are a few elderly women who are poor operative risks and have a limited life span, and these represent the main indication for pessary treatment. With modern anesthesia (local, block, and low spinal), such easily performed procedures as the Le Fort operation are usually preferred; but there is a small number of cases in which operation is not feasible or desirable. Pessaries are utilized for such women, but these have certain definite unpleasant aspects, as will be discussed.

The Vaginal Pessary

Because of the safety of modern-day surgery, various vaginal plastic and other reparative procedures are performed with relative impunity. At the same time it should be recalled that the old fashioned pessary still plays a role in the treatment of current gynecological procedures. It is no panacea, for it frequently leads to leukorrhea despite daily douches, and frequent removal and cleansing are necessary. An improperly fitted, too large pessary may induce urinary retention,

whereas a pessary that is too small may slip out. Lastly, there are a few women who, because of individual structural deviations, just cannot be satisfactorily fitted with any of the standard types of pessary. Nevertheless the pessary has very definite uses and should not be discarded from our gynecological armamentarium, although long-term usage of pessaries is usually undesirable.

Indications. The two main indications for employment of a pessary are *prolapse* and *retrodisplacement*, in certain cases only and under certain conditions.

PROLAPSE. It is impossible to set any arbitrary age beyond which appropriate surgical correction should not be accomplished. The actual birth date is no criterion of physical age, and we see many 70-year-old "youngsters" whose activity and physical condition belie their true age, just as we have a number of decrepit 50-year-old women, aged before their time. Obviously medical contraindications to surgery must be considered, but in this era there is only a rare woman who cannot tolerate some form of vaginal operation, which may be performed under a variety of specialized anesthesias.

For the patient who is not a candidate for surgery, a *ring pessary* is probably most suitable, for it tends to take up slack in the vagina as well as form a kind of cradle under the cervix. Hard rubber or plastic are less malleable but preferable to the soft rubber, "doughnut" type of pessary, which becomes foul rapidly and leads to leukorrhea, ulceration, and bleeding. As to the size of the pessary, individualization is necessary, for it must be large enough to stay in and small enough to allow for removal and cleansing. Trial and error are sometimes necessary, but it must be remembered that too tight a pessary can cause severe ulceration.

RETRODISPLACEMENT. Asymptomatic retropositions require no treatment, but when a patient with either a congenital or postpartum backward displacement of the uterus complains of cramps, rectal or back pressure, or prolonged dribbling menstruation, a pessary deserves con-

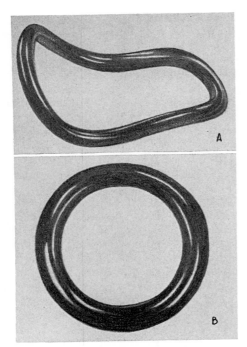

FIG. 13.19. Types of pessary for ordinary use. *A*, the Albert Smith pessary especially valuable in the treatment of retrodisplacements; the Hodge instrument is a modification of this, having a concave posterior arm and a somewhat broader anterior arm. *B*, the ordinary ring pessary of hard rubber employed especially in cases of prolapse.

sideration. It is important to emphasize that the uterus must first be manually restored to its normal anterior position, for a pessary, merely shoved in, accomplishes nothing. Sometimes the uterus, even when it is free, is boggy and tender, so that light anesthesia is necessary for proper application of the pessary.

As a general rule the *Smith-Hodge* or *Findley folding pessary* (in which a small segment at each end is of soft rubber for easier insertion) is preferable. After the fundus is pushed upward by combined pressure in the posterior fornix, along with downward and backward pressure on the cervix, the pessary is applied (Fig. 13.20). The pessary should fit snugly with its front end up under the pubic arch; but if this is too snug retention of urine may follow because of suburethral

pressure. The back end encompasses the cervix, and fits snugly against the posterior fornix and uterosacral ligaments, and it is probably the latter leverage that maintains the replaced uterus in its normal position. A hard rubber pessary, if immersed in hot water, can be easily molded to fit the specific anatomy of the individual patient.

Contraindications and Complications of Pessaries. (1) A fixed retroposition such as may occur with inflammatory disease or endometriosis is a contraindication, for if the uterus cannot be mobilized anteriorly, a pessary will be worthless. A trial under anesthesia will often bring anterior what has seemed to be a fixed uterus, merely due to relief from discomfort and spasm.

(2) Marked outlet relaxation with cystocele and rectocele frequently finds the tissues so atonic and flabby that a pessary does no good. Although prolapse and retrodisplacement frequently coexist, they are still amenable to pessary treatment, but an appropriate pessary may not be easy to find except by much "trial and error."

(3) Severe vaginitis or cervical infection militate against usage of a pessary. Actually, despite daily douches and occasional (every 6 to 8 weeks) removal of the instrument for cleansing, long continued wearing of a pessary is invariably followed by some irritative trauma to the vaginal epithelium, especially where there is a pasty-thin postmenopausal vagina. Actually the neglected pessary may become encrusted and literally burrow its way into the submucosal tissues; indeed, in past generations frequent use of a special instrument (the "pessariotome") was necessary to cut the pessary out. This complication is rare but by no means unheard of in this enlightened generation of patients and gynecologists.

(4) A recent publication by a British colleague is actually entitled "The Dangerous Vaginal Pessary." He refers to 13 patients, all of whom had been noted to have serious pelvic complications following prolonged usage of a pessary.

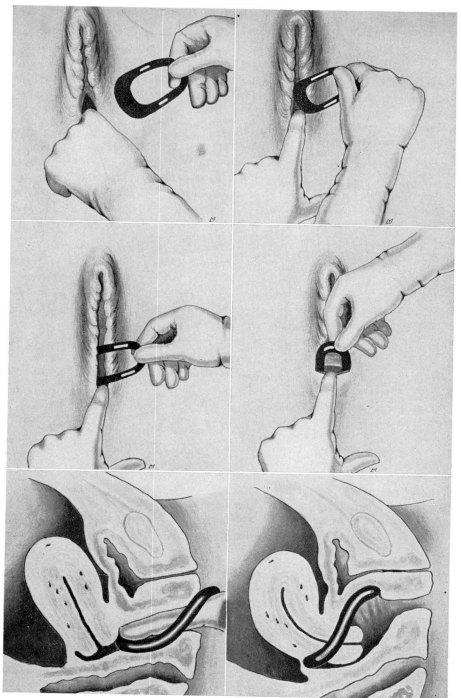

FIG. 13.20. Diagram showing the successive steps in the introduction of a pessary. (From Davis, C. H. (Editor): *Gynecology and Obstetrics*. W. F. Prior Company, Inc., Hagerstown, Md., 1933.)

Primary cancer, severe infections, fistulas, etc., are recorded. Indeed, of 8 cases of primary vaginal cancer, 6 women had worn a pessary for many years. Admittedly this is not a valid reason for discontinuance of the application of a pessary; the gynecologist should be wary of undue prolonged irritation, and consider biopsy where there is suspicion.

Practical Use of Pessaries. The rational clinician will use pessaries infrequently, but they are of extreme service in the following groups of cases.

(1) In the occasional elderly, bad medical risk.

(2) For the immediate postpartum uterus with a boggy, retroflexed uterus. Often a pessary properly applied will permit the attenuated ligaments to "take up slack" so that after a few months the instrument may be removed, and the uterus will stay anterior. Routine use of the so-called "knee-chest" exercises are also helpful.

(3) In the habitual aborter, where the uterus falls back and can actually become incarcerated in the pelvis. If the pessary is worn until the uterus becomes large enough to rise above the pelvic brim, it can then be safely removed.

(4) As a therapeutic test to determine whether suspension operation is indicated. As noted earlier, the current gynecologist would prefer to avoid any surgery until the family has been completed, after which he is free to perform such definitive surgery as vaginal hysterectomy and repair. There are, however, the occasional young women with marked retropositions who have bitter complaints, and it should be mandatory that the first step is application of a pessary. If this is followed by relief of symptoms, which later recur after subsequent removal of the pessary and retroposition, then it would seem likely that the faulty position of the uterus is the cause of the symptoms. Patients so tested will generally profit by a suspension operation, and it is a shame that this procedure, so helpful in properly selected cases, has acquired a bad name as a result of indiscriminate usage. A pessary is not

a good long term investment in the young woman, and we prefer to use it primarily as a therapeutic test or in any case as a temporary stop-gap pending more appropriate treatment.

As we have indicated, we believe that Smith-Hodge and ring pessaries, both of which may be obtained in various sizes, are all that the average doctor needs for this type of therapy. We would emphasize that pessaries are employed only occasionally, but still have very definite indications, particularly where operation would be attended by considerable risk. As Bantock remarked in 1905, "I am not aware that there is on record a single case in which a woman has lost her life through the use, or even the abuse, of a vaginal pessary."

REFERENCES

Beecham, C. T. (Editor): Complications of gynecologic surgery. Clin. Obstet. Gynec., *5:* 501, 1962.

Blaikley, J. B.: Colpocleises for difficult vesicovaginal and rectovaginal fistulas. Amer. J. Obstet. Gynec., *91:* 589, 1964.

Brunschwig, A., and Frick, H. C.: Urinary tract fistulae after radical cancer surgery. Amer. J. Obstet. Gynec., *72:* 479, 1956.

Carter, B., Palumbo, L., Creadick, R. N., and Ross, R. A.: Vesicovaginal fistula. Amer. J. Obstet. Gynec., *63:* 479, 1952.

Collins, C. G., and Jones, F. B.: Preoperative cortisone for vaginal fistulae. Obstet. Gynec., *9:* 533, 1957.

Conger, G. T., and Keettel, W. C.: The Manchester-Fothergill operation; its place in gynecology. Amer. J. Obstet. Gynec., *76:* 634, 1958.

Counseller, V. S., and Symmonds, R. E.: Vesicourethral suspension for urinary stress incontinence. Amer. J. Obstet. Gynec., *75:* 525, 1958.

Diaz-Bazan, N.: Cervical carcinoma with procidentia in El Salvador. Obstet. Gynec., *23:* 281, 1964.

Everett, H. S., and Mattingly, R. F.: Urinary tract injuries as a result of pelvic surgery. Amer. J. Obstet. Gynec., *71:* 503, 1956.

Everett, H. S., and Mattingly, R. F.: Vesicovaginal fistula. Amer. J. Obstet. Gynec., *72:* 712, 1956.

Falk, H. C., and Bunkin, I. A.: Management of vesicovaginal fistula following abdominal total hysterectomy. Surg. Gynec. Obstet., *93:* 404, 1951.

Frank, R. T.: Study of anatomy, pathology and treatment of uterine prolapse, rectocele and cystocele. Surg. Gynec. Obstet., *24:* 42, 1917.

Gainey, H.: Personal communication.

Graben, E. A., O'Rourke, J. J., and McElrath, T.: Iatrogenic bladder damage during hysterectomy. Obstet. Gynec., *23:* 267, 1964.

Gray, L. A.: Place of vaginal hysterectomy in gynecologic surgery. Western. J. Surg., *67:* 153, 1959.

Gray, L. A.: Prolapse of uterus and vagina. Postgrad. Med., *30:* 207, 1961.

Green, T. H.: Development of a plan for the diagnosis and treatment of urinary stress incontinence. Amer. J. Obstet. Gynec., *83:* 632, 1962.

Hesselberg, E.: Cancer of the cervix associated with procidentia. South Afric. J. Obstet. Gynec., *46:* 589, 1963.

Hodgkinson, C. P., Doub, H. P., and Kelly, W. T.: Urethrocystograms: metallic bead chain technique. Clin. Obstet. Gynec., *1:* 668, 1958.

Hodgkinson, C. P., and Kelly, W. T.: Urinary stress incontinence in the female. Obstet. Gynec., *10:* 493, 1957.

Jeffcoate, J. N. A.: Posterior colpoperineorrhaphy. Amer. J. Obstet. Gynec., *77:* 490, 1959.

Kelly, H. A.: *Operative Gynecology.* Appleton-Century Crofts, Inc., New York, 1928.

Kinzel, G. E.: Enterocele: study of 265 cases. Amer. J. Obstet. Gynec., *81:* 1166, 1961.

Latzko, W.: Postoperative vesicovaginal fistulas. Amer. J. Surg., *58:* 211, 1942.

Lund, C. J. (Editor): Symposium on urinary incontinence in the female. Clin. Obstet. Gynec., *6:* 125, 1963.

Lynch, F. W.: Retroversions of uterus following delivery. Trans. Amer. Gynec. Soc., *47:* 177, 1922.

Marchetti, A. A., Marshall, V. F., and Shultis, L. D.: Simple vesicourethral suspension. Amer. J. Obstet. Gynec., *74:* 57, 1957.

McCall, M. L.: Posterior culdoplasty. Obstet. Gynec., *10:* 595, 1957.

Mengert, W. F.: Vesicovaginal fistula; principles of closure. Amer. J. Obstet. Gynec., *84:* 1213, 1962.

Miller, N. F., and George, H.: Lower urinary fistulas in women. Amer. J. Obstet. Gynec., *68:* 436, 1954.

Moir, J. C.: Vesico-vaginal fistulae. Amer. J. Obstet. Gynec., *71:* 476, 1956.

Moir, J. C.: Injuries of bladder. Amer. J. Obstet. Gynec., *82:* 124, 1961.

Phaneuf, L.: Surgical management of prolapse of uterus and vagina; a report of 730 personal operations. Surg. Gynec. Obstet., *77:* 209, 1943.

Porges, R. F.: Classification of pelvic relaxations. Surg. Gynec. Obstet., *117:* 769, 1963.

Read, C. D.: Enterocele. Amer. J. Obstet. Gynec., *62:* 743, 1941.

Reich, W. J., and Nechtow, M. J.: Ligation of internal iliac (hypogastric) arteries; life-saving procedure for uncontrollable gynecological and obstetrical hemorrhage. J. Internat. Coll. Surgeons, *36:* 157, 1961.

Ricci, J. V.: *The Cystocele in America.* Blakiston Company, Division of McGraw-Hill Book Company, Inc., New York, 1950.

Russell, J. K.: The dangerous vaginal pessary. J. Obstet. Gynaec. Brit. Comm., *69:* 405, 1962.

Shaw, W. F.: Treatment of prolapsus uteri, with special reference to Manchester operation of colporrhaphy. Amer. J. Obstet. Gynec., *26:* 667, 1933.

Siegel, P., and Mengert, W. F.: Internal iliac ligations in obstetrics and gynecology. J. A. M. A., *178:* 1059, 1961.

Symmonds, R. E., and Pratt, J. H.: Vaginal prolapse following hysterectomy. Amer. J. Obstet. Gynec., *79:* 899, 1960.

TeLinde, R. W.: *Operative Gynecology,* Ed. 3. J. B. Lippincott Company, Philadelphia, 1962.

Tompkins, P.: In defense of suspension of the uterus in treatment of infertility. Fertil. Steril., *7:* 317, 1956.

Tyrone, C. H.: Procidentia of uterus. Ann. Surg., *145:* 963, 1957.

Uhlenhuth, S., and Nolley, G. W.: Vaginal fascia, a myth. Obstet. Gynec., *10:* 349, 1957.

Ullery, J. C.: *Stress Incontinence in the Female.* Grune & Stratton, Inc., New York, 1953.

Ward, G. G.: Pelvic floor injuries, rectocele and enterocele. In *Obstetrics and Gynecology,* edited by A. H. Curtis. W. B. Saunders Company, Philadelphia, 1933.

Wharton, L. R., Jr., and TeLinde, R. W.: An evaluation of fascial sling operation for urinary incontinence in female patients. J. Urol., *82:* 76, 1959.

14

HYPERPLASIA OF THE ENDOMETRIUM AND ENDOMETRIAL POLYPS

HYPERPLASIA

The condition designated as hyperplasia of the endometrium was, at one time, rather distinctively linked up with the syndrome of functional uterine bleeding, but we now know that this association is frequent but far from invariable. Actually, (dys)functional bleeding is purely a clinical term, and endometrial hyperplasia a pathological classification. Although the latter represents the chief cause of functional bleeding, this may occur from any type of endometrium.

Histological Pattern. The histological pattern of hyperplasia is produced by *persistent estrogen stimulation in the absence of progesterone*, as has been shown by its experimental production in such animals as the monkey or hamster (Figs. 14.1 and 14.2). This implies that it is associated with the anovulatory type of cycle. The follicle not only fails to rupture, but continues to grow and to function beyond the usual ovulation period, so that an abnormal growth effect is produced upon the endometrium. In other cases a group of follicles continues to mature to various levels and to produce estrogen, with a pronounced growth effect.

The *characteristic changes in the ovary*, therefore, are an absence of functioning corpora lutea, and the presence of either a single, large, persistent, functioning follicle or a considerable group of smaller, functionally active follicles. In the latter case, the ovaries may be grossly cystic, but the small cysts are lined with an intact granulosa. There is a thick cortex with infrequent corpora lutea, and, indeed, there is a close resemblance to the so-called Stein-Leventhal ovary. Where a single large follicle appears to dominate the picture, it may present clinically as a follicle cyst of considerable size, although here again there is a well preserved granulosa-theca zone and an active estrogenic function.

The factor which checks the growth and continued function of the follicles is believed to be an inhibition of the anterior pituitary gonadotropins by increased amounts of estrogen (the "feedback" mechanism), resulting in withdrawal of the stimulus to follicle growth, rapid regression, withdrawal of estrogen, and thereby a bleeding phase. This is in conformity with what has been said in previous chapters as to the importance of hormone withdrawal in the causation of uterine bleeding.

Microscopic Appearance of Hyperplasia. This, in the frank case, is extremely distinctive. The most characteristic feature

282

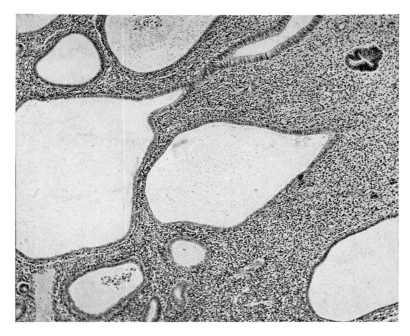

Fig. 14.1. Typical Swiss-cheese pattern of hyperplasia of endometrium

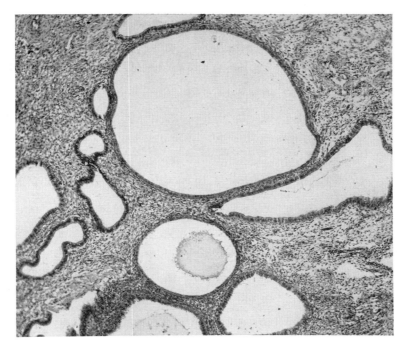

Fig. 14.2. Another example of hyperplasia with characteristic Swiss-cheese pattern

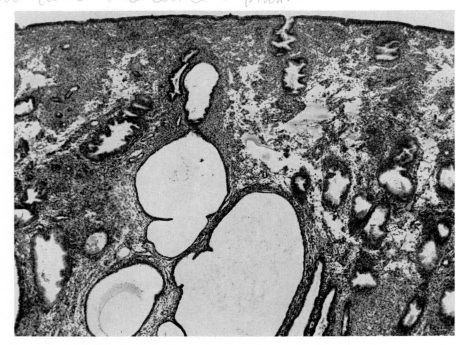

FIG. 14.3. "Focal hyperplasia" in center flanked by typical progestation endometrium

is the gland pattern, which is commonly spoken of as the *Swiss-cheese type*, because of the disparity in size of the gland lumina. Some are large and cystic, while others, perhaps in the same microscopic field, are small in caliber. The epithelium is cuboidal or cylindrical, with heavily stained nuclei, and in the small glands it may even show some stratification. The stroma is abundant and compact. Mitoses are numerous in the epithelium, and not infrequent in the stroma. The epithelium shows an *absence of the secretory activity* produced by progesterone, since the secretion of the latter is in abeyance.

Focal Hyperplasia. Occasionally patches of hyperplastic endometrium may be found in conjunction with a general secretory reaction. It must be borne in mind that the basalis endometrium is not responsive to the biphasic hormonal stimulus. Where an intact endometrium is available for study as in a hysterectomy specimen, one must conclude that there are occasionally patches of superficial tissue of the immature basal type that have not acquired the capacity of response to progesterone (Fig. 14.3).

Gross Appearance of the Endometrium. This is variable; in some cases it may be enormously thickened and polypoid, so that the large amounts removed by curettage may lead the surgeon to assume the likelihood of cancer. In such cases, the polypoid overgrowth presents a sharp line of demarcation at the internal os from the cervical mucosa, which lacks the great responsiveness of the endometrium to the estrogenic hormone. It is this condition of *polypoid* hyperplasia (Fig. 14.5) which formerly was wrongly spoken of as polypoid endometritis. In other cases, and with the same microscopic pattern, the endometrium is of normal thickness, or it may even be thinner than normal.

Proliferative Varieties of Hyperplasia. In a great majority of cases the microscopic pattern of hyperplasia is a frankly benign one. In a small proportion, however, markedly proliferative and adenomatous pictures are produced,

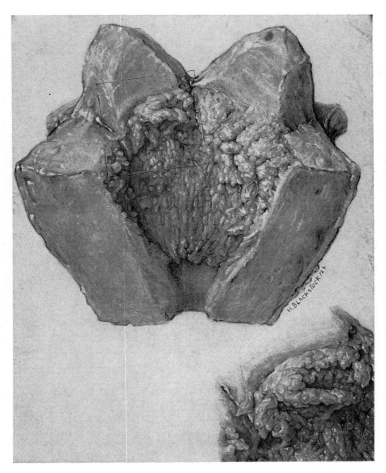

Fig. 14.4. Gross appearance of benign polypoid hyperplasia of endometrium. Note the physiological line of demarcation at the internal os.

sometimes diffusely involving the whole endometrium but more often in certain focal area, and these have often been mistaken for cancer. The percentage of these doubtful cases, however, is very small. When there is serious doubt, the safe plan is that expressed in the dictum of Halban, "Nich Karzinom, aber besser heraus!" (Not carcinoma, but better out!) In the milder degrees of proliferative overactivity, however, there is rarely any difficulty in excluding malignancy, and conservative treatment is indicated. A study of the atypical proliferative varieties of hyperplasia has been made by Novak and Rutledge, to whose paper the interested reader may be referred. The

differential diagnosis and relationship of atypical hyperplasia and endometrial adenocarcinoma is discussed in Chapter 15, with consideration of estrogen as a causative agent.

Differentiation of Progestational and Hyperplastic Endometrium. McKay *et al.* have carried out extensive studies on endometrial histochemistry in normal, atrophic, hyperplastic (cystic and adenomatous), and malignant tissues. Ribonucleoprotein, acid and alkaline phosphatase, and glycogen content were studied by appropriate stains. For details, the reader is referred to their publications, but in essence this work suggested that the earlier stages of endometrial cancer

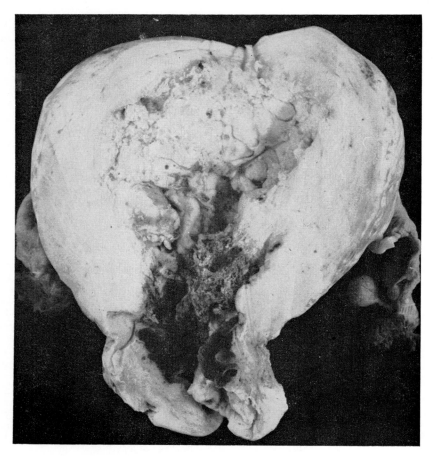

Fig. 14.5. Marked polypoid hyperplasia (histologically benign) following prolonged estrogen therapy. (Courtesy of Dr. Derek Tacchio, New Castle, England.)

showed a progestational pattern. This would, of course, help to explain certain secretory changes that seem to occur in low grade adenocarcinoma, but is difficult to reconcile with the frequent postmenopausal status of the patient. It is likewise difficult to reconcile with the presumed estrogen role in certain hyperplasias and possibly adenocarcinoma unless we assume an altered metabolic background, "a long continued estrogen plus progesterone stimulation." The possibility of convertability of the steroids at either the site of production or the end organ is currently under wide discussion.

Whatever the mechanism, it may on occasion be extremely difficult to distinguish between certain progestational endometria and various forms of proliferative hyperplasia. Both exhibit abundant evidence of secretory activity, considerable infolding and intraluminal tufting by tall pale-staining cells, and considerable proliferation of the glands. Both may justifiably be called a secretory endometrium, but this does not necessarily imply that ovulation has occurred (Fig. 14.8).

The report of a "secretory" endometrium in a woman over 50 years of age, especially if there is abnormal bleeding, should suggest the patient may be anovulatory (although this is not absolute). If a well developed decidual-like stroma is present, there is considerable support for recent ovulation and pro-

Iperplasia dell'endometrio e polipi –

L'iperplasia si associa spesso (insieme) all'emorragia
disfunzionale anovulatoria –.
Causa: ~~eccesso~~ stimolazione estrogenica
prolungata, non bilanciata da
progesterone –

An. Pat.: (ovaio) Nessuna così luteri funzionanti
(ecco perché manca il progesterone) con
una o più cisti follicolinica (somiglianza
con SF (eventuale) – L'ipercumulo d'estrogeni
blocca l'ipofisi, le cisti cessano di crescere,
diminuisce gli estrogeni, quindi prid'tr'
eurotica –
endometrio) : epitelio cuboidale (come nel
luteale) con nuclei ipocolorati; ghiandole dilatate
a fessure bifisseno, senza segni di secrezione
ghiandolare (manca il progesterone !)–
Talvolta l'iperplasia è focale: questo succede sul
l'endometrio basale, quella cioè che poggia nella
muscolatura che non risponde al progesterone –
talvolta si aniste ad una iperplasia dell'endometrio

fenomeni secretori e iperplastici (cioè
che ghiandole oltre che dilatarsi si moltiplicano
nel numero). — Queste forme d'iperplasia sono
atipiche e difficili da distinguere dal carcinoma. Per l'anno secretorio si pensa che il progesterone
si formi fa una trasformazione degli stromi o
arrestando l'ovulazione —
Gli stromi nella fot - menopausa si formerebbero
dalle Enzimatically Active Stromal Cells —
Terapia: la perdita ematica da iperplasia
endometriale (di tipo cioè anovulatorio) si
cura con il raschiamento nelle giovani,
con l'isterectomia nei casi anziani o atipici.
(pag. 633)
—
Polipi endometriali : se sono tipo riproduttivo
o il tipo normale ciclo o' endometrio o quello
iperplastico, spesso frequente. Nelle giovani
non in incontri a degenerazione nel tum,
mentre è frequente nella fotmenopausa
(10 - 15%), nella quale si richiede a
raso cautelativo l'isterectomia —

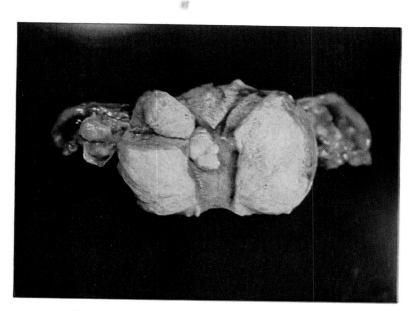

PLATE XIV.I. Endometrial polyp of moderate size

Quando si riscontra una iperplasia dell'endometrio con note di attività secretoria in una donna di 50 anni, o riconsideriamo l'ovulazione per spiegare questa influenza progestinica o la consideriamo una iperplasia atipica, dal momento che l'iperplasia tipica non si accompagna a fenomeni secretori (pag 284). L'iperpl. in fase secretiva è considerata precursore o coesistente con l'adenocarcinoma.

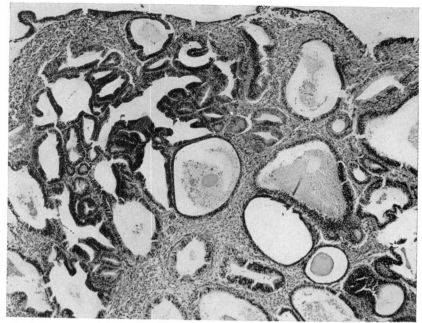

FIG. 14.6. An example of a proliferative type (*left*) with associated cystic hyperplasia

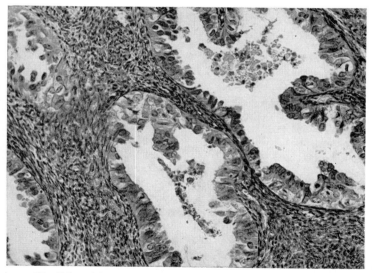

FIG. 14.7. Areas like this, with pale-staining epithelium not unlike that seen in the tube, may occasionally be seen with hyperplasia and may lead to the diagnosis of adenocarcinoma.

gesterone influence. If not, one must be concerned about an atypical hyperplasia, especially if there are associated areas of the benign-cystic ("Swiss cheese") variety. This matter of distinction is of more than academic importance, for these proliferative endometrial patterns seem to be a precursor to adenocarcinoma, or coexist in conjunction with a true malignancy.

Postmenopausal Hyperplasia. It is now well known that the urine of post-

di tipo più "secretorio" e con notevole proliferazione ghiandolare

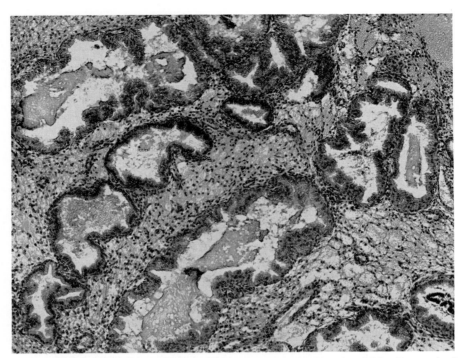

Fig. 14.8. Endometrium of a 54-year-old woman with only occasional bleeding and almost certainly not ovulating. Note obvious similarities to progestational pattern despite monophasic temperature chart.

menopausal women, even of those many years beyond the menopause, may, at times, show the presence of estrogenic hormone. The source of this is not known, although there is some support of the adrenal cortex as a probable source of the hormone. Unpublished studies of our own utilizing histochemical techniques would suggest frequent steroidal function of hilus cells (both estrogenic and androgenic) as well as by ovarian stromal cells.

There is some evidence, however, that hyperplastic ovarian stromal cells not only look like, but act like, theca cells in an ability to secrete estrogen, even in the postmenopausal era. Scully has recently commented on certain ovarian stromal cells which are enzymatically active (EASC) and a presumed source of steroidogenesis in ovaries of all ages. However, Bulbrook and Greenwood have found estrogen in the urine of women with breast cancer who have had oophorectomy, adrenalectomy, and hypophysec-

tomy. What source this might evolve from is speculative, but estrogen intake in the diet must be suspect with possible conversion from cholesterol and similar substances. Indeed it was years after this hypothesis that cholesterol was first noted as an intermediate biosynthetic product in androgen or estrogen formation. It is not surprising, therefore, that hyperplasia, formerly looked upon as exclusively a lesion of reproductive life, may at times be found in women far beyond the menopause, and that it may occasionally cause postmenopausal bleeding.

Novak and Yui have found postmenopausal hyperplasia not infrequently in association with adenocarcinoma. There is suggestive evidence that in the menopausal and postmenopausal woman, hyperplasia, especially proliferative, may progress to adenocarcinoma. The hyperplasia of reproductive life, on the other hand, appears to have no relation to the

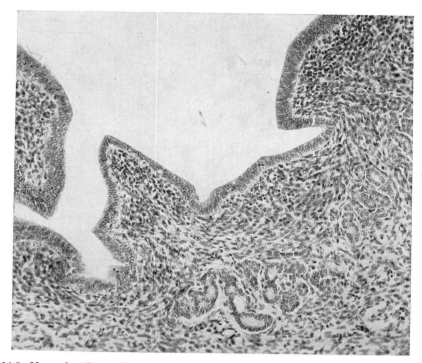

FIG. 14.9. Normal endometrium of hamster before estrogen administration. (Courtesy of Dr. R. A. Bacon, Department of Anatomy, Johns Hopkins Medical School, Baltimore, Maryland.)

development of cancer. A study of post-menopausal endometria by Novak and Richardson revealed the frequent occurrence of active and even hyperplastic endometria in women at times many years after the menopause.

No present day discussion of this topic would be complete without calling attention to the fact that hyperplasia of the endometrium, sometimes of atypical variety, is often the result of *excessive and prolonged administration of estrogens* in the treatment of menopausal symptoms (see Chapter 15).

Management of Hyperplasia. Endometrial hyperplasia in the menstrual era is usually an innocuous and self-limited process, and this is fully discussed in the chapter on functional bleeding. Where hyperplasia is constantly recurrent in the aging endometrium, in general or in a polyp, it is somewhat more ominous in respect to the later development of fundal adenocarcinoma, especially if the

woman concerned is in the menopausal age bracket. Indeed we are convinced that recurrent hyperplasia, especially if it is *increasingly* atypical or proliferative does not warrant conservatism because of the higher incidence of subsequent endometrial cancer. The continued pattern of a sustained stimulus (probably estrogen) suggests that hysterectomy is a well warranted prophylaxis against the advent of carcinoma of the endometrium. Nevertheless we refrain from such terms as adenocarcinoma Stage O or in situ since there are no set histological criteria and since certain markedly adenomatous lesions occasionally regress spontaneously or can be made to regress with progesterone (see following chapter).

Cause of Bleeding in Hyperplasia. The hormonal factors in the bleeding, as already discussed, are brought about by the reciprocal interplay of the pituitary and ovaries. As for local factors, Schröder believes that these consist of small

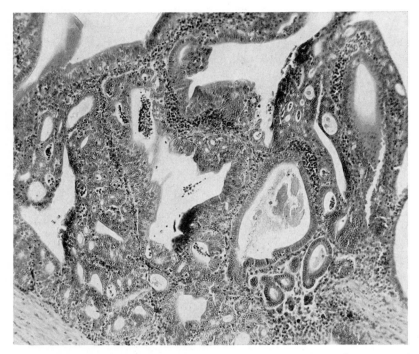

Fig. 14.10. Endometrium of hamster after long course of estrogen. (Courtesy of Dr. R. A. Bacon, Department of Anatomy, Johns Hopkins Medical School, Baltimore, Maryland.)

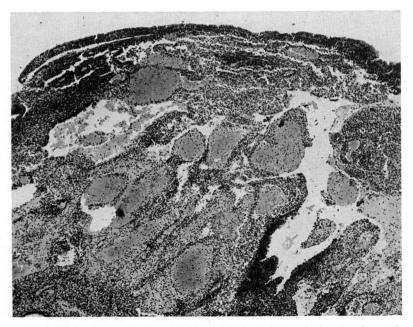

Fig. 14.11. Thromboses in an area of necrobiosis in hyperplasia of endometrium

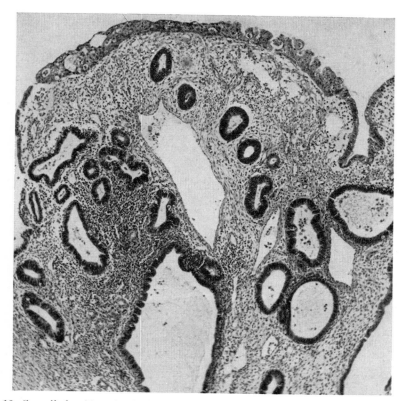

FIG. 14.12. So-called epidermization or squamous metaplasia, a benign process, seen either on the surface or in the glands in the occasional case of hyperplasia.

localized areas of necrobiosis, from which the blood has its source. Others, while conceding the presence of such small areas of necrosis, do not believe that these are sufficient to explain the frequently profuse hemorrhage, and are inclined to attribute the chief role to changes in the blood vessels, with increased permeability of their walls. Sippe describes various sinus-like vascular channels with a rather superficial position that may be the source of profuse bleeding.

Clinical Characteristics and Treatment. These are fully discussed in Chapter 32, "Functional Bleeding."

ENDOMETRIAL POLYPS

The term polyp is a clinical one, referring to tumors attached by a stem or pedicle. Thus a polypoid tumor within the uterus may be a myoma, carcinoma, or sarcoma, or it might be made up of retained placental tissue (placental polyp). The common *endometrial polyp* is one made up of endometrial tissue. Such polyps may be single or multiple, small, or large enough to fill the uterine cavity. The pedicle may become so long that the growth projects beyond the cervix, and, in rare cases, beyond the vaginal introitus.

Microscopic Structure. The microscopic structure of these polyps is like that of the endometrium from which they spring, with some qualification on the basis of the functional or nonfunctional type of the constituent epithelium. In some polyps the endometrial tissue shows a functional cyclical response paralleling that of the general uterine mucosa. When the latter exhibits a progestational picture, for example, so does the endometrium of the polyp. In a far larger proportion of cases, however, the polyp is made up of an immature or unripe

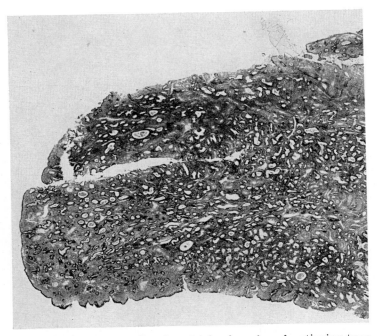

FIG. 14.13. Typical small endometrial polyp of nonfunctioning type

type of endometrium like that seen in the basalis, and not responsive to progesterone. Such polyps, therefore, show a proliferative picture, with often a typical Swiss-cheese hyperplasia pattern, at all phases of the menstrual cycle, even when the surrounding endometrium is in a progestational phase. Schröder's concept of an origin from the basalis portion of the endometrium with a surrounding mantle of more superficial and responsive tissue seems particularly rational.

Clinical Characteristics. Unless they become large enough to protrude from the cervix, or unless secondary degenerative or ulcerative changes develop, endometrial polyps are apt to be entirely symptomless. As a matter of fact a large proportion are not discovered until uteri removed for other indications are opened, while others are brought away in the course of curettage for diagnostic or other indications.

In the larger polyps or those which obtrude into the cervical or vaginal canals, *bleeding* is almost always a symptom, because of the secondary ulcerative changes which develop. As a rule it is of metrorrhagic type and moderate degree, but, in some cases, it may be quite profuse. Through interference with the blood supply in the pedicle, the larger polyps may undergo necrosis and sloughing, with the production of an offensive discharge as well as bleeding.

Premalignant Potentialities of Endometrial Polyp. It has generally been assumed that endometrial polyps have little tendency to be associated with or to evolve into fundal adenocarcinoma, and there seems little doubt that this view is correct as regards women during menstrual life. In the menopausal and postmenopausal eras, however, there would seem to be considerable question as to whether such lesions can be regarded with complete equanimity. A study by Peterson and Novak would indicate that polyps in postmenopausal women must be regarded with a certain degree of suspicion, because of associated malignancy. Although the polyp itself rarely undergoes malignant degeneration (0.5 to 1%), more recent work by Wolfe and Mackles

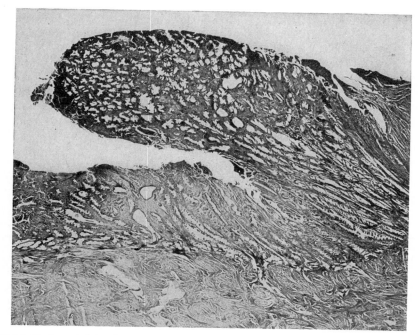

FIG. 14.14. Endometrial polyp of functioning type showing premenstrual secretory activity of glands similar to that in surrounding endometrium.

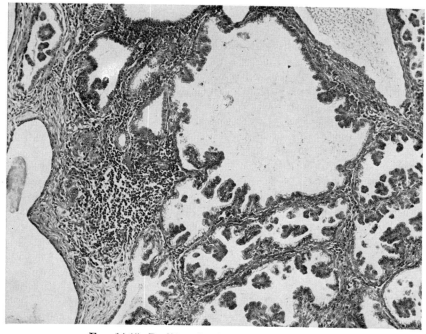

FIG. 14.15. Proliferative hyperplasia in a polyp

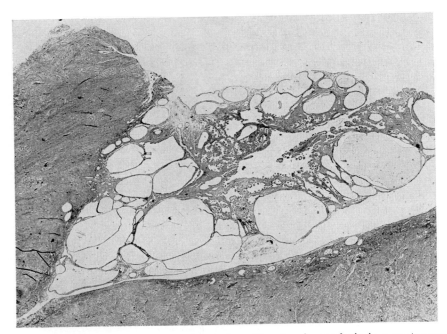

FIG. 14.16. Polyp with both retrogressive and proliferative hyperplasia in a postmenopausal patient.

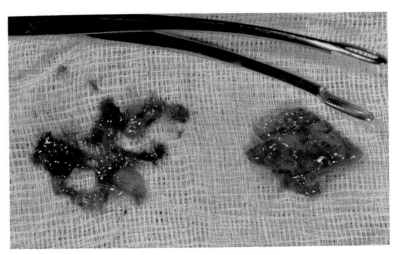

FIG. 14.17. Polyp forceps

would seem to confirm our impressions that polyps in the climacteric must be viewed with certain misgivings.

Indeed, analysis of some 1100 polyps in our clinic revealed that 10 to 15 % were *associated* with malignancy in postmenopausal women. Of particular interest were those polyps which exhibited an active hyperplasia after cessation of menstrual life. These appeared to represent a focal patchy form of hyperplasia which deserves the same consideration as a diffuse postmenopausal hyperplasia (discussed in this chapter). Adenomatous or recurrent atypical polypoid lesions should not be viewed too conservatively, for they may be associated with or be forerunners of endometrial cancer.

Treatment. The polyps which manifest themselves by protrusion through the cervical canal are readily diagnosed, although it is not always easy to be sure whether they spring from the cervix or from the endometrium. The distinction is not usually of practical importance, as the method of treatment is the same for both types. For the endometrial growths, especially those of larger size, the cervix should be dilated and the growth removed, followed by curettage, to make sure that other small polyps are not present. It is wise to follow any curettage with the introduction of a long narrow forceps to "fish around" for a possibly overlooked polyp. This may easily happen despite the most thorough uterine scraping.

REFERENCES

Bulbrook, R. D., and Greenwood, F. C.: Persistence of urinary estrogen excretion after oophorectomy and adrenalectomy. Brit. Med. J., 1: 662, 1957.

Bulbrook, R. D., and Greenwood, F. C.: Effects of hypophysectomy on urinary estrogen in breast cancer. Brit. Med. J., 1: 666, 1957.

Holmstrom, E. G.: Functional uterine bleeding. J. Iowa Med. Soc., 47: 376, 1957.

Israel, S. L., and Weber, L. L.: Postmenopausal uterine bleeding. Obstet. Gynec., 7: 286, 1956.

Kupperman, H. S., Epstein, J. A., Blatt, M. H. G., and Stone, A.: Induction of ovulation in the human; therapeutic and diagnostic significance. Amer. J. Obstet. Gynec., 75: 30, 1958.

Lambeth, S. S., and Kinter, E. P.: Endometrial hyperplasia. Obstet. Gynec., 5: 692, 1955.

Larson, J. A.: Estrogens and endometrial carcinoma. Obstet. Gynec., 3: 1, 1954.

Masters, W. H.: Sex steroid influence on the aging process. Amer. J. Obstet. Gynec., 74: 733, 1957.

McBride, J. M.: Premenopausal cystic hyperplasia and endometrial carcinoma. J. Obstet. Gynaec. Brit. Comm., 66: 288, 1959.

McKay, D. G., Hertig, A. T., Bardawil, W. A., and Velardo, J. T.: Histochemical observations on endometrium. II. Abnormal endometrium. Obstet. Gynec., 8: 140, 1956.

Meyer, R.: Über seltenere gutartige und zweifelhafte Epithelveränderungen der Uterus-schleimhaut in Vergleich mit den ihnen ähnlichen Karzinomformen. Arch. Gynaek., 115: 394, 1922.

Munnell, E. W., and Flick, F. H.: Surgical diagnosis and management of dysfunctional uterine bleeding. Surg. Gynec. Obstet., 106: 321, 1958.

Novak, E. R.: Relationship of endometrial hyperplasia and adenocarcinoma of the uterine fundus. J. A. M. A., 154: 217, 1954.

Novak, E., and Richardson, E. H., Jr.: Proliferative changes in senile endometrium. Amer. J. Obstet. Gynec., 42: 564, 1941.

Novak, E., and Rutledge, F.: Atypical proliferative hyperplasia of endometrium. Amer. J. Obstet. Gynec., 55: 46, 1948.

Novak, E., and Yui, E.: Relation of hyperplasia to adenocarcinoma of uterus. Amer. J. Obstet. Gynec., 32: 674, 1936.

Overstreet, E. W.: Clinical aspects of endometrial polyps. Surg. Clin. N. Amer., 42: 1013, 1962.

Peterson, W. F., and Novak, E. R.: Endometrial polyps. Obstet. Gynec., 8: 40, 1956.

Randall, C. L., Birtsch, P. K., and Harkins, L. L.: Ovarian function after the menopause. Amer. J. Obstet. Gynec., 74: 719, 1957.

Randall, L. M.: Management of dysfunctional uterine bleeding during adolescence. J. Louisiana Med. Soc., 110: 160, 1958.

Roddick, J. W., and Greene, R. R.: Endometrial changes and ovarian morphology. Amer. J. Obstet. Gynec., 75: 235, 1958.

Schröder, R.: Endometrial hyperplasia in relation to genital function. Amer. J. Obstet. Gynec., 68: 294, 1954.

Scott, R. B.: The elusive endometrial polyp. Obstet. Gynec., 1: 125, 1953.

Scully, R. E., and Cohen, R. B.: Oxidative-enzyme activity in normal and pathological human ovaries. Obstet. Gynec., 24: 667, 1964.

Sippe, G.: Endometrial hyperplasia and uterine bleeding. J. Obstet. Gynaec. Brit. Comm., 69: 1015, 1962.

Taylor, H. C.: Endometrial hyperplasia and carcinoma of body of uterus. Amer. J. Obstet. Gynec., 23: 309, 1932.

Turnbull, A. C.: Radium menopause or hysterectomy. J. Obstet. Gynaec. Brit. Comm., 62: 176, 1955.

Wall, J. A., and Jacobs, W. M.: Dysfunctional uterine bleeding in the premenopausal and menopausal years. Amer. J. Obstet. Gynec., 74: 985, 1957.

Waschke, G.: Beitrag zur Frage der Bezihung zwischen der Hyperplasia des Endometrium und dem Korpuskarzinom. Geburtsh. Frauenheilk., 15: 568, 1955.

Wolfe, S. A., and Mackles, A.: Malignant lesions arising from benign endometrial polyps. Obstet. Gynec., 20: 542, 1963.

15

ADENOCARCINOMA OF THE CORPUS UTERI

Adenocarcinoma of the body of the uterus is much more frequent than adenocarcinoma of the cervix, but less common than epidermoid cervical cancer. In past years it was felt that fundal adenocarcinoma was only one-fifth or one-sixth as frequent as squamous cell cancer of the cervix, but more recent observations suggest that endometrial adenocarcinoma is of almost equal incidence, particularly in communities where there is a high proportion of white private patients. As indicated earlier by Novak and Villa Santa, a hospital having a large number of colored patients will have a high ratio of cervical cancer, whereas corpus cancer increases with a restricted white clientele. Obviously, geographical, racial, and ethnic status are influential factors and deserve careful evaluation; however, the increased life expectancy of the American female probably allows more endometrial cancers to develop.

Gross Pathology. Adenocarcinoma may arise from any portion of the uterus, and may present in either of two chief forms, which, however, are not always sharply separable.

DIFFUSE FORM. In the so-called diffuse form a large portion of, or perhaps the entire, endometrial surface is diffusely involved in the growth, which appears as a polypoid or fungoid overgrowth, with much surface ulceration and necrosis. In the advanced stages the muscular wall may show extensive involvement, and the disease may penetrate even to the serosa, forming nodules on the surface. On the other hand, even extensive surface involvement may be associated with little or no demonstrable penetration of the deeper layers. In the more advanced cases the myometrial involvement causes great increase in the size of the uterus, even to several times its normal size. As a matter of fact, the *size of the uterus* has been used as the chief criterion in the usual clinical classification of the disease, although other methods of classification are currently being utilized.

CIRCUMSCRIBED FORM. The adjective circumscribed may seem to be a poor one when applied to a malignant process, but there are certain cases in which adenocarcinoma, aside from the stage of the disease, appears to be limited to a comparatively small area of the endometrium. This may be true even in the presence of extensive invasion of the musculature. As a matter of fact, in certain early forms the cancer may present as a small polypoid growth. It is in cases of this latter sort that the curette may remove all the gross disease, so that examination of the uterus, after its removal, may show no evidence of the cancerous process which had been clearly demonstrable in the microscopic examination of the curettings. A considerable group of such cases has been reported.

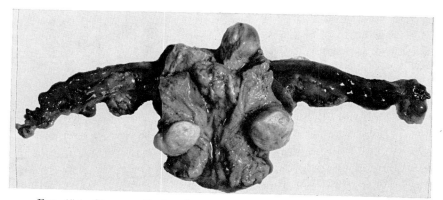

FIG. 15.1. Circumscribed endometrial cancer with coincidental myoma

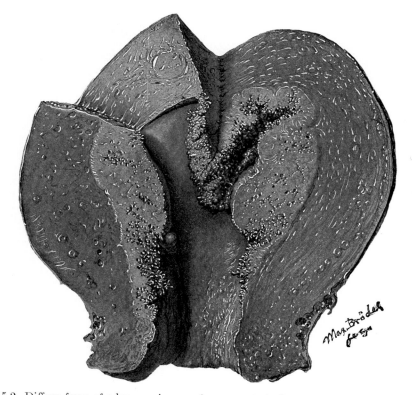

FIG. 15.2. Diffuse form of adenocarcinoma of corpus uteri. (From Cullen, T. S.: *Cancer of the Uterus*. Appleton-Century-Crofts, Inc., New York, 1900.)

Clinical Classification of Endometrial Adenocarcinoma. The most recent report by the editorial committee of the International Federation of Gynecology and Obstetrics has amended the classifications for staging endometrial cancer as follows.

Stage O. Histological findings suspicious of malignancy but not proven.

Stage I. The carcinoma is confined to the corpus.

Stage II. The carcinoma has involved the corpus and the cervix.

Stage III. The carcinoma has extended

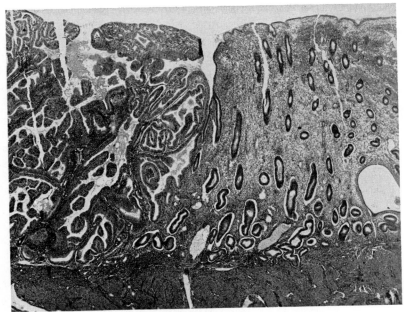

Fig. 15.3. Microscopic picture of adenocarcinoma (*left*) as contrasted with normal endometrium (*right*).

outside the uterus but not outside the true pelvis.

Stage IV. The carcinoma has extended outside the true pelvis or has obviously involved the mucosa of the bladder or rectum.

While this method of staging would appear to permit too much latitude in Stage I, its approval by such an august organization will probably lead to its general usage and abandonment of such other plans as indicated earlier by Miller Gusberg, and others. Extent of the disease is the most important single prognostic factor.

Microscopic Diagnosis. *Histological gradation* of cancer is the other factor involved in classifying adenocarcinomas. The microscopic diagnosis is made on the basis of two chief criteria, *viz.*

(1) The Pattern or Architecture. Whereas in the normal endometrium at any phase of menstrual or postmenstrual life the gland pattern is a uniform one, in adenocarcinoma there is marked departure from this orderly arrangement of the glands, which show not only a marked increase in number, but also varying de-

grees of atypicalness, with often highly intricate convolution, branching, and such cell proliferation as to obliterate the gland pattern.

(2) Individual Cell Changes. The normal endometrium shows an epithelium made up of fairly uniform cells of mature type, which during reproductive life may show marked functional activity. The nuclei are fairly uniform, and mitoses are found only in those cyclical phases characterized by rapid but normal proliferative activity, chiefly the late postmenstrual and early interval phases. In adenocarcinoma, on the other hand, the cells show varying degrees of immaturity and dedifferentiation and reveal abnormal pleomorphic nuclei; many of the latter show hyperchromatosis, normal or abnormal mitotic activity, and other evidences of anaplasia. Various degenerative changes with the production of lipoid-like and "foam" cells may be found. The epithelium is often stratified, and in some cases the lumina may be solidly full of cells. Very rarely a mesonephric adenocarcinoma may present as a primary endometrial lesion. In discussing this unusual

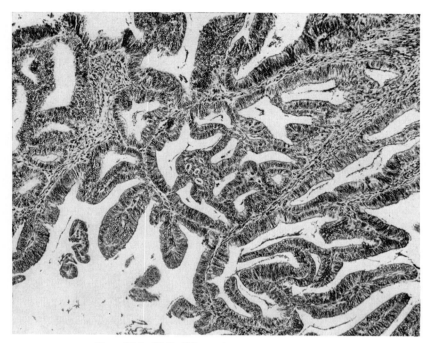

FIG. 15.4. Well differentiated adenocarcinoma

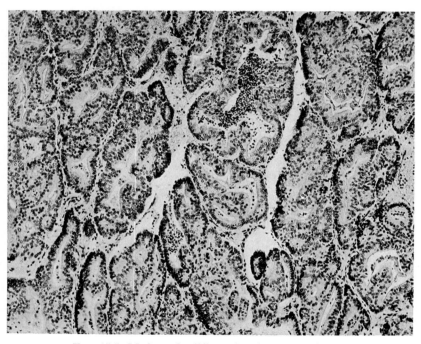

FIG. 15.5. Moderately differentiated adenocarcinoma

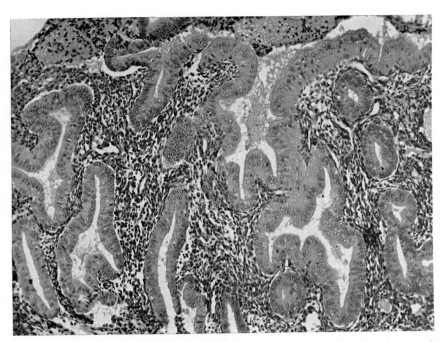

FIG. 15.6. Atypical adenomatous hyperplasia which might be mistaken for adenocarcinoma

entity Villa Santa questions whether this is due to degenerative changes of an adenocarcinoma or whether this is derived from celomic mesenchyme.

Differential Microscopic Diagnosis. While the microscopic diagnosis of adenocarcinoma is often simple enough, there is at least one endometrial lesion which may offer great difficulty in this respect. We refer to the *atypical proliferative or adenomatous varieties of hyperplasia* which have been described in a preceding chapter (Chapter 14). Where the atypical changes are of mild degree the differentiation is simple enough. When the lesion is a very adenomatous one, with marked epithelial proliferation, the simulation of low grade carcinoma is so perfect that pathologists will differ in their diagnostic interpretation.

As a matter of fact, there is a small group in which we do not believe that any pathologist can be absolutely sure. In any form of hyperplasia mitoses are present, often in large numbers, so that these are not helpful in the microscopic differentiation. In the lower grade adenocarcinomas there is likely to be little dedifferentiation

of the epithelial cells, while in either the benign or malignant lesion the epithelial layer may be stratified. Again, a large proportion of adenocarcinomas will show only minimal or no invasion of the myometrium. As a matter of fact, there is usually far more invasion of the muscle in the entirely benign adenomyosis than is seen in many adenocarcinomas.

Endometrial Adenocarcinoma "in Situ." This unfortunate term has considerable vogue in current gynecological parlance and literature, and we deplore its wide usage for all kinds of minor deviation from typical endometrial hyperplasia. Although cervical cancer in situ has certain definite standard requirements, such as full thickness replacement of the lining epithelium by abnormal, undifferentiated, basal cells, there are no such rigid criteria for a definition of adenocarcinoma in situ of the endometrium. While cognizant of what such excellent gynecological pathologists as Hertig and Brewer mean to imply by the appellation, we dislike it, for it has stimulated a too frequent improper diagnosis of "intraepithelial adenocarcinoma." Often the lesion in question is cystic glandular hyperplasia; occasionally normal secretory patterns are suspect, and if this seems absurd, let us admit that occasionally this can be a problem. There is the common intraluminal tufting and budding by tall, pale-staining secretory or pseudosecretory cells. In many instances it appears that this intraglandular secretion represents mucin rather than glycogen. Salm has pointed out that this occurs in the normal endometrium or well differentiated carcinomas.

In any case, many genuine proliferative hyperplasias are evanescent and self-limited, so that it seems unwise to regard them as even a Stage ICO cancer. At the same time there is little doubt that a certain number do seem to progress into true adenocarcinoma, but the terminology should suggest a potentially precancerous role rather than an in situ status.

The clinically malignant nature of the true adenocarcinoma, as indicated by its extension to lymphatic glands, is proof that its cells do actually break through the basement membrane, and in certain cases this penetration is easily demonstrable, as well as its extension to the muscularis. It thus appears that there is a whole series of gradations, a species of histological stepping stones, between atypical hyperplasia and adenocarcinoma, and there is no sure criterion as to the point at which the lesion assumes actually malignant characteristics. In the doubtful group the safe clinical plan is to treat them as potential cancer, which is usually easy in that most such patients are in the incipient menopausal era and have completed their family.

PROLIFERATIVE HYPERPLASIA IN THE YOUNG WOMAN

Only occasionally are younger women so afflicted, but these represent a greater problem. If the diagnosis is not 100 % certain following curettage it would seem that another confirmatory curettage several months later is warranted before any definitive therapy, and with no real risk to the patient. Jackson and Dockerty have indicated the frequent finding of low grade adenoacanthoma with clinical and pathological findings in the ovary suggesting a Stein-Leventhal syndrome. We admit this may occur, but as an infrequent occurrence, although Stein himself has never seen such a coincidence in 25 years of experience. Perhaps his diligence in treating this problem early has prevented this sequel, and prompt treatment of this syndrome might be considered a form of prophylaxis against endometrial adenocarcinoma (Fig. 15.7).

Kaufman, Abbott, and Wall suggest that varied forms of abnormal endometrium are associated with the Stein-Leventhal ovary. The pattern is frequently proliferative or hyperplastic, occasionally adenomatous, but wedge resection of the ovary is often followed by reversion to normal. The importance of a curettage along with wedge resection is emphasized, with careful follow-up of the woman with a hyperplastic endometrium, especially if there are proliferative adenomatous tendencies. At a certain indeterminant point there may be not regression to normal but progression into adenocarcinoma.

ESTROGEN THERAPY

It is important to remember that various pseudomalignant lesions may follow the *injudicious and prolonged administration of estrogens* in postmenopausal or other women. Indeed, routine history of the postmenopausal bleeder should include direct questioning as to estrogen therapy, and where this is found in conjunction with equivocal curettings repeat curettage may be performed after discontinuance of the hormone (Fig. 15.8).

Histological Grading of Adenocarcinoma. In keeping with the accepted rule that the greater the degree of unripeness and dedifferentiation of the cells the greater the clinical malignancy of the tumor, systems of grading these tumors have been suggested by various authors, that most popular being the plan suggested by Broders. According to this, four grades are distinguished. In Grade I, the least malignant, the proportion of dedifferentiated cells is relatively small, not exceeding

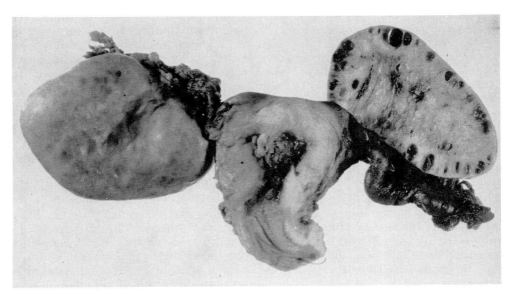

FIG. 15.7. Polycystic ovaries associated with endometrial carcinoma in a 15-year-old girl (Courtesy of Dr. R. Greenblatt, Augusta, Georgia).

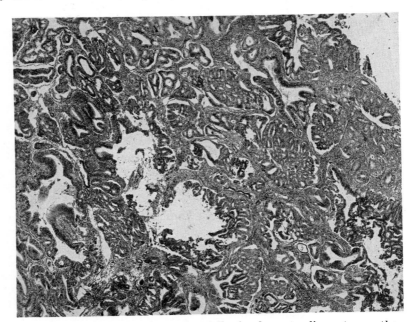

FIG. 15.8. Postmenopausal endometrium following long-standing estrogen therapy

25%. In this type the atypicality of the gland pattern is not nearly so marked as in the more malignant grades. This variety is often spoken of as *adenoma malignum*. At the other extreme, Grade IV malignant cells are present in 75 to 100%.

In this last group the pattern is extremely atypical, and many of the gland lumina may, because of extreme epithelial activity, appear quite solid, so that such areas may be difficult to distinguish from solid epidermoid carcinoma. Examination

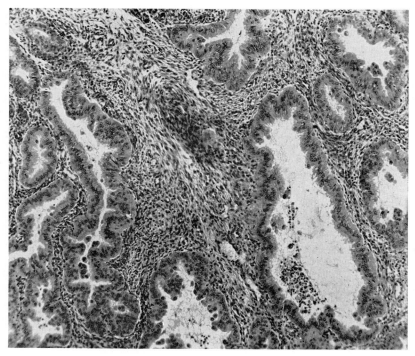

Fig. 15.9. Interpreted as proliferative hyperplasia at menopause, age 50; x-ray induction of menopause instituted.

of other areas will almost always show the gland pattern and thus permit of proper classification. Actually, such qualifying terms as "differentiated, intermediate, and undifferentiated" are of equal service in histologically grading adenocarcinoma. It seems quite apparent that microscopic grade generally parallels myometrial invasion and ultimate prognosis in many cases. In other words a well differentiated tumor is much less apt to invade or metastasize, and should offer a much better prognosis. Nolan and Darden, as well as the Mayo group, would appear to afford suggestive evidence that such is exactly the case.

Adenoacanthoma of Uterus. This is an interesting and not infrequent type of adenocarcinoma in which there is an associated "squamous metaplasia" of certain so-called indifferent cells just beneath the epithelium. More recently, Novak and Nalley have suggested that there is a direct transformation from metaplastic endometrial lining cells as evidenced by all intermediate transition forms. Be that as it may, one may find in either the benign hyperplasia of the endometrium or, much more frequently, in adenocarcinoma, extensive areas of squamous epithelium adjoining the gland lumina, often forming large plaquelike fields between them (Fig. 15.11). Such pictures have often led to the erroneous diagnosis of combined adenocarcinoma and squamous cell carcinoma. It should be remembered, however, that it is the gland carcinoma alone which is important, and that the squamous elements, while giving the lesion a different and unusual histological appearance, do not in themselves show any evidence of malignancy. Indeed they are highly differentiated and often spinal.

This is borne out by the relatively favorable results in the treatment of such cases, although certain British authors cite an increased malignancy. Occasionally true epidermoid cancer can arise high in the canal and involve the endometrial

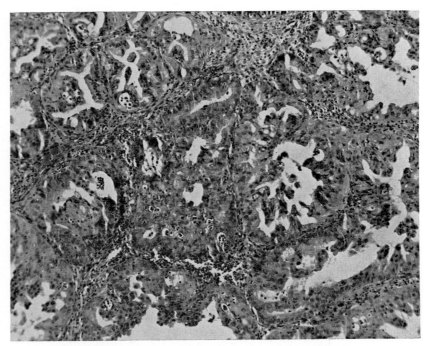

Fig. 15.10. Evolvement of frank adenocarcinoma 7 years later

surface. Rarely does true epidermoid cancer arise in the corpus, as noted by Peris, Jernstrom, and Bowers. These are both very different entities from true adenocanthomas, where benign squamous metaplasia occurs in conjunction with low grade, generally favorable, adenocarcinomas.

Relationships of Endometrial Hyperplasia to Adenocarcinoma. Although it seems probable that myomata and adenomyosis are rather frequent concomitants of fundal cancer, there is no definite evidence that these have more than a casual relationship, although estrogen would seem a possible common denominator. Similarly endometrial hyperplasia *during the menstrual era* appears of no particular import and often seems to be a rather transient and self-limited affair.

On the other hand, hyperplasia *around and after the menopause*, especially where it is recurrent and assumes an adenomatous proliferative pattern, is considerably more worrisome: (1) Such atypical microscopic varieties may be encountered

as to make differentiation from early neoplasm utterly impossible, even though some extremely adenomatous patterns may be completely benign and followed by no malignant trends. It is important to emphasize that these equivocal histological architectures may be a sequel to exogenous estrogen (frequently given without indication or discrimination) or may be spontaneous. (2) Adenocarcinoma is frequently preceded by these intensely hyperplastic patterns, which may occur during either the menstrual or postmenopausal era. In the latter instance, one may only conjecture as to the source of estrogen, which is known to be the usual stimulus to hyperplasia. The adrenal gland has been proved capable of estrogen production, but in recent years there has been considerable speculation about the function of the postmenopausal ovary. Some feel that hyperplastic stromal cells (morphologically indistinguishable from theca cells and often taking up fat avidly) may be a source of estrogen despite disagreement by Roddick and Greene. In any case numerous publica-

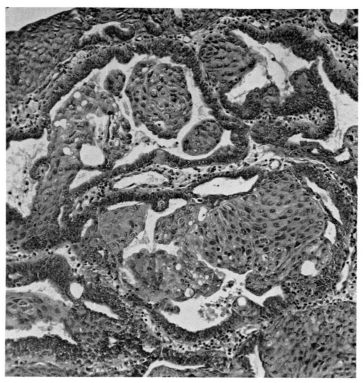

Fig. 15.11. Adenoacanthoma of uterus. This is distinguished by the presence of plaques of well differentiated, obviously benign, squamous cells in association with adenocarcinoma.

tions have stressed the frequency with which corpus cancer is preceded by an atypical endometrial hyperplasia.

Since estrogen is the normal cause of endometrial hyperplasia, and since estrogen therapy has been observed to produce hyperplastic patterns indistinguishable from adenocarcinoma, it is only logical that this steroid has been under considerable suspicion as a possible factor in the evolution of fundal cancer. Admittedly there is not final proof that estrogens are carcinogenic, although we find it difficult to accept statements (Wilson) "that estrogen and progesterone are prophylactic to breast and genital cancer to an unknown degree." Wilson enlarges on his point by advocating that women be kept endocrine rich and thereby cancer poor by elimination of the menopause. We would urge all readers to be cautious before accepting this astonishingly different approach to reality.

The recent review by Andrews affords additional evidence to the possible role of estrogen in the etiology of endometrial cancer. Of equal importance, however, is the belated admission by a senior statesman, Dr. L. A. Emge that "I, for one, believe that such hazards as long term estrogenization in the post-menopausal woman are real and deserve serious consideration." If a critical gynecologist of this stature could make such a statement, it behooves all of us to be attentive.

Until recently, however, it has been impossible to produce adenocarcinoma in experimental animals by huge doses of estrogens, although Meissner, Sommers, and Sherman have been able to produce in certain strains of rabbit unequivocal adenocarcinoma which, even after cessation of the steroid, went on to metastasize and kill the animal. Estrogen must be regarded as possibly carcinogenic because of many different observations, no one of

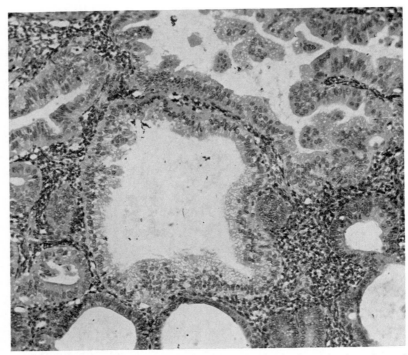

Fig. 15.12. Endometrium of postmenopausal woman who had received prolonged estrogen therapy with resultant bleeding. Repetition of curettage 6 weeks later showed normal senile endometrium with complete regression of the atypical hyperplasia after stoppage of estrogens. (Courtesy of Dr. D. Dickson, Santa Barabara, California.)

which is conclusive; but *in toto* they seem highly suggestive. These may only be summarized as follows.

Late Menopause. Repeated observations have noted that women with adenocarcinoma have a history of a protracted late menopause and, since anovulation at this era is common, the opportunity for prolonged unopposed estrogen is present. This deserves reevaluation, for most clinicians believe that today's woman is apt to menstruate and ovulate longer.

"Bloody Menopause." With adenocarcinoma patients have a high incidence of premenopausal bleeding, necessitating curettage, which shows hyperplasia or an anovulatory pattern in a high percentage of cases.

Castration. Repeated observations have noted the rarity of endometrial cancer following bilateral oophorectomy, a not uncommon procedure until recent years.

The study by Cianfrani reporting 12 cases of cancer developing after castration might seem to negate this thesis but the reader must recall the frequent difficulty in ablating all ovarian tissue in certain cases (pelvic inflammatory disease, endometriosis, etc.) or the confusion in microscopically diagnosing early cases.

Feminizing Ovarian Tumors. Many granulosa-theca cell tumors which are capable of estrogen production have been frequently noted as coexisting with endometrial cancer in a much higher ratio than the laws of chance would allow. This frequent association (15 to 20% in most series) has been called the "spontaneous biological experiment" and would seem to afford a real basis for concepts of estrogen as a profound proliferative stimulus.

Estrogen Therapy. There has been a number of cases reported with the sequence of prolonged estrogen therapy and later adenocarcinoma and, although no

CHECKLIST
GYNECOLOGIC HISTORY AND EXAMINATION

PATIENT'S NAME_____ AGE_____

THE GYNECOLOGIC HISTORY

I PRELIMINARY DATA

A. Age
B. Gravidity and Parity

II CHIEF COMPLAINT

III PRESENT ILLNESS

IV MENSTRUAL HISTORY

A. Adolescent menstrual history
   1. Age of menarche
   2. Regularity of initial cycles
   3. Amount and duration of bleeding
   4. Associated symptoms
   5. Medical management

B. Customary menstrual pattern
   1. Interval between "normal" periods
   2. Amount and duration of typical flow
   3. Total number of boxes of pads or tampons used during entire period
   4. Associated discomforts (dysmenorrhea, headache, premenstrual symptoms)

C. Recent menstrual data
   1. Dates and description of last normal menstrual period and last menstrual period
   2. Excessive menstrual flow (menorrhagia)
   3. Intermenstrual spotting or bleeding
   4. Bleeding following contact (intercourse or douching)
   5. Amenorrhea
   6. Relationship of irregularities to recent medication (estrogens, progestins)

V PAST HISTORY

A. Serious illnesses

B. Obstetric history. Includes term and premature birth, early and late abortion, hydatid mole; recorded in chronologic order with sex and weight of the fetus and dates of birth.
   1. Any puerperal complications?
   2. Number of children now alive
C. Surgical history. List each operation (including tonsillectomy) chronologically. Record:
   1. Surgeon and hospital
   2. Diagnosis
   3. What was done?
   4. Did it improve the patient's health?

VI FAMILY HISTORY

VII MARITAL HISTORY

THE GYNECOLOGIC EXAMINATION

I BREASTS
   A. Inspection and palpation
   B. Masses
      1. Cystic or solid
      2. Fixation
   C. Bloody discharge from the nipple
   D. Palpation of axilla

II ABDOMEN
   A. Inspection
   B. Percussion
         ascites versus cyst
   C. Palpation

III PELVIC EXAMINATION
   A. External genitalia
   B. Cytologic smear
   C. Cervix and vagina
   D. Internal genitalia
   E. Rectovaginal examination

CHECKLIST
GYNECOLOGIC HISTORY AND EXAMINATION

PATIENT'S NAME_____ AGE_____

THE GYNECOLOGIC HISTORY

I PRELIMINARY DATA

A. Age
B. Gravidity and Parity

II CHIEF COMPLAINT

III PRESENT ILLNESS

IV MENSTRUAL HISTORY

A. Adolescent menstrual history
   1. Age of menarche
   2. Regularity of initial cycles
   3. Amount and duration of bleeding
   4. Associated symptoms
   5. Medical management

B. Customary menstrual pattern
   1. Interval between "normal" periods
   2. Amount and duration of typical flow
   3. Total number of boxes of pads or tampons used during entire period
   4. Associated discomforts (dysmenorrhea, headache, premenstrual symptoms)

C. Recent menstrual data
   1. Dates and description of last normal menstrual period and last menstrual period
   2. Excessive menstrual flow (menorrhagia)
   3. Intermenstrual spotting or bleeding
   4. Bleeding following contact (intercourse or douching)
   5. Amenorrhea
   6. Relationship of irregularities to recent medication (estrogens, progestins)

V PAST HISTORY

A. Serious illnesses

B. Obstetric history. Includes term and premature birth, early and late abortion, hydatid mole; recorded in chronologic order with sex and weight of the fetus and dates of birth.
  1. Any puerperal complications?
  2. Number of children now alive
C. Surgical history. List each operation (including tonsillectomy) chronologically. Record:
  1. Surgeon and hospital
  2. Diagnosis
  3. What was done?
  4. Did it improve the patient's health?

VI FAMILY HISTORY

VII MARITAL HISTORY

THE GYNECOLOGIC EXAMINATION

I BREASTS
A. Inspection and palpation
B. Masses
  1. Cystic or solid
  2. Fixation
C. Bloody discharge from the nipple
D. Palpation of axilla

II ABDOMEN
A. Inspection
B. Percussion
    ascites versus cyst
C. Palpation

III PELVIC EXAMINATION
A. External genitalia
B. Cytologic smear
C. Cervix and vagina
D. Internal genitalia
E. Rectovaginal examination

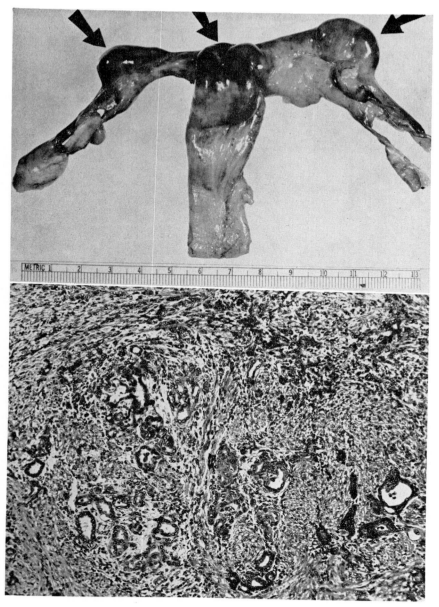

FIG. 15.13. *Top*, tumor nodules in bicornuate rabbit uterus after prolonged stilbestrol. *Bottom*, microscopic cancer. The cancer depicted in the lower figure metastasized and led to death even after cessation of the steroid stimulation. (Courtesy of Dr. Sheldon Sommers, Boston, Massachusetts.)

one can state positively that this is a matter of cause and effect, discriminating gynecologists are rather reluctant to utilize prolonged unopposed estrogens. Of particular interest in certain of these cases is the finding of all degrees of endometrial proliferation up to frank adenocarcinoma in the same specimen. Gusberg and Hall

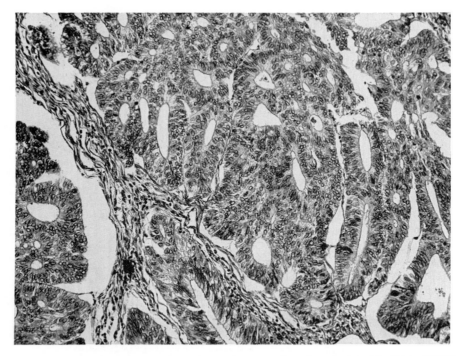

FIG. 15.14. High power of more proliferative areas in polyp depicted in Plate XV.II

note 23 patients in a 20-year span who had received exogenous estrogens for over a year.

Association of Hyperplasia and Adenocarcinoma. This association was first noted by Taylor in 1932 and Novak and Yui in 1936, and there has been considerable confirmation by more recent authors. Not only may adenocarcinoma coexist with hyperplasia, but it is not infrequently preceded by it around the menopausal era. Extremely atypical proliferative degrees of hyperplasia may be found, and indeed all variants of simple and adenomatous hyperplasia may be found along with adenocarcinoma.

Postmenopausal Hyperplasia. Hyperplasia in the menstrual era rarely has any dire sequelae and is often a transient innocuous process unlike hyperplasia in the climacteric woman. A recent publication by Novak points out the similarities between women with *postmenopausal* hyperplasia and malignant adenocarcinoma in regard to such features as obesity, hypertension, diabetes, nulliparity, prolonged menstruation, bloody menopause, etc., all of which have been repeatedly noted as occurring commonly with adenocarcinoma. Indeed it is hard to avoid the impression that postmenopausal hyperplasia and adenocarcinoma are mere variants of a similar generalized metabolic or endocrine process with carcinoma an exaggerated and extreme end-stage if there is a continuance of the stimulus (perhaps *estrogen*).

The high incidence of ovarian stromal hyperplasia in association with endometrial endocarcinoma has been noted by Woll *et al.*, Novak and Mohler, and most recently by Marcus who has reviewed the literature and discussed the pros and cons of this controversial subject. Sherman and Woolf, however, are more concerned with hyperplasia of the hilus cells and their production of a bisexual steroid ("sexagen") that may induce adenocarcinoma. During the menstrual era the function of the hilus cell is suppressed by the ovarian hormones; with impaired postmenopausal gonadal function and in-

Prendu l
muncline avolente
adiminto dinbete

300 | 36
40 91,1

    77 | 36
   300 86 %
   278
   = 220
     216

35 00 | 36
32 4 97 %
= 2 6 0
  2 5 2
  = 80

Pour 80 more bro 24 cisti di Bebeli

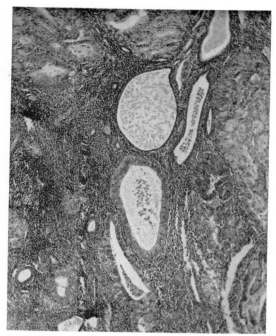

FIG. 15.15. Adenocarcinoma of uterus associated with postmenopausal hyperplasia

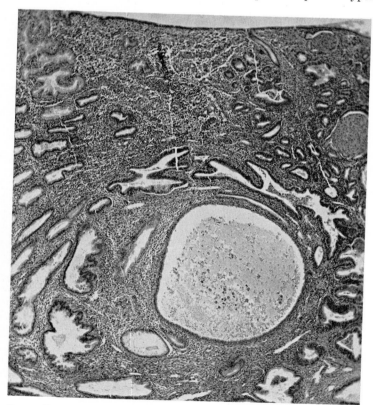

FIG. 15.16. Generally progestational (*left*) response with focal area showing only estrogen effect. (Note benign squamous metaplasia on *right*.)

creased follicle-stimulating hormone (FSH) there is stimulation of the hilus cells with production of a steroid (estrogenic) that incites later adenocarcinoma. If there is incomplete suppression during the menstrual era, the hilus cell may manufacture an androgenic steroid that provokes the Stein-Leventhal picture.

The recent study by Varga and Henriksen would seem to question the validity of the above concept. They note marked variation in LH excretion, and no significant response to progesterone therapy in patients with endometrial cancer or a control group. A decrease in the LH excretion following progesterone therapy is an integral part of Sherman and Woolf's theory due of course to the reciprocal and inhibitory mechanism of the ovarian and pituitary hormones. At this writing their concepts, while highly stimulating, are far from being critically acceptable. That the hilus cell may be a potent producer of steroids on occasion seems likely, however, as suggested by unpublished studies of our own on the histochemical qualities of postmenopausal ovaries.

One must be cognizant of the occasional young women who develop adenocarcinoma in the face of a biphasic cycle with obvious evidence of ovulation. The pathologist, however, frequently finds patches of hyperplasia in association with a generally progestational endometrium, and it is felt that these foci represent unripe undifferentiated endometrium which may be incapable of response to progesterone and thereby subject to *protracted unopposed estrogen stimulation* (Fig. 15.16). These areas may occur in a polyp or in the endometrium, but show a common incapability of response to progesterone. This would seem a very logical answer to those who deride the "estrogen theory" by quoting small groups of women with adenocarcinoma associated with a corpus luteum or a generally secretory endometrium or both. Carcinoma in the young ovulating woman appears a different and infrequent type of adenocarcinoma, and the usual variety would make it difficult to discount the important role of estrogen. Genetic pre-disposition to cancer is likewise of considerable import.

Clinical Characteristics. More than two-thirds of all cases occur in women beyond the menopause, the proportion being roughly 75 % postmenopausal, 15 % menopausal, and 10 % still menstruating, according to compiled reports. Obesity, hypertension, diabetes, and a history of previous curettage are frequent concomitants. There is often a history of sterility or poor fertility. The question of whether an irradiation menopause is a causative factor is speculative, despite much suggestive evidence that irradiation in general must be regarded as under some suspicion as far as the genesis of certain malignancy is concerned (Novak and Woodruff).

By far the most frequent and most important symptom is *abnormal bleeding*, commonly in the form of *metrorrhagia*. In the case of women still in the menstruating age, *menorrhagia* is frequently observed. Next to bleeding, the most significant symptom is an *abnormal discharge*, at first watery, but soon admixed with blood. As with cancer elsewhere, *pain* is not a symptom until the later invasive stages of the disease. The same statement

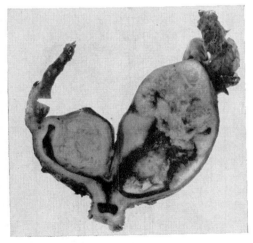

Fig. 15.17. Extensive endometrial adenocarcinoma in right (facing) horn of bicornuate uterus; adenomyosis on other side. (Courtesy of Dr. A. S. Duncan and A. H. John, Cardiff, Wales.)

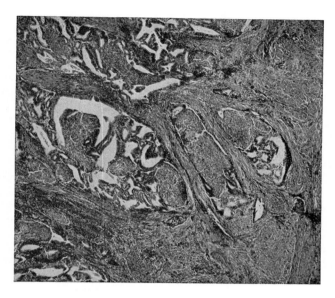

FIG. 15.18. Adenocarcinoma invading uterine musculature

can be made with reference to *loss of weight* and *general debility*, although *anemia* may become marked if there is any pronounced blood loss.

On occasion there may be no abnormal bleeding, but pressure symptoms due to a uterus massively distended by blood which cannot escape due to some obstruction in the lower genital tract. Arrata and Zarou find that in about one-third of their cases of postmenopausal hematometra, there is an endometrial carcinoma.

Diagnosis. The first thought of every physician when confronted with a case of postmenopausal bleeding should be of cancer of the uterus, either of the cervix or of the body. Cervical cancer can usually be eliminated by careful inspection and office smears and biopsy.

Assuming, however, that a cervical or vaginal source for the bleeding can be eliminated, an intrauterine source may be safely assumed. As a matter of fact, it is often possible to observe a blood-stained discharge or a trickle of blood escaping from the cervical canal. Even then, it is by no means certain that adenocarcinoma exists, this being found in less than 10% of all cases of postmenopausal bleeding. Other possible causes are benign polyps or

hyperplasia, submucous myoma, senile endometritis, etc. Payne, Wright, and Fetterman have indicated the frequent role of estrogen in the causation of postmenopausal bleeding, as well as the infrequency (25%) of malignant disease.

There is only one decisive way to make the diagnosis, and this diagnostic procedure should be standard. We refer to *curettage and microscopic examination.* It is in such cases that curettage has its clearest and most important application. Vaginal cytology with maturation index (MI) should never be neglected (where there is not excessive bleeding) although its accuracy in detecting endometrial cancer perhaps approaches only 80 to 85%. Aspiration or lavage of the endometrial cavity do not approach the efficacy of curettage.

If curettage yields only extremely scant tissue from the uterine cavity, it is probable that cancer will not be found on microscopic examination, but Beutler, Dockerty, and Randall have noted that adenocarcinoma in conjunction with an atrophic endometrium is often missed.

If a submucous myoma is the cause of the bleeding, the cervix is often somewhat patulous, the uterine cavity longer than normal and irregular in outline, and the curette will often serve indirectly to outline the projecting tumor as it passes over and around the latter.

If abundant tissue is brought away, and the uterus is enlarged, the gynecologist will be suspicious especially if the woman is well beyond the menopause, and if the removed tissue is polypoid, necrotic, and friable. Appropriate intracavitary radium should be available, and where the gross curettings are suggestive, this should be utilized pending "frozen" or "rush" sections of the endometrium. If carcinoma is revealed, the intracavitary radium is retained until the requisite cancerocidal dosage is achieved. If there is no malignancy, the radium is removed after a much shorter time, sufficient usually to take care of the ordinary case of benign bleeding. Many gynecologists omit preoperative irradiation if there is a small uterus and only scant endometrium obtained at curettage.

When the patient is still in the menstruating age, the significance of abundant curettings is much less, for such a finding is frequent with such conditions as benign hyperplasia and unsuspected incomplete abortion, to mention only the most important. With the latter, the experienced gynecologist can often, although not by any means always, make a reasonably safe diagnosis from the chunky nature of the removed particles, their characteristic placental appearance, and the presence of large thrombotic areas. In the case of very early abortions, or those which had occurred many weeks or even months previously, the microscope is necessary for diagnosis.

The abundant polypoid tissue obtained in some cases of hyperplasia may easily mislead the inexperienced, but the distinction can often be made with reasonable certainty with the naked eye from the firmness of the polypoid growth, the smoothness of the covering mucosa, and the absence of the necrosis and friability which would ordinarily be found in an adenocarcinoma yielding a corresponding amount of tissue.

Extension of Adenocarcinoma. This is the most favorable type of uterine cancer by virture of its tendency to remain confined to the surface. Myometrial extension may occur, and increased degrees impair the prognosis. Ovarian involvement by tubal or lymphatic extension occurs in 10 to 15 % of our own cases. Vaginal, especially suburethral, tumor was frequent in the pre-irradiation days. A recent review by Boutselis, Ullery, and Bain confirms the relative infrequency of vaginal metastasis in irradiated patients. The prognosis where the vagina is involved is poor, perhaps because this type of lesion is generally quite undifferentiated.

It is our own feeling that this form of uterine cancer only occasionally travels by way of the lymphatics, chiefly those accompanying the ovarian vessels. Javert in particular has stressed the frequency with which endometrium is found in the lymph nodes in both endometriosis and corpus cancer. In the latter disease Javert feels that nodal involvement is more common than adnexal extension, and therefore argues for more radical surgery.

Gland Involvement. Different studies regarding gland involvement show considerable variation. Javert's 28 % must be regarded as an extreme degree of nodal involvement. Some authors note a considerably lower figure, although Miller *et al.* concur with other authors that if the cervix shows extension of endometrial cancer, nodal involvement is proportionately more frequent. Such patients are suggested as candidates for Wertheim hysterectomy despite medical complications, unless one believes (as we do) that the deep pelvic nodes are responsive to external irradiation.

Much more logical is Beck and Latour's negative approach as to the value of pelvic lymphadenectomy. In studying 36 cases of endometrial cancer coming to autopsy they conclusively show that where there is deep myometrial invasion or pelvic lymph node involvement, there is a high (over 90%) association of extrapelvic metastasis. As Javert has indicated, the 5-year survival of patients with positive nodes is zero. Thus, why increase morbidity by lymphadenectomy if it is of no value, as would appear to be the case. We cannot stress too strongly that lymphadenectomy which is suggested so blithely by many gynecologists is followed by a not inconsiderable number of serious complications.

No one will deny that lymph node as well as adnexal spread of the disease can occur and frequently parallels the extent of myometrial spread. Yet there are few clinics that routinely advocate a radical procedure including node dissection on these frequently elderly, obese, hypertensive, and diabetic patients when results with conservative treatment are rather good. Indeed, it is difficult to reconcile the reputed high lymph node involvement of endometrial cancer with the frequent cure by total hysterectomy without any kind of lymph node dissection.

In advanced cases the peritoneum may be the seat of implantation. The cancerous disease may, especially in growths involving the lower part of the corpus, extend into the *cervix*, and metastasis or extension to the *vagina* may occur. Carcinoma involving the corpus and endocervix has a worse prognosis and is a distinct entity requiring special treatment such as irradiation to corpus and cervix (Thompson and Graham) or radical surgery. *Distant metastases* to such locations as the liver or lungs may likewise be noted in the later stages, as may any form of extracorporeal extension.

In attempting evaluation of metastatic disease, one must be cognizant of Bailar's observations that almost 5% of women with endometrial cancer had another extrauterine malignancy. Breast cancer is much more frequent, and lower bowel lesions are disproportionately common. The astute clinician should be mindful of this possibility.

Treatment. One of the most controversial points that may arise at any meeting attended by the best gynecologists is the method by which endometrial cancer should usually be treated. All are agreed that a small proportion of women have such serious medical handicaps that they can tolerate no form of major surgery,

and irradiation therapy alone must be utilized. Most are likewise agreed that where the preliminary curettings are scant and of low grade activity, and the uterus is small and free, simple total hysterectomy and adnexectomy will probably suffice. However, the prognosis decreases where extrauterine extension or significant myometrial involvement has occurred, and of course these are factors which do not always become apparent until after laparotomy. Three main approaches to the treatment of corpus cancer are utilized which may be merely summarized as follows.

(1) *Irradiation.* There are very few American gynecologists who would prefer this as the sole means of therapy in the medically fit patient, although it has been the usual method of treatment in Stockholm. No one would deny that there is a certain salvage, in the nature of slightly less than 50%; and in the poor risk woman or the one who for various reasons has a limited life expectancy, it deserves consideration, as it does in the treatment of vaginal recurrences. X-ray plus some means of radium therapy, preferably by the Heyman multiple capsules, rather than a simple tandem, are employed. A vaginal source seems to be of value in minimizing recurrence in that area. Indeed, Dieckmann, McCartney, and Carpenter advocate irradiation as routine treatment in some patients, with repeated recurettage and additional radiotherapy where residual cancer is found.

(2) *Surgery.* Few would question that the operation of total hysterectomy and adnexectomy is the most important part of the usual therapy of corpus cancer, a disease frequently characterized merely by surface extension, minor degrees of myometrial involvement, and rare nodal spread. The abdominal approach is routine, although Bastianse and Pratt, Symmond, and Welch advocate a vaginal hysterectomy, which we utilize only in the occasional poor risk, obese patient. Such excellent American gynecologists as McKelvey and McLennan utilize surgery alone, and this is the usual form of therapy by many European gynecologists. Pre-

alcune della stessa efficacia

liminary suture of the cervix is the rule in unirradiated patients to militate against manipulation leading to vaginal recurrence.

There are a few enthusiastic gynecologists who advocate radical Wertheim operations plus lymphadenectomy as a standard form of surgery. It is difficult to accept this routine, for lesser operations achieve as high as 90 to 95% salvage, with none of the attendant risks entailed in radical surgery, particularly where the patients are so frequently obese and of poor medical quality. We have often labored long and hard to remove the total uterus, and in such patients the risk attendant to an upper vaginectomy and lymphadenectomy would seem prohibitive, especially if we consider that nodal disease is usually fatal, irrespective of the degree of surgery. Even the most ardent radical surgeon admits this to be a fact, and the recent studies of Barber, Dockerty, and Pratt involving 85 lymphadenectomies of which 17 showed positive nodes, yielded only one long term survivor. Just what the morbidity is cannot be stated, but it is considerable.

(3) *Irradiation plus Surgery.* Dispassionate observers seem uniform in agreeing that for all stages of fundal adenocarcinoma, a combined treatment gives the best results, while admitting that if there is still localized disease, irradiation is not necessary. Yet it is impossible to state dogmatically what the extent of the disease may be from prehysterectomy examination and evaluation of the curettings.

A seemingly optimal approach to the bleeding postmenopausal woman whose cervix is proved normal by biopsy, is to plan curettage with radium available. Should the removed endometrium be abundant, grayish, necrotic, and fungoid in nature, the likelihood of endometrial cancer is good, although hyperplasia may occasionally present an identical appearance. Radium can, however, be inserted, and "rush sections" obtained, so that even if the gross diagnosis is wrong, a very minor radiation dosage may be utilized. If, however, cancer is revealed, the full cancerocidal dosage of radium may be given. Preoperative x-ray, as practiced by Miller at the University of Michigan, seems at least as effective, and perhaps more rational in dealing with potential tumor outside the uterus, for it must be remembered that radium has a very limited (2 cm. from the source) cancerocidal effect on cancer cells.

As to just why irradiation should be so effective, there is considerable speculation, for in many independent observations the removed uterus has evidenced a significant (over 50%) evidence of tumor. Histologically, the criteria for what is *viable* tumor are extremely tenuous, and one must conclude that, although irradiation may not obliterate all neoplasm, it creates an environment designed to make subsequent implantation and extension less likely.

However, it is difficult to argue with well constructed statistics such as those of Kimbrough, who compared two very large compilations of many reports dealing with patients treated (1) by surgery alone and (2) by combined therapy, with a 15% difference in favor of the latter method of treatment. Actually the results are even more impressive, for the more favorable patients were treated surgically, with irradiation an adjuvant only if the lesion were found to be more advanced. In an earlier personal communication Kimbrough adds: "I have no doubt that preoperative radiation by a multiple source method, particularly including vaginal vault radiation, will yield better results than ever."

The usual plan has been to allow an interval of about 6 weeks between irradiation and surgery—enough time for the edema and vascularity to subside without permitting the tumor to spread. Decker has suggested earlier surgery with the logical argument that, once delivered, the irradiation effect will persist. Although we have utilized this in only a few cases, with no major complications, the patients have occasionally had a markedly adhesive vaginitis (due to surgery plus irradiation effect) so that subsequent postoperative examinations were difficult.

£ d '6 felt.

Above all, this short interval between irradiation and surgery might allow insufficient time for fibrosis and scarring of the lymphatics, which we think impedes dissemination of the tumor at the time of hysterectomy.

Javert and Renning find a tendency to less frequent preoperative irradiation, but a greater incidence of postsurgical x-ray as dictated by the extent of tumor extension. It seems that this is a very logical premise, and their salvage would indicate little difference regardless of the modality of irradiation. Beck, Latour, and Bourne likewise feel that in medically fit patients without advanced disease, surgery alone is as effective as combined treatment.

Drug Therapy. Kelly and Baker have utilized progesterone in large doses (500 mgm. twice a week) in women with recurrent and advanced endometrial cancer. Whether this is a guarding effect against a possible estrogenic stimulus is uncertain, but their results in about one-third of treated patients suggest striking remissions if not a cure. We can record only a few personal cases, but one was a patient who had a biopsy-proven chest lesion following pelvic surgery and irradiation. Following progesterone treatment the thoracic lesion melted away, and has been quiescent for over 1½ years. Similar results (29.6% of 27 patients) have been reported by Kennedy.

Of considerable interest if less dramatic are those women who have the earliest forms of endometrial adenocarcinoma, wherein progesterone has seemingly arrested the course of the disease. In a discussion of 40 patients with adenomatous hyperplasia and 10 with early adenocarcinoma, Kistner enlarges on this, meanwhile quoting Gusberg's comments that atypical hyperplasia, adenomatous hyperplasia, carcinoma in situ, and Stage 0 cancer are histologically similar. Although we might disagree to the extent that the first two are merely premalignant, Kistner has demonstrated that temporary regression of a hyperactive endometrial pattern may be obtained while stressing that this should not be the usual treatment in the older parous patient even with a low-grade histological tumor. Recent observations have indicated more extensive use of progesterone in many stages of endometrial cancer, especially where surgery is not feasible.

Even more recent observations have suggested that clomiphene can lead to regression of the early forms of endometrial cancer (Wall and his associates). How long this remission may last is uncertain.

Salvage. There is nothing more difficult than assessing the salvage of adenocarcinoma as reported by different clinics using different and often varied methods of treatment. One great drawback is the fact that some clinics report and treat as early adenocarcinoma many cases of what we believe to be merely benign proliferative hyperplasia, and the reader must be mindful of this possibility in evaluating statistics. The over-all 5-year salvage noted in the *Twelfth Annual Report of the Results of Treatment in Carcinoma of the Uterus* is 63.9%.

Where only the endometrium is involved, surgery alone or in conjunction with irradiation should afford close to 100% salvage. Where the superficial myometrium is involved, the salvage begins to decrease in proportion to the degree of myometrial involvement, but even where this is widespread, salvage should be upwards of 50%. Where extrauterine extension or metastasis occurs, salvage becomes markedly decreased. A recent report by Gusberg and his associates summarizes most studies. Among 1383 women treated by hysterectomy alone, the cure rate was *64%*; where preoperative radium was utilized in 1146 patients, the figure was over *76%*. Such statistics on large series make it difficult to belittle the importance of radium. Obviously endometrial cancer is a more favorable disease than the cervical variety, although Miller believes that we are overly enthusiastic in assessing results.

REFERENCES

Andrews, W. C.: Estrogen and endometrial carcinoma. Obstet. Gynec. Survey, *16:* 747, 1961.

Annual Report on the Results of Treatment in Carcinoma of the Uterus, Vol. 12. Stockholm, 1963.

Arrata, W. S., and Zarou, G. S.: Postmenopausal hematometra. Amer. J. Obstet. Gynec., *85:* 959, 1963.

Bailar, J. C.: Multiple tumors with uterine cancer. Cancer, *16:* 842, 1963.

Bamforth, J.: Carcinoma of body of uterus and its relationship to endometrial hyperplasia. J. Obstet. Gynaec. Brit. Comm., *63:* 415, 1956.

Barber, K. W., Jr., Dockerty, M. B., and Pratt, J. H.: A clinicopathologic study of surgically treated carcinoma of the endometrium with nodal metastases. Surg. Gynec. Obstet., *115:* 568, 1962.

Bastianse, M. A.: Carcinoma of the body of the uterus. J. Obstet. Gynaec. Brit. Comm., *49:* 611, 1952.

Beck, R. P., and Latour, J. P. A.: Necropsy reports on 36 cases of endometrial carcinoma. Amer. J. Obstet. Gynec., *85:* 307, 1963.

Beck, R. P., Latour, J. P. A., and Bourne, H. B.: Treatment of endometrial carcinoma reassessed. Amer. J. Obstet. Gynec., *88:* 178, 1964.

Beutler, H. K., Dockerty, M. B., and Randall, L. M.: Precancerous lesions of the endometrium. Amer. J. Obestet. Gynec., *86:* 433, 1963.

Boutselis, J. G., Ullery, J. C., and Bain, J.: Vaginal metastases following treatment of endometrial carcinoma. Obstet. Gynec., *21:* 622, 1963.

Brewer, J. I.: Carcinoma in situ of endometrium. Southern Med. J., *51:* 554, 1958.

Brewer, J. I., and Foley, T. J.: Endometrial cancer and cirrhosis. Obstet. Gynec., *1:* 67, 1953.

Broders, A. C.: The grading of carcinoma. Minnesota Med., *8:* 726, 1925.

Chanen, W.: A clinical and pathological study of adenoacanthoma of the uterine body. J. Obstet. Gynaec. Brit. Comm., *67:* 287, 1960.

Cianfrani, T.: Endometrial cancer after bilateral oophorectomy. Amer. J. Obstet. Gynec., *69:* 64, 1955.

Corscaden, J. A., Fertig, J. W., and Gusberg, S. B.: Carcinoma subsequent to radiotherapeutic menopause. Amer. J. Obstet. Gynec., *51:* 1, 1946.

Corscaden, J. A., and Towell, H. M.: Management of carcinoma of the fundus. Amer. J. Obstet. Gynec., *68:* 737, 1954.

Decker, W. H.: Endometrial cancer; early post-radiation surgery. Amer. J. Obstet. Gynec., *76:* 20, 1958.

Dieckmann, W. J., McCartney, C. P., and Carpenter, J. W.: The treatment of endometrial carcinoma by means of repeated applications of intracavitary radium. Amer. J. Obstet. Gynec., *70:* 1258, 1955.

Dockerty, M. B., Lovelady, S., and Foust, G.

T., Jr.: Carcinoma of corpus uteri in young women. Amer. J. Obstet. Gynec., *61:* 966, 1951.

Emge, L. A.: Geriatric aspects of primary endometrial cancer. J. Amer. Geriat. Soc., *11:* 553, 1954.

Emge, L. A.: The estrogen-cancer hypothesis in reference to protracted estrogen substitution. Obstet. Gynec., *20:* 915, 1962.

Fahlund, G. R. R., and Broders, A. C.: Postmenopausal endometrium and its relation to adenocarcinoma of corpus uteri. Amer. J. Obstet. Gynec., *51:* 22, 1946.

Finn, W. F.: Transtubal spread of tumor cells in carcinoma of body of uterus. Surg. Gynec. Obstet., *103:* 332, 1956.

Fraser, A. C.: The symptoms of premenopausal carcinoma of the uterine body. J. Obstet. Gynaec. Brit. Comm., *70:* 125, 1963.

Gardner, W. U.: Tumors in experimental animals receiving steroid hormones. Surgery, *16:* 8, 1944.

Garnett, J. D.: Constitutional stigmas associated with endometrial cancer. Amer. J. Obstet. Gynec., *76:* 11, 1958.

Giammalvo, J. T., and Kaplan, K.: The incidence of endometriosis interna in 120 cases of carcinoma of the endometrium. Amer. J. Obstet. Gynec., *75:* 161, 1958.

Gore, H., and Hertig, A. T.: Premalignant lesions of the endometrium. Clin. Obstet. Gynec., *5:* 1148, 1962.

Greene, J. W.: Feminizing mesenchynomas and endometrial carcinoma. Amer. J. Obstet. Gynec., *74:* 31, 1957.

Greene, R. R., and Peckham, B. M.: Carcinogenic cells in ovary. Amer. J. Obstet. Gynec., *61:* 637, 1951.

Gusberg, S. B.: Precursors of corpus carcinoma, estrogens and adenoamtous hyperplasia. Amer. J. Obstet. Gynec., *54:* 905, 1947.

Gusberg, S. B., and Hall, R. E.: Precursors of corpus cancer. III. Appearance of cancer of endometrium in estrogenically conditioned patients. Amer. J. Obstet. Gynec., *80:* 374, 1960.

Gusberg, S. B., and Hall, R. E.: Precursors of corpus cancer. IV. Adenomatous hyperplasia as stage 0 carcinoma of the endometrium. Amer. J. Obstet. Gynec., *87:* 662, 1963.

Gusberg, S. B., Jones, H. C., and Tovell, H. M. M.: Selection of treatment for corpus cancer. Amer. J. Obstet. Gynec., *80:* 374, 1960.

Gusberg, S. B., and Yannopoulos, D.: Therapeutic decisions in corpus cancer. Amer. J. Obstet. Gynec., *88:* 157, 1963.

Harris, H. R.: Foam cells in the stroma of carcinoma of the body of the uterus. J. Clin. Path., *11:* 19, 1958.

Hertig, A. T., and Sommers, S. C.: Genesis of endometrial carcinoma. I. Study of prior biopsies. Cancer, *2:* 946, 1949.

Jackson, R. L., and Dockerty, M. B.: Stein-

Leventhal syndrome and endometrial cancer. Amer. J. Obstet. Gynec., 73: 161, 1957.

Javert, C. T., and Hoffman, K.: Endometrial adenocarcinoma. Cancer, 5: 485, 1952.

Javert, C. T., and Renning, E. L.: Endometrial cancer survey of 610 cases treated at Woman's Hospital. Cancer, 16: 1057, 1963.

Kaufman, R. H., Abbott, J. P., and Wall, J. A.: The endometrium before and after wedge resection of the ovaries in the Stein-Leventhal syndrome. Amer. J. Obstet. Gynec., 77: 1271, 1959.

Kelly, R. M., and Baker, W. H.: Progesterone for endometrial cancer. New England. J. Med., 264: 216, 1961.

Kennedy, B. J.: A progesterone for treatment of advanced endometrial cancer. J. A. M. A., 184: 102, 1963.

Kimbrough, R. A.: Personal communication.

Kistner, R. W.: Treatment of carcinoma in situ of the endometrium. Clin. Obstet. Gynec., 5: 1166, 1962.

Kottmeier, H. L.: Place of radiation therapy and of surgery in treatment of uterine cancer. J. Obstet. Gynaec. Brit. Comm., 62: 737, 1955.

Kottmeier, H. L.: Carcinoma of the corpus uteri; diagnosis and therapy. Amer. J. Obstet. Gynec., 78: 1127, 1959.

Larson, J. A.: Estrogens and endometrial carcinoma. Obstet. Gynec., 3: 1, 1954.

Liggins, G. C., and Way, S.: A comparison of the prognosis of adenoacanthoma and adenocarcinoma of the corpus uteri. J. Obstet. Gynaec. Brit. Comm., 67: 294, 1960.

Mansell, H., and Hertig, A. T.: Granulosa-theca cell tumors and endometrial carcinoma. Obstet. Gynec., 6: 385, 1955.

Marcus, C. C.: Ovarian cortical stromal hyperplasia and carcinoma of the endometrium. Obstet. Gynec., 21: 175, 1963.

McBride, J. M.: Functional activity of genital tract in postmenopausal endometrial carcinoma. J. Obstet. Gynaec. Brit. Comm., 61: 574, 1955.

McBride, J. M.: Premenopausal cystic hyperplasia and endometrial hyperplasia. J. Obstet. Gynaec. Brit. Comm., 66: 288, 1959.

McLennan, C. E.: Argument against preoperative radium for endometrial cancer. Western J. Surg., 66: 193, 1958.

Meissner, W. A., Sommers, S. C., and Sherman, G.: Endometrial hyperplasia, endometrial carcinoma and endometriosis produced experimentally by estrogen. Cancer, 10: 500, 1957.

Miller, M. C., Robertson, G. T., Swanson, W. C., and Walker, J.: Gynecologic malignant disease in the eastern region of Scotland. 1. Malignant disease of the body of the uterus. J. Obstet. Gynaec. Brit. Comm., 69: 553, 1962.

Miller, N. F.: Carcinoma of the endometrium. Obstet. Gynec., 15: 579, 1960.

Montgomery, J. B., Lang, W. R., Farrell, D. M., and Hahn, G. A.: End results in adenocarcinoma of the endometrium managed by preoperative irradiation. Amer. J. Obstet. Gynec., 80: 972, 1960.

Nolan, J. F., and Darden, J. S.: Treatment failures in Stage I carcinoma of the uterine corpus. Amer. J. Obstet. Gynec., 83: 949, 1962.

Novak, E. R.: Uterine adenocarcinoma in patient receiving estrogens. Amer. J. Obstet. Gynec., 62: 688, 1951.

Novak, E. R.: Relationship of endometrial hyperplasia and adenocarcinoma of the uterine fundus, J. A. M. A., 154: 217, 1954.

Novak, E. R.: Postmenopausal endometrial hyperplasia. Amer. J. Obstet. Gynec., 71: 1312, 1956.

Novak, E. R., and Mohler, D. I.: Ovarian stromal changes in endometrial cancer. Amer. J. Obstet. Gynec., 65: 1099, 1953.

Novak, E. R., and Nalley, W. B.: Uterine adenoacanthoma. Obstet. Gynec., 10: 396, 1957.

Novak, E. R., and Villa Santa, U.: Factors influencing the ratio of uterine cancer. J. A. M. A., 174: 1395, 1960.

Novak, E. R., and Woodruff, J. D.: Post-irradiation malignancy. Amer. J. Obstet. Gynec., 77: 667, 1959.

Novak, E., and Yui, E.: Relation of endometrial hyperplasia to adenocarcinoma of the uterus. Amer. J. Obstet. Gynec., 32: 674, 1936.

Parsons, L., and Cesare, F.: Therapy for endometrial cancer. Surg. Gynec. Obstet., 108: 582, 1959.

Payne, F. L., Wright, R. C., and Fetterman, H. H.: Postmenopausal bleeding. Amer. J. Obstet. Gynec., 77: 1216, 1959.

Peel, J. H.: Etiology and treatment of corpus cancer. Amer. J. Obstet. Gynec., 71: 706, 1956.

Peris, L. A., Jernstrom, P., and Bowers, P. A.: Primary squamous cell carcinoma of uterine corpus. Amer. J. Obstet. Gynec., 75: 1019, 1958.

Pratt, J. H., Symmond, R. E., and Welch, J. S.: Vaginal hysterectomy for carcinoma of the fundus. Amer. J. Obstet. Gynec., 88: 1063, 1964.

Renning, E. L., and Javert, C. T.: Analysis of a series of cases of carcinoma of the endometrium treated by radium and operation. Amer. J. Obstet. Gynec., 88: 171, 1964.

Roddick, J. W., and Greene, R. R.: Ovarian stromal hyperplasia and endometrial cancer. Amer. J. Obstet. Gynec., 75: 1015, 1958.

Rutledge, F. N., Tan, S. K., and Fletcher, G. H.: Vaginal metastases from adenocarcinoma of corpus uteri. Amer. J. Obstet. Gynec., *75:* 167, 1958.

Salm, R.: Mucin production of normal and abnormal endometrium. Arch. Path., *73:* 42, 1962.

Sandberg, E. C., and McLennan, C. E.: Surgery alone for endometrial carcinoma. Obstet. Gynec., *9:* 670, 1957.

Schmitz, H. E., Smith, C. J., and Fetherston, W. C.: The effect of preoperative irradiation on adenocarcinoma of the uterus. Amer. J. Obstet. Gynec., *78:* 1048, 1959.

Schwartz, A. E., and Brunschwig, A.: Radical panhysterectomy and pelvic node excision for carcinoma of corpus uteri. Surg. Gynec. Obstet., *105:* 675, 1957.

Shaw, W., and Dasteur, B.: Association of certain ovarian cells with endometrial cancer. Brit. Med. J., *2:* 113, 1949.

Sherman, A. I., and Woolf, R. B.: Endocrine basis for endometrial carcinoma. Amer. J. Obstet. Gynec., *77:* 233, 1957.

Speert, H.: Corpus cancer; clinical, pathological, and etiological aspects. Cancer, *1:* 584, 1948.

Speert, H.: The premalignant phase of endometrial carcinoma. Cancer, *5:* 927, 1952.

Stander, R. W.: Irradiation castration. Obstet. Gynec., *10:* 223, 1957.

Stowe, L. M.: Histologic study of effect of irradiation on adenocarcinoma of endomtrium. Amer. J. Obstet. Gynec., *51:* 57, 1946.

Te Linde, R. W., Jones, H. W., and Galvin, G. A.: What are the earliest endometrial changes to justify a diagnosis of endometrial cancer? Amer. J. Obstet. Gynec., *66:* 953, 1953.

Thompson, N. J., and Graham, J. B.: Carcinoma of corpus and endocervix. Obstet. Gynec., *24:* 144, 1964.

Tweeddale, D. N., Grothey, R. L., Harvey, H. E., and Tanner, F. H.: Cervical *vs.* endometrial cancer; relative incidence. Obstet. Gynec., *2:* 623, 1953.

Varga, A., and Henricksen, E.: Urinary excretion assays of pituitary luteinizing hormone (LH) related to endometrial cancer. Obstet. Gynec., *22:* 129, 1963.

Villa Santa, U.: Tumors of mesonephric origin in the female genital tract. Amer. J. Obstet. Gynec., *89:* 680, 1964.

Wall, J. A., Franklin, R. R., and Kaufman, R. H.: Reversal of benign and malignant endometrial changes with clomiphene. Amer. J. Obstet. Gynec., *88:* 1072, 1964.

Wall, J. A., and Mastrovito, R.: Malignant neoplasms in the endometrium. Amer. J. Obstet. Gynec., *74:* 866, 1957.

Washke, G.: Beitrag zur Frage der Beziehung zwischen der Hyperplasia des Endometrium und dem Korpuskarzinom. Geburtsh. Frauenheilk., *15:* 568, 1955.

Way, S.: Vaginal metastases of carcinoma of body of uterus. J. Obstet. Gynaec. Brit. Comm., *58:* 558, 1951.

Way, S.: Etiology of carcinoma of body of uterus. J. Obstet. Gynaec. Brit. Comm., *61:* 46, 1954.

Wilson, R. A.: The roles of estrogen and progesterone in breast and genital cancer. J. A. M. A., *182:* 101, 1962.

Woll, E., Hertig, A. T., Smith, G. V., and Johnson, L. C.: Ovary in endometrial carcinoma. Amer. J. Obstet. Gynec., *56:* 617, 1948.

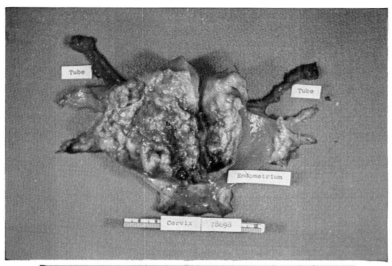

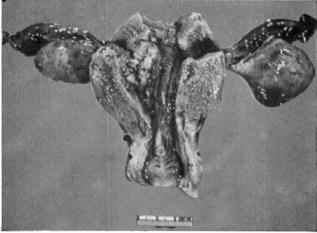

PLATE XV.I. *Top*, diffuse extensive cancer extending through myometrium; *bottom*, polypoid adenocarcinoma associated with corpus luteum.

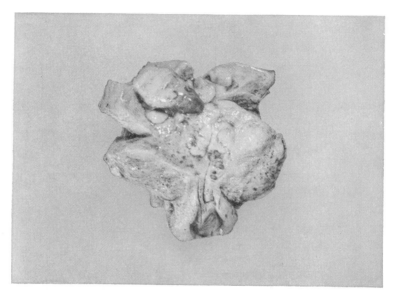

PLATE XV.II. Fundal cancer after estrogen therapy for 11 years. Note the thick myometrium with endometrial proliferation and the polypoid adenocarcinoma at left cornu.

16

MYOMA OF THE UTERUS

General Characteristics. By far the most common tumor of the uterus is the myoma. Other benign tumors of this organ (lymphangioma, mesothelioma, hemangiopericytoma, hemangioma, lipoma, etc.) are so rare that they need only scant discussion. It is estimated that fully 20% of all women over 35 years of age harbor uterine myomas, although frequently without symptoms and without the patient's knowledge of their existence. For unknown reasons the incidence of myoma is much higher in the colored than the white race. The greatest incidence is between the ages of 30 and 45, but myoma is not infrequent between 20 and 30. New tumors rarely develop after the menopause, and already existing growths diminish in size, although they do not disappear. Postmenopausal increase in size is practically always indicative of secondary degeneration of one sort or another, and should lead to the suspicion of sarcomatous change, although more innocuous degenerative changes may be found.

Myomas are frequently spoken of as *fibroids*, but it is definitely established that they are of muscle cell origin and are not derived from fibrous tissue elements. The term *fibroid* is now so thoroughly entrenched in popular use that it would be difficult to dislodge, and actually we use the terms more or less interchangeably. Myomas of the uterus may be single or, more frequently, multiple. They may be of microscopic size, or they may reach mammoth proportions, filling almost the entire abdominal cavity and weighing as much as 100 pounds or more. They are of dense structure, well encapsulated, and form small or large nodules which can be peeled out from the surrounding muscular wall of the uterus. On cutting into such a tumor its surface is seen to be of a glistening white color, and to present a characteristic whorl-like trabeculation, so that it stands out in sharp contrast to the surrounding muscularis.

Location. The location of the tumors may be *cervical* or *corporeal*, the former being much less common. When they reach very large size, as they occasionally do, they impinge on the bladder and may bring about urinary retention through blockage of the urethra. Such large cervical tumors not infrequently become impacted in the pelvic cavity, and the technical difficulty in their removal are apt to be much greater than with the more movable tumors of the corpus uteri.

Types. From the standpoint of their position as regards the various layers of the uterine wall, myomas are divided into three groups.

A) *Submucous tumors,* developing just beneath the uterine or cervical mucosa, push the latter before them as they grow. They constitute about 5% of all myomas,

319

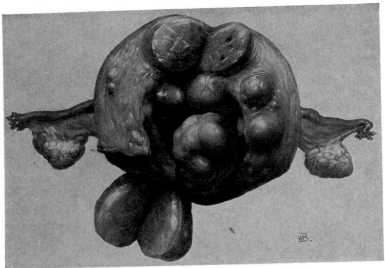

FIG. 16.1. Gross appearance of myoma, chiefly interstitial and submucous. (From Kelly, H. A.: *Operative Gynecology*. Appleton-Century-Crofts, Inc., New York, 1928.)

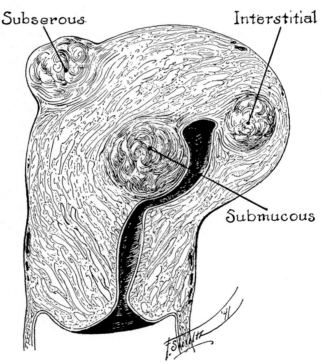

FIG. 16.2. Cut surface of myoma showing characteristic whorl-like appearance

and they are much more likely than either of the other two varieties to cause profuse bleeding and require hysterectomy, even though small. Their presence can usually be detected by feeling the curette "bump" over the protruding surface, although they are generally too firmly embedded to be removed by the curette. The hazard

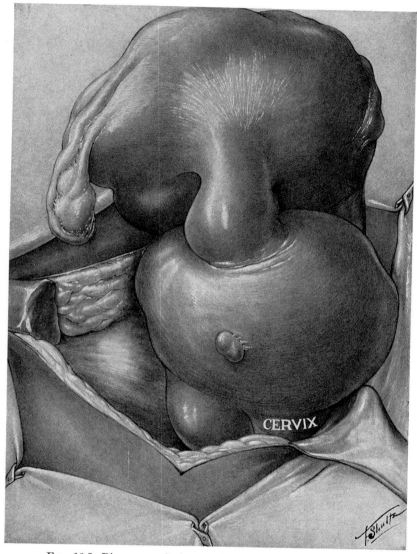

FIG. 16.3. Bizarre cervical myoma displacing corpus upward

of sarcomatous degeneration is likewise greater with this group. The covering mucous membrane becomes thin and atrophic, and frequently ulceration and infection supervene. This may penetrate deep into the underlying tumor, with resultant suppuration and sloughing.

While some submucous tumors, even of large size, are sessile, others become pedunculated as a result of the expulsive action of the uterine muscle. When the pedicle of such a *myomatous polyp* becomes long, it may protrude from the cervix or even from the vagina. The surface of such tumors frequently becomes ulcerated, with infection almost always occurring. Moreover, the circulatory impairment not infrequently brings about extensive necrosis and even gangrene. Certain myomas, especially of the pedunculated submucous variety may be associated with inversion of the uterus although this unusual entity is most common in the puerperal woman.

2) *Interstitial* or *intramural* myomas are those situated in the muscular wall, with no close propinquity to either the mucosa or serosa. When small they bring about no external change in uterine contour, but when larger and multiple, they cause marked uterine enlargement and a nodu-

lar contour and consistency. The tendency, however, is to grow toward the mucous membrane or the serous surface.

3) *Subserous* or *subperitoneal* tumors, like the submucous, may be sessile or they may become pedunculated. On occasion large veins overlying the surface of the fibroid may rupture with massive intraperitoneal bleeding; Saidi has tabulated 26 cases, a few of which have occurred during pregnancy. Often subserous tumors grow out between the folds of the broad ligament (*intraligamentary* myoma), even impinging on the ureter and iliac vessels, and sometimes giving rise to difficult problems in diagnosis and operative treatment. All manner of bizarre shapes may occur, with adhesions to surrounding organs, especially to the omentum. In such cases the tumor receives more and more blood supply from the omental vessels and less and less from the uterine vessels. Gradually the tumor may be weaned away from the uterus entirely, the pedicle becoming thinner and thinner and finally disappearing. Such *parasitic* myomas are rare, but when they occur they may give rise to interesting diagnostic problems.

Microscopic Structure. The characteristic histological picture of myoma

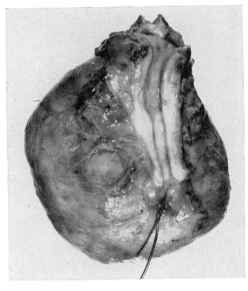

Fig. 16.4. Large myoma arising from posterior surface of cervix (end of probe at cervix).

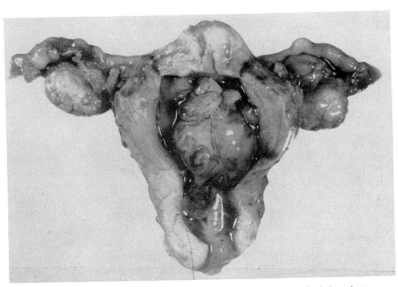

Fig. 16.5. Myomatous uterus to show large submucous myoma bulging into opened cavity with associated endometrial polyps.

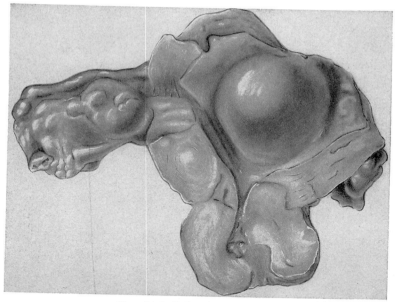

FIG. 16.6. Submucous myoma

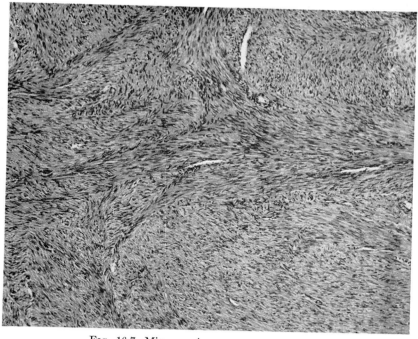

FIG. 16.7. Microscopic appearance of myoma

is that of spindle cell involuntary muscle cells arranged in an interlacing or whorl-like pattern. The cells are uniform in size, if one makes allowance for the different angles at which they are cut. Between the muscle bundles there is found a variable amount of connective tissue, and this may, indeed, be more abundant in some tumors than the muscle tissue. There is no definite capsule about the myomatous elements,

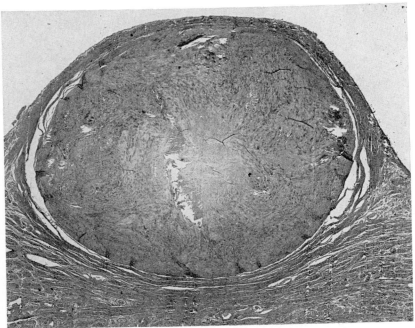

Fig. 16.8. Hyaline change in small myoma

but they are usually sharply marked off from the surrounding uterine musculature by a pseudocapsule of light areolar tissue.

Intravenous Leiomyomatosis. One may rarely find intravenous extension of benign myomatous tumor into the pelvic veins. In noting this infrequent occurrence Harper and Scully note the difficulty in distinguishing this from certain malignant processes as (endometrial) sarcoma or stromatosis, but indicate a favorable prognosis. Idelson and Davids describe benign but metastasizing myoma and review the literature on this infrequent problem; it would seem difficult to exclude the possibility of sarcoma in some area of the tumors despite the extensive studies by the authors to establish this fact. Wolfe and Mackles have described certain uncommon tumors of the generative tract, and note various blastomatous lesions, as well as neoplasms containing striated muscle, perhaps a variant of the mixed mesodermal tumor (see Chapter 18).

Secondary Changes in Myoma. A considerable number of secondary changes may occur, and these may alter the his-

tological picture very profoundly. The following may be described.

(1) Hyaline Degeneration. This, the most common of all secondary changes, is seen to some degree in almost all myomas, except those of very tiny size. The hyaline change may involve broad areas of the tumor, or it may occur in long intercommunicating strands and columns which appear to tease apart the muscle bundles.

(2) Cystic Degeneration. The tendency of hyaline degeneration is toward liquefaction, and small or large cystic cavities may thus be produced. Indeed, in extreme cases practically all of the original tumor is thus involved, being converted into a large cystic cavity. The clinical impression may thus simulate pregnancy or an ovarian cyst. Extreme edema and engorgement of the lymphatics may occur and simulate a lymphangiomatous pattern.

(3) Calcification. This is especially apt to occur where there is some circulatory disturbance, as in the myomas of old women. Where extreme, the myoma may be converted into a hard, stony mass, the

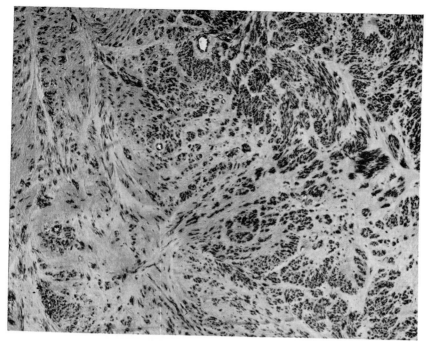

FIG. 16.9. Hyaline degeneration of myoma (microscopic)

"wombstone" of the older writers. Preoperative flat plate may reveal multiple foci of calcium deposits.

(4) *Infection and Suppuration.* This is most common in the submucous variety of myoma, which is so prone to thinning and ulceration of the overlying mucosa, thus giving access to organisms from the uterine canal.

(5) *Necrosis.* This is commonly due to impairment of the blood supply or to severe infection. Pedunculated tumors may become necrotic through torsion of the pedicle. An interesting form of necrosis is the so-called *carneous* or *red degeneration,* seen most often but not always in association with pregnancy. Its cause is not definitely known, although many believe it to be explained by an aseptic degeneration associated with hemolysis or a local tissue ischemia.

(6) *Fatty Degeneration.* This is rare, but may occur with advanced hyaline degeneration. In other cases large areas of genuine fat in the substance of a myoma are probably due to the fact that the tumor is of mixed variety.

(7) *Sarcomatous Degeneration.* This important type of change is discussed in Chapter 18, "Sarcoma of the Uterus," but it would be wise to simply note that malignant change is so rare as to in no way influence our manner of handling myomata.

Etiology and Histogenesis. Nothing of a definite nature is known as to the etiology of uterine myomas, although it is established that they are of muscle histogenesis. Most investigators accept Meyer's view that the source is not from mature muscle elements, but from cells of an immature type. Miller's work with tissue culture is provocative but preliminary. Schwarz's ideas suggest an origin from the perivascular muscle fibers, and the case report by Marshall and Morris seems confirmatory of this as an occasional occurrence.

There has been some discussion as to the possible role of the *ovarian hormones* in the causation of uterine myoma, but the evidence for this theory is far from convincing. No explanation has been suggested as to why they occur in some

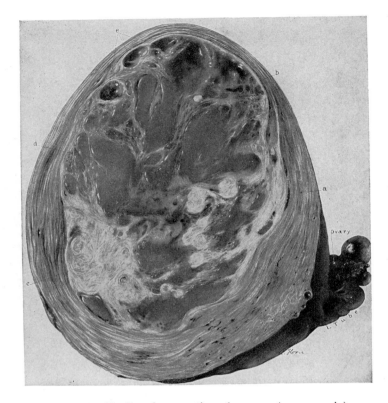

FIG. 16.10. Hyaline degeneration of myoma (macroscopic)

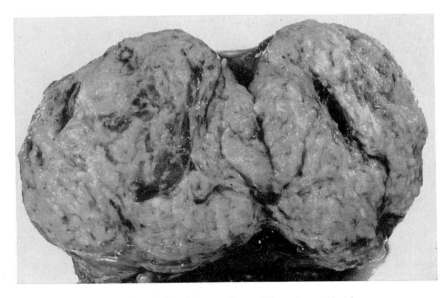

FIG. 16.11. Extensive degeneration with early cystic changes

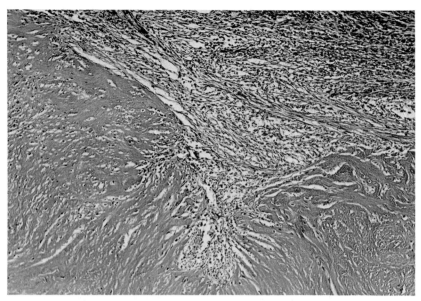

Fig. 16.12. Margin of myoma undergoing necrosis

women and not in others, since estrogen is produced in practically all women during the reproductive period of life and sometimes beyond. Furthermore, a good many women with myomas ovulate, producing progesterone, supposedly more or less antiestrogenic and antitumorigenic. The experimental production of fibroid tumors has been reported by a number of observers but, with one or two exceptions, these artifically produced tumors do not resemble the common form of uterine myoma either histologically or in their topographical distribution. Especially provocative has been the work of Lipschutz, who has been able by means of estrogens to produce in guinea pigs fibromatous tumors, not only on the surface of the uterus but also in various extragenital locations throughout the abdomen. This fibromatogenic effect of estrogen could be prevented by the simultaneous administration of progesterone or testosterone propionate. Interesting as this work is, its bearing upon the etiology of uterine myoma is not clear, and certainly cannot be assumed.

Symptoms and Physical Signs. The mere presence of myoma does not necessarily produce any symptoms, and every practitioner knows that even large growths may be entirely symptomless.

Palpable Mass. In a considerable proportion of cases the patient is impelled to seek advice because she has noticed a lump in the lower abdomen or, in the case of large tumors, a general enlargement of the abdomen. Sometimes a mass of which the patient had been unaware is noticed by the physician in the course of an abdominal examination made for other indications.

Bleeding. The symptom which is, in the minds of most physicians, most characteristically linked up with fibroids is excessive or prolonged menstruation. This, however, is frequently lacking. Moreover, even when bleeding is present, it does not by any means follow that it is produced by an existing myoma. The abnormal bleeding usually takes the form of hypermenorrhea (excessive menstruation), but intermenstrual bleeding or bloody leukorrhea may also be noted. In the latter case, one must always be on the alert for an associated lesion, such as adenocarcinoma, polyp, or a functional factor. In a large proportion of cases there is no doubt that dysfunction of the ovaries is the responsible factor in the

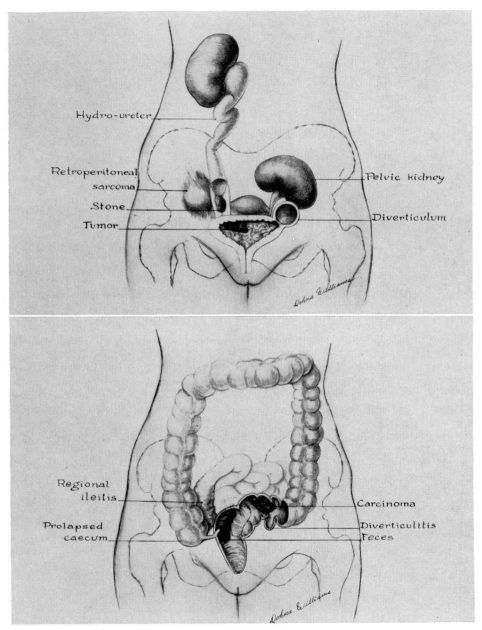

FIG. 16.13. *Top*, urinary disorders leading to lower abdominal pain with associated myoma. *Bottom*, gastrointestinal causes of pain which may coexist with myoma.

bleeding, and this is suggested by the frequent existence of hyperplasia of the endometrium in myomatous uteri.

The type of myoma most likely to cause bleeding is the submucous. Interstitial growths may or may not cause menstrual excess, the mechanism in such cases being probably an interference with uterine contractility. Subserous growths in themselves probably never produce abnormal hemorrhage.

The frequency of bleeding with the submucous tumors is thought to be due to the rupture during menstruation of ves-

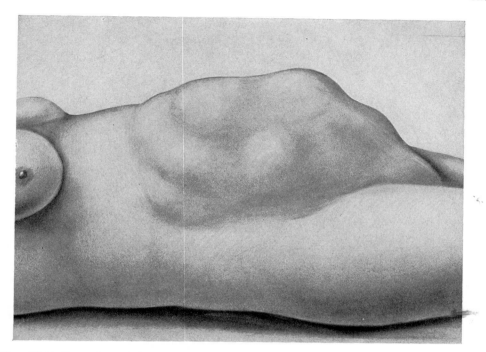

FIG. 16.14. Irregular nodular contour of abdomen produced by a huge myoma in a thin patient. (From Kelly, H. A., and Cullen, T. S.: *Myomata of the Uterus*. W. B. Saunders Company, Philadelphia, 1909.)

sels in the venous plexus just beneath the uterine mucosa. Sampson many years ago demonstrated by his injection experiments that it is from this venous network that the bleeding of myoma has its source, and these observations have been more recently confirmed by Faulkner. Other factors in the bleeding of submucous tumors are the frequency of ulceration, with direct opening up of blood vessels, and the venous stasis so often present in the polypoid tumors because of compression of the pedicle. Another menstrual symptom not infrequently seen is a shortening of the menstrual interval (*polymenorrhea*) possibly due to the effect of the associated hyperemia upon the function of the ovary.

Pain. Pain is certainly not a characteristic symptom of myoma, although it is often present. Concomitant pelvic inflammatory disease or endometriosis, as well as various genitourinary or gastrointestinal causes of pain must be considered (Fig. 16.13). The most frequent form seen with the larger tumors is a *sensation of weight and bearing-down.* More common is *dysmenorrhea*, which may be produced by even small interstitial or submucous growths.

The development of pain and tenderness in large, previously painless myomas is generally due to circulatory disturbances, with perhaps local necrosis, or to inflammatory change, with adhesions to surrounding structures, such as the omentum or intestine. In the rare cases in which pedunculated subserous myomas undergo torsion of the pedicle, the pain may be acute, and accompanied by nausea and vomiting. Finally, in very large growths, or in those firmly impacted in the pelvis, pain may be the result of pressure upon nerve trunks, and in such cases it may radiate to the back and lower extremities.

Pressure Effects. The larger myomas often make pressure upon the bladder, producing *bladder irritability, increased frequency of urination,* and possibly *dys-*

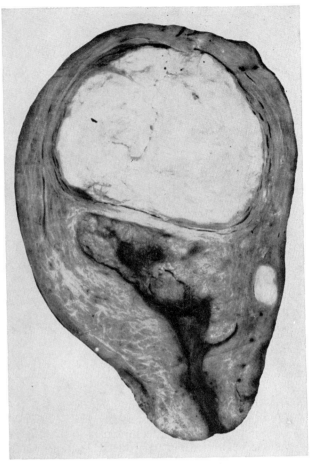

FIG. 16.15. Myoma with associated endometrial cancer. (Courtesy of Prof. Robert J. Kellar, Edinburgh.)

uria. When impacted in the pelvis they may bring about *retention of urine* through blockage of the urethra. When of sufficient size and appropriately located, hydro-ureteronephrosis may ensue, along with a real possibility of damage to the urinary tract at operation. The pressure effects upon the rectum are less conspicuous, although *constipation* and occasionally *pain on defecation* may be produced. Very large growths which extend into the upper abdomen may produce *digestive disturbances,* and in extreme cases pressure upon the vena cava or iliac veins may even cause *edema* of the lower extremities.

Secondary Symptoms. *Anemia* with *weakness, lassitude, headache,* and *short-*

ness of breath may occur. There was formerly much discussion of the so-called *"fibroid heart,"* referring to a form of myocardial degeneration supposedly characteristically associated with uterine myoma. It is now generally agreed that no such characteristic cardiac condition exists. When genuine cardiac disease is present, it is coincidental, while functional cardiac disturbances are often explainable by the pressure and circulatory disturbance produced by large tumors. A few cases of erythrocytosis have been attributed to myomata which are generally large (Rothman and Rennard).

Myoma and Pregnancy. There is a considerable difference of opinion as to the role of myoma in the production of infertility. No one would doubt that even very large myomata are perfectly compatible with uncomplicated pregnancy and normal delivery. On the other hand, most students, such as the late Isadore Rubin, feel strongly that fibroids may on occasion be a factor in impairing fertility, and consequently mandate myomectomy, *after other causes for sterility are excluded.* Indeed it is not difficult to envision how a myoma might produce such a distortion of the cavity or malposition so that failure to implant or early abortion might be a sequel.

At the same time there are those who insist that the myoma *per se* is not the important factor. Repeated anovulation has been proposed as the actual cause of sterility, and sustained estrogen, unopposed by progesterone, is suggested as an etiological agent for myomatous development. If this be so, it is difficult to reconcile with the surgical results following myomectomy. As Rubin has noted, the incidence of pregnancy following myomectomy is 25 to 40%, far higher than nonoperated sterile women might achieve, even after prolonged marital relationships. The size, number, and location of fibroids in relation to the cornua and endometrial cavities are obvious variables so that no guarantee can be given to any woman in whom myomectomy is contemplated. Rubin suggests that it be considered "an alternative to hysterectomy in order to improve the chances of parenthood," and a more recent review by Ingersoll summarizes the indications for and results with myomectomy.

A patient should never be promised myomectomy before operation; the surgeon may find it desirable or even necessary to remove the uterus, for on occasion there may be considerable bleeding. The careful clinician will assure the woman that he is cognizant of her wishes and will do his best to abide by them, but the ultimate decision must be his. He should likewise point out that myomectomy will not assure pregnancy, but there is a definite possibility, 15 to 25% as noted by Brown, Chamberlain, and TeLinde,

that subsequent hysterectomy may be required. If, however, within that interim a pregnancy or two should intervene, most women will gladly accept a second operation.

Should the patient with a myoma become pregnant it is possible that there will be no problems of any kind throughout the gestation. On the other hand, there seems no doubt that, in addition to producing infertility, myomas may be a factor in causing a disproportionately high incidence of abortion, generally in the first trimester.

In the second trimester pain and tenderness may occur in a previously asymptomatic myoma, with fever, leukocytosis, and development of a surgically acute abdomen. This is generally due to carneous (red) degeneration, a curious phenomenon of pregnancy which is probably related to impaired or inadequate circulation in the fibroid, although other degenerative changes or causes of an acute abdomen must be considered. Should expectant conservative treatment not avail, exploration with myomectomy is reluctantly carried out. Curiously enough most of these surgically-treated women do not go into labor or even bleed, and we can recall such bland behavior even when the uterine cavity was entered. Nevertheless many obstetricians will elect to give large doses of prophylactic progesterone. Similarly, many will later elect cesarean section, although it is our own opinion that myomectomy itself would not always contraindicate delivery from below, unless there are other factors to be considered.

In the third trimester and at delivery a fibroid may cause premature bleeding, uterine inertia, or mechanical blockage to normal passage through the birth canal. Postpartum hemorrhage due to an atonic uterus and infection of the endometrium and adjacent myoma is more common after vaginal delivery. Cesarean section with hysterectomy is performed frequently these days, and is probably easier and preferable to multiple myomectomy when procreative desires are complete. Total hysterectomy immediately following cesarean section is generally simple for the well trained gynecologist. Although the tissues are quite vascular, planes of cleavage are extraordinarily good. At operation the cervix is so soft that it is difficult to feel within the vagina; if a subtotal hysterectomy is first accomplished, the operator's finger can then be placed down into the endocervical canal, allowing for easy identification and removal of the cervix.

The clinician should recall, however, that small myomas may increase remarkably in size during the course of pregnancy, and yet regress when it is terminated. Whether this is due to an increased hormonal stimulus or simply to a better blood supply is uncertain, although the latter seems likely. Full consideration of the temporary but evanescent growth of fibroids should precede any final decision to perform hysterectomy at the time of cesarean section.

Physical Signs. *Abdominal Palpation.* In some cases a presumptive diagnosis of uterine myoma can be made by palpating the tumor through the abdominal wall, especially when the latter is not too obese. Such tumors present as large or small masses springing from the pelvis and growing upward into the abdominal cavity. They are hard, generally of irregular nodular contour, movable unless so large that they fill most of the abdomen, and not tender.

Bimanual Pelvic Examination. In many cases the diagnosis of myoma is extremely easy, especially when bowel and bladder are empty. One or more nodular outgrowths on the uterine surface can be felt between the examining fingers within the vagina and the external hand. The size and number of the outgrowths vary from a tiny, insignificant, single protuberance to many large nodules which may increase the aggregate size of the uterus enormously. Usually the uterine origin of the nodules is obvious from their direct continuity with the uterine surface.

The problem, however, is not always so simple, and examination under anesthesia is occasionally necessary. In the case of obese or highly nervous women, where the uterus is hard to outline, it may be difficult to determine whether a firm globular mass felt behind the cervix is a myoma of the posterior wall or merely a rather large retroflexed fundus. Again, when a firm, solid mass is felt laterally, it is not always easy to decide between a pedunculated subserous myoma and a solid tumor of the ovary. The latter is apt to be much more freely movable, and careful palpation will ordinarily permit of its definite separation from the uterus, with a clear interval between the tumor and the mass. It must be remembered, however, that adnexal masses, either inflammatory or neoplastic, may be so firmly adherent to the uterus that they may simulate uterine myoma quite perfectly. Even a thick-walled ovarian cyst may be readily mistaken for myoma, especially as some myomas are rather soft because of secondary degeneration. Culdoscopy may on occasion be decisive, if there is no indication for laporotomy.

One of the most important diagnostic problems presented to the gynecologist is to differentiate between myoma and early pregnancy, or to decide whether or not pregnancy exists in an obviously myomatous uterus. Nowadays the problem has been much simplified because of the accuracy of even early "quick" pregnancy tests, and it is desirable to obtain such tests whenever there is any suspicion of pregnancy.

In spite of the greatest care and expertness on the part of the gynecologist, a certain inevitable proportion of errors will be made in attempting to differentiate myoma from other pelvic conditions. Where there is any question that the intrapelvic tumor is ovarian rather than uterine in origin, laparotomy should be performed because of the dismal nature of many ovarian lesions.

The submucous variety of myoma presents special difficulties in diagnosis, being concealed within the uterus, they may show no appreciable enlargement or irregularity. In such cases *diagnostic curettage* is indicated in an effort to determine the cause of the patient's bleeding, which may be due to any one of a number of causes, such as submucous myoma, incomplete miscarriage, polyp, adenocarcinoma, or to a functional factor. The decision is often based on the palpatory findings of the curette as well as on the gross and miscroscopic examination of the tissue removed by the curette, and we feel that the use of hysteroscopy or hysterograms adds little. A submucous myoma can usually be diagnosed by careful manipulation of the curette, which reveals a moundlike eminence at some point of the uterine surface, with often marked distortion of the uterine cavity. Radium therapy is strongly contraindicated in submucous tumors because of the possibility of infection.

Myometrial Hypertrophy. The condition of an enlarged symmetrical uterus (in the absence of adenomyosis) has been in a sense a "dumping ground," dignified by such nomenclature as "fibrosis uteri, chronic subinvolution, chronic passive congestion, etc." While in many instances the terminology may represent an attempt by an overenthusiastic surgeon to sneak a normal parous uterus by an alert tissue committee, we believe that on occasion the grossly, but diffusely enlarged uterus may represent a valid symptom-producing entity which Lewis, Lee, and Easler have chosen to speak of as *myometrial hypertrophy.*

They arbitrarily utilize a weight of more than 120 gm. as a diagnostic index, and point out that the increased size is due to hypertrophic smooth muscle hypertrophy. It is suggested that over 5% of uteri removed warrant this designation which is associated with excessive menstrual bleeding. Although the authors seem loath to assign a cause-effect basis, it would seem that the mere increase in size of the uterus might be expected to incur more profuse periods, aided in part by an overstretched if hypertrophic myometrium that might be incompetent and unable to exhibit adequate contraction, so that the periods are prolonged and heavy. Certainly any uterus weighing more than 200 gm. should be considered abnormally large. Even if there is no demonstrable lesion, the pathologist should not be critical of the surgeon who removes a uterus in which abnormal bleeding persists after several curettages and trials of hormone therapy.

TREATMENT

In general, any one of three plans of treatment is indicated when uterine myoma has been diagnosed, *viz.*

(1) Expectant Treatment, with Periodic Examination. Not all myomas call for active treatment, but since they all present some degree of potentiality for subsequent problems, the selection of an expectant plan of treatment should always be combined with the advice that periodic examination be sought at regular 6-month intervals. When menstrual function ceases, a myoma rarely causes difficulty, often involuting. Thus, in the immediately premenopausal woman simple observation is all the treatment that an only slightly symptomatic myoma warrants. In every case age, procreative desires, the likelihood of an incipient menopause, etc., should be factors to consider, even when symptoms suggest surgery.

We feel it unwise, however, to allow even an asymptomatic myoma to grow longer than a 10-week pregnancy, particularly when the woman is young and the tumor has a long time to grow extremely large, or when there is evidence of rapid growth. Very large myomas can be difficult surgical problems, and when ultimate hysterectomy seems inevitable it is best performed before the possibility of operative complications is increased. If a conservative plan is contemplated for a growing myoma, it is wise to obtain pyelograms as a means of assaying any dilatation of the upper urinary tract.

In the postmenopausal era a myomatous uterus is rarely symptomatic. However, any postclimacteric growth of a myoma suggests either sarcomatous change or the possibility that the supposed uterine tumor is really ovarian; in either case exploration is indicated.

(2) Radiotherapy. In this era of improved surgical techniques, an irradiation menopause is utilized only in bad risk patients, and the fibroid must be smaller than a 3-month pregnancy, not submucous, not associated with inflammatory disease, or impinging on the rectum. Today's gynecologist will find rare indications for an irradiation menopause, much preferring abdominal or vaginal hysterectomy. It is our own preference to reserve vaginal hysterectomy for small tumors because morcellation of large or multiple myomas can be extremely bloody. Even serious medical complications can be safely handled with current anesthesia methods, drugs, etc., so that major surgery may be denied only a very few women.

An exceedingly important preliminary to radiation, and one never to be omitted, is *diagnostic curettage*, and microscopic examination of the endometrium. *The mere fact that a patient with uterine myoma has abnormal bleeding is no proof that the myoma is the cause of the bleeding*, which may be due to entirely different factors, and sometimes to malignant intrauterine disease. Indeed, there is some controversy as to whether an irradiation menopause may incite endometrial cancer in the postmenopausal era. Obviously radiotherapy should be avoided in the young woman lest an artificial menopause is produced.

In discussing radiotherapy in the treatment of uterine myoma, reference is made to both radium and deep x-ray therapy, both of which have a place, and both of which are highly effective. Radium has the advantage of requiring only a single treatment, and this can often be applied at the time of the diagnostic curettage. As for ultimate results, our experience has been that these are just as satisfactory with the use of deep x-ray, although termination of the bleeding is not so rapid. A recent article by Montgomery and Long covers all phases of radiation therapy in the treatment of myomas.

(3) Surgical Treatment. This is the only treatment to be considered in the case of pedunculated submucous tumors, which are usually easily removable through the vagina. The vaginal approach is all the more important where sloughing and infection are present, because of the greater danger of peritonitis were an abdominal operation done in such cases.

Myomectomy has its great field in the removal of tumors in cases where the preservation of reproductiveness is of great importance. Even when the tumors are multiple and of considerable size, myomectomy is often feasible, and Rubin has been one of the great disciples of multiple myomectomy, as noted earlier in this chapter. However, there are disadvantages to be considered, such as the development of extensive adhesions, the weakening of the uterine wall produced by the removal of large tumors, and subsequent tumor formation. Israel and Mutch have summarized the indications and techniques of myomectomy.

In spite of these risks, definitely greater than with a clean-cut hysterectomy, the operation is often indicated when the patient is extremely anxious for the possibility of pregnancy. Many such women are more than willing to assume such risks as have been mentioned, and the possibility of later hysterectomy, if they can be given a chance for pregnancy, and they are often rewarded by materialization of their hopes. On the other hand, in the presence of large and numerous myomatous nodules, the chances for the patient to bear children are so slight, and the risks of subsequent trouble so real, that hysterectomy is unquestionably the wiser procedure. The course in each case will be determined by a consideration of the individual existing circumstances, and by the conservative or radical trends of the individual surgeon. Myomectomy should always be preceded by diagnostic curettage if there has been abnormal bleeding, as the latter may be due to an intrauterine lesion, like adenocarcinoma, and not to the myoma (Fig. 16.15).

When hysterectomy is performed upon women still in the menstruating age, there

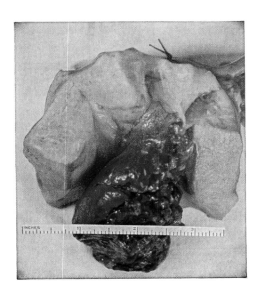

PLATE XVI.I. Sloughing submucous myoma

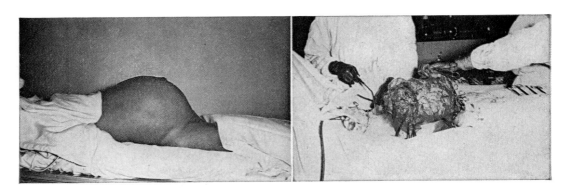

PLATE XVI.II. *Left*, gross distortion of abdomen in 110-pound patient by otherwise asymptomatic myoma. *Right*, part of 30-pound tumor as viewed at operation, some being deep in pelvis.

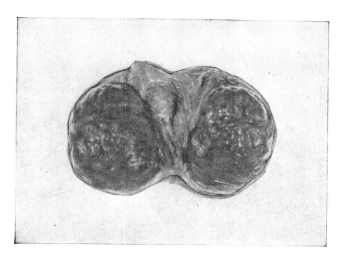

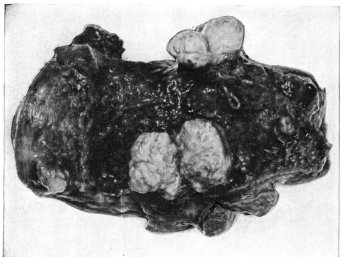

PLATE XVI.III. *Top*, red or carneous degeneration of myoma. *Bottom*, submucous myoma in uterus removed by Porro Cesarean section.

is no question as to the *advisability of leaving one or both ovaries*. In addition to preventing development of a precipitate menopause, there is some question as to what role the postmenopausal gonad may play in guarding against the development of coronary and generalized atherosclerosis. Actually, there is considerable evidence that the postmenopausal ovary is not to be regarded as a functionless, useless organ. In discussing pathology found in postsurgical preserved ovaries, Randall, Hall, and Armenia agree that there is a certain risk of subsequent neoplasm but indicate that conservation of ovarian tissue is worth the risk, even where the previous operation was done for ovarian disease.

The qualified gynecologist will of course perform total hysterectomy in something more than 95 % of all cases. The realistic clinician will admit, however, that an occasional case, complicated by extensive inflammatory disease or endometriosis, is best treated by a subtotal operation. He should be praised rather than criticized for his discrimination, and we do not instruct our residents to *always* perform a complete operation in the face of medical or other complicating factors. Where conservation of the cervical stump seems likely, preoperative smear and biopsy are mandatory.

REFERENCES

Abithol, M. M.: Submucus fibroids complicating pregnancy, labor, and delivery. Obstet. Gynec., *10:* 529, 1957.

Barter, R. H., and Parks, J.: Myoma uteri associated with pregnancy. Clin. Obstet. Gynec., *1:* 519, 1958.

Brandfass, R. T., and Everts-Suarez, E. A.: Lipomatous tumors of the uterus. Amer. J. Obstet. Gynec., *70:* 359, 1955.

Brown, A. L., Chamberlain, R. W., and Te Linde, R. W.: Myomectomy, Amer. J. Obstet. Gynec., *71:* 759, 1956.

Counseller, V. S., Hunt, W., and Haigler, F. H., Jr.: Carcinoma of ovary following hysterectomy. Amer. J. Obstet. Gynec., *69:* 538, 1955.

Everett, H. S.: Effect of uterine myomas on the urinary tract. Clin. Obstet. Gynec., *1:* 429, 1958.

Faulkner, R. L.: Blood vessels of myomatous uterus. Amer. J. Obstet. Gynec., *47:* 185, 1944.

Faulkner, R. L.: Red degeneration of myomas. Amer. J. Obstet. Gynec., *53:* 474, 1947.

Gerbie, A. B., Greene, R. R., and Reis, R. A.: Heteroplastic bone and cartilage in the female genital tract. Obstet. Gynec., *11:* 573, 1958.

Harper, R. S., and Scully, R. E.: Intravenous leiomyomatosis of the uterus. Obstet. Gynec., *18:* 519, 1961.

Henriksen, E.: Lipoma of uterus; report of 3 cases. Western J. Surg., *60:* 609, 1952.

Idelson, M. G., and Davids, A. M.: Metastasis of uterine fibromyomata. Obstet. Gynec., *21:* 78, 1962.

Ingersoll, F. M.: Myomectomy and fertility. Fertil. Steril., *14:* 596, 1963.

Israel, S. L., and Mutch, J. C.: Myomectomy. Clin. Obstet. Gynec., *1:* 455, 1958.

Kanter, A. E., and Zummo, B. P.: Lipomas of gynecologic interest. Amer. J. Obstet. Gynec., *71:* 376, 1956.

Kelly, H. A., and Cullen, T. S.: *Myomata of the Uterus.* W. B. Saunders Company, Philadelphia, 1909.

Kimbrough, R. A.: General considerations in the treatment of myoma uteri. Clin. Obstet. Gynec., *1:* 437, 1958.

Lardaro, H. H.: Extensive myomectomy. Amer. J. Obstet. Gynec., *79:* 43, 1960.

Lewis, P. L., Lee, A. B. H., and Easler, R. E.: Myometrial hypertrophy. Amer. J. Obstet. Gynec., *84:* 1032, 1962.

Lipschutz, A.: *Steroid Hormones and Tumors,* Ed. 1. The Williams and Wilkins Company, Baltimore, 1950.

Marshall, J. F., and Morris, D. S.: Intravenous leiomyomatosis of the uterus and pelvis; case report. Ann. Surg., *149:* 126, 1959.

Meyer, R.: Die pathologische Anatomie der Gerbarmutter. In *Handbuch der spezielle pathologische Anatomie und Histologie,* edited by F. Henke and O. Lubarsch, Vol. 7, Part 1. Julius Springer, Berlin, 1930.

Miller, N. F., and Ludovici, P. P.: Investigation into origin and development of uterine myomas. Amer. J. Obstet. Gynec., *70:* 720, 1955.

Miller, N. F., Ludovici, P. P., and Douta, E.: Problem of the uterine fibroid. Amer. J. Obstet. Gynec., *66:* 734, 1953.

Montgomery, J. B., and Long, J. P.: Radiation therapy for myoma uteri. Clin. Obstet. Gynec., *1:* 445, 1958.

Novak, E. R.: Benign and malignant changes in uterine myomas. Clin. Obstet. Gynec., *1:* 421, 1958.

Pedowitz, P., Felmus, L. B., and Grayzel, D. M.: Vascular tumors of uterus. I. Benign vascular tumors. II. Malignant vascular tumors. Amer. J. Obstet. Gynec., *69:* 1291, 1309, 1955.

Pedowitz, P., Felmus, L. B., and Grayzel, D.
M.: Vascular tumors of the uterus. Amer.
J. Obstet. Gynec., *71:* 1256, 1956.

Plaut, A.: Lymphangiocystic fibroma of
uterus. Amer. J. Obstet. Gynec., *51:* 842,
1946.

Randall, C. L., Hall, D. W., and Armenia, C.
S.: Pathology in the preserved ovary after
unilateral oophorectomy. Amer. J. Obstet.
Gynec., *84:* 1233, 1962.

Rothman, D., and Rennard, M.: Myoma-
erythrocytosis syndrome. Obstet. Gynec.,
21: 102, 1962.

Rubin, I. C.: Uterine fibromyomas and sterility. Clin. Obstet. Gynec., *1:* 501, 1958.

Sabbagh, M. L.: Lipoma of the uterus. Obstet.
Gynec., *4:* 399, 1954.

Saidi, F., Constable, J. D., and Ulfelder, H.:
Massive intraperitoneal hemmorhage due
to uterine fibroids. Amer. J. Obstet.
Gynec., *82:* 367, 1961.

Sampson, J. A.: Blood supply of uterine myomata. Surg. Gynec. Obstet., *14:* 215, 1912.

Schwarz, O.: Benign diffuse enlargement of the
uterus. Amer. J. Obstet. Gynec., *61:* 902,
1951.

Sitaratra, A., and Sarna, V.: Fundal fibromyoma of the uterus causing nonpuerperal
inversion. Antiseptic, *59:* 435, 1962.

Stander, R. W.: Irradiation castration. Obstet.
Gynec., *10:* 223, 1957.

Stout, A. P.: Hemangiopericytoma. Cancer,
2: 1027, 1949.

Taylor, H. C., Jr.: Endocrine factors in origin
of tumors of uterus. Surgery, *16:* 91, 1944.

Wolfe, S. A., and Mackles, A.: Uncommon
myogenic tumors of the female generative
tract. Obstet. Gynec., *22:* 199, 1963.

17

ADENOMYOSIS OF THE UTERUS

Adenomyosis of the uterus is characterized by histologically benign invasion of the uterine musculature by the endometrium, which normally is found only lining the uterine cavity. It has in the past been frequently spoken of as adenomyoma, but the suffix "oma" has reference to a tumor, and adenomyosis is not a tumor in the proper sense of the word, any more than is endometriosis. As a matter of fact, there would seem to be many points of similarity between adenomyosis and pelvic endometriosis, although adenomyosis characteristically affects the 40-year-old, parous woman, and endometriosis the younger, sterile patient. In both, however, we deal with ectopic growth of endometrial tissue. For that matter, adenomyosis was at one time spoken of as *endometriosis interna*, to distinguish it from endometriosis externa or pelvic endometriosis.

It is true that in some locations definite tumor masses may occur which are made up of muscle tissue and endometrium, and to these the term *adenomyoma* is more properly applied. Such tumor nodules, for example, not infrequently develop on the round and broad ligaments, but as a rule the process is too diffuse to be considered as a discrete tumor. With adenomyosis of the uterus we apparently deal with an exaggerated growth activity of the endometrium, which pushes down into the underlying muscle. With this endometrial invasion is combined a marked, generalized overgrowth of the muscle elements.

Pathology. The enlargement of the uterus produced by adenomyosis is a diffuse one, and not nodular, as in the case of myoma. There is often enormous thickening of the uterine wall, usually asymmetrical, the posterior wall being more often and more extensively involved than the anterior. In some cases, however, the enlargement may be quite uniform. Never, however, does the uterus reach the large proportions seen in many cases of myoma, rarely being larger than a large orange. It should not be forgotten, however, that myoma and adenomyosis often coexist.

The distinctive *microscopic* characteristic is the presence of islands of typical endometrial tissue scattered throughout the muscle, often far beneath the endometrial surface, and sometimes extending to the peritoneal surface. The endometrial glands in the ectopic tissue are surrounded by typical endometrial stromal cells. Occasionally the endometrium is of functioning type, menstruating just as does the normal surface endometrium. In such cases collections of chocolate-colored menstrual blood are seen throughout the wall, constituting miniature uterine cavities.

Far oftener the endometrium is of the

337

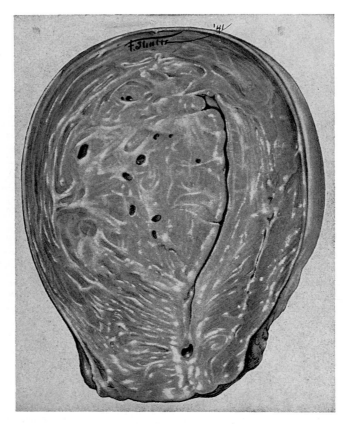

FIG. 17.1 Gross appearance of uterus with diffuse adenomyosis, in sagittal section

immature, nonfunctioning type, often presenting a typical Swiss-cheese hyperplasia pattern. When the endometrium penetrates to the peritoneum, it may continue to propagate itself, sometimes producing extensive pelvic endometriosis. In such cases the uterus is often densely adherent to the rectum and other surrounding organs. The muscle tissue shows marked hyperplasia, with a whorl-like tendency not unlike that seen in myoma. Pregnancy may bring about decidual changes in the invading endometrium quite like those noted in the uterine mucosa proper.

Sandberg and Cohn have indicated that superficial adenomyosis rarely shows decidual changes whereas this is relatively frequent in the more extreme degrees of myometrial invasion. It strikes us that the logical explanation is that continued growth has allowed the aberrant endo-

metrium to mature and achieve the faculty of progesterone response, and indeed this is one of several possibilities noted by the authors.

It would thus seem that adenomyosis may be compared to an inverting polyp, and may be made up of a mature responsive form of endometrium or more often of an immature juvenile tissue completely incapable of response to progesterone. Hyperplasia in conjunction with a biphasic cycle is common and proliferative forms are not rare. Actual *adenocarcinoma* developing in these aberrant islands has been reported on a few occasions (Novak and Woodruff). Perhaps this origin is more common than appreciated. Extension of any malignant spread of adenomyosis would almost certainly traverse up the lines of least resistance, the glandular channels, and involve the endometrial surface. Symptoms such as bleeding would

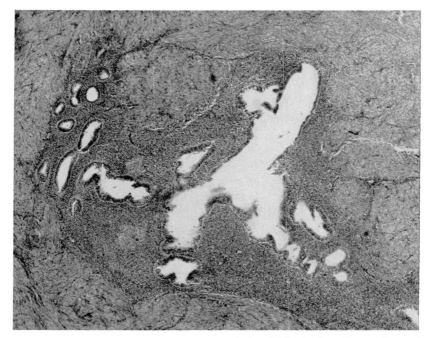

FIG. 17.2. Microscopic appearance of adenomyosis in which the invading endometrium is of functioning (secretory) type.

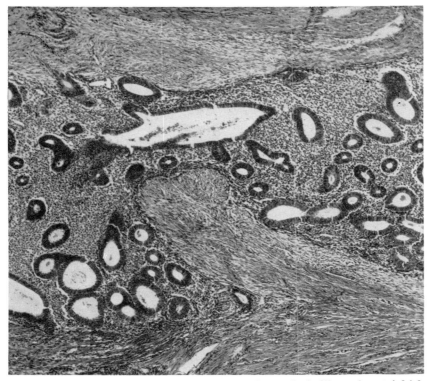

FIG. 17.3. Adenomyosis showing a nonfunctioning hyperplasia-like endometrial island

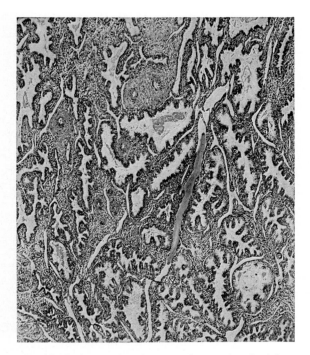

FIG. 17.4. Decidual changes in adenomyosis associated with pregnancy

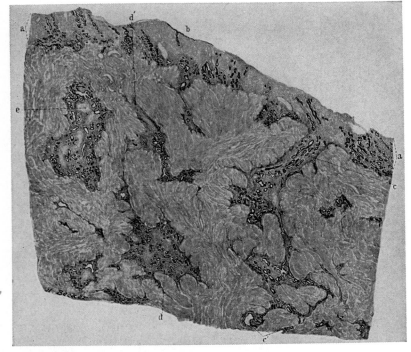

FIG. 17.5. Low power section of wall of uterus showing manner of invasion of uterine musculature by endometrium.

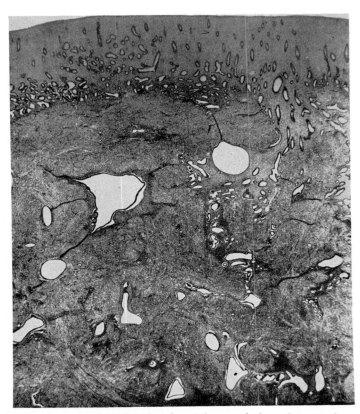

FIG. 17.6. Showing how glands of basal endometrium push down into uterine muscle in case of adenomyosis.

often be produced only at this time, but when hysterectomy is finally accomplished the pathological diagnosis is "endometrial adenocarcinoma with myometrial extension." For a recent review, the reader is referred to the article by Colman and Rosenthal, as well as the excellent resume by Emge.

In any case a very real problem to the pathologist is distinction between well differentiated endometrial adenocarcinoma with early invasion and superficial malignancy with associated adenomyosis. That the latter sequence is common we are well aware of, and insofar as differential diagnosis is concerned, we too are often uncertain. If, however, there is no observed evidence of direct invasion with reaction on the part of the invaded myometrium or if the ectopic endometrium is obviously better differentiated than the

surface adenocarcinoma, it is probable that there is merely associated adenomyosis.

Histogenesis. The histogenesis of aberrant endometrium was formerly widely discussed, but it is now clearly established, as a result of the work of Cullen and others, that it has its source from downward growth of the surface endometrium. Histological studies often show the direct continuity of the deep islands with the surface mucosa, although the overgrowth of muscle elements may nip off the connecting endometrial process.

Stromal Adenomyosis or Endometriosis. Robertson *et al.* have called attention to a form of adenomyosis in which the invading tissue is altogether stromal, with no gland elements, and which some designate as stromal endometriosis, although a better designation

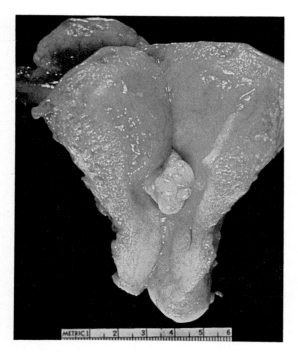

Fig. 17.7. Benign stromatosis; compare lack of invasion with that shown in Fig. 17.9. (Courtesy of Dr. D. Nichols, Buffalo, New York.)

would seem to be stromal endometrios is or adenomyosis, in spite of the absence of gland elements. While such stromal invasion occurs, it is relatively rare, and it should not be assumed unless the stu dy of many sections demonstrates an actu al absence of glands. The above-mentioned authors speak of benign and malignant forms, but the latter is better looked upon as akin to a low grade endometrial sarcoma (see Chapter 18, "Sarcoma of the Uterus").

Recent publications on the subject of this lesion, frequently referred to as *stromatosis*, have clarified many of its pathological and clinical characteristics, although its comparative rarity suggests the need for only a short discussion. It has been suggested that there are three categories of cases, with all intermediate gradations. (1) The simplest is identical with ordinary adenomyosis except that the invading endometrium is made up entirely of stroma, with no glands. It is clinically entirely benign. (2) In this

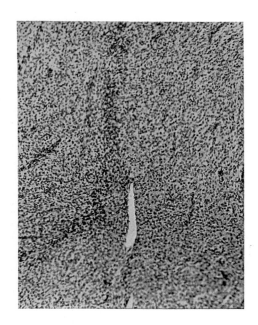

Fig. 17.8. Stromal adenomyosis. The invading stroma in this case showing malignant characteristics.

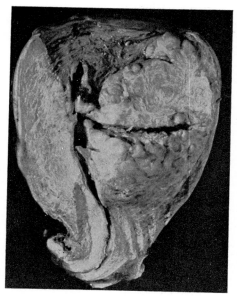

FIG. 17.9. Gross appearance of uterus with malignant stromatosis; compare with benign stromatosis in Fig. 17.7. (Courtesy of Harper Hospital, Detroit.)

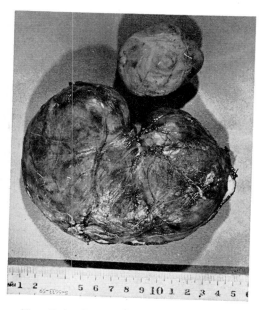

FIG. 17.10. Intraligamentary hemangiopericytoma (*below*) with myoma. (Courtesy of Dr. Albert Brown, Saskatoon, Canada.)

group the endometrial stroma invades not only the musculature but may also exhibit endolymphatic and intravascular penetrativeness, growing in a rubbery, wormlike fashion into both lymphatics and veins. It may thus become at least locally invasive, pushing into the broad ligaments, but it has no tendency to distant metastases. According to Henderson, cases of this kind can often be temporarily cured even if the removal of tumor tissue is not altogether complete, although death may occur from local extension. (3) The definitely malignant group, speaking histologically, is also malignant clinically. For this reason, we ourselves classify such cases as *endometrial sarcoma*, in spite of the fact that the morphological characteristics of the sarcoma cells are remindful of the stroma from which they arise. The histological differences between these three types are exceedingly tenuous, and there is considerable logic in accepting only benign stromatosis or a malignant type which is a low grade variant of endometrial sarcoma.

Hemangiopericytoma. On occasion the pathologist may encounter difficulty in distinguishing between stromal endometriosis and *hemangiopericytoma*, a vascular lesion closely related to a glomus tumor, and a rather new addition to gynecological pathology. Histologically it is characterized by a concentric arrangement of pericytes around capillaries, but such special stains as Massons, silver, and reticulum are often necessary. Grossly one may find a tumor much like a vascular myoma, generally unlike the wormlike buds of stromatosis. Hemangiopericytoma is generally regarded as a low grade (20 to 25%) malignant tumor.

Clinical Characteristics of Adenomyosis. The two symptoms are *menorrhagia* and *dysmenorrhea*, generally increasingly severe in the older (fifth decade) woman who has borne children. The former may be partly explained by *menorrhagia* the increased amount of endometrium, but is often due to the ovarian dysfunction so often associated. The dysmenorrhea is typically of colicky nature, being due to the painful contractions of the uterine muscle, induced by the menstrual swelling of the endometrial islands. When pelvic endometriosis is present, it often involves the uterosacral ligaments, and the · menstrual swelling of the endometrium in the region produces *pain* referred to the rectum or the lower sacral region. Where endometriosis is present there may be some intermenstrual discomfort, but this is not nearly as characteristic as the menstrual symptoms.

Novak and De Lima indicate that pelvic endometriosis and adenomyosis coexist with relative frequency. Benson states that pelvic endometriosis occurs in only 13 % of cases of adenomyosis; he also adds that surface endometrial hyperplasia is a rare accompaniment. Fibroids are common, occurring in 44 % of all cases in Emge's series.

Diagnosis. While the diagnosis is not usually made until after pathological examination, there is a group of cases in which at least a strongly presumptive diagnosis can be made clinically. When one finds a moderately and diffusely enlarged uterus firmly fixed in the pelvis, with one or more small nodules palpable in the region of the uterosacral ligaments, and when these findings are combined with menorrhagia and a colicky dysmenorrhea referred to the rectum or lower sacral or coccygeal regions in a parous woman, there will be little doubt of the presence of adenomyosis probably combined with endometriosis. In a large proportion of cases, however, pelvic endometriosis does not coexist, and preoperative diagnosis is often not possible. A symmetrically enlarged uterus with the proved absence of pregnancy in a 40-year-old woman with increasing dysmenorrhea and menorrhagia should be highly suggestive of adenomyosis.

Treatment. Since, like myoma, this disease is usually dependent on continued ovarian function, minor symptoms in the premenopausal woman require only palliative treatment. Where symptoms are extreme, however, the proper treatment is surgical; in many cases the operation is performed on the incorrect diagnosis of myoma, pelvic inflammatory disease, or a combination of the two. Hysterectomy is indicated, the fate of the ovaries being decided on the basis of such factors as the age of the patient and the presence or absence of ovarian or general pelvic endometriosis.

For a discussion of adenomyosis involving various extrauterine locations, see Chapter 22.

REFERENCES

Adamson, T. L., Brown, R., and Myerscough, P. R.: Postmenopausal bleeding. J. Obstet. Gynaec. Brit. Comm., *64:* 566, 1957.

Benson, R. C., and Smeeden, V. D.: Adenomyosis; a reappraisal of symptomatology. Amer. J. Obstet. Gynec., *76:* 1044, 1958.

Colman, H. I., and Rosenthal, A. H.: Carcinoma developing in areas of adenomyosis. Obstet. Gynec., *14:* 342, 1959.

Cope, E.: Adenocarcinoma of the endometrium with malignant stromatosis. J. Obstet. Gynaec. Brit. Comm., *65:* 58, 1958.

Cullen, T. S.: *Adenomyoma of Uterus.* W. B. Saunders Company, Philadelphia, 1908.

Cullen, T. S.: Distribution of adenomyomata containing uterine mucosa. Arch. Surg., *1:* 215, 1920.

Emge, L. A.: Problems in the diagnosis of adenomyosis uteri. Western J. Surg., *64:* 291, 1956.

Emge, L. A.: Elusive adenomyosis of uterus; its historic past and its present state of recognition. Amer. J. Obstet. Gynec., *83:* 1541, 1962.

Giammalvo, J. T., and Kaplan, K.: Endometriosis interna and endometrial carcinoma. Amer. J. Obstet. Gynec., *75:* 161, 1958.

Harper, R. S., and Scully, R. E.: Intravenous leiomyomatosis of the uterus. Obstet. Gynec., *18:* 519, 1961.

Henderson, D. N.: Endolymphatic stromal myosis. Amer. J. Obstet. Gynec., *52:* 1000, 1946.

Hunter, W. C.: Benign and malignant (sarcoma) stromal endometriosis. Surgery, *34:* 258, 1953.

Hunter, W. C., and Lattig, G. J.: Stromal endometriosis and uterine adenomyosis. Amer. J. Obstet. Gynec., *75:* 258, 1958.

Hunter, W. C., Smith, L. L.: and Reiner, W. C.: Adenomyosis. Amer. J. Obstet. Gynec., *53:* 663, 1947.

Kumar, D., and Anderson, W.: Malignancy in endometriosis interna. J. Obstet. Gynaec. Brit. Comm., *65:* 435, 1958.

Novak, E., and De Lima, O. A.: A correlative study of adenomyosis and pelvic endometriosis, with special reference to the hormonal reaction of ectopic endometrium. Amer. J. Obstet. Gynec., *56:* 634, 1958.

Novak, E. R., and Woodruff, J. D.: Postirradiation malignancy of the pelvic organs. Amer. J. Obstet. Gynec., 77: 667, 1959.

Park, W. W.: Stromatosis. J. Obstet. Gynaec. Brit. Comm., 56: 755, 1952.

Pedowitz, P., Felmus, L. B., and Grayzel, D. M.: Vascular tumors of the uterus. Amer. J. Obstet. Gynec., 69: 1291, 1955.

Pedowitz, P., Felmus, L. B., and Grayzel, D. M.: Benign vascular tumors. Amer. J. Obstet. Gynec., 69: 1309, 1955.

Robertson, T. B., Hunter, W. C., Larson, C.

P., and Snyder, G. A. C.: Benign and malignant stromal endometriosis. Amer. J. Clin. Path., 12: 1, 1942.

Sandberg, E. C., and Cohn, F.: Adenomyosis in the gravid uterus at term. Amer. J. Obstet. Gynec., 84: 1457, 1962.

Scott, R. B.: Adenomyosis and adenomyoma. Clin. Obstet. Gynec., 1: 413, 1958.

Stearns, H. C.: Study of stromal endometriosis. Amer. J. Obstet. Gynec., 75: 603, 1958.

Stout, A. P.: Hemangiopericytoma. Cancer, 2: 1027, 1949.

18

SARCOMA OF THE UTERUS

Sarcoma of the uterus is far less common than carcinoma; however, any precise statistics are difficult to assemble, for many clinics designate as low grade sarcomas what we personally would consider as merely cellular myomas. Obviously, this discrepancy affects not only salvage but also the incidence. In a study from our own laboratory (Novak and Anderson) 59 instances of sarcoma were encountered in a period of 25 years, while during this same period 1263 cases of uterine cancer of all varieties (excluding only chorionepithelioma) were observed. Sarcomas therefore constituted less than 5% of all uterine malignant tumors.

Pathology and Classification. It is now generally accepted that sarcoma of the uterus may arise from any of the connective tissue elements of the uterine structure, and that it may be of myogenic origin as well. Thus it may arise from the myometrium, endometrium, blood vessels, or a myoma. Whether any lesion should be categorized as a leiomyosarcoma (of smooth muscle origin) or a fibromyosarcoma (of connective tissue variety) seems of purely academic interest as compared to whether it is malignant or benign.

Ober, as well as others, has attempted to classify sarcoma on a histogenetic basis, and he proposes the following scheme

(which is presented here only in outline form).

(1) Leiomyosarcoma
(2) Mesenchymal sarcoma
    (a) Pure homologus as endometrial sarcoma *bnf 343*
    (b) Pure heterologous as rhabdomyosarcoma
    (c) Mixed homologous as carcinosarcoma
    (d) Mixed heterologous as carcinosarcoma plus other heterologous elements
(3) Blood vessel sarcomas
(4) Lymphomas
(5) Unclassified
(6) Metastatic

There are numerous subclassifications which are not necessary for a simple workable means of dividing these lesions. It is often difficult enough to distinguish them from various epithelial tumors without specific regard to their precise histogenesis.

SARCOMA

(1) Although *leiomyosarcoma* is a very infrequent complication of myoma, in the nature of 0.2% or less, the prevalence of myomata still makes this the most common form of uterine sarcoma. Because of the rarity of malignant degeneration, however, the clinician tends to disregard this in his treatment of myomata. Sudden

346

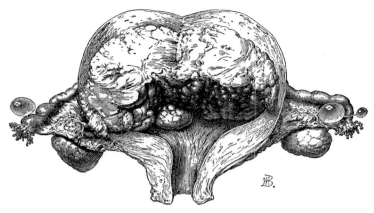

Fig. 18.1. Sarcoma of body of uterus. (From Kelly, H. A.: *Operative Gynecology.* Appleton-Century-Crofts, Inc., New York, 1928.)

accelerated growth of a previously static tumor or postmenopausal enlargement will always suggest the possibility of sarcoma, and indicate surgery despite symptoms; actually most cases will ultimately show only degenerative changes, but the clinician cannot afford to procrastinate.

The diagnosis of this particular lesion is rarely made preoperative, because the symptoms and physical findings are attributed to the myomata; indeed surgery itself only rarely affords a clue, for in many instances the malignant change will involve only the central area of the tumor so that the surface is not abnormal. On occasion the myoma may be somewhat softer, cystic, and yellowish, and thus quite different from the firm nodular consistency usually found.

If the tumor be cut open after its removal, one will find an absence of the symmetrically whorled white, firm surface, the "raw pork" appearance described by Cullen, or when necrotic changes are marked, a more pultaceous appearance with cystic and hemorrhagic degeneration. Although this may represent merely degenerative phenomena, it should impel the surgeon to increase the scope of his operation; *i.e.*, removal of, rather than ovarian conservation, hysterectomy rather than myomectomy, etc.

(2) *Endometrial sarcoma* is less common and less malignant than leiomyosarcoma.

It not infrequently assumes a polypoid architecture, and this is likewise true of growths originating from the mucosa of the cervix. However, benign polyps are generally smoother and less friable than these endometrial lesions, which histologically show complete overgrowth of abnormal stroma although an infrequent abnormal and distorted gland may be found. On occasion both connective tissue and epithelium are stimulated to malignancy with the development of a *carcinosarcoma.* This should be regarded merely as a variant of endometrial sarcoma; Williams and Woodruff have discussed its relationship to benign polyp and endometrial adenocarcinoma.

Since this is a surface lesion, it frequently produces bleeding so that subsequent curettage may make the diagnosis, or if the lesion protrudes out the cervical os, simple biopsy may suffice. This of course is in contrast to leiomyosarcoma; if diagnosis is made, our preference is to employ preoperative irradiation, for it seems much more radiosensitive than leiomyosarcoma.

There are all degrees of histological and clinical malignancy with endometrial sarcoma. On occasion it may be very difficult to make a distinction between this and the locally invasive but nonmetastasizing *stromal endometriosis*, or *stromatosis* (see Chapter 17) which may be a rather com-

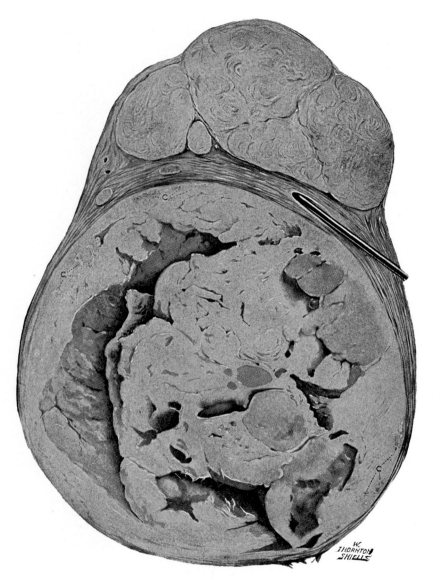

FIG. 18.2. Sarcoma of body of uterus. (From Kelly, H. A.: *Operative Gynecology*. Appleton-Century-Crofts, Inc., New York, 1928.)

pletely benign process or locally malignant with venous and lymphatic extension but rarely distant metastasis. (The rare hemangiopericytoma may histologically be a very difficult diagnostic problem.) More malignant degrees of stromal endometriosis or adenomyosis (stromatosis) merge imperceptibly into the patterns of an endometrial sarcoma.

The recent publication by Woodruff and Williams summarizes our own experiences with the rare highly malignant *mixed mesodermal tumor*. These have been considered to be of a teratomatous nature, containing a variety of mesodermal elements, such as cartilage, striped muscle, or mucoid tissue. Such tumors had been thought by many to be explained by the

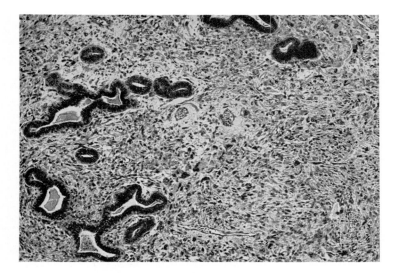

FIG. 18.3. Endometrial sarcoma

pulling down of mesodermal tissue by the Wolffian duct during the period of its embryologic descent.

More recently, Taylor has reemphasized that all of the elements are of stromal (Müllerian) origin, with abnormal differentiation being responsible for the component bone and cartilage formation. With this current view we are in complete accord. The frequency of *preceding irradiation* has been noted in most reports of these tumors. A recent case in association with bilateral thecoma has been reported by Laurian and Monroe. The prognosis is poor with, frequently, metastases to distant parts of the body, and Taylor has noted only 6 survivors in 40 patients studied.

Certain of these lesions seem to involve the cervix and vagina even in adults. There seems a close kinship between these and the *sarcoma botryoides* of vagina and cervix, seen primarily in children, although the histogenesis is not necessarily the same (see Vagina).

(3) *Mural sarcomas* may at times also arise as nodular and fairly circumscribed tumors, so that it may be difficult to be sure whether or not the tumor was preceded by a benign myoma. More often, however, they are much more diffuse in their growth, so much so that they may

produce a fairly uniform enlargement of the uterus, which may even resemble an early pregnancy. The same thing is true of the diffuse varieties arising from the endometrial stroma.

(4) *Lymphomas.* The various lymphoid malignancies are rare in the uterus, but still more commonly found than in the ovary. Ober and Tovell have noted occasional cases of lymphosarcoma which present primarily in the uterus with no apparent evidence of this disease in other areas of the body. Leukomoid deposits may likewise involve the genital tract, but generally in connection with an extensive spread of infiltrates so that the prognosis is very poor. In any case the outcome with any pelvic lymphoma is guarded.

Leiomyosarcoma. With reference to the much discussed question of the *incidence* of sarcomatous changes in myomas, the wide discrepancy of figures quoted suggests that there is as yet incomplete uniformity in recognition of the histological criteria of malignancy. The most common error is to mistake very cellular but benign myomas for spindle cell sarcoma, so that in some series an incidence of as much as 10% of malignancy is reported. It would seem that mere cellularity in the absence of in-

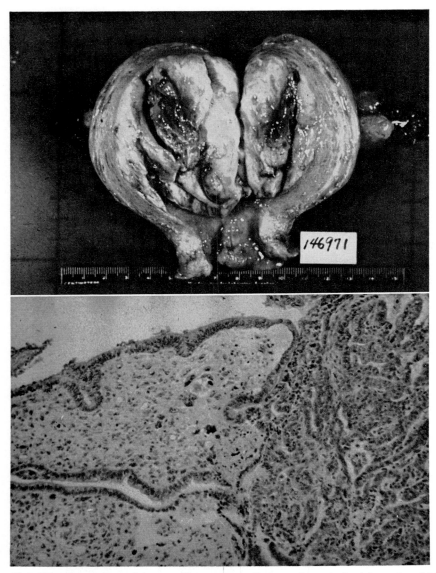

FIG. 18.4. Mixed mesodermal tumor. *Top*, gross pathology characterized by polypoid lesions arising from endometrial surfaces. *Bottom*, histologically, various sarcomatous and carcinoid elements of mesodermal origin may be noted.

creased mitoses and abnormal and giant cells should not warrant the diagnosis of even a "low-grade sarcoma." Such is not the rule, however, and this might account for the high incidence of sarcoma in some clinics, as well as a high salvage, for these lesions rarely cause difficulties in the postoperative era. At least two mitotic figures per high power field should be encountered before considering a diagnosis of sarcoma. Such descriptive terms as round, giant, or spindle are occasionally utilized.

It is not always easy to be sure whether or not sarcoma is secondary to benign myoma. The mere presence of myomas does not justify this assumption and, moreover, it must be remembered that sarcoma may arise as a rather nodular

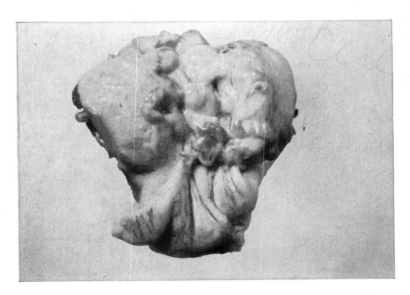

PLATE XVIII.I. Endometrial sarcoma

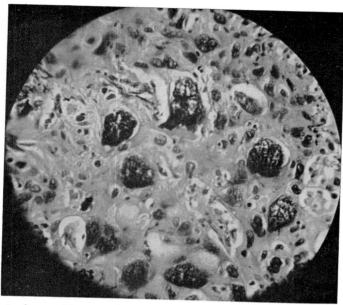

FIG. 18.5. Note abnormal forms and mitotic figures which are of extreme importance in assessing the malignancy of sarcoma. (Courtesy of Dr. N. Diaz-Bazan, San Salvador.)

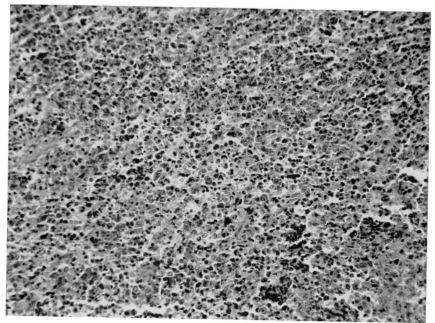

FIG. 18.6. Round cell sarcoma of uterus (with secondary infection)

growth which might simulate a sarcomatous myoma. On the other hand, when a sarcoma is found developing in the interior of a myoma in which one can still find abundant evidence of the original benign tumor, the origin from such a tumor seems clear. In the late stages of the disease, however, such aids in deter-

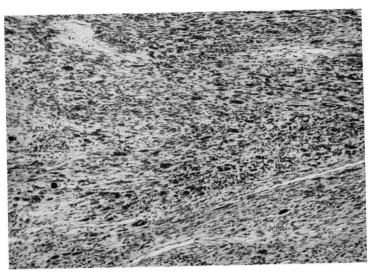

FIG. 18.7. Spindle cell sarcoma of uterus

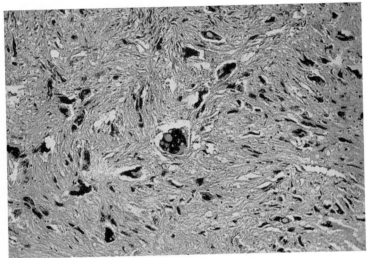

FIG. 18.8. Giant cells of symplasmic type due to degenerative process

mining the origin of the tumor are not available, and one can only speculate on this point.

In our own series of 59 cases, it was considered that in 39, or 66.1 %, the sarcoma was secondary in myomas. This gives an incidence of 0.56 % of sarcomatous degeneration in the 6981 myomas comprised in our material, a figure somewhat lower than the 1.2 % of Kelly and Cullen in an earlier study from the same laboratory. Certainly, however, the incidence would seem less than 1 % according to accrued statistics, but one must always be mindful of "what constitutes a sarcoma." Such interpretation obviously dictates the salvage; for example, a recent article by Radman and Korman notes 17 of 19 patients alive following treatment for sarcoma. It would seem that their cases must include certain lesions of low grade activity, or else other figures are extremely pessimistic. The usual salvage lies in the 25 to 30 % bracket, although Corscaden and Singh, in reporting at most a 0.13 % incidence of malignant change in myomas, indicate that salvage with true sarcoma is very low.

In a group of 41 women who had all their treatment at the Mayo Clinic, Aaro and Dockerty note a surprisingly high 46 % 5-year survival. It is likewise apparent from their study that mitosis count is a frequently helpful method of assessing the prognosis. A recent unpublished study from Johns Hopkins (Montague and Woodruff) on sarcoma arising in myoma suggests a nearly 50 % salvage of patients treated.

Clinical Characteristics. The disease most frequently affects women during the middle period of life, our own series showing the highest incidence during the fifth decade. On the other hand, the rare grape-like sarcoma of the cervix and vagina occurs characteristically in infancy. Any portion of the uterus may be the seat of the tumor, although the body is far more frequently involved than is the cervix. The greater frequency of corporeal as compared with cervical myomas will no doubt explain in part at least the predilection of sarcoma for the corpus uteri.

The *symptomatology* is not distinctive, and is usually that of myoma in which most sarcomas arise. The diagnosis is not made until operation; or even more frequently, not until the pathological examination. *Abnormal bleeding* may be entirely absent, especially when the endometrium is not involved. On the other hand, it may be of great significance, especially when it occurs after the menopause, and particularly when in these postmenopausal cases the uterus is the seat of presumably myomatous enlargement. In younger women there may be either menstrual excess or intermenstrual bleeding, or both. Needless to say the hemorrhage is in any event only suggestive of possible malignancy, and carcinoma will more frequently be found to be its cause than sarcoma.

Certain tumors arise *retroperitoneally* and, although they are generally not of pelvic origin, must be considered in differential diagnosis. Clinically they may present as a pelvic mass of considerable size with no associated menstrual abnormality. Pratt has pointed out the surgical difficulties with these lesions which are usually lymphomas or sarcomas.

Abnormal discharge may likewise be a symptom, as in carcinoma. In the earlier stages it is likely to be thin and watery, but sooner or later serosanguineous. Still later it may, as a result of necrosis and ulceration, become quite foul, and may even contain sloughing particles or shreds of tissue. *Rapid increase in the size of myomatous tumors*, especially when this is associated with bleeding, should likewise suggest the possibility of sarcoma. *Pain* may be a symptom, although often not until the later infiltrative stages of the disease, when it may be intense and continuous. In these late stages, profound *anemia*, *cachexia*, and *weakness* may be noted, necessitating extensive preoperative preparation. Although recurrence and metastases with a fatal outcome are usually rapid, there are such exceptions as that noted recently by Drake and Dobben. They report a case with probable recurrence 18 years after complete operation and recovery, and their publication, with microscopic sections, would seem to suggest that it is a recurrent rather than a new malignancy.

Extension of the disease is by direct continuity, by the blood stream, and less commonly by the lymphatics. The hematogenous route is most important in metastasis, which therefore is more characteristically systemic rather than regional. Among the organs most frequently involved are the lungs and liver. Chest x-ray is routine when uterine sarcoma is diagnosed.

Treatment. Because of the difficulties of diagnosis, the treatment of sarcoma is often a matter of expediency rather than of deliberate planning. Surgery has been, and still is, the backbone of treatment, especially as so large a proportion of sarcomas are not discovered until operation for supposed myoma, or until the laboratory examination of such supposedly benign tumors. The possibility of sarcomatous change in myomas must always be borne in mind by the surgeon, and it is a wise precaution to cut into the tumor masses as soon as the uterus is removed, for a presumptive diagnosis of sarcoma can sometimes be made from the gross appearance of the cut surface.

Occasionally sarcoma is found after myomectomy has been performed or, more frequently in earlier days, when subtotal hysterectomy was the operation of choice. Although a secondary complete operation seems desirable in such instances, many patients were cured with no further treatment. It would seem that the patient's salvation lies in the fact that so many of the sarcomas developing in myomas are comparatively early and of a relatively low degree of malignancy, i.e., cellular myoma. Certainly we would hesitate to reoperate to remove a conserved ovary with an unsuspected sarcoma, preferring to believe that the adnexa retained will not be the sole site of infiltrative or recurrent disease.

Even the most extensive surgery and the most complete radiotherapy will fail to cure the more malignant types of sarcoma when these have reached an advanced stage, as they unfortunately often do, before the patient comes to operation. These advanced cases are poor operative risks as a result of such factors as extreme anemia, cachexia, and early extension and metastasis. The preferable plan of treatment is panhysterectomy followed by deep roentgenization, although there is considerable question as to how effective deep x-ray may be. As mentioned previously, endometrial sarcoma appears more radiosensitive. Chemotherapy is generally ineffectual.

REFERENCES

Aaro, L. A., and Dockerty, M. B.: Leiomyosarcoma of the uterus. Amer. J. Obstet. Gynec., 77: 1187, 1959.

Carelton, C. C., and Williamson, J. W.: Osteogenic sarcoma of the uterus. Arch. Path., 20: 121, 378, 1961.

Cope, E.: Adenocarcinoma of the endometrium with malignant stromatosis. J. Obstet. Gynaec. Brit. Comm., 65: 58, 1958.

Corscaden, J. A., and Singh, B. P.: Leiomyosarcoma of uterus. Amer. J. Obstet. Gynec., 75: 149, 1958.

Crawford, E. J., and Tucker, W.: Sarcoma of the uterus. Amer. J. Obstet. Gynec., 77: 286, 1959.

Drake, E. T., and Dobben, G. D.: Leiomyosarcoma of the uterus with unusual metastasis. J. A. M. A., 170: 1294, 1959.

Finn, W. F.: Sarcoma of uterus. Amer. J. Obstet. Gynec., 60: 154, 1950.

Goodfriend, M. J., and Lapan, B.: Carcinoma sarcoma of uterus. New York J. Med., 50: 1139, 1950.

Greene, R. R., and Gerbie, A. B.: Hemangiopericytoma of the uterus. Obstet. Gynec., 3: 150, 1954.

Hahn, G. A.: Gynecologic considerations in malignant lymphoma. Amer. J. Obstet. Gynec., 75: 673, 1958.

Hardy, J. A., and Moragues, W.: Mixed mesodermal tumors of the uterus. Amer. J. Obstet. Gynec., 63: 307, 1952.

Herman, L., and Barrows, D. N.: Sarcoma of uterus. Obstet. Gynec., 6: 18, 1955.

Hill, R. P., and Miller, F. N.: Combined mesenchymal sarcoma and carcinoma (carcinosarcoma) of the uterus. Cancer. 4: 803, 1951.

Hughesdon, P. E., and Cocks, D. P.: Endometrial sarcoma complicating cystic hyperplasia. J. Obstet. Gynaec. Brit. Comm., 62: 567, 1955.

Hunter, W. C.: Benign and malignant (sarcoma) stromal endometriosis. Surgery, 34: 258, 1953.

Hunter, W. C., Nohlgren, J. S., and Lancefield, S. M.: Stromal endometriosis or endometrial sarcoma. Amer. J. Obstet. Gynec., 72: 1072, 1956.

Kelly, H. A., and Cullen, T. S.: Myomata of the Uterus. W. B. Saunders Company, Philadelphia, 1909.

Laurain, A. R., and Monroe, T. C.: Mixed mesodermal sarcoma of the corpus uteri with associated bilateral thecoma. Amer. J. Obstet. Gynec., 78: 613, 1959.

Marcella, L. C., and Cromer, J. K.: Mixed meosdermal tumors. Amer. J. Obstet. Gynec., 77: 275, 1959.

McElin, J. W., and Davis, H., Jr.: Mesodermal mixed tumors. Amer. J. Obstet. Gynec., 63: 605, 1952.

Meyer, R.: Uterossarkome. In Handbuch der spezielle pathologische Anatomie und Histologie, edited by F. Henke and O. Lubarsch, Ch. 24. Julius Springer, Berlin, 1930.

Montague, A., Schwarz, D. P., and Woodruff, J. D.: Leiomyosarcoma originating in myoma. Amer. J. Obstet Gynec., in press.

Novak, E., and Anderson, D. F.: Sarcoma of uterus. Amer. J. Obstet. Gynec., 34: 740, 1937.

Ober, W. B.: Uterine sarcomas; histogenesis and taxonomy. Ann. N. Y. Acad. Sci., *75:* 568, 1959.

Ober, W. B., and Jason, R. S.: Sarcoma of the endometrial stroma. Arch. Path., *56:* 301, 1953.

Ober, W. B., and Tovell, H. M.: Mesenchymal sarcomas of the uterus. Amer. J. Obstet. Gynec., *77:* 246, 1959.

Ober, W. B., and Tovell, H. M.: Malignant lymphomas of the uterus. Bull. Sloane Hosp., *5:* 65, 1959.

Pratt, J. H.: Some surgical considerations of retroperitoneal tumors. Amer. J. Obstet. Gynec., *87:* 956, 1963.

Radman, H. M., and Korman, W.: Sarcoma of the uterus. Amer. J. Obstet. Gynec., *78:* 604, 1959.

Retikas, D. G.: Hodgkin's sarcoma of the cervix. Amer. J. Obstet. Gynec., *80:* 1104, 1960.

Rubin, A.: Histogenesis of carcinosarcoma of the uterus. Amer. J. Obstet. Gynec., *77:* 269, 1959.

Scheffey, L. C., Levinson, J., Herbut, P. A., Hepler, T. K., and Gilmore, G. H.: Osteosarcoma of the uterus. Obstet. Gynec., *8:* 444, 1956.

Schiffer, M. A., and Mackles, A.: Stromal endometriosis. Obstet. Gynec., *7:* 531, 1956.

Schiffer, M. A., Mackles, A., and Wolfe, S. A.: Reappraisal of diagnosis in uterine sarcoma. Amer. J. Obstet. Gynec., *70:* 521, 1955.

Symmonds, R. E., and Dockerty, M. B.: Sarcoma and sarcoma-like proliferations of the endometrial stroma. Surg. Gynec. Obstet., *100:* 232, 322, 1955.

Symmonds, R. E., Dockerty, M. B., and Pratt, J. H.: Sarcoma and sarcoma-like proliferation of the endometrial stroma. Amer. J. Obstet. Gynec., *73:* 1054, 1957.

Taylor, C. W.: Mixed mesodermal tumors of the female genital tract. J. Obstet. Gynaec. Brit. Comm., *65:* 177, 1958.

Thornton, W. N., Jr., and Carter, J. P.: Sarcoma of uterus, a clinical study. Amer. J. Obstet. Gynec., *62:* 294, 1951.

Webb, G. A.: Uterine sarcoma. Obstet. Gynec., *6:* 38, 1955.

Williams, T. J., and Woodruff, J. D.: Similarities in malignant mixed mesenchymal tumors of the endometrium. Obstet. Gynec. Survey, *17:* 1, 1962.

Wilson, L. A., Graham, L. J., Thornton, W. N., Jr., and Nokes, J. M.: Mixed mesodermal tumors of uterus. Amer. J. Obstet. Gynec., *66:* 718, 1953.

Wolfe, S. A., and Pedowitz, P.: Carcinosarcoma of uterus. Obstet. Gynec., *12:* 54, 1958.

Zeigerman, J. H., Imbriglia, J., Makler, P., and Smith, J. J.: Ovarian lymphosarcoma. Amer. J. Obstet. Gynec., *72:* 1357, 1956.

19

ACUTE PELVIC INFLAMMATORY DISEASE

The rationale of separate chapters for acute and chronic pelvic inflammatory disease is that the former is (with certain exceptions) almost exclusively a medical problem, whereas most cases of chronic recurrent infection almost inevitably culminate in some type of surgical procedure.

The advent of the more recent and improved antibiotic agents has been attended by a significant decrease in the more serious forms and complications of infection of the generative tract. Probably pelvic infection is almost as frequent, but prompt treatment and response would seem to have led to a considerable reduction of such formerly frequent sequelae as tubo-ovarian or pelvic abscess, pelvic peritonitis, or even permanently closed tubes.

Pelvic inflammatory disease is usually secondary to infection and upward migration of various bacteria introduced at a lower level, although in its incipient form there may be remarkably little in the way of symptomatology. In any case the course of the disease is dependent on the strain and virulence of the particular organisms involved, as well as the individual body resistance to the offending bacteria. Although in most cases the tubes seem to bear the primary impact of the infectious process, there is a strong tendency for extension to the ovaries and pelvic peritoneum as a result of the propinquity of these structures to the uterus and tubes, and the intimacy of the lymphatic and vascular supply of all the pelvic organs.

Thus, the syndrome produced by genital infection is frequently a composite one, produced by various degrees of tubal involvement, with or without extension to the ovaries and pelvic peritoneum. As a rule the uterus itself is more or less immune to the inflammatory impact, for although there may be a very definite pathological involvement of the endometrial surface, this contributes little to the general symptomatology. This composite clinical syndrome is usually designated as pelvic inflammatory disease, and although there are many exceptions, the usual tendency is to begin with a rather acute episode, followed by either complete resolution or else gradual subsidence into a more chronic process characterized by not infrequent acute or subacute resurgence.

Etiology. From an etiological as well as from a clinical standpoint, one may distinguish three types of pelvic inflammatory disease.

(1) *Gonorrheal*, due to infection by the Gonococcus, and comprising the largest proportion, about 60% of all cases, although recent studies by Lukasik find the Gonococcus much less frequent than intestinal bacilli in tubal cultures. This should not imply any decrease in gonorrheal disease, for frequently culture is negative in cases of undoubted gonococcal tubo-ovarian abscess.

(2) *Pyogenic*, due to infection by any one of a number of organisms, most fre-

quently the Streptococcus (aerobic or anaerobic) or Staphylococcus. It is this variety of infection with which we are chiefly concerned in the frequent cases of puerperal and postabortive infection.

(3) *Tuberculous*, the result of infection by the tubercle bacillus, and embracing approximately 5% of the cases of pelvic inflammatory disease in areas where poverty and malnutrition abound. This form of pelvic infection is of chronic nature, and is discussed in Chapter 21.

GONORRHEAL TYPE

Pathology. The immediate focus in cases of infection of the upper genital tract is a gonorrheal involvement of the cervix, from which site the organisms make their way by surface invasion along the endometrium to the tubes and often beyond this to the peritoneum and ovaries. An acute gonorrheal infection of the urethra or vulvovaginal glands may constitute the primary focus.

Acute Endometritis of Gonorrheal Type. This form is rather rarely encountered in the pathological laboratory, inasmuch as both curettage and hysterectomy are usually contraindicated in the course of acute gonorrheal infections. It is characterized grossly by edema and hyperemia of the mucosa, and microscopically by hyperemia and infiltration by large numbers of polymorphonuclear leukocytes. Its tendency is toward spon-

taneous resolution, because of the usually good drainage of the uterine canal, and even more because of the monthly desquamation of menstruation with gradual attenuation in each cycle. The endometrium may thus be completely purged of all infection even though there is extensive chronic tubal or tubo-ovarian infection. There are, however, numerous exceptions to this, because of the frequent occurrence of reinfection.

Acute Salpingitis. This may be an almost immediate sequel of acute gonorrheal infection of the lower genital tract, or it may not occur until long afterward, perhaps many months or even years after the original infection. Since the organisms reach the tube by way of the mucous membrane, it is not surprising that the latter is the primary seat of the pathological changes. It becomes reddened and swollen, and soon gives forth an exudate which, except in the mildest cases, is purulent. This type of involvement is unfortunate for the patient, in that later occlusion and distention of the tube so frequently occur, with sterility a frequent result. The exudate may escape from the still open end of the tube, producing *acute pelvic peritonitis* and sometimes *pelvic abscess*.

The inflammatory process is rarely limited to the endosalpinx alone, the whole tube being swollen, hyperemic, and reddened, while acute *perisalpingitis* may

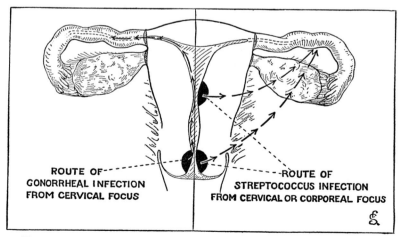

FIG. 19.1. Schematic drawing of two chief routes of pelvic infection

i) nell's forma cronica linfociti e plasmacellule (frog. 368)

[handwritten notes at top of page]

manifest itself by a fibrinous exudate on the tubal peritoneum, with light adhesions to surrounding structures. Occlusion of the fimbriated orifice or of other parts of the lumen may occur, with the production of a *pyosalpinx*, although this is more often encountered in an acute exacerbation of the chronic form. As already mentioned, pelvic abscess may result from bacterial invasion or even escape of purulent exudate into the pelvis. Finally, and most frequently, the subsidence of the acute infection leaves a residue of chronic salpingitis of one form or another.

The *microscopic characteristics* of acute gonorrheal salpingitis are like those of acute inflammation in general. The chief features are infiltration with polymorphonuclear leukocytes, hyperemia, and edema. In the milder cases the epithelium may be intact, but in the more severe forms it shows degeneration and often is lost over considerable areas. The inflammatory reaction is rarely limited sharply to the mucosa, and commonly involves the muscular and serous coat to a greater or less extent.

A very important characteristic of acute gonorrheal salpingitis, and one which has great bearing on the practical treatment of such cases, is the tendency of the infecting organisms to disappear within a short time, ordinarily about 10 days. While, therefore, acute salpingitis may leave in its wake a pathologically wrecked tube, often distended with pus, and no longer of value from the standpoint of childbearing, the bacteriological examination of the tube and its contents often shows these to be sterile. This was pointed out years ago by the bacteriological studies of Curtis and others, and has been confirmed more recently by Blinick.

SEPTIC OR PYOGENIC TYPE

The pyogenic form of acute salpingitis usually follows *childbirth* or *abortion*, the latter especially of the criminal type. The infecting organism, generally the Streptococcus or Staphylococcus, reaches the tube by a route quite different from that followed by the Gonococcus (Fig. 19.1), and the resulting changes in the tube are likewise quite different from those de-

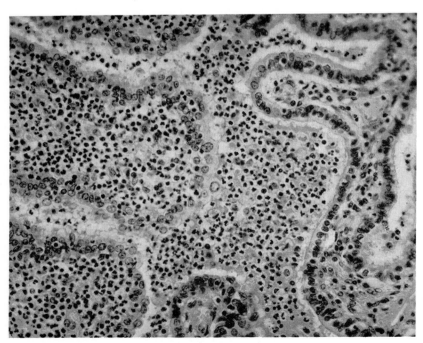

FIG. 19.2. Acute salpingitis

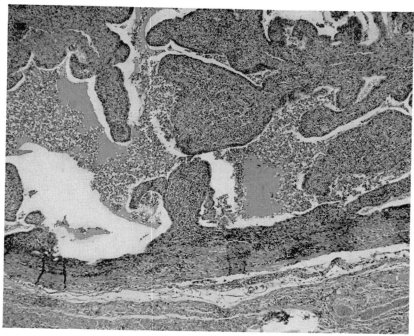

FIG. 19.3. Subacute salpingitis

scribed for the gonorrheal variety. From portals of entry in the lower genital canal, usually the cervix, the organisms are disseminated outward through the veins and lymphatics of the broad ligaments. Thrombophlebitis and periphlebitis, lymphangitis and perilymphangitis, with cellulitis and even abscess of the broad ligaments are frequent results.

It might be appropriate to note that Sarma, writing from India, has tabulated a list of exotic diseases which may cause infection in the gravid or normal woman. Kala-azar, bilharziasis, malaria, and other diseases rarely seen in this country deserve consideration in various pelvic disorders seen in certain tropical areas.

Acute Endometritis. In the milder forms of infection, the endometrium may be merely hyperemic and edematous, but in the more virulent infections, it may show extensive necrosis. The microscopic picture is that of acute inflammation, with varying degrees of necrotic change. With this one also finds in most cases degenerated villi and decidual tissue, and not infrequently extensive hemorrhage and

thrombosis. On occasion a postabortal infection may be due to the *Clostridium welchii*, and women harboring this organism may be critically ill with general sepsis, shock, and renal failure. Massive antibiotics and such heroic measures as dialysis or an artificial kidney may not suffice; Rabinowitz *et al.* suggest the desirability of hysterectomy, and in a small group of cases this seemed to produce better results, especially if combined with a massive dosage of drugs.

Acute Salpingitis. As already stated, the infection reaches the tube from the outside, so to speak, and this explains why the resulting salpingitis is of predominantly interstitial type, with often little or no involvement of the mucosa. The cross section of such a tube characteristically shows an enormously thickened and infiltrated mesosalpinx, with great thickening of the tubal wall, but with a lumen which is quite normal and which is lined by an intact or almost intact mucosa. This is in sharp contrast to the gonorrheal form, in which the destructive force of the infection is vented upon the mucosa

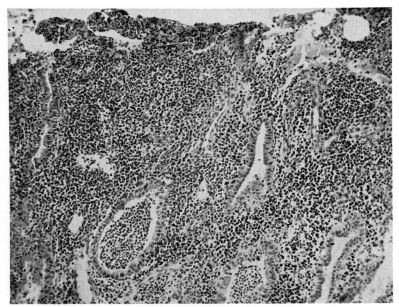

FIG. 19.4. Acute endometritis. Note the purulent exudate in the glands

primarily, with frequent occlusion of the lumen and subsequent sterility.

On the other hand, the prognosis as to childbearing following pyogenic infection of the tubes is much better, and one not infrequently observes later pregnancies in cases of extensive pelvic inflammation of the pyogenic type. This is of course not always the case, for the tubal orifices are sometimes closed by the extensive pelvic peritonitis which may accompany any acute infection of the pelvic organs.

The *microscopic picture* of acute pyogenic salpingitis, as might be expected from what has been said, is that of a normal or only slightly infiltrated mucosa, with great thickening of the muscularis as a result of edema and leukocytic infiltration, and with usually some degree of acute fibrinous peritonitis of the tubal serosa.

Acute Ovaritis or Oophoritis. The ovary not infrequently participates in acute pelvic inflammatory processes, but rarely except as a penalty of its proximity to the tube. However, one only rarely observes oophoritis except in association with salpingitis; while on the other hand, the ovary is frequently uninvolved even in the presence of severe tubal inflammation, either acute or chronic. The fact remains, however, that acute oophoritis, and even ovarian abscess, is at times found as a part of acute pelvic inflammatory disease, although abscesses are also often seen in association with longstanding chronic inflammation. Pelvic abscesses are often tubo-ovarian, representing the merging of tubal and ovarian cavities. *Ovarian abscess* with normal tubes is occasionally seen as a sequel to posthysterectomy infection which apparently spreads along lymphatic routes. Wilson and Black point out that this most commonly follows vaginal hysterectomy.

Acute Pelvic Peritonitis. In either the gonorrheal or pyogenic forms of infection acute pelvic peritonitis is a common concomitant. This manifests itself most frequently in the form of serous or fibrinous exudates with early development of adhesions between any of the adjoining pelvic structures, or between these and the small intestine, sigmoid, or rectum. In the acute stage these are light and fibrinous, but with increasing organization they later become dense and fibrous.

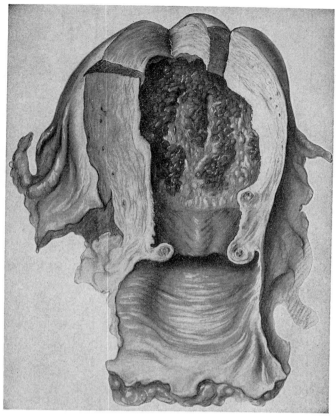

FIG. 19.5. Acute necrotic endometritis. (From Watson, B. P.: In *Obstetrics and Gynecology*, edited by A. H. Curtis. W. B. Saunders Company, Philadelphia, 1933.)

As a result of exudation of infected material from the tube, or perhaps more frequently through the virulence of the peritoneal infection itself, *pelvic abscess* frequently results. It is not always easy to distinguish clinically between large abscesses within the tube or ovary (tubo-ovarian abscesses) and the extratubal variety, in which the pus is situated in the pelvic cavity proper, generally in the cul-de-sac, in which case its upper wall is usually formed by the matted and adherent intestinal coils. The usual location of the pelvic abscess in the region of the cul-de-sac points the way to its easy evacuation by incision through the posterior vaginal vault (*posterior colpotomy*), the operation which is frequently indicated. Occasionally this is utilized in the postsurgical patient in whom there has

been persistent slight bleeding; this may localize in the cul-de-sac and, if secondarily infected, may form a pelvic hematocele, amenable to drainage.

SYMPTOMS AND SIGNS

Gonorrheal Form. The gonorrheal form may follow this infection in the lower genital canal, or at times its nature can be assumed if there is a history of recent gonorrheal infection in the marital partner. In a large proportion of cases, however, the history is of little help, the assumption of gonorrheal causation being based chiefly on the absence of any factor likely to produce pyogenic infection, such as recent childbirth, spontaneous miscarriage, criminal abortion, instrumentation, or operations upon the cervix.

In many cases, although not by any

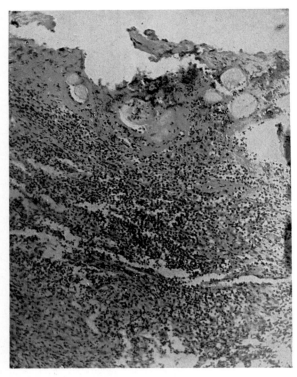

F<small>IG</small>. 19.6. Acute puerperal endometritis. (From Watson, B. P.: In *Obstetrics and Gynecology*, edited by A. H. Curtis. W. B. Saunders Company, Philadelphia, 1933.)

means all, the acute symptoms appear during or immediately after a menstrual period. This is explained by the greater vulnerability of the uterine cavity to gonorrheal invasion at the time of menstrual desquamation. Severe *pain* in the pelvic and lower abdominal region, *muscular rigidity*, and *tenderness, abdominal distention, nausea and vomiting, fever, leukocytosis, rapid pulse*, with considerable *prostration* in the severe cases, are the common symptoms. The fever may reach 103° or even higher, with a marked leukocytosis and increased pulse rate. The abdomen is usually tense and tympanitic, with marked tenderness and rigidity in the lower quadrants. In the severe forms which are associated with the formation of large tubal or tubo-ovarian abscesses, it may be impossible to palpate even large masses on examination because of the tenderness and rigidity of the ab-

dominal walls incurred by the pelvic peritonitis.

Pelvic Examination. This may be difficult and unsatisfactory, because of the patient's pain, tenderness, and rigidity, but usually the desired information is obtainable. When the uterus can be outlined between the examining hands, it is apt to be rather fixed, and efforts to move it by manipulation of the cervix or fundus cause much pain. There is extreme tenderness in both sides of the pelvis, but often in the acute stage no definite mass or enlargement of the adnexa can be made out. When the fever and pelvic pain persist, accompanied often by rectal pressure and pain, examination may reveal increasing induration, with later fluctuation and even bulging, in the region of the cul-de-sac, at times extending into the sides of the pelvis and perhaps downward along the posterior vaginal wall to a level which may be considerably lower than the cervix. Such findings leave no doubt as to the presence of a *pelvic abscess*, calling for evacuation through the posterior vaginal fornix (posterior colpotomy).

Postpartum and Postabortive Types. In these cases the patient is often very weak and septic, and there may be considerable local trauma in the perineum and vagina, so that much gentleness is necessary in the examination, ideally performed with sterile technique. The cervix is apt to be lacerated and infected, especially if the pelvic infection follows full term delivery. The uterus in such cases is large and uninvoluted, while in the case of early criminal abortions, it is only slightly enlarged. Even gentle manipulation of the uterus may be quite painful. One must always be cognizant of the possibility of uterine perforation and other trauma associated with criminal abortion.

Where the infection has invaded the broad ligaments the latter may be enormously thickened and infiltrated, so that the adnexa themselves cannot be made out (*broad ligament cellulitis*). Where broad ligament abscesses are present, as they often are at a later stage, the lateral masses are even larger. In some cases,

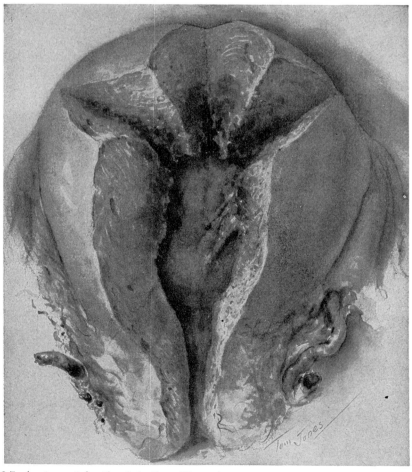

Fig. 19.7. Acute postabortive infection. Uterus large and edematous. Necrosis of uterine wall at placental site. Remnant of retained placental tissue. Bilateral thrombosis of uterine veins. (From Danforth, D. W.: In *Obstetrics and Gynecology*, edited by A. H. Curtis. W. B. Saunders Company, Philadelphia, 1933.)

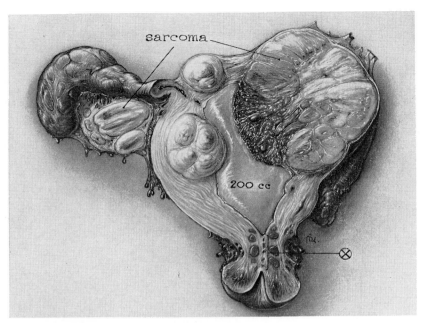

Fig. 19.8. Cervical stenosis with degenerating submucous myosarcoma with resultant pyometra. (Courtesy of Dr. Erle Henricksen, Los Angeles, California.)

however, the broad ligaments show little involvement, and the enlarged and inflamed adnexa may be palpated as irregular, tender masses in the sides of the pelvis. Marked thickening, infiltration, and tenderness of the broad and uterosacral ligaments is a frequent manifestation of the *parametritis* so commonly present.

Pyometra. Where there is any blockage of the canal, as may occur particularly with senile changes in the cervix or upper vagina, pus may accumulate, with the formation of a pyometra. This is particularly common with a uterine malignancy, especially after irradiation, and is *not* a sequel to acute endometritis in the usual young woman. Surprisingly, despite the massive accumulation of pus, there may be little systemic reaction. Misdiagnosis is rather frequent for the overdistended softened uterus suggests an ovarian cyst.

DIAGNOSIS

Gonorrheal Infection. A history of gonorrhea in either the patient or her husband is of great value in diagnosis, but this aid is lacking in the great majority of cases. The occurrence of severe lower abdominal pain, usually bilateral, during or just after menstruation, with lower abdominal tenderness and rigidity, moderate tympanites, fever, often nausea and vomiting, rapid pulse, leukocytosis, leukorrhea, and marked pelvic tenderness on bimanual examination, will usually suffice to make the diagnosis reasonably certain. When acute cervicitis or urethritis is present, gonococci are occasionally demonstrable in the discharges.

In discussing the current status of gonorrhea, Simpson and Brown deplore the efficacy of past methods in detecting and treating gonorrhea. They suggest that use of the fluorescent antibody technique as noted by Deacon will disclose that a considerable number of promiscuous although asymptomatic women may harbor the Gonococcus. Due to varying degrees of drug resistance, massive dosage of penicillin is sometimes required to obliterate the disease.

Postpartum and Postabortive In-

fection. Here the history of onset following delivery or abortion is of obvious importance. The symptomatology is similar to that described for the gonorrheal group except that in the more virulent cases, usually of streptococcal type, prostration is more marked, and chills not infrequently occur. The symptoms may manifest themselves within 6 or 8 hours or not for a number of days following the delivery or abortion. Where a definite history of criminal induction of abortion through instrumentation is obtained, the appearance of such symptoms as described leaves little doubt as to the origin of the infection. In many cases, even those of very virulent type, there is very little pain, although the systemic intoxication may be profound. There is a tendency to localization in the pelvis, with often a residue in the form of a large pelvic inflammatory mass or a broad ligament cellulitis or abscess. Unlike the gonorrheal cases, the fever in cases of this group is apt to be persistent, dragging along for weeks and even months. The importance of blood cultures, both aerobic and anaerobic, cannot be too strongly emphasized.

Many clinicians are beginning to feel that evacuation of the necrotic uterine contents will decrease the fever much sooner and thus avoid prolonged hospitalization. Massive dosage of antibiotics for less than 24 hours is followed by curettage, a procedure undreamed of for the febrile patient heretofore. Yet preliminary results indicate no ill effects, and make possible great financial and time saving to the patient. Considerable care must be exercised not to perforate the soft edematous uterus.

DIFFERENTIAL DIAGNOSIS

Acute Appendicitis. Although the initial pain in acute appendicitis may be diffuse, it soon tends to localize in the right lower abdomen, and this is even more true of the tenderness, which is sharply limited to the McBurney area. There is only slight fever, with a leukocytosis which in proportion to the fever

is much higher than with pelvic inflammation. The problem is more difficult and sometimes impossible in the case of a perforative appendicitis with peritonitis. Under such conditions the abdominal pain, tenderness, and rigidity, like that of acute pelvic inflammation, involve the whole lower abdominal zone. Moreover, fever may be quite high and the pulse rapid, with considerable prostration. Nausea and vomiting are apt to be more severe than with pelvic inflammation and usually abdominal distention is much more pronounced. The history, especially that of an onset with original localization in the right lower quadrant, as well as a record of previous attacks of appendicitis, is of the greatest value. Finally, while pelvic examination may show some tenderness even in cases of appendiceal peritonitis, it is rarely as clear-cut and pronounced as in the severe case of acute pelvic inflammation, while in some cases of the latter definite adnexal enlargement, or possibly even a pelvic abscess, may be palpable.

Acute Pyelitis. Although the kidneys are situated far above the pelvic level, the fact remains that severe acute pyelitis can at times produce a clinical picture not unlike that of acute pelvic inflammatory disease. High fever, accelerated pulse, abdominal pain, tenderness and distention, nausea and vomiting, and high leukocytosis are all frequent symptoms. The pain of pyelitis usually involves chiefly the upper abdominal zone, although sometimes it is general over the entire abdomen. Palpation over the kidney region may show marked tenderness in the costovertebral angle. With pyelitis there may be a high fever and some pain, but patients do not appear as ill or distressed as with salpingitis or appendicitis.

As a rule the abdominal pain of pyelitis is preceded or accompanied by pain in the lumbar region, radiating along the flanks, and there is likely to be increased frequency of urination, with some dysuria and tenesmus, although in a surprising proportion of cases such symptoms are not elicited. Of obvious importance is microscopic examination of the catheterized urine, which in pyelitis is likely to reveal large numbers of pus cells, often in clumps. Because of edema and ureteral blockage with poor drainage, however, the urine may be entirely negative for considerable periods of time.

Suppurating Ovarian Cyst. The occurrence of infection or torsion of an ovarian cyst gives rise to symptoms quite like those of acute pelvic inflammatory disease, but there may be a history of a previously existing tumor or on examination the rounded elastic unilateral tumor can be felt on pelvic and often on abdominal examination.

TREATMENT

Bed rest is preferable and usually easily enforced simply because the patient prefers this regimen and often spontaneously assumes a Fowler position because of the increased comfort due to relaxed abdominal muscle. This should be encouraged for it promotes gravitation of the infection to the pelvis; meals should be soft or liquid as determined by the presence of nausea or vomiting, and should these latter be prominent, intravenous fluids may be necessary. Fluids should be forced, the bowels regulated, and such analgesics or sedatives as aspirin and codeine or the barbiturates may be utilized.

Although there may be those individuals who consider douches or sitz baths inadvisable, we feel that heat in any form increases comfort and promotes resolution of the inflammatory process. Diathermy seems an expensive and cumbersome means of achieving the same effect, and this is rarely used.

In this day and age of high powered antibiotics it is well to remember that the much less expensive sulfonamides are frequently effective, and such drugs as Gantrisin or Kynex are usually tolerated well without toxic effects. A multitude of oral penicillin compounds are available, and these are also effective. A combination of the sulfonamides and penicillin seems of synergistic value, and this is frequently given for 4 to 7 days. Our own preference is to utilize these drugs initially, the more expensive broad spectrum antibiotics being held in reserve.

When strains of the disease resistant to sulfonamide-penicillin therapy are found, most of the antibiotics may be utilized with occasional good results. Streptomycin, chloromycetin, and tetracycline are a few of the many such agents available. Should there be no clinical response, the possibility of an acid-fast origin must be considered as well as such complications as a localized abscess or suppurative thrombophlebitis. Cortisone has been suggested by Collins for its antifibrotic tendencies.

Surgery during Acute Stage. Generally speaking, surgery should be avoided during the acute stage, but as mentioned previously there is a growing tendency to early curettage in conjunction with massive antibiotic treatment where bleeding is a problem.

In other cases, especially of the Streptococcus variety most common after criminal abortions, examination may show enormous thickening and infiltration of the broad ligaments, with a continuing septic type of fever and, later, a suspicion of broad ligament abscess. Most of these cases are more safely drained through a gridiron incision just above Poupart's ligament than through the vagina, the latter carrying with it some risk of injury to the ureter or the uterine artery. A pelvic abscess, when sufficiently soft and pointing low in the rectovaginal septum, deserves posterior colpotomy. In rare instances, rupture of a tubo-ovarian abscess may occur during this acute stage, and this may produce symptoms of shock which may even simulate those seen with rupture of a tubal pregnancy. When there is a strong suspicion of this complication, pelvic laparotomy is indicated; otherwise morbidity and mortality are high. Generally complete pelvic "clean-cut" is preferable to unilateral adnexectomy, as noted by Vermeeren and Te Linde. Pedowitz and Bloomfield note 100% mortality in the early days of conservative therapy,

1) nella posizione di Fowler, il paziente ha la testa più in alto dei piedi-

with a current figure of less than 4 % with more extreme degrees of surgery, combined with massive antibiotic therapy. It must be stressed that a ruptured tuboovarian abscess is a serious complication with considerable morbidity and some mortality.

Attention may also be called to the frequent simulation of mechanical obstruction in cases of acute pelvic peritonitis, associated as it may be with an adynamic or paralytic ileus. In most cases it is advisable to institute such nonsurgical measures as intestinal decompression as promptly as possible, but one should not delay too long if improvement does not occur, because of the real possibility of obstruction of a mechanical type.

Finally, there is an occasional but inevitable case in which there is doubt between an acute salpingitis and an acute appendicitis. Although it should be an infrequent occurrence, it is better to err on the side of safety and to remove an occasional appendix unnecessarily than to run the hazard of appendiceal perforation and peritonitis.

REFERENCES

Blinick, G.: Gonorrheal disease in the female. Clin. Obstet. Gynec., 2: 492, 1959.

Collins, C. G., Davidson, V. A., and Mathews, N. M.: Use of cortisone in pelvic cellulitis. New Orleans Med. Surg. J., 104: 389, 1952.

Collins, C. G., and Jansen, F. W.: Treatment of pelvic abscess. Clin. Obstet. Gynec., 2: 512, 1959.

Collins, C. G., Nix, F. G., and Cirha, H. T.: Ruptured tubo-ovarian abscess. Amer. J. Obstet. Gynec., 71: 820, 1956.

Deacon, W. E.: Flourescent antibody tests for detection of gonococcus in women. Public Health Rep., 75: 125, 1960.

De Alvarez, R. R., and Figge, D. C.: Antibiotics in pelvic inflammatory disease. Obstet. Gynec., 5: 765, 1955.

Frisch, A. W.: Postpartum infections. J. Clin. Obstet. Gynec., 5: 684, 1962.

Girardet, R., and Enquist, I. F.: Differential diagnosis between appendicitis and acute pelvic inflammatory disease. Surg. Gynec. Obstet., 116: 212, 1963.

Hedberg, E., and Spetz, S. O.: Acute salpingitis; views on prognosis and treatment. Acta Obstet. Gynec. Scand., 37: 131, 1958.

Hesseltine, H. G.: Pelvic inflammatory disease. Surg. Clin. N. Amer., 33: 269, 1953.

Kanter, A. E., Zummo, B. P., and Horwitz, C.: Erythromycin in acute pelvic inflammatory disease. Obstet. Gynec., 6: 541, 1955.

Lukasik, J.: A comparative evolution of the bacteriological flora of the uterine cervix and the fallopian tubes in cases of salpingitis. Amer. J. Obstet. Gynec., 87: 1028, 1963.

Pedowitz, P., and Bloomfield, R. D.: Ruptured adnexal abscess (tubo-ovarian) with generalized peritonitis. Amer. J. Obstet. Gynec., 88: 721, 1964.

Rabinowitz, P., Schiffer, M. A., Pomerance, W., and Friedman, I. S.: Management of postabortal infections complicated by acute renal failure. Amer. J. Obstet. Gynec., 84: 780, 1962.

Sarma, V.: Gynecologic and obstetric aspects of tropical diseases. Medioscope, 45: 181, 1961.

Schwartz, O., and Dieckmann, W. H.: Puerperal infection due to anaerobic Streptococcus. Amer. J. Obstet. Gynec., 13: 467, 1927.

Simpson, W. G., and Brown, W. J.: Current status of the diagnosis and management of gonorrhea. J. A. M. A., 182: 173, 1962.

Smith, H. A., and Greene, R. R.: Physiologic endosalpingitis. Amer. J. Obstet. Gynec., 72: 174, 1956.

Vermereen, J., and Te Linde, R. W.: Intra-abdominal rupture of pelvic abscesses. Amer. J. Obstet. Gynec., 68: 402, 1954.

Wilson, J. R., and Black, J. R.: Ovarian abcess. Amer. J. Obstet. Gynec.. 90: 34, 1964.

20

CHRONIC PELVIC INFLAMMATORY DISEASE

Even a single attack of acute pelvic inflammation used to leave some residue of chronic disease and this was likely to be marked by repeated reinfection and exacerbations. The peritoneal involvement was indicated by the development of pelvic adhesions involving the uterus, tubes, and ovaries. Currently, it would appear that the newer antibiotics may completely cure salpingitis without the usual residue of "closed tubes" and sterility. Unquestionably, this is a factor in the increased Negro birth rate.

Chronic Endometritis. This is a relatively common lesion, although much less so than was once believed. Even in the presence of extensive chronic adnexitis, the endometrium may be entirely normal, due to the usually good drainage of the uterine canal, and also because of the monthly desquamation of menstruation. For example, the Gonococcus is a frequent invader of the endometrium, over which the infection travels upward to the tube. Acute forms of endometrial infection are rather rarely encountered in laboratory material, for as the endometritis becomes chronic it is attenuated with each menstrual desquamation, so that after two or three cycles the endometrium is rather completely purged of its infection. Reinfections from the cervix, however, are very frequent.

The *microscopic characteristics* of chronic salpingitis are similar to those of chronic inflammation elsewhere. The chief feature is a more or less extensive infiltration with round and plasma cells.

One of the most common forms of chronic endometritis is the *postabortive*. Retention of placental tissue is frequent after either full term delivery or abortion, especially the latter. Even in spontaneous abortion, the uterine cavity is soon invaded by organisms from the cervix and vagina, so that one may expect to find chronic endometritis in all the very numerous cases of incomplete miscarriage in which operative removal of the retained placental tissue is necessary. So frequent is this association that it is a good rule in all cases of chronic endometritis to examine the microscopic slides for chorionic villi and other evidences of recent pregnancy.

When villi are found they may be well preserved or they may show marked degeneration with fibrosis or hyalinization (ghost or shadow villi). Not infrequently the retained villi may form a polypoid mass of grumous material firmly attached to the uterine wall. The finding of villi is absolutely diagnostic of preceding pregnancy. Decidual cells are also often found. When they are well preserved, and have the typical appearance of large polygonal cells put together in mosaic fashion, there can be little doubt of preceding pregnancy. However, since decidual cells are of maternal origin, they cannot be considered as decisive in diagnosis as the fetal villi, and they may at times be

1) la freaus des joueures ha scalor frequente pulin c'è il dreuaggio
" da serum pingeri = + frequente, specie postabortiva -

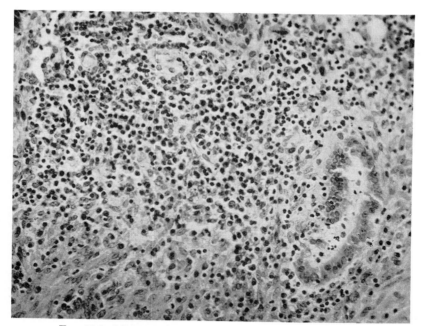

FIG. 20.1. Microscopic appearance of chronic endometritis

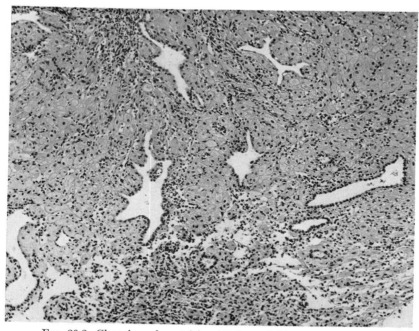

FIG. 20.2. Chronic endometritis with large field of decidual cells

simulated by other cells, such as those of certain types of epidermoid cancer. Some degree of myometritis may be a concomitant of endometritis.

Subinvolution of Uterus. Subinvolution of the uterus, as the term indicates, refers to the condition in which postpartum or postabortum involution is incom-

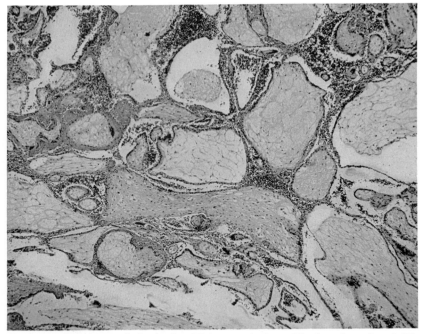

FIG. 20.3. Degenerated chorionic villi in association with chronic endometritis

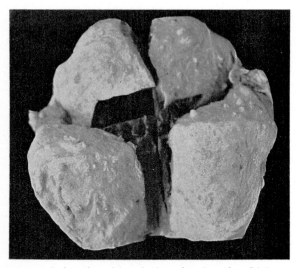

FIG. 20.4. Gross picture of chronic subinvolution showing the thickness of the uterine wall and the bumpy appearance due to enlarged blood vessels.

plete. The term, however, is not merely a clinical one, for Schwarz and his coworkers, as well as other writers, have shown that it is characterized by distinctive histological changes. Whereas normally involution is complete in 8 or 10 weeks after delivery, the subinvoluted uterus may show, many months later, a persistent moderate enlargement and congestion, especially when it is retrodisplaced, as it so commonly is. The syndrome of "pelvic congestion" as described by Taylor seems to us to be a rather nebulous dumping ground for all kinds of vague psychosomatic problems, and a frequent excuse in attempting justification of questionable hysterectomies before tissue committees (see "Myometrial Hypertrophy," p. 333).

The chief *microscopic* feature appears to be an increased amount of elastic tissue around the vessels and between the muscle bundles as a result of incompleteness of absorption of this tissue following delivery. Another characteristic finding is the formation of new blood vessels in the lumina of the degenerated and obliterated original vessels.

Chronic Salpingitis. This may be present either in the form of a diffuse chronic inflammation of the tubal wall (chronic interstitial salpingitis) or of certain sequelae of the inflammatory process, marked by overdistention of the tube with retained exudate (pyosalpinx or hydrosalpinx).

An interesting special variety of chronic salpingitis is the so-called *salpingitis isthmica nodosa*, in which the residue of a sustained chronic inflammatory process is limited chiefly to the isthmic portion of the tube. In such cases marked nodulation of the tubal isthmus is seen, the nodules being sometimes so large as to simulate small cornual fibroid tumors. The remainder of the tube may seem fairly normal, and the fimbriated end may be open, although in other cases the entire tube is thickened and the end closed and bulbous.

Microscopic examination in such cases presents a curious picture, in that there may appear to be many small lumina instead of just one. The original isthmic lumen may or may not be still recognizable, but in addition to this, many epithelium-lined glandlike cavities are scattered throughout the muscularis. Such cases are often mistaken for adenomyosis of the tube, but they differ from the latter in that the lining epithelium is tubal rather than uterine, that endometrial stroma is lacking, and that the muscle shows various degrees of round cell infiltration. Occasionally, however, distinction is very difficult.

Hydrosalpinx. Gonorrheal infection especially is prone to cause inflammatory

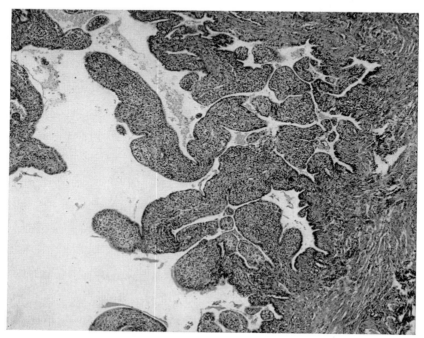

FIG. 20.5. Microscopic appearance of chronic interstitial salpingitis

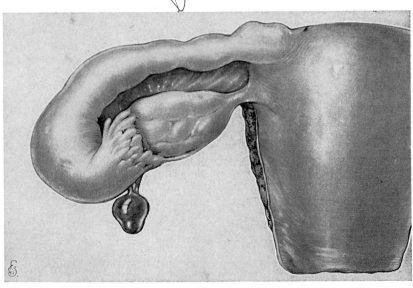

FIG. 20.6. Salpingitis isthmica nodosa

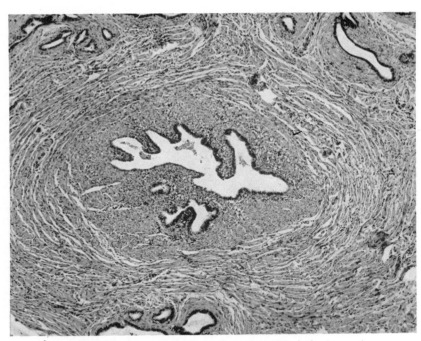

FIG. 20.7. Microscopic appearance of salpingitis isthmica nodosa

obstruction at various points in the tube, especially the uterine and fimbriated ends. Purulent material is retained between the obstructed areas, with often enormous distention of the tube, constituting *pyosalpinx*. Mention has already been made of the fact that the invading organisms tend to disappear within a short time, with the ultimate formation of a *hydrosalpinx;* and either may present as a large adherent mass frequently mistaken for an ovarian cyst. Various tubo-ovarian inflammatory masses may occur.

The microscopic picture of *pyosalpinx*

il gonococco distrutto primo, provoca formazione di pus, da istinto (non dreno, sparke quindi (hidrosalpingx) – (pyosalpinx) is that of chronic inflammatory infiltration of the thickened walls, adhesions on the peritoneal surface, round and plasma cell infiltration of the tubal folds, degeneration and sometimes loss of considerable areas of the covering epithelium, and the presence of a large amount of pus within the lumen.

Two types of *hydrosalpinx* are described, *simplex* and *follicularis*. In the former the lumen on cross section is seen to consist of a single thin-walled cavity. In the follicular variety, on the other hand, it is divided into a number of, sometimes many, small compartments by *trabeculae* representing the fused tubal folds. In this variety, the overdistention of the lumen is preceded by a follicular salpingitis, in which this same matting together and fusion of adjacent folds takes place.

As to the cause of hydrosalpinx, there would seem to be little doubt that the condition is the frequent end result of longstanding pyosalpinx, in which the purulent elements have been resorbed and

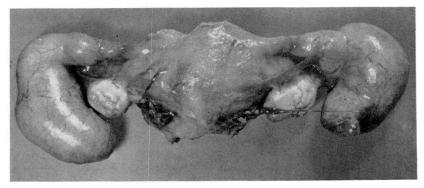

Fig. 20.8. Large bilateral pyosalpinx

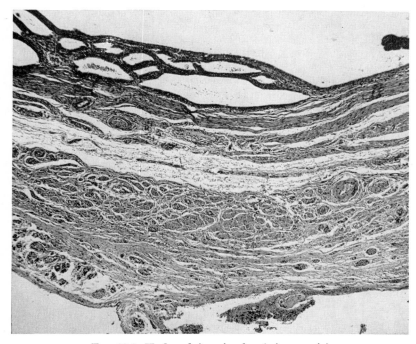

Fig. 20.9. Hydrosalpinx simplex (microscopic)

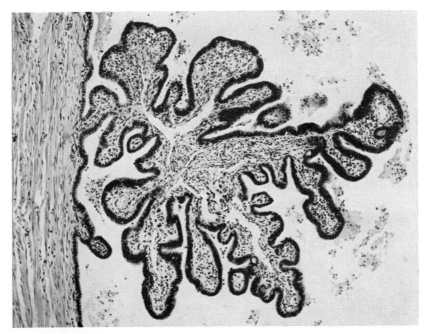

FIG. 20.10. Wall of large hydrosalpinx simplex showing persistence of stunted tubal folds

a clear fluid left. This is confirmed by the fact that hydrosalpinx is rarely found unless the history indicates that the pelvic disease has been of long duration.

The *microscopic* appearance of hydrosalpinx simplex shows a clear cystic central cavity, with a flattened tubal mucosa whose folds have been ironed out and almost or entirely obliterated although, usually an occasional small fold can be seen here and there. The thinned-out wall of the tube often shows little or no evidence, in the form of inflammatory change, of the infection which had occurred perhaps many years previously.

In hydrosalpinx follicularis, as mentioned in the gross description, the distended lumen presents a multilocular appearance, each locule being a cross section of a gutter-like subdivision of the lumen. As in the simple variety, there is apt to be little microscopic evidence of the infectious storm which had passed over the tube long before.

Chronic Oophoritis and Periooph-oritis. The ovaries may be extensively involved in chronic pelvic inflammatory disease, but on the whole much less frequently than the tubes. In most cases the ovarian involvement is secondary to that of the adjacent tube. Infection may enter the ovary through the portals of ruptured follicles, and either a chronic oophoritis or an abscess thus result. In the former the ovarian stroma may show considerable inflammatory infiltration; in the latter large accumulations of pus may develop, not infrequently merging with an adjacent pyosalpinx to form a *tubo-ovarian abscess*. The so-called cystic degeneration of the ovary is not infrequent, presumably from an exaggeration of the process of atresia folliculi as a result of the inflammatory hyperemia. Various "tubo-ovarian inflammatory cysts" may be formed.

Perhaps the most frequent of all ovarian lesions in chronic pelvic inflammatory disease is *chronic perioophoritis*, which is practically always found when the ovarian substance is involved, and in addition is often present when the ovary itself is comparatively normal. The surface involvement of the ovary is expressed

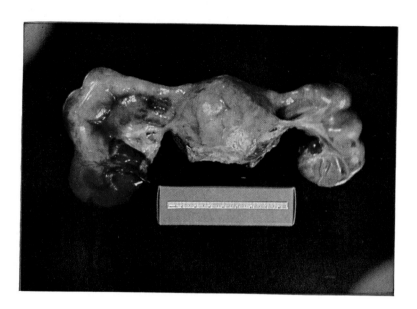

PLATE XX.I. Typical appearance of chronic salpingitis

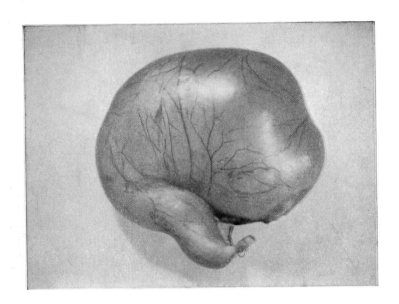

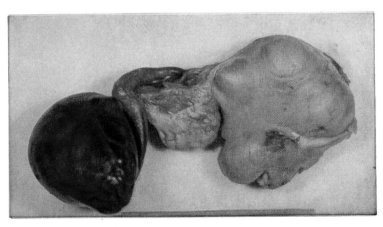

PLATE XX.II. *Top*, large thin-walled hydrosalpinx. *Bottom*, moderate-sized hydrosalpinx which has undergone torsion in its distal portion.

uterus may be in normal position, but is often retroverted or retroflexed, and often much less movable than normally. Efforts to move it about by manipulation of the cervix or fundus may cause much pain, and drawing the cervix forward will also make the patient complain of pain, which not infrequently is referred to the rectum. The uterosacral ligaments are often thickened and sensitive, but not nodular as in endometriosis. Examination under anesthesia is frequently helpful, especially in the tense patient.

DIFFERENTIAL DIAGNOSIS

Among the pelvic conditions which may be mistaken for chronic pelvic inflammatory disease, and *vice versa*, is *ectopic pregnancy*. In the latter condition there is likely to be a history of slight delay, in menstruation, followed by persistent slight bleeding of a "spotting" character. Sometimes, on the other hand, the flow may be anticipated by a number of days. In pelvic inflammatory disease the menstrual rhythm is often not disturbed. With ectopic pregnancy the pain is likely to be colicky, severe, and one-sided, with not infrequently associated nausea and attacks of faintness. The latter are lacking in chronic pelvic inflammation, and the pain is most often bilateral and of heavy bearing-down or aching character. Pelvic examination in cases of tubal pregnancy shows a unilateral tender mass, with no tenderness in the opposite side. Culdoscopic examination is generally decisive, and this simple endoscopic method of visualizing the pelvic organs is highly recommended in the study of many pelvic complaints.

Evaluation of tubal disease is often facilitated by examination under anesthesia along with curettage which may on occasion reveal a tuberculous disease. We likewise feel that a Rubin's test may be of assistance in the distinction of inflammatory disease and endometriosis. Sweeney rightly emphasizes the possibility of false negative or positive tests, but gives us the impression that insufflation is just about as useful as hysterograms,

especially if proper techniques and interpretation are not to be had. We feel that evaluation of hysterosalpingograms is not always completely reliable; for example, a recent patient with an apparent complete cornual blockage in her only remaining tube subsequently became pregnant.

Pelvic endometriosis is another condition which may be difficult to distinguish from chronic pelvic inflammatory disease. In either, there may be a history of pelvic pain, increasing dysmenorrhea, dyspareunia, and involuntary sterility, and in either the pelvic examination may reveal the adnexa to be enlarged and adherent to the posterior surface of a retroplaced uterus. The presence of one or more nodules in the uterosacral ligaments is always highly suggestive of endometriosis, but this physical sign is often absent. Of circumstantial value is the fact that endometriosis is more likely to occur in the higher types of patient, while pelvic inflammatory disease is more apt to be seen in the dispensary group. In the presence of severe symptoms of the type enumerated above, surgery is likely to be indicated with either disease, so that failure to make an accurate preoperative diagnosis works no hardship on the patient.

Ideopathic retroperitoneal fibrosis is placed in this chapter with certain misgivings, for it is by no means certain that this represents an inflammatory process. Actually it is a rather new entity in gynecological journals, and it is only in the last 5 years that this ill defined disease has been recognized by us, although such urologists as Ormond noted it earlier.

Clinically the symptoms are rather vague, consisting primarily of nondescript pain with occasional nausea, anorexia, low grade fever, and urinary symptoms. Pelvic examination may suggest varying degrees of induration or the presence of a mass, and pyelography often shows bilateral ureteral obstruction with a tendency towards medial displacement of the ureters.

The cause is highly speculative; infections of various types including tuberculosis, collagen disorders, hypersensitivity reaction, and a host of other etiological factors have been suggested. That it is an infection of the pelvis (admittedly retroperitoneal) with subsequent lymphangitis and fibrosis seems most likely. Treatment has generally consisted of lysis of the obstructed ureter, occasionally with intraperitoneal fixation, although x-ray and cortisone have also been suggested as therapeutic measures.

TREATMENT

The trend of recent years in the management of chronic pelvic inflammatory disease has been definitely a conservative one, although there are still many cases in which surgery must be invoked. It should be remembered, first of all, that the disease is rarely a life-endangering one, so that efforts at conservative treatment are not fraught with any real danger to the patient, as is the case with certain other gynecological diseases.

In women with large tubo-ovarian masses and with often a retrodisplaced uterus firmly fixed to the rectum, and with troublesome symptoms which can not be relieved by palliative measures, surgery is fully justified. This is true even in the case of younger women, especially when repeated tubal patency tests have shown the tubes to be closed. If pregnancy is to be denied such women, the next best thing is to restore them to health, as can be done in most cases by surgery. The results of plastic procedures to restore tubal patency are notoriously poor, but they are justified if the patient is exceedingly anxious for even the slightest possibility of success, and if the slimness of her chances in this respect is honestly put before her.

It must also be remembered that women with chronic pelvic inflammatory disease must run the risk of acute exacerbations as a result of reinfection from the cervix or from an infected sex partner. This is probably the usual explanation of such exacerbations, rather than the assumption of a flare-up in a dormant tubal infection (Curtis). In any event, if exacerbations occur rather frequently in spite of treatment of lower genital foci and efforts to prevent marital reinfection, surgery may be indicated, but it should be done in a quiescent period of the disease. Abdominal operation is always contraindicated in the acute stage, and should ordinarily be deferred for a number of weeks after subsidence of the acute symptoms.

On the whole, however, conservative treatment is indicated when the patient gets along quite comfortably, with perhaps no discomfort other than slight dysmenorrhea or occasional slight bearing-down in the pelvic region, or perhaps not even these symptoms. Even if the symptoms are much more pronounced, there is no urgency in recommending surgical treatment, and conservative treatment should be given a trial. This consists of such simple measures as enforcing a reasonable amount of rest, moderation in sexual intercourse, the eradication of any foci of infection in the cervix, urethra, or vulvovaginal glands, the avoidance insofar as possible of reinfection, and the use of hot douches or sitz baths. Some have advocated the use of some form of cortisone (for its antifibrotic effect) in conjunction with antibiotics.

When, on the other hand, the patient becomes increasingly miserable because of pain in the lower abdomen, severe dysmenorrhea, menstrual irregularities, and sometimes even a condition of semiinvalidism, elective operation is ordinarily indicated. In the same way, the nature and extent of the operation must be decided on an individual basis. In most cases, unfortunately, both tubes are involved and both must often be removed. If one tube is still patent and the patient exceedingly anxious for children, she will usually be willing to run the risk of a possible second operation later on, if she can be honestly told that she has at least some chance of pregnancy.

Even if both tubes are closed, some form of plastic operation such as salpingostomy, resection and tubouterine anastomosis, or cornual implantation of the ovaries is justified in the occasional case in which the woman is desperately anxious for motherhood, with full explanation of the very small percentage of successful results in such cases, probably not over about 5%.

Results with tuboplastic surgery following tubal sterilization are somewhat better, for one is not dealing with a basically diseased tube. Indeed operation on infected closed tubes may often restore patency but not the vital physiological and peristaltic action of the oviduct. Siegler and Hellman have recently reviewed the prerequisites for and results with tubal plastic surgery in 50 patients. Hanton, Pratt, and Banner report 18 pregnancies among 75 women treated by a variety of tuboplastic procedures; however, 74% of those studied had patent tubes immediately postoperative although in those studied later, tubal patency was present in 55%.

When both tubes are so hopelessly involved that their removal is necessary, opinion is uniform that hysterectomy is advisable. There is no reason to preserve the uterus when pregnancy cannot ensue, but of course the woman should be advised as to what hysterectomy will entail. The true facts are apt to be very different from what she had heard in the beauty parlor or her bridge club. Only in the youthful, unrealistic woman who cannot be convinced of the unimportance of continued menstruation should the uterus be preserved. Total hysterectomy is the operation of choice, but it is preferable to leave the cervix should removal pose a threat to the integrity of ureter, bladder, or bowel. When the discriminating surgeon suspects he may have a difficult operative case, he will perform office biopsy and smear. If these are negative the decision to abstain from removal of the cervix is made much more simple.

Finally, the *importance of conserving ovarian tissue* whenever possible cannot be too strongly emphasized. Practically all operations for pelvic inflammatory disease are done on women in the reproductive age for the cessation of menstruation seems to uniformly end the stimulus to "flare-ups" even when infection has been present. Entirely aside from the question of pregnancy, and even when this is obviously impossible, the retention of ovarian tissue may spare the woman many of the possible discomforts of an artificial menopause. It is perfectly true that even complete ablation of both ovaries in young women may cause only slight menopausal disturbance, but in a small proportion the symptoms are sufficiently severe that, in the woman's own mind, her lot is far worse than before operation. Where one tube is closed but not hopelessly distorted, it seems preferable on occasion to preserve the entire adnexa. Removal of the tube alone, especially where adherent, is often attended by marked cystic changes in the ovary. In any case preservation of some ovarian tissue can usually be accomplished.

REFERENCES

Bayly, M. A., and Satlin, A. H.: Residues of pelvic inflammatory disease and abnormal uterine bleeding. Amer. J. Obstet. Gynec., *82:* 505, 1961.

Curtis, A. H. (editor): Gonorrheal disease of female genitalia. In *Obstetrics and Gynecology*, Vol. 2, Ch. 52. W. B. Saunders Company, Philadelphia, 1933.

Curtis, A. H.: Hypertrophy of uterus. Amer. J. Obstet. Gynec., *50:* 748, 1945.

Dumoulin, J. G., and Hughesdon, P. E.: Chronic endometritis. J. Obstet. Gynaec. Brit. Common., *58:* 222, 1951.

Gardner, G. H.: Management of chronic pelvic infection. Surg. Gynec. Obstet., *70:* 370, 1940.

Gordon, C. A.: Management of chronic pelvic inflammations. Amer. J. Surg., *13:* 484, 1931.

Greenhill, J. P.: Present status of plastic operation on fallopian tubes. Amer. J. Obstet. Gynec., *72:* 516, 1956.

Hanton, E. M., Pratt, J. H., and Banner, E. A.: Tubal plastic surgery at the Mayo Clinic. Amer. J. Obstet. Gynec., *89:* 934, 1964.

Harrow, B. R., and Sloane, J. A.: Ideopathic retroperitoneal fibrosis. J. A. M. A., *182:* 148, 1962.

Hesseltine, H. C.: Pelvic inflammatory disease. Surg. Clin. N. Amer., *33:* 269, 1953.

Hurtig, A.: Cortisone in obstetrics and gynecology. In *Year Book of Obstetrics and Gynecology, 1963–1964*, edited by J. P. Greenhill, p. 369. Year Book Medical Publishers, Inc., Chicago, 1964.

Hüter, K. A., and Hartman, P.: Antiphlogistic corticosteroids in combination with tetracycline in the treatment of inflammations of the female genital tract. Geburtsh. Frauenheilk., *18:* 1223, 1958.

Jones, H. W.: Discussion of above paper. Obstet. Gynec. Survey, *14:* 279, 1959.

Josey, W. E., Thompson, J. D., and Te Linde, R. W.: Ten years' experience with culdoscopy; analysis of 594 cases. Southern Med. J., *50:* 713, 1957.

Magruder, C. J.: Surgical management of chronic pelvic inflammatory disease. Obstet. Gynec., *13:* 591, 1959.

Ormond, J. K.: Bilateral ureteral obstruction due to envelopment and compression by an inflammatory retroperitoneal process. J. Urol., *59:* 1072, 1948.

Phaneuf, L. E.: Pelvic infection in women. New Eng. J. Med., *209:* 334, 1933.

Schwarz, O.: Benign diffuse enlargement of the uterus. Amer. J. Obstet. Gynec., *61:* 902, 1951.

Siegler, A. M., and Hellman, L. M.: Tubal plastic surgery. A retrospective study of 50 cases. Amer. J. Obstet. Gynec., *86:* 448, 1963.

Sweeney, W. J.: Pitfalls in present-day methods of evaluating tubal function. Fertil. Steril., *13:* 124, 1962.

Symmonds, R. E., Dahlin, D. C., and Engel, S.: Ideopathic retroperitoneal fibrosis. Obstet. Gynec., *18:* 591, 1961.

Taylor, H. C.: Pelvic pain based on vascular and autonomic nervous system disorder. Amer. J. Obstet. Gynec., *67:* 1177, 1954.

21

TUBERCULOSIS OF FEMALE GENERATIVE ORGANS

Whereas any portion of the female genital tract may be invaded by the tubercle bacillus, there is almost uniformly initial pelvic involvement of the tubes, although there are exceptional cases of primary cervical tuberculosis in which the sexual partner has been thought to be the source of infection. With the exception of these few instances, in which infection is incurred by intercourse with a male having tuberculosis epididymitis, tubal involvement is almost 100% in the woman with pelvic tuberculosis.

By the same token, peritonitis is almost always secondary to pelvic (tubal) tuberculosis, although it is often difficult to establish this. Certainly involvement of the peritoneum without a real tuberculous endo- (not just peri-) salpingitis is unusual. With the routine pasteurization of milk and the disappearance of bovine tuberculosis, primary gastrointestinal acid-fast disease is rare, and the tubes seem to be about the only logical focus for both pelvic and intraabdominal tuberculosis, at least in the United States.

Modes of Infection. In almost all cases tuberculous involvement of the female genitalia is secondary to pulmonary tuberculosis, although it is rare to find that this lesion is currently active. Occasionally pelvic tuberculosis may be a part of a generalized miliary tuberculous disease, but we have been so impressed by the infrequent association of urinary and genital tuberculosis as to speculate as to whether involvement of one system may tend to immunize the other. However, pulmonary disease is the usual primary site and the probable route of dissemination is almost certainly hematogenous. It is difficult to explain why it is the tubes that usually receive the primary impact of this blood stream involvement. It is likewise difficult to understand how pelvic tuberculosis can occur in the absence of an active pulmonary lesion, unless we assume that a clinically undetected lung disease has undergone spontaneous healing *after* there has been some type of bacteremia to which the tubes alone are singularly responsive. In any case chest x-ray usually shows evidence of only an old primary complex.

TUBERCULOSIS OF TUBES

As already stated, the tubes constitute the initial seat of genital tuberculosis in the overwhelming majority of cases, the bacilli reaching them by any one of the routes mentioned above. Tuberculous salpingitis is not by any means rare, forming approximately 5% of all cases of salpingitis in some areas of the world where disease and malnutrition are present, although it is much less common in this country.

Pathology. The *gross* appearance of the tuberculous tube varies in different cases, but as a rule is not different from that of the various forms of chronic gonorrheal salpingitis. The tube may resemble a pyosalpinx, occasionally hydrosalpinx, frequently chronic interstitial salpingitis, and not infrequently salpingitis isthmica nodosa. In the form associated with miliary tuberculous peritonitis, numerous tubercles may stud the surface, just as they do the pelvic peritoneal cavity. Far more frequently, however, no tubercles are visible externally, although they may be present in advanced stages of the hematogenous variety. Greenberg and others have called attention to the so-called tobacco-pouch or mail-pouch appearance of the fimbriated extremity, produced by the eversion of the fimbriae (see Fig. 21.2). This is in contrast to the closed bulbous fimbriated extremity so characteristic of the gonorrheal variety. This feature, however, is by no means a constant one. As a matter of fact the diagnosis of tuberculous salpingitis is usually not made until microscopic examination has been carried out.

Microscopic. The microscopic diagnosis is easy in the frank, advanced case, but it may be difficult in the early phases of the disease or in the late reparative phase, which is not infrequently noted. Many blocks may have to be taken from various parts of the tube before the telltale evidence, in the form of tubercles and giant cells, can be demonstrated. Acid-fast stains are more specific; even when these are negative, a positive culture may be obtained.

The above emphasizes the difficulty of eliminating a primary site in the tubes in cases of tuberculosis of other parts of the genital canal. In the early stages one often finds a markedly proliferative, adenomatous-looking pattern in the folds. This should always excite suspicion, and it *should not be mistaken for adenocarcinoma*, as it has often been. In the more outspoken cases, one finds numerous tubercles, many with giant cells, and chronic inflammation. The tubercles may be limited to the mucosa, or they may be

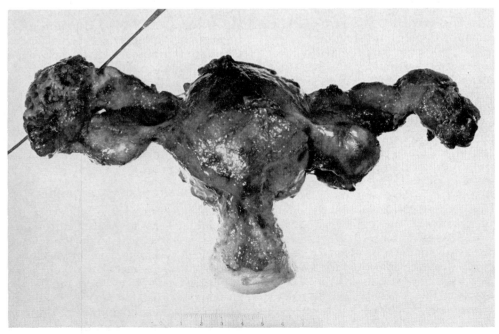

FIG. 21.1. Tubal tuberculosis. Note probe protruding out patent fimbria at reader's left

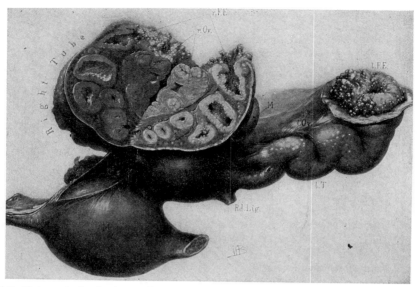

FIG. 21.2. Tuberculosis of tubes and ovaries; note everted condition of fimbriated end of tube

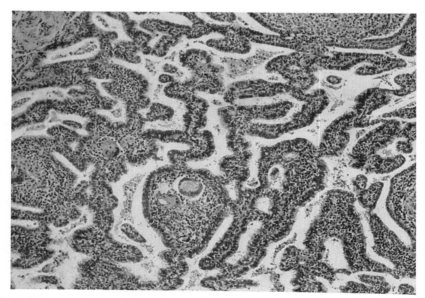

FIG. 21.3. Microscopic appearance of tubal tuberculosis with typical tubercles and giant cells and marked proliferation of tubal folds.

scattered throughout the muscularis and on the peritoneal coat. In advanced stages, extensive caseation is common.

TUBERCULOSIS OF THE ENDOMETRIUM

As noted by Greenberg, this is always secondary to tubal involvement, occur-ring in about 50% of patients with tuberculous salpingitis. Although Knauss, in performing bilateral salpingectomy, has found residual endometritis in 80% of all women; most of these patients also had a tuberculous peritonitis, a further testimony to the high association of tubal and peritoneal disease. The presence of acid-fast endometritis is presumptive evidence of tubal disease, but the absence of tubercles in removed endometrium by no means excludes a specific tuberculous adnexitis. Actually, sterility work-ups have disclosed an unsuspected tuberculous endometritis in nearly 5% of cases, and such writers as Sharman conclude that latent tubal tuberculosis is a not infrequent factor in the production of sterility.

The *pathology* of tuberculous endometritis is characterized by the presence of typical tubercles with epithelioid and giant cells, involving the endometrium alone or with occasional extension into the myometrium. In early cases it may be difficult to find tubercles in curettings, but the finding of a chronic endometritis should always prompt a thorough search for evidence of the acid-fast bacillus. In advanced stages there are extensive tubercles with many giant cells and varying degrees of caseation, but even in advanced disease there are no specific gross findings. Acid-fast culture of the endometrium is positive in only about 75% of all cases, and acid-fast stains are often unsuccessful. As a rule pelvic tuberculosis behaves like tuberculosis anywhere.

TUBERCULOSIS OF THE OVARIES

This practically never occurs in the absence of tubal involvement, and when present, it generally consists of a rather marked perioophoritis rather than a real ovarian involvement. This tends to heal spontaneously following removal of the tube so that preservation of at least one ovary can generally be accomplished even in very extensive pelvic tuberculosis afflicting a young woman (see section on "Treatment"). The recent study by Francis would seem to affirm ovarian conservation in the young woman.

TUBERCULOSIS OF THE CERVIX

This has already been discussed in Chapter 11, "Cervicitis and Cervical Polyp."

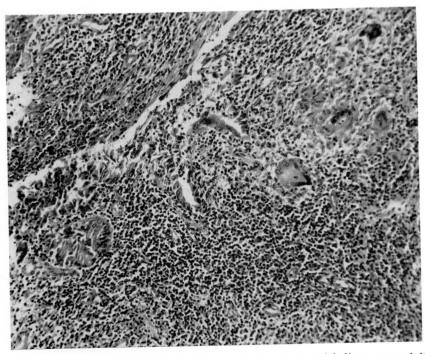

Fig. 21.4. Typical tuberculosis involving the cervix (squamous epithelium, *upper left*, barely distinguishable).

The final diagnosis of pelvic tuberculosis is often not made until laparotomy is performed, and may not be apparent even at the operating table. Careful histological study is necessary; frequently it is necessary to cut many blocks and make many sections of the tube before the characteristic lesions can be found. Care must be taken to exclude various granulomatous processes and foreign body giant cell reaction. Where tuberculosis is found unequivocally in one tube, we have always been able to find it in the other, although theoretically this might not be true. Bilateral tubal involvement seems, however, to be almost the uniform rule.

TREATMENT

In past years the treatment of diagnosed pelvic tuberculosis was almost entirely surgical plus the usual regimen of rest, fresh air, good nutrition, etc. Tuberculous peritonitis was treated by paracentesis or laparotomy with simple exposure to air, and although the morbidity and mortality rates were high, some of the patients did well. Recent advances in the fields of antibiotics and chemotherapy in the last 15 years have equipped us with a number of effective antituberculous drugs. At this writing there are three main effective antituberculous drugs, but extensive work on the development of others is currently under way.

One must not infer that surgical procedures have been completely abandoned, for this is certainly not true. Chemotherapy is used only in those patients who have patent tubes, are desirous of further pregnancy, and have little or no discomfort. Persistent, painful adnexal masses, continued fever, and elevated sedimentation rate, ascites, and failure to respond to medical treatment are indications for a surgical replacement for any existent medical mode of treatment. In many instances operation is made technically less difficult and attended by a lower morbidity rate with preoperative antituberculous therapy, utilized for several months prior to surgery. In some instances there is such a striking response to medical therapy that surgery can be deferred for as yet undetermined periods of time.

Medical Treatment. Of the three main available drugs, the first to be used was (dihydro) *streptomycin*, and it is still widely utilized today if sensitivity tests indicate that the organism to be treated will respond. Streptomycin must be given intramuscularly, and generally 1 gm. daily is given for several weeks. Dosage is gradually decreased to 1 gm. biweekly, and the patient may be maintained on this dosage for many months, or until toxicity is noted. This consists primarily of evidence of eighth nerve damage, both acoustic and cochlear branches being susceptible, with resultant deafness, vertigo, nausea, etc. These toxic effects are by no means universal and actually afflict only a few patients. However, once toxic effects appear, they are very slow to disappear even after cessation of the offending drug; therefore, the physician is wise to be alerted for the incipient signs of toxicity.

Frequently utilized in conjunction with streptomycin has been *para*aminosalicylic acid (PAS) which, while only mildly bactericidal, has seemed to enhance the effect of streptomyocin. PAS must be taken orally and in large dosage, generally 3 gm. four times a day. Not a few, but a great many, patients have such severe gastrointestinal disorders as to mandate discontinuance of this drug. Profound anorexia, nausea, vomiting, and diarrhea can be expected in a considerable proportion of those patients taking PAS, so that this medication simply must be stopped.

The most recent addition to antituberculous chemotherapy has been isonicotinic acid (INH). This has the advantage of oral administration and in small doses has been considered to be nontoxic. Dosage has varied according to body weight, 5 mg. per kg. of body weight, which generally approximates 300 to 400 mg. daily. More recent unpublished work, however, suggests that there are some patients who metabolize INH very rapidly with uncertain therapeutic effect. For this reason, very large dosages of INH (1000 to 1500 mg.) have been tried in a few individuals with promising if preliminary results. Where large doses of INH are being used, it is important to accompany this by ample doses of pyridoxine (200 mg. daily) to guard against the most important toxic effect, peripheral neuritis.

Thus, there are three main drugs available for the medical treatment of tuberculosis of the female generative tract. It would seem that no one drug is nearly as effective as a combination of any two, but any combination of two is just about as effective as any other. PAS and INH can of course be taken orally, and no physician-administered injection of streptomycin is thereby necessary for the woman who is treated on an outpatient basis. Equally good results may be obtained by combinations of streptomycin and INH, which will of course obviate the unpleasant gastrointestinal disorders incurred by PAS although a twice weekly intramuscular injection is necessary. Fortunately, none of the drugs utilized need serious consideration in regard to expense, all being reasonably priced. Chemotherapy is generally continued for about 18 months.

Following diagnosis and medical treatment the patient must be kept under close observation. Pelvic tuberculosis is still a potentially serious disease, and miliary or various forms of extragenital tuberculosis can arise. If a patient has been treated because of a curettage-proved tuberculous endometritis, repeat curettage is in order every 6 months for several years. Should the endometritis persist or recede only to recur later, surgery is indicated.

Surgical Treatment. Persistent or recurrent endometritis is only one of several indications for prompt surgical intervention. We are in complete accord with Zummo, Sered, and Falls who feel that patients with the more advanced forms of pelvic disease are to be considered as candidates for surgery. They further state that despite early diagnosis and initial response to available drugs, subsequent surgical intervention is still necessary. They find indications to consist of adnexal masses, abscesses, prominent thickenings, and ascites, and with such tenets these authors are in full accord.

As a matter of fact, if it can be determined that the tubes are definitely unequivocally closed, there is not much justification for prolonged medical therapy. In other words, medical therapy should be reserved primarily for those individuals who have patent tubes and are anxious for further pregnancies, with the prospect of surgery should the chemotherapeutic regimen show the slightest sign of recurrent activation, drug resistance, or other such features. The extensive review from Liverpool (Francis) would suggest confirmation of a surgical approach where the tubes are occluded or where there is persistent extensive disease. A highly enlightening discussion by Schaefer and Sutherland clarifies the indications for surgical treatment and emphasizes the necessity of preoperative drug therapy. Certain minor differences may be noted in the American and English approach to pelvic tuberculosis, but basically their thoughts are similar to our own.

Should a patient have extensive pelvic tuberculosis initially or such other indications as noted above, it is probable that her interests are best served by operation. It must be understood that pelvic tuberculosis was formerly treated by surgery alone, and that these operations were often the most difficult a surgeon would be asked to perform. The tissues were edematous and friable, adhesions were multiple and cartilaginous, and the patients were often in poor general health. Morbidity was high in the days of surgical treatment alone for extensive tuberculosis, with a considerable proportion of such complications as fistulas, wound disruption, bowel obstruction, and even death.

It has been conclusively shown that

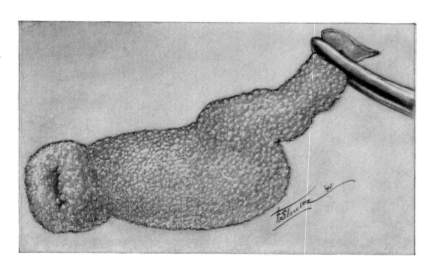

PLATE XXI.I. Tuberculosis of tube associated with tuberculous peritonitis

a preoperative course of chemotherapy will cause enough tissue improvement to make operation technically less difficult and fraught with fewer complications. Following drug treatment there seems to be a subsidence of edema, and a marked improvement of tissue induration. Some combination, then, of drugs should precede surgery for several months at least; indeed chemotherapy has been advocated for many months preoperative unless there is evidence of drug resistance. Our belief is that with extensive pelvic involvement, a prolonged course of drugs is desirable, but where there is a freely mobile uterus without adnexal masses (but with closed tubes and with biopsy proven acid-fast disease of the endometrium), only a token 1 week course of drugs is sufficient. Subsequent chemotherapy for another 18 months is usually recommended.

As to the type of surgery, there has been considerable change in our thinking processes in the last two decades. It used to be stated that simple removal of the tubes was sufficient operation, and this removal of the primary pelvic focus would then permit the lower genital tract to purge itself of the disease. Part of the rationale of this thinking may have been influenced by the lesser facilities for major surgery 20 years ago, for it has been conclusively shown that there is a high incidence of tuberculous endometritis following simple salpingectomy. Similarly Schaefer, Brown, Gilbert, and Te Linde, and Stallworthy find that the greatest incidence of tuberculous cervicitis has been in those cases in which only subtotal hysterectomy has been performed.

The British take an even grimmer view and Stallworthy points out that the tuberculous uterus is treated "like the malignant one with a corpus carcinoma." The cervix is packed and sutured to avoid spillage and total hysterectomy with bilateral salpingo-oophorectomy is performed. Opinion is uniform that total hysterectomy is desirable, with removal of the tubes and frequently both ovaries in case of extensive disease. Even where frank tuberculous abscesses are encountered with free spillage of the necrotic caseous contents, drainage is to be avoided because of the very real possibility of fistula formation.

Many American clinicians feel that in the case of young women it is perfectly permissible to conserve an ovary and thereby avoid a premature menopause. Obviously this is not feasible in cases in which there is a frank tuberculous tubo-ovarian abscess, but there are many instances in which cursory inspection suggests considerable ovarian involvement. Yet more careful appraisal will show only a thickened adherent capsule, and the pathological nature of adnexal tuberculosis, we must remember, is to involve not the ovarian substance, but only the capsule. It has always been our policy to practice this conservative surgery, when feasible, on the young woman, and we cannot recall a case in which a retained ovary caused any further difficulty in perpetuating or activating the acid-fast process.

PREGNANCY AND TUBERCULOSIS

It has been noted that there is a rather large number of women, outwardly healthy and with no other complaint than infertility, who are found to have endometrial tuberculosis. Sharman estimates these to comprise about 5% of all patients appearing at a Sterility Clinic, but he also believes that a much truer index of pelvic tuberculosis would be 10%, since the endometrium is involved in only about 50% of patients with tubal disease. Greenhill is inclined to feel that this figure is much higher than the likely incidence in the United States, and does not believe that a significant number of cases with acid-fast disease is being overlooked in our own clinics.

Once a diagnosis of tuberculous endometritis has been established in the young woman desiring pregnancy, how then shall she be handled? If there is no other contraindication to pregnancy such as closed tubes, if there are no palpable adnexal masses, fever, or ascites, and if the patient is cooperative, medical therapy is instituted, and actually these cases represent the main indication for drug therapy as far as the treatment of pelvic tuberculosis is concerned. It seems only fair to warn the woman that although her disease can be controlled in most instances, there may be exceptional drug-resistant cases which culminate in hysterectomy. At the same time she should be advised that the chances of a normal intrauterine pregnancy are relatively slim (as will be discussed subsequently).

The woman is then placed on one of the plans for medical therapy and is curetted (with culture) about twice a year. Should there be no recurrence of endometrial tuberculosis and no palpable evidence of incipient adnexal masses or induration, there is no reason not to continue conservative management for years. Yet it is a mistake to think that the antituberculous drugs are a panacea, for resistant strains occur. Also apparently it is possible to obliterate the disease in the endometrium without really curing the primary site, the tubes. Although these are open, for some reason the disease appears to flourish and to be difficult to eradicate in this location.

Despite the good medical results following treatment of asymptomatic pelvic tuberculosis, only a very few women have normal intrauterine pregnancies that go to term.

The report by Snaith and Barnes records six full term pregnancies among 158 treated patients, and Stallworthy records an 18% conception rate with 10% term pregnancy. Kreibich's 2.2% figure for normal pregnancy seems more realistic.

Schaefer has critically analyzed cases of full term pregnancy following genital tuberculosis where such an analysis was possible. His careful critique makes it seem apparent that in many reported cases the initial diagnosis of tuberculosis was far from absolute, and without histological or culture proof of acid-fast disease. Schaefer states that "less than 100 of 7357 patients with genital tuberculosis had full term intra-uterine pregnancies. The exact number is difficult to ascertain." The author adds that in the infrequent cases of pregnancy following genital tuberculosis, the end result is usually an abortion or an ectopic pregnancy. He further emphasizes the failure of tubal plastic surgery after antituberculous therapy, and points out that extensive degrees of genital infection lead to permanent infertility. This scholarly review should emphasize the extreme infrequency of normal term pregnancy in the woman with treated pelvic tuberculosis, and the patient should be appraised of this fact before institution of therapy.

Studdiford has published a rather extensive review of the simultaneous occurrence of pregnancy and pelvic tuberculosis. Fortunately the combination is rare, because the acid-fast disease is generally associated with intractable sterility. Where pregnancy occurs, however, there is a high incidence of spontaneous abortion which causes a drastic flare-up of the latent pelvic tuberculosis. Actually 3 out of Studdiford's 6 patients had a fatal outcome, prompting his statement that "in the rare event that uterine pregnancy should occur in a recently recognized case of pelvic tuberculosis, radical removal of the pelvic organs might be seriously considered." Before embarking on any plan for radical surgery one may well consider that a number of Studdiford's patients were treated before present day drugs were available, and Schaefer's more recent study is much more encouraging.

Even where pelvic tuberculosis has been treated and is quiescent, a not inconsiderable number of the small group of women becoming pregnant have the pregnancy terminated with spontaneous abortion. *Tubal pregnancies* are likewise disproportionately common. An excellent review of the subject is that of Halbrecht, who reported his material from Israel where constant warfare with resultant poor nutrition and hygiene have made pelvic tuberculosis unusually common. Halbrecht notes the important role that drugs and antibiotics play in controlling tubal infection, but states that they

la prondmesa ussoge consumenule (2.2% Kreibish) e c'e 1 un possibilita su 4 che gresta giunga a termine - l'un spesso si trus in aborto o in prondan to tubarica.

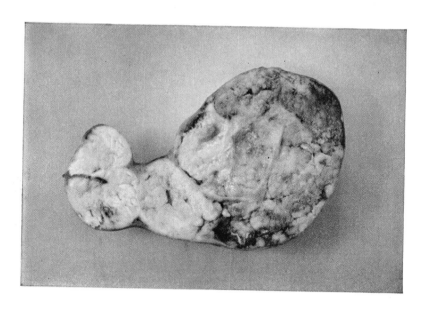

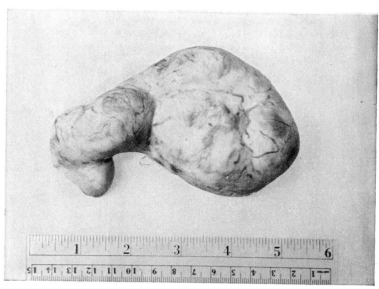

PLATE XXII.I. Primary carcinoma of tube

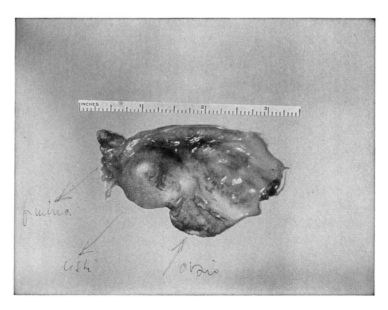

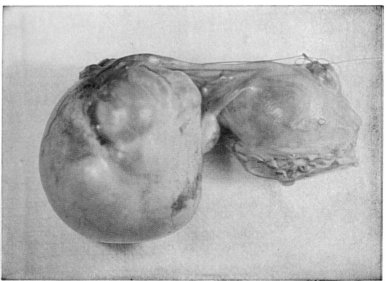

PLATE XXII.II. *Top*, small parovarian cyst; note its position between ovary and end of tube. *Bottom*, rather large parovarian cyst which might be mistaken for ovarian; note, however, the separateness of the ovary from the growth.

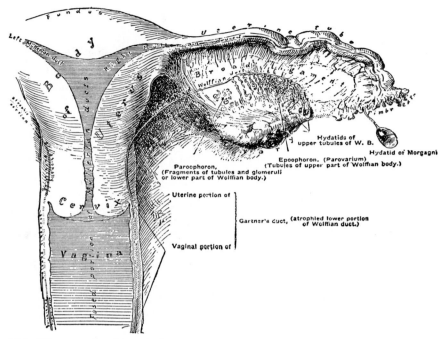

FIG. 22.6. Diagram showing relations of parovarian and Gartner's duct to pelvic organs. (From Cullen, T. S.: Bull. Johns Hopkins Hosp., 7: 112, 1896.)

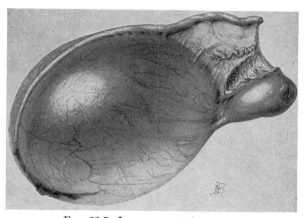

FIG. 22.7. Large parovarian cyst

other conditions. On the other hand, parovarian cysts may reach a very large size, although rarely as large as many cysts of the ovary itself. They are usually easily recognizable as of parovarian origin by their position, the ovary being intact and separate from the tumor, and the tube being stretched across the upper circumference of the cyst. The walls are very thin and the cavity contains a clear fluid. A papillomatous tendency is often noted on the inner wall of the cysts, more particularly in the smaller growths. Microscopically the cyst is lined by a single layer of cuboidal or flat epithelium.

The symptoms of parovarian cyst are like those of the more common ovarian cysts, for which they are usually mistaken

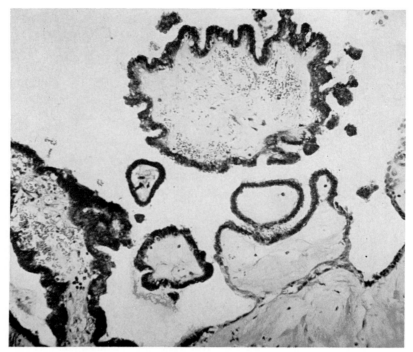

FIG. 22.8. Microscopic appearance of wall of parovarian cyst showing a low columnar epithe lium and often, as in this case, a papillary tendency.

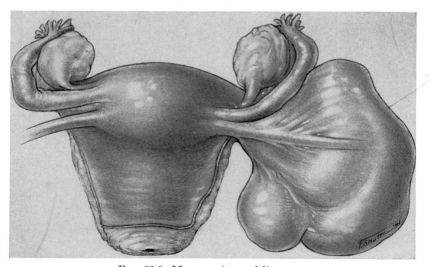

FIG. 22.9. Myoma of round ligament

preoperatively. There is no tendency to malignancy, and treatment is surgical.

TUMORS OF THE ROUND LIGAMENTS

Like the uterus, the round ligaments are made up of smooth muscle. *Myoma* is therefore fairly common, presenting the same histological structure as does uterine myoma, but confusing the situation at operation by grossly distorting and occasionally replacing the round ligament or dissecting under the bladder. Another tumor which is not extremely

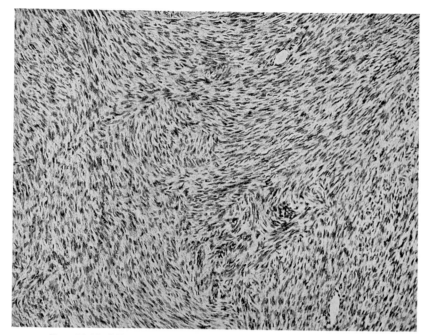

FIG. 22.10. Microscopic structure of myoma of round ligament

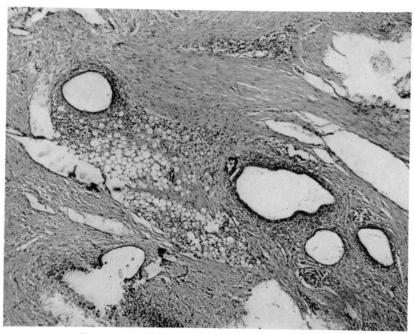

FIG. 22.11. Adenomyoma of uterosacral ligament

rare is *adenomyoma*, which histologically consists of endometrial tissue islands embedded in a matrix of involuntary muscle. *Sarcoma* is exceedingly rare.

TUMORS OF THE BROAD LIGAMENTS

While not very common, *myoma* may develop from the involuntary muscle normally included in the structure of the broad ligaments. *Cysts* may likewise be encountered, arising from that portion of Gartner's duct (vestigial remains of Wolffian duct) which courses along the lateral margin of the uterus. Imperfect obliteration and cystic distention of portions of this duct give rise to cysts, usually small but sometimes quite large.

Novak, Woodruff, and Novak have pointed out that an identical tumor may be found at any level of the genital tract where *remnants of the mesonephric duct* may be found. In the cervix, vaginal fornices, broad ligaments, or region of the ovary may be found a histologically similar tumor. This may be similar to the ovarian mesonephroma of Schiller or the so-called clear cell adenocarcinoma, but admixtures are frequent. In the broad ligament region it is of low grade malignancy and appears quite similar to ovarian mesonephroma (see Chapter 24).

TUMORS OF THE UTEROSACRAL LIGAMENTS

While *myoma* occurs, the most common tumor of the uterosacral ligaments is *adenomyoma*. In cases of pelvic endometriosis these ligaments are frequently the seat of endometrial "implants." These consist often of very superficial islands of endometrial tissue but in some cases the ectopic endometrium excites a marked local muscular reaction, producing nodular adenomyomas which must be considered definitely neoplastic. These nodules vary in size from a few millimeters to several centimeters in diameter. They are often multiple. Because of the respon-

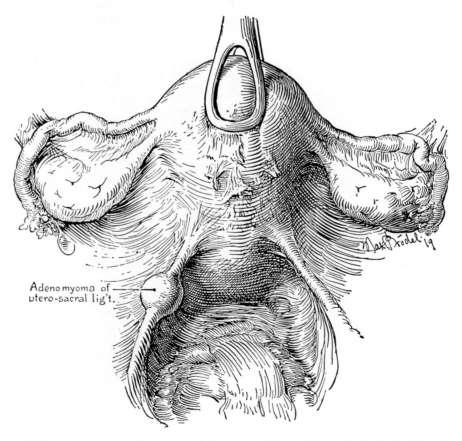

Adenomyoma of utero-sacral lig't.

Fig. 22.12. Adenomyoma of uterosacral ligaments. (From Cullen, T. S.: Bull. Johns Hopkins Hosp., 7: 112, 1896.)

siveness of the contained endometrium to the ovarian hormones, the growths are usually dark, bluish red. The same menstrual responsiveness gives rise to menstrual pain, which is referred to the rectum or the lower sacral or coccygeal regions. This symptom, coupled with the presence of palpable nodules in the uterosacral regions, justifies a presumptive diagnosis of pelvic endometriosis, although it is often impossible to know if this represents diffuse external endometriosis or an extension of internal (adenomyosis) disease. In any case, both represent examples of misplaced uterine mucosa.

The adenomyomatous growth may involve the adjoining rectal wall and may infiltrate the rectovaginal septum (*adenomyoma of rectovaginal septum*). When such growths are encountered as a part of the picture of extensive pelvic endometriosis, as they so often are, complete removal of ovarian tissue leads to their regression. Adenomyosis or endometriosis of the upper vagina can be distinguished only by biopsy from the unusual case of posthysterectomy prolapse of the tube, as noted by Bobrow and Friedman.

REFERENCES

Abrams, J., Kazal, H. L., and Hobbs, R. E.: Primary sarcoma of fallopian tube. Amer. J. Obstet. Gynec., 75: 180, 1958.

Bobrow, M. L., and Friedman. S.: Tubal prolapse following abdominal hysterectomy. Obstet. Gynec., 11: 646, 1958.

Brewer, J. I., and Guderian, A. M.: Diagnosis of uterine-tube carcinoma by vaginal cytology. Obstet. Gynec., 8: 664, 1956.

Cavallero, G., and Rossi, R.: Contribution to the study of malignant mixed tumors of the Fallopian tube (carcinosarcoma). Pathologica, 51: 443, 1959.

Cron, R. S., and Claude, J. L.: Primary papillary carcinoma of uterine tube. Obstet. Gynec., 13: 734, 1959.

Cruttenden, L. A., and Taylor, C. W.: Primary carcinoma of fallopian tube; report of case superimposed on tuberculous salpingitis. J. Obstet. Gynaec. Brit. Comm., 57: 937, 1950.

Cullen, T. S.: Adenomyoma of round ligament. Bull. Johns Hopkins Hosp., 7: 112, 1896.

Dede, J. A., and Janovski, N. A.: Lipoma of the uterine tube—a gynecological rarity. Obstet. Gynec., 22: 461, 1963.

Emge, L. A.: Six cases of primary carcinoma of fallopian tube. Western J. Surg., 56: 334, 1948.

Frankel, A. W.: Primary carcinoma of the fallopian tube. Amer. J. Obstet. Gynec., 72: 31, 1956.

Gardner, G. H., Greene, R. R., and Peckham, B.: Tumors of the broad ligament. Amer. J. Obstet. Gynec., 73: 563, 1957.

Green, T. H., Jr., and Scully, R. E.: Tumors of the fallopian tube. Clin. Obstet. Gynec., 5: 886, 1962.

Grimes, H. G., and Kornmesser, J. G.: Benign cystic tumor of the oviduct. Obstet. Gynec., 16: 85, 1960.

Hayden, G. E., and Potter, E. L.: Primary carcinoma of the fallopian tube. Amer. J. Obstet. Gynec., 79: 24, 1960.

Hu, C. V., Taylor, M. L., and Hertig, A. T.: Primary carcinoma of the tube. Amer. J. Obstet. Gynec., 59: 58, 1950.

Hurlbutt, F. R., and Nelson, H. B.: Primary carcinoma of the uterine tube. Obstet. Gynec., 21: 730, 1963.

Israel, S. L., Crisp, W. E., and Adrian, D. C.: Preoperative diagnosis of primary carcinoma of the fallopian tube. Amer. J. Obstet. Gynec., 68: 1589, 1954.

Larsson, E., and Schooby, J. L.: Positive vaginal cytology in primary carcinoma of the fallopian tube. Amer. J. Obstet. Gynec., 22: 1369, 1956.

McQueeney, A. J., Carswell, B. L., and Sheehan, W. J.: Malignant mixed Mullerian tumor primary in uterine tube. Obstet. Gynec., 23: 338, 1964.

Novak, E., Woodruff, J. D., and Novak, E. R.: Mesonephric origin of certain female genital tumors. Amer. J. Obstet. Gynec., 68: 1222, 1954.

Picton, F. C. R.: Primary carcinoma of the fallopian tube. J. Obstet. Gynaec. Brit. Comm., 66: 663, 1959.

Riggs, J. A., Wainer, A. S., Hahn, G. A., and Farell, D. M.: Extrauterine tubal choriocarcinoma. Amer. J. Obstet. Gynec., 88: 637, 1964.

Scheffey, L. C., Lang. W. R., and Nugent, F. B.: Clinical and pathological aspects of primary sarcoma of uterine tube. Amer. J. Obstet. Gynec., 52: 904, 1946.

Taussig, F. J.: Sarcoma of round ligament of uterus, Surg. Gynec. Obstet., 19: 218, 1914.

Teel, P.: Adenomatoid tumors of the genital tract. Amer. J. Obstet. Gynec. 75: 1347, 1958.

Wharton, L. R., and Krock, F. H.: Primary carcinoma of the fallopian tube. Arch. Surg., 18: 848, 1929.

Williams, T. J., and Woodruff, J. D.: Malignant mixed mesenchymal tumor of the uterine tube. Obstet. Gynec., 21: 618, 1963.

23

BENIGN TUMORS OF THE OVARY

In a recent dissertation on the origin of ovarian tumors, McKay has emphasized the concepts of histological examination, the use of logic, knowledge of ovarian embryology, as well as other data. With these doctrines we are in full accord, and we might stress the importance of a knowledge of ovarian histology in the neonatal and infant years, as described by Curtis. A brief resume of a practical classification of ovarian tumors follows. This is our own but by no means the only classification.

OVARIAN TUMORS

BENIGN

Cystic
  Nonneoplastic: follicle, lutein, Stein-Leventhal, inclusion, as well as endometrial and inflammatory
  Neoplastic: pseudomucinous, serous, and dermoid
Solid: fibroma, Brenner (rarely malignant), etc.

MALIGNANT

Cystic: pseudomucinous, serous, and others
Solid: carcinoma, adenocarcinoma, and mesonephroma

OTHER RARE MALIGNANT

Sarcoma, lymphoma, teratoma, etc.

ENDOCRINE POTENTIAL

Virilizing or feminizing: mesenchymomas or gonadal stromal tumors (arrhenoblastoma, granulosa-theca cell); sometimes inert. Dysgerminoma, generally inert
Rare hilus and adrenal: usually virilizing

METASTATIC OR BY EXTENSION
Pattern similar to primary
Krukenberg

BENIGN CYSTS

By far the most frequent of all ovarian tumors are the cysts, most of which are not genuine neoplasms. This applies particularly to the smaller cystic structures which are so frequently found in the ovary and which are to be looked upon as functional retention cysts originating in the follicles or corpora lutea. Many cysts, on the other hand, are true neoplasms, whose constituent cells are capable of independent autonomous growth, and such cysts may reach enormous size. On the basis of this distinction, therefore, the benign cysts of the ovary may be divided into two groups: (1) the nonneoplastic cysts, and (2) the neoplastic cysts.

Nonneoplastic (Functional) Cysts of the Ovary

Follicle Cysts. These arise from simple cystic overdistention of follicles during the process of atresia folliculi (see Chapter 3). Every month a considerable number

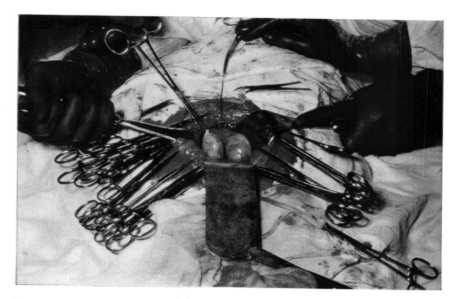

PLATE XXIII.I. Bilaterally-enlarged, smooth, oyster-white ovary; note small uterus

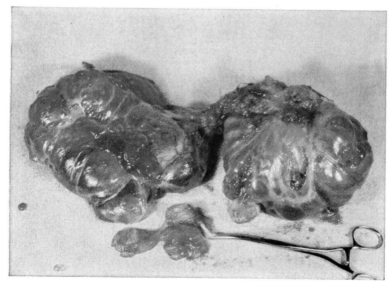

PLATE XXIII.II. Pseudomucinous cyst, which ruptured and produced pseudomyxoma peritonei and mucocele of appendix, the latter being seen in the lower part of the picture (author's case).

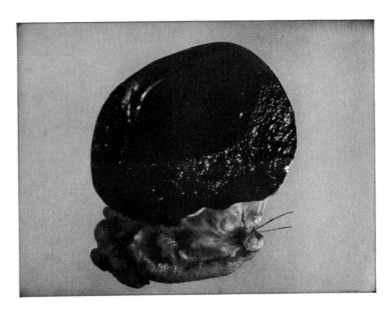

PLATE XXIII.III. Torsion of pedicle of small ovarian cyst showing dark gangrenous picture produced by interference with circulation.

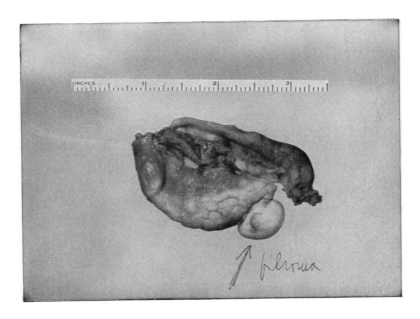

PLATE XXIII.IV. Small fibroma on surface of ovary

therapy is indicated over the course of 8 to 10 weeks before deciding on laparotomy; in the middle age group, evaluation should not be so prolonged, and in the postmenopausal patient, any adnexal enlargement warrants prompt laparotomy.

TREATMENT. In the rare case in which

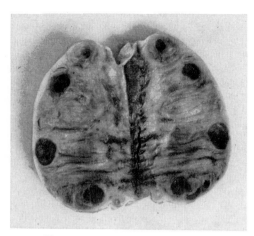

FIG. 23.5. Follicular hematomas

operation is indicated because of definite symptoms, or in the numerous cases in which follicular cysts are revealed at operation for other indications, they are best treated by either simple puncture (needling) or excision, depending upon their size. The involution of the smaller cysts is undoubtedly hastened by simple evacuation of the contained fluid by needle puncture. When the cyst is larger, it can be shelled out, often intact, with conservation of the normal ovarian tissue.

Lutein Cysts. In the first place it should be remembered that many functionally normal mature corpora lutea contain a considerable amount of fluid. This is especially true of the corpus luteum of pregnancy, which at times forms a cystic structure comprising as much as half the ovarian bulk. The term "lutein cyst" is generally used collectively, although it is important clinically to consider the possibility of pregnancy lest removal of the cyst increase the chances of abortion. Actually this does

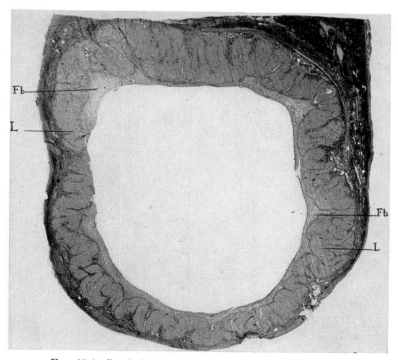

FIG. 23.6. Cystic but functionally normal corpus luteum

not occur often; indeed, bilateral oophorectomy may be followed by a normally progressing pregnancy. Lutein cysts may, of course, occur in the absence of pregnancy.

The origin of the true lutein cyst is in most cases from a corpus luteum hematoma. The latter, in turn, is brought about by an exaggeration of the hemorrhage which normally takes place into the corpus cavity in the so-called stage of vascularization. When the bleeding is excessive, a large *corpus luteum hematoma* is produced, characterized chiefly by a thinned out, bright yellow lutein wall about the blood-filled central cavity. Gradually, however, there is a resorption of the blood elements, leaving a clear or slightly bloody fluid. At the same time a layer of fibroblastic tissue is deposited along the inner margin of the lutein layer, so that in old corpus luteum cysts the lutein cells may be buried beneath a heavy layer of cicatricial tissue.

SYMPTOMS. The symptoms of lutein cysts cannot always be correlated with their histological appearance. In the most interesting group, the symptoms resemble those of early tubal pregnancy. Menstruation is apt to be slightly delayed, followed by persistent slight bleeding, with often pain in one or the other of the lower quadrants, and with the presence on pelvic examination of a small tender swelling in the corresponding side of the pelvis. This represents the characteristic symptomatology of early tubal pregnancy, and yet not infrequently in place of the latter one may find at operation a lutein cyst instead.

As a matter of fact there are some who believe that in such cases one is actually dealing with very early abortion of a fertilized but as yet unimplanted egg, although there is no direct evidence to substantiate this view. Others look upon the syndrome as identical with that of the so-called *corpus luteum persistens*, in which, for some unknown reason, the normal regression of the corpus is deferred, with persistence of the progestational phase in the endometrium, through a mechanism which may be similar to

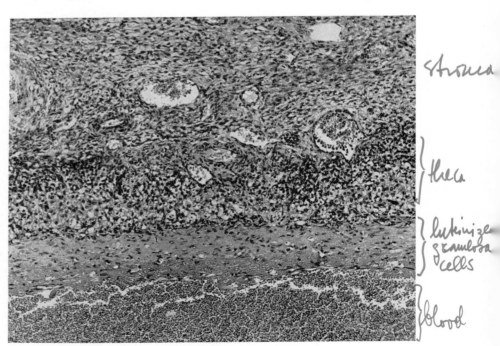

FIG. 23.7. Wall of lutein cyst

the pseudopregnancy observed in some of the lower animals.

A rare type of lutein cyst is that which is found in some cases of hydatidiform mole and chorionepithelioma. In some cases of this sort the wall of the cyst is formed by luteinized granulosal cells, but usually the cyst is composed of paralutein (theca-lutein) cells of connective tissue rather than epithelial origin.

DIAGNOSIS. The diagnosis of lutein cysts is obviously difficult, and in the majority of cases their presence is not suspected before operation, especially as they so often produce no symptoms. When they are of considerable size they can of course be palpated, but this gives no clue as to their histological nature. In a small group of cases the presence of a cyst of this character can be at least suspected when a symptom complex like that of tubal pregnancy is produced. When such a problem arises pregnancy tests may be of service, for they are often positive in tubal gestation, and negative in the corpus luteum cysts. Culdoscopy of course is more conclusive.

TREATMENT. The treatment of lutein cysts or hematomas consists of observation, for most of them undergo spontaneous disappearance. In the case of hemorrhagic cysts of considerable size, however, excision is the proper treatment. At times the yellowish shimmer of the wall gives a clue to the lutein character of the cyst, and in such cases the surgeon should, before removal of the cyst, consider the possibility of very early gestation, as has already been mentioned. In a large proportion of cases the lutein character of the cyst is not suspected before laboratory examination.

Stein-Leventhal Ovary. Dr. Irving Stein in 1928 focused attention on a group of patients who experienced such features as hirsutism, sterility, obesity, and oligoamenorrhea. The clinical picture of this so-called Stein-Leventhal syndrome will be dealt with fully in Chapter 31.

At the same time Stein was careful to point out that the validity of the "Stein-Leventhal" syndrome is dependent upon a certain gross pathological appearance of the ovaries, and that this is mandatory for proper diagnosis. Indeed, such operative treatment as wedge resection of the ovary demands this characteristic ovarian architecture if any benefits are to be hoped for. Although this "S.L." type of ovary is perhaps not an ovarian tumor, it seems advisable to mention the pathological details of the ovary in this chapter.

Bilateral enlargement of the ovaries must be present, and the ovarian surface is smooth, oyster-gray, and without evidence of a corpus luteum. Frequently the ovaries are larger than hen's eggs, and although there is a predominance on one side, almost uniformly both ovaries are enlarged. If wedge resection is carried out the operator will find the cortex extremely thick and fibrotic. Allen and Woolf feel that the ovarian medulla is culpable by virtue of excessive androgen secretion, and they perform medullary resection with good results. However, the cause must be regarded as uncertain.

Microscopically there is a thickened, fibrotic, almost hyalinized tunica beneath which there may be many follicles in all stages of maturation and atresia (Fig. 23.9), but without evidence of frequent corpora lutea, although old corpora albicantia may be present. A single corpus luteum should not neces-

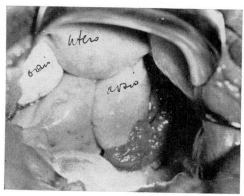

FIG. 23.8. Small uterus anterior with bilateral Stein-Leventhal ovaries. (Courtesy of Dr. Albert Brown, Saskatchewan, Canada.)

sarily negate the diagnosis if all other features of an "S.L." ovary are present. Frequently there is marked proliferation of the theca interna in the follicle wall (Fig. 23.10), and there are some who contend that these proliferative theca cells are the agent for producing the virilizing effects. Others feel this hyper-

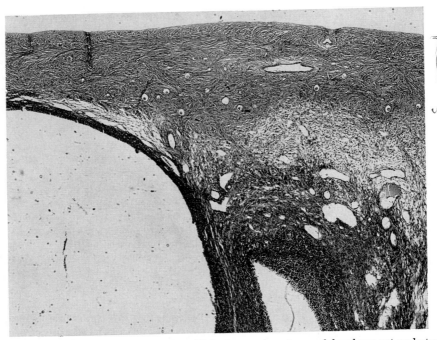

corteccia

FIG. 23.9. Thickened cortex with many follicles in varying stages of development and atresia

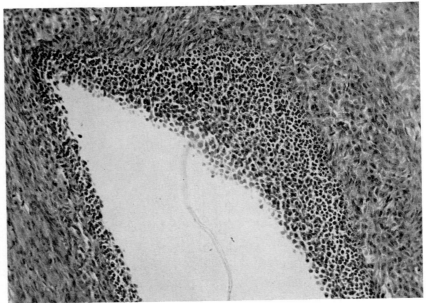

FIG. 23.10. Follicle lined by granulosa cells with marked proliferation of theca layer

Il cisto adenoma seroso degenera verso la
malignità nel 25% dei cani, quello
pseudomucinoso nel 5-10% e
la cisti dermoide nel 1-3% –
— pag. 428

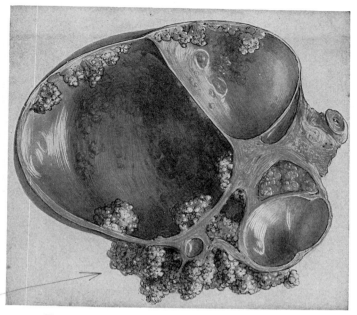

FIG. 23.17. Papillary serous cystadenoma of ovary

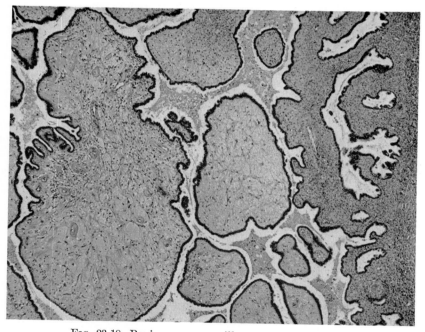

FIG. 23.18. Benign serous papillomatous cystadenoma

epithelium, which likewise is made up of ciliated and nonciliated columnar cells. In other tumors, or in other parts of the same cyst wall, the epithelium may be cuboidal or peg-shaped. The stroma is fibrous, with often such hydropic degeneration as to resemble the jelly of Wharton of the umbilical cord. Rather characteristic of this variety of cyst is the frequent presence of small calcareous granules, the so-called *psammoma bodies,* an end product of the tumor implants (Fig. 23.19).

When the epithelium is of the above type, and arranged in a single layer, there is no doubt of the benign nature of the cyst, at least from a histological standpoint. However, departures from this clearly benign pattern are very common, with stratification of the epithelium and evidence of epithelial over-activity. This entails frequent difficulty in microscopic diagnosis, and it is not always easy to determine whether one is dealing with a benign serous cystadenoma or a papillary cystadenocarcinoma.

HISTOGENESIS. While there is some difference of opinion as to the origin of pseudomucinous cysts, there would seem to be little doubt as to the origin of the serous type from the surface epithelium of the ovary. It is possible to demonstrate microscopically all stages of transition from simple invagination of the germinal epithelium, to invagination plus slight papillary formation, to the typical serous papillomatous cyst.

Small surface papillomas of the ovary are not infrequent, but *solid papillomas* of the same germinal epithelial origin may reach large size, filling the entire pelvis, with at times no discernible cystic tendency. More often the germinal epithelium by its invagination forms increasingly large cystic cavities, with the characteristic papillary ingrowths. In view of this mechanism it is easy to see why papillary excrescences may be found on either the external or internal surface of a serous cyst.

Fibroadenoma and Cystadenofibroma. While the former of these is not a cystic

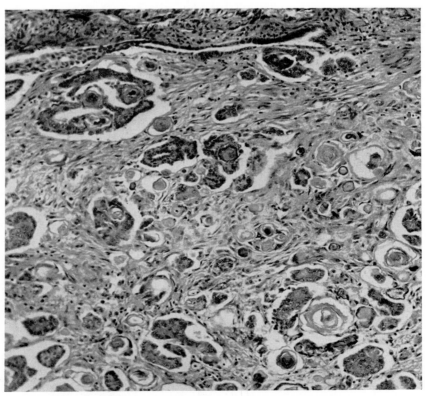

FIG. 23.19. Psammoma bodies showing transition between recognizable papillae and acellular calcified bodies.

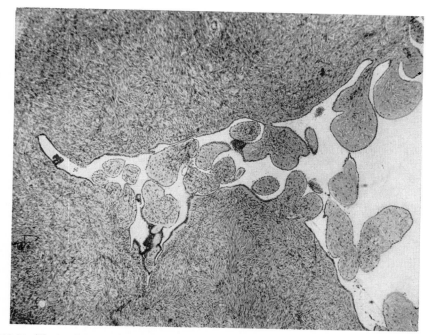

FIG. 23.20. Photomicrograph showing how invagination of the surface epithelium with a papillomatous tendency brings about the development of what is essentially an early papillary serous cystadenoma.

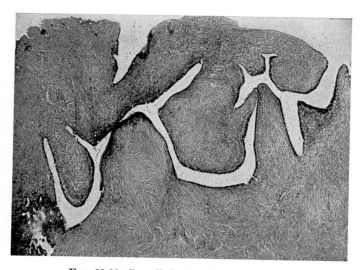

FIG. 23.21. So-called adenofibroma of ovary

tumor, and the latter only partly so, they are properly considered here because their histogenesis is so closely allied to that of serous cystadenoma. Like the latter, they arise from the surface epi-thelium of the ovary, which undergoes invagination, with the formation of long, cleftlike tubules surrounded by fibrous tissue, so that the picture is very similar to that of the ordinary fibroadenoma of

La cisti dermoide diventa maligna nel 1-3%
dei casi -

the breast. Such lesions are therefore designated as *fibroadenoma of the ovary*. They are usually of small size, and may be found only on microscopic examination.

On the other hand, the invaginations often become cystic and may attain large size, as shown in Figure 23.23. Such tumors, designated as *cystadenofibroma*, are usually partly cystic and partly solid, in varying proportions. When small they form dense whitish, partly cystic nodules near the surface, but when large they may replace all or nearly all the ovarian

substance. They are benign, but in rare cases may become malignant.

Dermoid Cysts. These tumors represent a (benign cystic) subdivision of ovarian teratoma and comprise the most common type of ovarian tumor found in the young girl. They are distinguished from the more serious solid tumors chiefly on the basis of their cystic character, their nonmalignant nature, and the fact that the foreign elements which they exhibit are dominantly ectodermal, with at times considerable mesodermal ad-

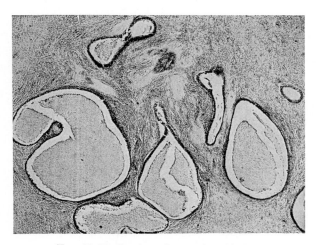

FIG. 23.22. Section of cystadenofibroma

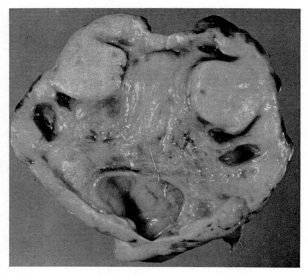

FIG. 23.23. Gross appearance of rather large cystadenofibroma

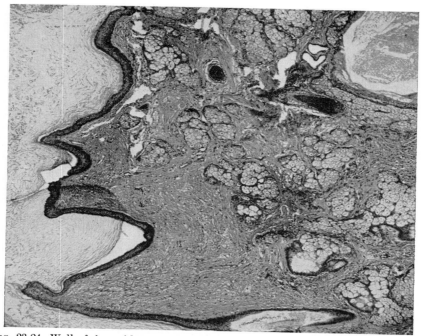

FIG. 23.24. Wall of dermoid cyst showing skin, sebaceous glands, and hair follicles

mixture, although elements of all three germ layers may occasionally be found. The solid teratomas always show a conglomeration of structures derived from all three fetal layers. The teratomatous elements of a dermoid cyst are always of mature differentiated type, with a high degree of differentiating potency, in contrast with the malignant teratoma, in which the elements are of immature variety.

It is this third criterion which, in our judgment, is most important, and which undoubtedly explains the benign nature of dermoid and the malignant nature of teratoma, made up as it is of unripe elements with consequently greater malignant potentiality.

Dermoid cysts rarely reach large size, but they are occasionally combined with cystadenomas of very large size, and generally of pseudomucinous type. They show a rather thick, opaque, whitish wall, and on cross section the dermoid nature is at once indicated by the presence of hair and a large amount of offensive, greasy, sebaceous material. At times

teeth (Fig. 23.29) and cartilaginous or osseous nodules are to be seen or felt in the cyst wall, and if these are found in preoperative x-ray the diagnosis is likely. However, Gerbie, Greene, and Reis have pointed out that calcification may be found in many areas of the pelvis. Dermoids are especially prone to occur in the younger patient, and Booth has indicated that this is the most common ovarian neoplasm seen in conjunction with pregnancy (about 1 in 600 pregnancies).

Microscopic examination shows skin-like stratified squamous epithelium lining the wall, but in the larger cysts this is often limited to a comparatively small raised area spoken of as the mamilla, from which arises also the hairy growth. Besides the stratified squamous epithelium and the hair follicles, we find sebaceous and sudoriferous glands, and often cartilage, the latter not infrequently in the wall of small ducts lined by ciliated epithelium, and resembling the trachea in structure. Entodermal elements, such as gastrointestinal mucous membrane, may also occasionally be found. A frequent

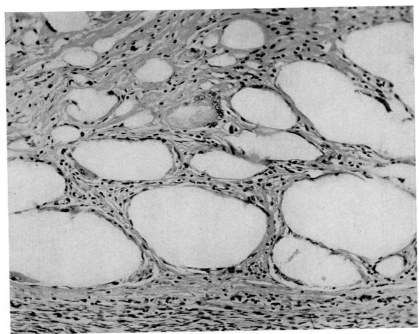

FIG. 23.25. Sievelike area in dermoid tumor showing foreign-body giant cells. Such areas are produced by the penetration of fatty material through the wall of the dermoid.

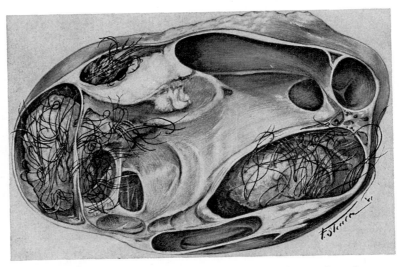

FIG. 23.26. Dermoid cyst of ovary containing hair and teeth

and characteristic finding in the vicinity of the wall is the presence of sievelike areas in which are scattered large *giant cells*, often polynuclear. These are of foreign body type, resulting from the penetration of the cyst wall by lipoid material. The wall of the cyst except at the mamillary area is often devoid of epithelium, and may show numerous endothelial leukocytes (pseudoxanthoma cells) as well as foreign body giant cells and cholesterol crystals. Considerable amounts of thyroid tissue (struma ovarii) may occur which can be thyrotoxic or undergo characteristic thyroid malignant degeneration.

Malignant degeneration can occur in primarily benign dermoid cysts. This sequence can be assumed when the unquestionably malignant lesion occurs in a definitely localized area of a dermoid which is otherwise entirely benign. Car-cinoma of the *epidermoid* type is seen in a small proportion of cases 1 to 3%. In one or two interesting personal observations we have even observed areas of typical *carcinoma in situ*. *Sarcoma* may also be seen, but is less frequent. A fine point of nomenclature is sometimes argued as to whether secondary malignant change in a benign dermoid justifies calling the tumor a malignant teratoma.

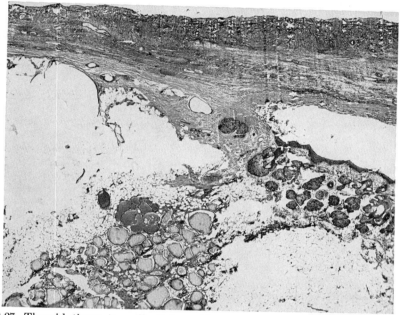

FIG. 23.27. Thyroid tissue in wall of dermoid cyst. (We have seen thyroid carcinoma)

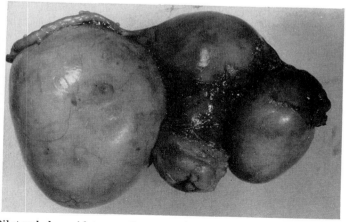

FIG. 23.28. Bilateral dermoid tumor "overriding" the uterus. An extreme anterior location suggests a dermoid tumor.

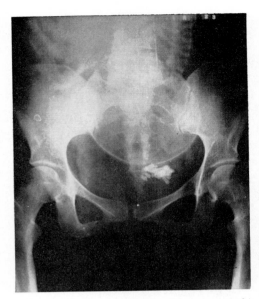

FIG. 23.29. Dermoid cyst (with many teeth) obstructing labor. (Courtesy of Dr. Albert Brown, Saskatchewan, Canada.)

This does not to us seem justified, the designation of malignant teratoma having a different connotation, as will be discussed in a later chapter (Chapter 24).

ORIGIN. There are two chief theories as to the origin of dermoids. One ascribes them to the imperfect development in later life of blastomeres which have lain dormant since early stages of embryonic development. The other, which is more popular, is that they arise from spurious developmental activity of the unfertilized ova which abound in the ovary, as noted in discussion of ovarian teratoma.

Symptomatology of Neoplastic Cysts. There is little of a characteristic nature in the symptomatology of cystadenomas of the ovary. For example, no distinctive influence is exerted on the *menstrual function*. At times menstruation may be rather free, probably as a result of the hyperemia produced by the tumor. In other cases, especially of large bilateral tumors, hypomenorrhea may result from the destruction of most of the ovarian parenchyma. Dysmenorrhea may or not be a symptom, but with the larger growths there is likely to be a sense of

heaviness or *pressure*, with often *dull aching pain*, in the affected side of the pelvis.

In a large proportion of cases, the first intimation of trouble comes when the patient herself notices a *mass* in the lower abdomen, often to one side of the midline. On the other hand, it is remarkable what size a tumor may attain before the patient suspects any abnormality. This is particularly true in stout women, whose only complaint even with huge cysts may be that the abdomen has become larger and harder.

With serous papillomatous tumors the presence of the ovarian cyst may be altogether unsuspected until *ascites* has developed, for this variety of cyst, even when histologically benign, can at times produce ascites. This is due to the fact that papillary tumors may implant themselves on the general peritoneal surface, producing irritation and exudation of serous fluid. Far more frequently, however, ascites is a feature of the malignant ovarian tumors. When ascites is pronounced, it may be impossible to palpate a mass in the lower abdomen until after paracentesis has been performed. Since there are many other possible causes of ascites, it is easy to understand that the problem of differential diagnosis may be difficult.

Complications. TORSION OF THE PEDICLE. Of the complications of ovarian cyst the most frequent is that of torsion or twisting of the pedicle, and the acute symptoms thus precipitated are not infrequently the first indication of the presence of an ovarian tumor. This complication is more common with tumors of small or moderate size than with the very large ones. A number of factors may be concerned in its production, the most important being the weight of the tumor, trauma in the form of sudden jolts, and the peristaltic movements of the intestine.

The twisting of the pedicle is generally in a clockwise fashion, and it may be slight or so extreme that several complete twists of the pedicle are demonstrable (Fig. 23.30).

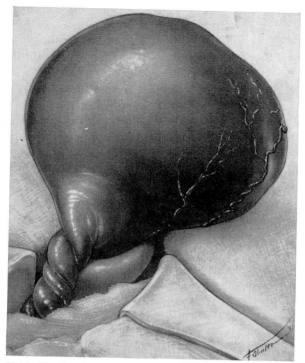

FIG. 23.30. Torsion of pedicle of ovarian cyst as seen at operation

The circulatory disturbance produced by the torsion usually affects the veins chiefly, with intense venous stasis, so that the cyst becomes dark bluish or even black. In extreme cases the arteries are also occluded, with gangrene of the cyst as a result. The cyst may even, if the condition is not recognized or is neglected, twist itself off completely, and cases are recorded in which rather large cysts have thus been severed from their attachment and undergo complete absorption.

The occurrence of torsion of the pedicle is associated with *pain* which may be sharp and persistent, but which in other cases may be only moderately severe and transitory. The latter is true when the twisting of the pedicle corrects itself, as it not infrequently does. A common history in cases of ovarian cyst of moderate size is that from time to time the patient has experienced attacks of sharp pain, with spontaneous disappearance after a short time. Such attacks are quite

certainly due to moderate and transitory twisting of the pedicle.

In a considerable proportion of cases, however, the symptoms produced by torsion of the pedicle are much more urgent. Sudden excruciating pain is experienced, usually referred quite definitely to one side or other of the lower abdomen. When the cyst is on the right side, the simulation of acute appendicitis may be made all the more perfect by the occurrence of *nausea and vomiting*, and by the development of tense *rigidity* over the right lower abdomen. The *pulse* is accelerated and the *temperature* elevated, although it rarely rises to more than perhaps 101°F. Examination of the blood shows a moderate *leukocytosis*. It is not surprising, therefore, that many patients with this condition are operated upon with the mistaken diagnosis of acute appendicitis.

If operation is for any reason delayed, the pain, tenderness, and rigidity persist, as well as the fever. This may continue for many days without the appearance of more alarming symptoms. In such neglected cases, however, secondary peritoneal inflammatory involvement always occurs, with extensive adhesions of the cyst to surrounding tissues, and with often suppuration of the cyst and even general peritonitis.

RUPTURE OF CYST. This is relatively infrequent, but may occur either spontaneously or as a result of trauma. In either case it is characterized by *pain*, often *nausea and vomiting*, and with a greater or lesser degree of *prostration* and at times actual *shock*. The latter is especially the case where the rupture is attended with marked intraperitoneal bleeding, as it is when large vessels are involved by the rupture. In such cases the peritoneal cavity may be filled with blood, with the rapid development of shock, characterized by rapid, thready pulse, subnormal temperature, air-hunger, and cold clammy skin. Such extreme bleeding, however, is rare, as in the majority of cases the rupture involves only an individual locule of the cyst. The initial pain and other symptoms may therefore subside after a few hours, although there may be much tenderness and rigidity over the lower abdomen for a number of days, with moderate fever. There is no doubt that spontaneous disappearance of the symptoms occurs in a considerable proportion of cases.

Rupture of small thin-walled locules no doubt often happens without producing any immediate symptoms. It carries with it the risk, however, of dissemination of the cyst contents into the general abdominal cavity, and of implantation of the cyst epithelium on the peritoneum. There is thus produced the rather rare *pseudomyxoma peritonei*, in which the abdomen may contain huge amounts of a gelatinous exudate. Evacuation of this exudate is followed by reaccumulation within a comparatively short time, because of the continued secretion of the peritoneal implants, and a fatal termination is noted in almost all cases.

An interesting lesion of the appendix,

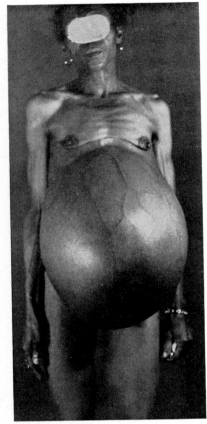

FIG. 23.31. Ovarian cyst weighing 73 pounds. (Case of Dr. Gordon Johnson, New Orleans.)

the so-called *mucocele*, is a frequent but not invariable occurrence with pseudomyxoma peritonei. The appendix may be enormously distended with gelatinous material, and large translucent gobs of the latter may be attached to the outer surface of the organ. The normal appendix epithelium in such cases is largely replaced by tall secretory epithelium identical with that seen in the wall of pseudomucinous cysts. Since mucocele can occur even in the absence of pseudomucinous cysts, it would seem that there must be a close kinship between pseudomucinous and intestinal epithelium, and this further suggests a probable teratomatous origin of pseudomucinous cysts, as mentioned in a previous part of this chapter.

SUPPURATION OF CYST. As already mentioned, secondary infection and suppuration of a cyst may follow torsion of its pedicle; but quite independently of the latter accident, infection of the cyst may occur through the hematogenous or lymphatic route, although often the mechanism may be obscure. Dermoid cysts appear to be more prone to infection that do the cystadenomas, possibly because of the irritating character of their content and the fact that the weight of such cysts is more apt to bring about predisposing circulatory disturbance. Secondary infection of an ovarian cyst is characterized clinically by symptoms not unlike those of the ordinary type of acute pelvic inflammatory disease, for which it is most frequently mistaken. *Pain, tenderness, rigidity, fever* which soon assumes a septic type, *nausea and vomiting,* not infrequently *chills,* marked *leukocytosis*—all these occur when suppuration of a cyst occurs. If operation is not resorted to, the symptoms persist, with increasing *weakness* and *prostration,*

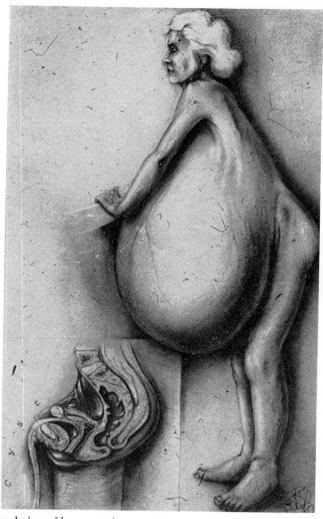

FIG. 23.32. Lateral view of large ovarian cyst. Insert shows displacement of abdominal viscera. (Courtesy of Dr. Erle Henricksen, Los Angeles.)

with the possibility of general peritoneal involvement. This chain of events, however, is by no means invariable, for in many of the smaller cysts subsidence of the inflammation occurs as with acute pelvic inflammatory disease in general.

MALIGNANT CHANGE. Secondary malignant change may occur with any of the benign neoplastic cysts. In some cases this sequence is easily demonstrable, as when a localized malignant area is found in the wall of a benign cyst. This is a not infrequent observation with *pseudomucinous cystadenoma*, in which, moreover, the histological differentiation between the benign and the malignant can be more sharply drawn than with the serous papillary cysts. From 5 to 10% of pseudomucinous cysts become malignant.

With the *serous papillomatous cystadenoma* the problem is a more difficult one, particularly because the histological differentiation between the benign and the malignant is much more difficult (see Fig. 23.33), and because even cysts which histologically are benign not infrequently exhibit essentially malignant characteristics such as implantation, infiltration of surrounding organs, recurrence, and ultimately the death of the patient. As a group the serous papillary cystadenomas unquestionably are more lethal than the pseudomucinous group. It is often impossible to be sure whether a malignant papillomatous growth has been so from the beginning or whether it has arisen secondarily in a previously benign serous cyst, although Meyer and others believe that the latter is the more frequent. At any rate, the incidence of malignant change in the serous papillary cyst is much higher than in the pseudomucinous variety, being commonly put at no less than 25%. Abel notes the ratio of serous to pseudomucinous malignancies as 4:1; Munnell, Jacox, and Taylor believe it is 7:1.

Woodruff and Novak point out the extreme difficulty in distinguishing between the benign and malignant and speak of a "borderline" group, charac-

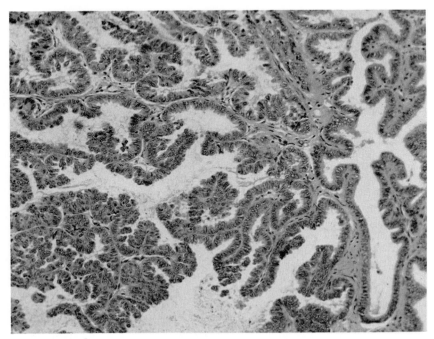

FIG. 23.33. Extremely papillary serous tumor, probably benign histologically, although it may exhibit malignant clinical trends.

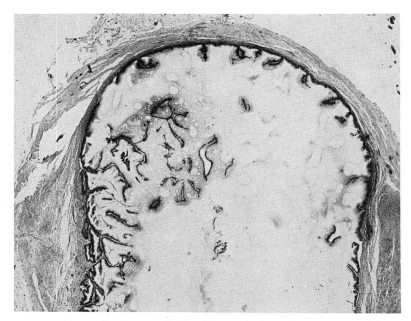

FIG. 23.34. Mucocele of appendix lined by typical pseudomucinous epithelium

terized by multiple papillae with early stratification of the lining epithelium. They emphasize the importance of multiple blocks to obtain a true composite picture of the tumor.

Malignant degeneration of *dermoid cysts* is relatively uncommon, 3% or less. It usually assumes the form of epidermoid or squamous cell carcinoma, but sarcoma may occasionally be seen (see above).

Differential Diagnosis. While the diagnosis of ovarian cyst is often easy, there are numerous cases in which the differentiation from other conditions is extremely difficult or impossible. Among the more important of these lesions which may simulate ovarian cyst, or *vice versa*, the following may be mentioned.

PREGNANCY. Either early or late gestation may be confused with ovarian cyst, or *vice versa*, as palpatory findings in themselves may not always be conclusive. Pregnancy tests, x-ray for a fetal skeleton, and auscultation for a fetal heart should be decisive.

ASCITES. Marked ascites may cause extreme enlargement of the abdomen not unlike that seen with the large cysts, although generally there is much more bulging in the flanks. The *history* of some such disease as hepatic cirrhosis or secondary peritoneal carcinomatosis may point to the probability of ascites. More important are the *percussion* findings. With the encysted fluid of ovarian cysts, percussion shows dullness anteriorly over the growth and tympany in the flanks. The reverse is the case with ascites, in which there is dullness over the flanks, with tympany over the front of the abdomen. *Palpation* of the abdomen in patients who are not too obese will often permit the definite outlining of the tumor mass in cases of ovarian cyst.

TUBERCULOUS PERITONITIS. While not very common, this disease can bring about a rather perfect simulation of ovarian cyst. This is due to the fact that the ascites of tuberculous peritonitis is frequently of the encysted variety, giving the exact feel of an ovarian cyst, as well as the same percussion findings. A history of pulmonary tuberculosis may be obtained, and there may be a slight evening elevation of temperature, while tuberculin tests may also be of some help. The encysted mass may be well above the pelvic zone, and the pelvic findings may be so normal as to suggest the probability of a cyst with an unusually long pedicle. However, tuberculous endometritis may coexist and be revealed by curettage (Chapter 22).

MYOMA OF UTERUS. Where this is large and easily palpable, mistakes are not likely to occur, but in smaller growths the diagnosis is not always easy, or even possible. A soft intraligamentary myoma, or a pedunculated uterine growth arising from the side of the uterus, gives palpation findings which may puzzle even the expert examiner. The decision between an ovarian and uterine growth is usually based upon the demonstrable separateness of the former from the uterus, and in the latter on its continuity with the uterine surface.

In the larger abdominal growths the diagnosis is usually easy. The large myoma is apt to be hard, nodular, and asymmetrical; the cyst is smoother in outline, of elastic feel, and in the case of moderate-sized tumors, situated to one side of the midline and more movable than the myoma. Where there is any doubt, however, exploration is indicated because of the malignant potential of ovarian tumors.

ABDOMINAL OBESITY. Certain types of obesity are characterized by huge abdominal deposits of fat which may lead to the suspicion of a large ovarian cyst. Elimination of the latter is usually easily made by percussion and pelvic examination. When the patient's abdominal wall is very thick and tense, palpation under anesthesia may be necessary to eliminate tumor, especially as such an examination will usually permit of clear outlining of the pelvic organs.

DIVERTICULITIS. This may be unassociated with gastrointestinal symptoms and may simulate perfectly a left ovarian tumor. Our own preference is to obtain barium enema whenever there is a left adnexal mass. An appendiceal abscess may cause confusion on the other side.

Treatment. The treatment of neo-plastic ovarian cysts is surgical. When the cyst manifests itself by acute symptoms due to some such complication as torsion of the pedicle, operation should be carried out as promptly as possible. In the absence of such acute symptoms surgical measures can be resorted to with much more deliberation, and at times may safely be deferred.

As a rule it is unwise to advise operation at once for symptomless cysts which are no larger, perhaps, than a lemon, because a considerable number of these are of follicular or corpus luteum type, and not infrequently undergo spontaneous shrinkage and disappearance, so that reexamination in even a few weeks may reveal an ovary of normal size. Certainly, however, reexamination should always be insisted upon, and in the case of the genuinely neoplastic cysts will show persistence and later gradual increase in the size of the tumor. With a 20-year-old patient, it is permissible to defer surgery for 2 or 3 months, although procrastination is not advisable in the postmenopausal woman. A general rule—the older the woman, the shorter the period of observation.

When cysts of considerable size or solid tumors are discovered, and whether or not they are producing symptoms, operation is almost always advisable. One may hesitate to give this advice to a patient who has had no symptoms whatsoever, but the reasonable certainty of increasing growth, and the ever present possibility of torsion of the pedicle as well as the more serious risk of malignant change, especially in women over 30, make this plan the proper one. There is no doubt that the malignant potentialities of ovarian growths are much greater as a group than, for example, is true of uterine fibroids. Furthermore, once ovarian cancer has developed, the patient's prospects of cure are slim under any method of treatment. A tactful and reassuring explanation will almost always ensure the patient's cooperation.

The type and extent of operation must depend upon the type of cyst and also upon the age of the patient and the importance or unimportance of preserving the possibility of pregnancy. The surgeon who possesses some knowledge of pathology enjoys a great advantage in the management of ovarian tumors. It is advisable to open the cyst immediately after removal before closure of the abdomen. If it is thin-walled, and especially if there is no papillomatous or solid ingrowth into the wall, one can be reasonably certain of its benign nature, so that conservative surgery is justified. On the other hand, even an innocuous appearing cystic tumor may reveal, on cut section, a vegetative, granular, or solid internal growth, so that there is a strong probability of malignancy, in which case the proper procedure would be removal of the entire uterus and the adnexa of both sides.

Serious problems of judgment often arise in the presence of unilateral papillomatous cysts in women of the child-bearing age, and in general the risks of conservatism with tumors of this group are definitely greater than with pseudo-mucinous or dermoid cysts. When such unilateral cysts are thin-walled, without discretely scattered papillomata on the surface or within the cavity, the uterus and the uninvolved adnexa may be left with reasonable safety. In the presence of extensively papillomatous growths, especially with infiltration of the surrounding tissues, complete operation is much the safer plan. With women beyond the menopause, the wiser policy with neoplastic cysts of any variety is the radical one of performing hysterectomy, with bilateral salpingo-oophorectomy. *Frozen section* is occasionally helpful.

OVARIAN TUMORS AND PREGNANCY. When small benign cysts are discovered in early pregnancy, most gynecologists are inclined to postpone their removal, for fear that the corpus luteum may be located in the ovary with the tumor, and that its removal might predispose to abortion, as Fraenkel found to be true in his early experiments on rabbits. While it has been clearly established that

the risk of abortion is far less in humans, it is still considered wise to defer operation until after the first trimester unless some more urgent indication should arise, such as torsion of the pedicle. By the same token, many gynecologists try to minimize the hazard of operations of this type by the substitutional administration of progesterone, although even without this the pregnancy will not usually be disturbed.

Whether or not an ovarian cyst should be removed promptly if discovered late in pregnancy should be decided on the basis of its size, its position, its rate of growth and the stage of gestation. If it is of moderate size, and riding high, its removal can often be deferred until after delivery. If the feel of the tumor suggests that it may possibly be malignant, its prompt removal is indicated. Only recently we have examined sections of a highly malignant papillary cystadenoma which had been treated expectantly until acute symptoms arose at the sixth month of pregnancy. It is evident, therefore, that each case must be judged on its individual merits, and mistakes can easily occur. Further discussion of specific ovarian tumors in conjunction with pregnancy will be noted in appropriate sections of the next two chapters.

Benign Solid Tumors of Ovary

Fibroma. This is a not uncommon tumor of the ovary, appearing sometimes as a small nodule on the surface or in the substance of the ovary, while in some cases it may attain huge size, filling most of the abdominal cavity and weighing many pounds. In the large tumors there may be nothing left of the normal ovarian parenchyma. The tumors are hard and solid, but in the larger ones large cavities may form as a result of cystic degeneration. The cut surface is whitish or yellowish white, and is of either homogeneous or trabeculated appearance.

Microscopically the structure is that of fibrous tissue of varying morphology. In some areas the cells are stellate or fusiform, with much intercellular tissue, so

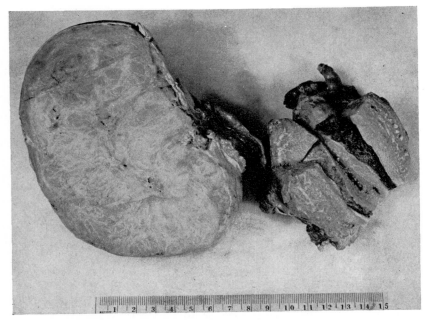

FIG. 23.35. Fibroma of ovary

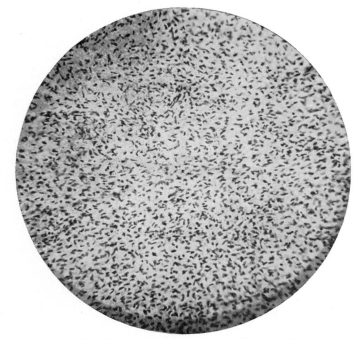

FIG. 23.36. Microscopic appearance of fibroma of ovary

that they resemble keloid tissue. In other areas, or in some tumors throughout, the cells are rather closely packed and spindle-shaped, and they may show an admixture of muscle cells (*fibromyoma*). In other tumors, areas of cartilage or bone may be found (*fibrochondroma* or *fibro-osteoma*), suggesting a teratomatous origin. Admixtures of theca cells are common if routine fat stains are performed.

The *symptoms* are those which one might suspect from the presence of a heavy pelvic mass, if the tumor is large. The small growths produce no symptoms. With those of larger size the patient herself notices the tumor sooner or later, and there is likely to be pain and heaviness in the affected side. There are no characteristic effects on menstruation, but menorrhagia and dysmenorrhea may be noted. Because of the heaviness of the growths, partial twisting or angulation of the pedicle may occur, with venous obstruction and, therefore, ascites.

Meigs called attention to a peculiar syndrome which may occur with these tumors, characterized by hydrothorax as well as ascites, and a considerable group of such cases has been described. The mechanism of this syndrome is not completely understood, but various lymphatics through the diaphragm seem the likely route for ascitic fluid into the chest. Contrary to an earlier belief, it is not distinctive of fibromas, as it has been noted with Brenner tumors, granulosal and thecomatous growths, and carcinoma, even in the absence of pleural metastasis. Meigs has recommended that the use of the term *"Meigs' syndrome"* be limited to only those cases in which the responsible tumors are of the benign solid type, such as fibromas and Brenner tumors, and that other tumors like the carcinomas be excluded, even though the hydrothorax is not produced by metastasis. Since the mechanism in both groups is presumably identical, it does not seem certain that the suggestion of Meigs will be adopted. The weight of the larger fibromas predisposes to torsion of the pedicle, so that the first warning of their presence may be the acute symptoms of the torsion, especially pain, nausea, and vomiting.

Since ascites is often combined with carcinoma of the ovary, and since the feel of a fibroma on bimanual examination is quite like that of some cancers, the *diagnosis* is not usually possible until operation. When a sharply defined solid unilateral ovarian tumor is encountered in a younger individual its fibromatous nature can at least be suspected, although even under these circumstances it may prove to be a Brenner tumor.

The treatment of fibroma is surgical, and this results in complete loss of chest and peritoneal fluid where there is a Meigs syndrome. As a matter of fact, operation is indicated in any solid tumor of the ovary, although distinction from a pedunculated fibroid is not easy.

Brenner Tumors of the Ovary. It is only in recent years that this interesting tumor form has been recognized, largely through the investigations of Robert Meyer. Its gross characteristics are not unlike those of fibroma, and, as will presently be discussed, a certain proportion of fibromas can be shown to be really Brenner tumors.

The *microscopic* structure of these tumors is characterized by the presence of *epithelial cell nests* or columns in a fibromatous matrix. The distribution of these cell nests throughout the stroma may at first suggest malignancy, but the cells show a remarkable uniformity, with not the slightest suggestion of anaplastic activity.

The characteristic cell nests often show a tendency to central cystic degeneration, the central cavity often containing a cytoplasmic mass which superficially resembles an ovum within a follicle. This indeed was the original interpretation, which led to the earlier designation of these tumors as "oophoroma folliculare."

Another interesting characteristic of some of these tumors is a tendency for *pseudomucinous transformation*, so the cyst may contain areas resembling pseudomucinous cystadenoma. Large cysts of the latter type may thus arise from Brenner tumors, although this is not the common origin of this type of cystadenoma, as described subsequently.

SYMPTOMS. Brenner tumors are rather rare, and they occur usually in older women, the majority of patients being beyond 50. They produce no characteristic symptoms, and the smaller ones are usually accidental findings in operations for other indications. The larger

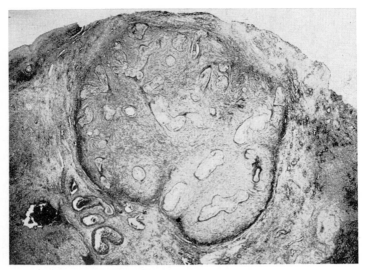

FIG. 23.37. Small Brenner tumor in cortex of ovary

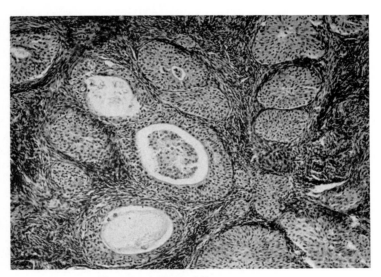

FIG. 23.38. Typical Brenner tumor

ones, however, may weigh up to 20 pounds (Averbach), with symptoms like those of large fibromas. The large size is attained by an enormous fibromatous overgrowth around the characteristic cell nests, and hence all presumably fibromatous tumors should be carefully studied for these characteristic cell nests. Bilaterality occurs in less than 10%.

While there is some doubt as to the *histogenesis* of Brenner tumors, the ex-

planation originally generally accepted was that suggested by Meyer, who believed that they arise from the so-called Walthard cell islets. These are collections of so-called indifferent cells, appearing as squamous plaques or as small clumps of gland acini, on or just below the surface of the ovary or on the tube or uterine ligaments. However, Greene and his coworkers have presented evidence that Brenner tumors may arise from other

peak of 4% at age 70, after which it decreases.

The *clinical grouping* of ovarian malignancies has not been emphasized as strongly as in the case of uterine, and especially cervical cancer, nor has there been any uniformity in the classification of ovarian cancers. Yet it is obvious that the clinical stage must have an important bearing on prognosis, and this is indicated in reports in which cases are thus subdivided. The classification usually employed is that of Helsel. According to this, *Group 1* comprises cancers limited to one ovary; *Group 2*, those cases in which the disease affects both ovaries or in which there is present a removable local extension; *Group 3*, cases in which there is locally irremovable extension or metastasis, or those in which there has been a rupture of the tumor at operation; and finally, *Group 4* would include the far advanced cases with a "frozen pelvis" or with distant metastasis. Other classifications do not differ materially from the above, and such descriptive terms as (1) completely, (2) incompletely operable, and (3) advanced would be as useful as any formal classification.

PRIMARY SOLID CARCINOMA OF OVARY

Types. The classification of solid primary ovarian cancer is also unsatisfactory from a pathological standpoint. We are obliged to have recourse chiefly to general pathological criteria of classification based chiefly on the growth pattern assumed by the tumors. An exception to this is seen in the case of a certain group of teratomatous and dysontogenetic lesions. Aside from these the following variations of pattern may be noted in primary solid carcinoma.

(1) *Adenocarcinoma*, the most common form, is characterized by its gland architecture. Like epidermoid carcinoma it may present various degrees of differentiation. In one type there is marked resemblance to endometrial adenocarcinoma, and Sampson has suggested that some of these tumors may actually arise from endometrial tissue in the ovaries.

Such an origin is not easy to establish, but this has been done in certain cases (see Chapter 26). In most of these, the adenocarcinoma arising in the endometrial cyst was of the type of adenoacanthoma, like a good many carcinomas arising in the uterine endometrium. Some adenocarcinomas are of papillary pattern and some nonpapillary.

(2) *Carcinoma*, also very frequent, is characterized by an absence of an adenomatous pattern. Various descriptive terms may be affixed, for example, papillary, medullary, alveolar, scirrhous, etc. Multiple blocks and microscopic sections are necessary for a solid pattern (Fig. 24.2) may coexist with a predominantly cystic one (Fig. 24.3).

Gross Characteristics. The size of solid ovarian carcinomas is very variable, although most of them give rise to symptoms which call for treatment before they have reached more than a moderate size. They may, however, attain sufficient size to fill the whole lower abdomen and to weigh many pounds. As a rule the external surface is smooth, but it may present many nodular thickenings or excrescences. On cutting into the tumor, the surface may be of grayish granular appearance, but often the tissue is brainlike and pultaceous, with not infrequently ragged looking cavities produced by extensive necrosis. In the smaller group of scirrhous tumors the consistency may be firm and fibrous. In the earlier stages the tumor is commonly unilateral, but there is an increasing tendency to bilaterality as the disease advances.

Mesonephroma of the Ovary. In 1939 Schiller published several articles concerning a certain type of ovarian lesion that he believed originated from mesonephric duct remnants. These tumors were tubular, and the lumina were lined by a flat, hobnail, cuboidal epithelium, with occasional intraluminal projections, strongly suggestive of primitive glomeruli. This pattern was considered a specific entity, and was referred to as "Schiller's mesonephroma."

* Il mesonefro è il dotto di Wolff con i suoi tubuli —

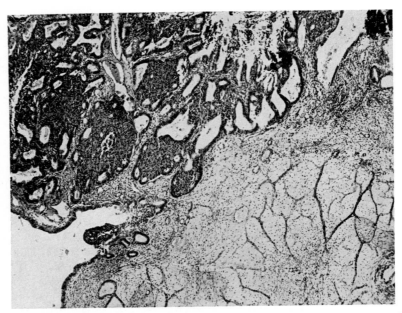

FIG. 24.1. Adenoacanthoma arising from endometrial cyst; endometrium below and to left

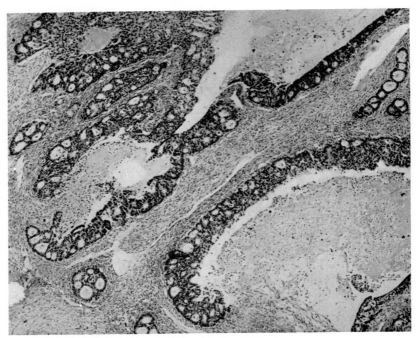

FIG. 24.2. Papillary carcinoma of ovary

Somewhat later Saphir and Lackner reported a few cases of clear cell adenocarcinoma of the ovary which they believed were identical to renal tumors. These hypernephromas or hypernephroid tumors of the ovary were thought to be of mesonephric origin, although we have never been able to find any cells in the

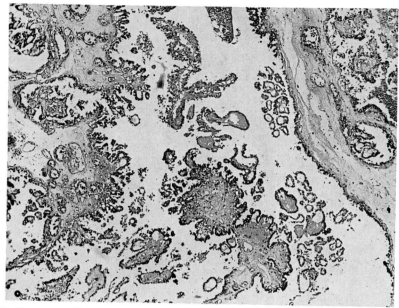

FIG. 24.3. Serous papillary cystadenocarcinoma of ovary. Other parts of this tumor show a much more solid and anaplastic pattern.

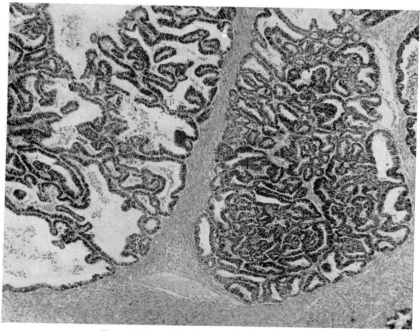

FIG. 24.4. Solid adenocarcinoma of ovary

primitive excretory system that might give rise to such tumors. Nevertheless this clear cell adenocarcinoma has been accepted by most gynecological patholo-gists and was previously referred to as hypernephroma, although it is indis-tinguishable from adrenal tumors in the ovary.

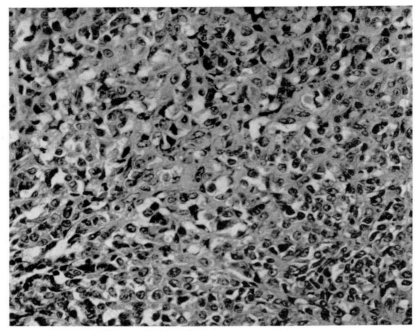

FIG. 24.5. Medullary carcinoma of ovary

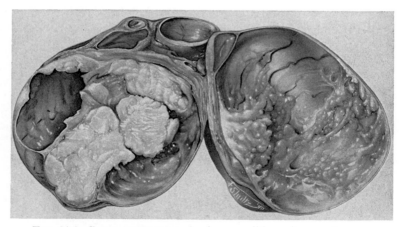

FIG. 24.6. Gross appearance of primary solid carcinoma of ovary

Separate publications by Novak, Woodruff and Novak, and Novak and Woodruff appear to have established two very important points. (1) Certain tumors may show various admixtures of both the Schiller pattern and the clear cell architecture. (2) Such lesions are found exclusively in areas where there are remnants of the mesonephric apparatus, and the tumors are identical irrespective of the level at which they occur. Such sites as the vagina, vaginal fornices, and broad ligament may be affected. Similarly, the ovary may be the seat of mesonephroma, although the lesion actually arises from extraovarian vestiges of the mesonephric tubules, with subsequent involvement of the gonad. An early publication by Novak et al. noted 13 cases of mesonephromas occurring in the lower genital tract; a more recent article concerns 35 ovarian mesoneph-

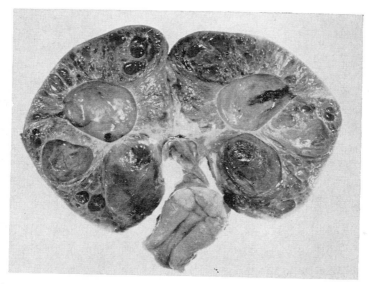

FIG. 24.7. Gross appearance of cut surface of large mesonephroma (other ovary previously removed).

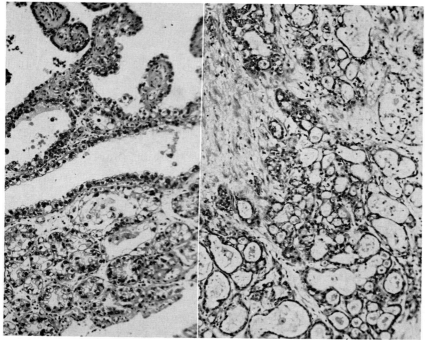

tubuli →

FIG. 24.8. Mesonephroma (different areas of the same tumor). *Right* portion shows tubular pattern lined by peglike epithelium; *left*, higher power to show clear cells lining tubules.

romas gathered from a files of the Ovarian Tumor Registry. Mesonephromas represent merely a variety of adenocarcinoma; they are usually partially cystic and solid.

Although histology is similar irrespective of the site at which they occur, ovarian mesonephromas appear to be considerably more lethal. Even where

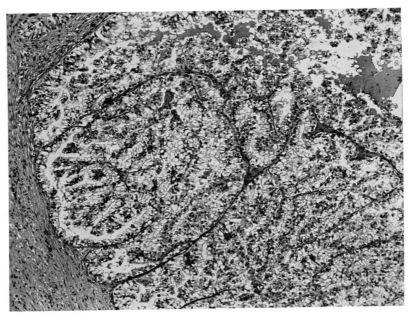

FIG. 24.9. Clear cell appearance of mesonephroma of ovary

the lesion is confined to the ovary, mortality approximates 50% despite any type of surgical and irradiation therapy. Where there is extraovarian extension there is practically no salvage. The high mortality rate, as compared to that of a similar tumor at a lower level, may well be a sequel of the intrapelvic location of the ovarian lesion where its presence is silent and not so apt to cause bleeding as vaginal and cervical mesonephromas. Wherever the tumor lies, it is endocrinologically inert.

Distinction of certain pure clear cell tumors of mesonephric origin from adrenal tumors is occasionally impossible; if there is any virilizing hormonal influence the lesion is apt to be adrenal. Certain other confused and confusing terms are often applied to these lipoid (or clear cell) growths, but we would suggest that such designations as masculinovoblastoma, hypernephroma, and luteoma should be reevaluated, with possibly the term "luteoma" being retained for such lesions as described by Scully and Sternberg. Distinction of such clear cell tumors as mesonephroma, hilus cell, or adrenal depends both on morphology

and any assistance the hormonal pattern may give. The papers of Novak and Woodruff are recommended for a more complete study of the tumors of mesonephric origin.

PRIMARY CYSTIC CARCINOMA OF OVARY

While a carcinoma of the ovary may arise as a cystic tumor, it can unquestionably develop in a previously benign cystadenoma of the ovary. As to the frequent occurrence of secondary carcinomatous changes in cystadenomas there can be no doubt. It is not rare, for example, to encounter carcinoma at some portion in the wall of benign cysts which have been known to be present for many years. Again, in many carcinomas large areas of entirely benign cystadenoma may still be observed. In any event, the adenocarcinomas of the ovary are to be looked upon as the malignant prototypes of the benign cystadenoma, arising from the same elements which gave rise to the latter. On the above basis we may distinguish three chief varieties of primary cystic ovarian carcinoma.

Pseudomucinous Cystadenocarcinoma. This is the malignant prototype of pseudomucinous cystadenoma, or arises from the same tissue elements which give rise to the latter. Only about 5 % of these undergo malignant degeneration; this occurrence is much less common than with the serous. The malignant disease may affect only a localized area of the cyst, but in most cases the latter is replaced by solid tumor.

The *microscopic examination* shows the typical picture of adenocarcinoma, but all degrees of differentiation are possible. The cells usually retain their mucoid tendencies to a greater or less extent, and hence one often finds large or small cavities filled with gelatinous material.

Serous Cystadenocarcinoma. This represents the malignant form of serous cystadenoma. It is much more common than the pseudomucinous variety, and is almost always characterized by a papillary architecture. The papillary growth is not infrequently present on the surface as well as within the cavity. All grades of transition may be seen between the picture of benign papillary serous cystadenoma and that characterized by almost solid papillary masses, with perhaps a

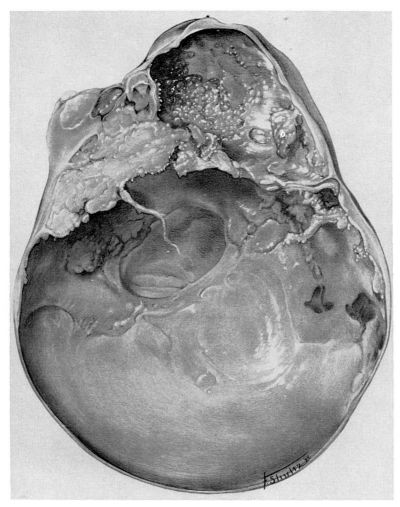

FIG. 24.10. Carcinoma of ovary developing in pseudomucinous cystadenoma

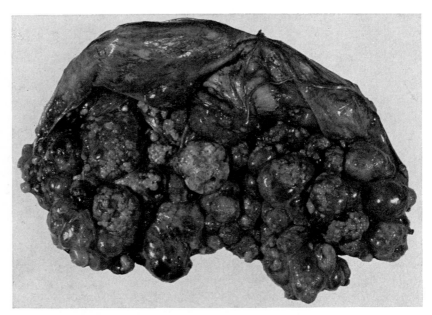

Fig. 24.11. Large pseudomucinous cystadenocarcinoma of ovary showing interior of large cyst cavity.

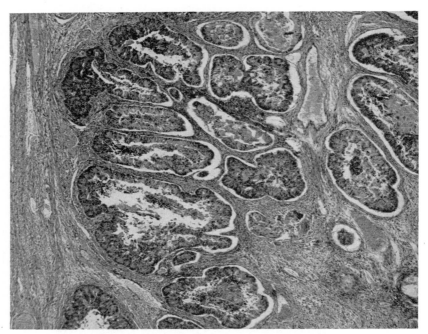

Fig. 24.12. Pseudomucinous cystadenocarcinoma of ovary

ragged cystic cavity here and there. Indeed, Woodruff and Novak have indicated that one must recognize a border-line low grade type of papillary malig- nancy characterized histologically by a marked papillary growth and a tendency to implant on peritoneal surfaces with the production of ascites (see preceding

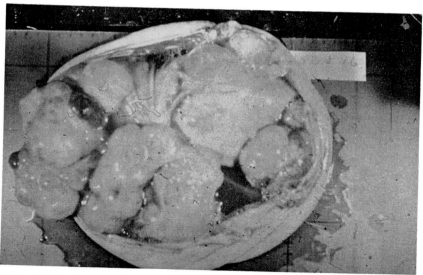

FIG. 24.13. Typical gelatinous appearance of opened pseudomucinous cystadenocarcinoma, multilocular and nonpapillary.

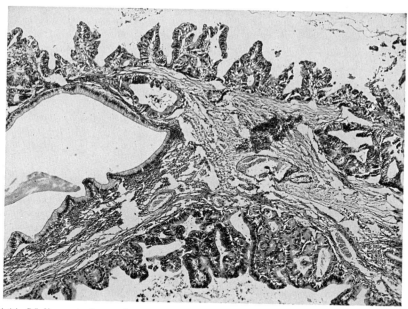

FIG. 24.14. Malignant change in a pseudomucinous cystadenoma (portion of wall of latter is seen at the *left*).

chapter). They have likewise stressed the importance of repeated pathological sections from many areas of the lesion, for an ovarian tumor can show a highly variegated appearance, from the extremely benign to the highly malignant.

The *microscopic examination* often pre-sents considerable difficulty, especially in the cases in which the gross appearance is much like that of the benign serous cysts and in which the epithelial elements present only moderate stratification and increase, and only a moderate and perhaps doubtful anaplastic activity. Even in the absence of very clear-cut evidence of histological malignancy, such tumors often exhibit clinical malignancy, especially as regards peritoneal implantation. It is usually safer, therefore, to err on the side of safety, and to consider them in the malignant group, with correspondingly radical treatment, which will usually include the removal of the adnexa of the opposite side, as well as the uterus.

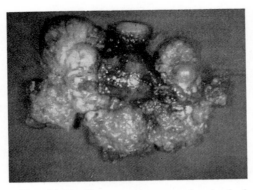

FIG. 24.15. Gross appearance of a typical serous cystadenocarcinoma of ovary.

In the majority of cases, however, the malignant nature of this group of tumors is more clearly defined, with many layers of epithelium, showing disparity in size and shape of the cells and especially the nuclei, hyperchromatosis and marked mitotic activity. Invasion of the stroma by the epithelium is likewise often evident. The structure is definitely papillary, and the epithelial tissue may or may not show a definitely glandular pattern.

Secondary Carcinoma in Dermoid Cysts. This is rare, occurring in only 1 to 3% of dermoid tumors (Blackwell) and assuming usually the form of epidermoid carcinoma, since it develops from the skinlike elements in such tumors. On several occasions we have seen a genuine intraepithelial pattern.

SECONDARY OR METASTATIC CARCINOMA OF OVARY

Carcinoma of almost any type may occur in the ovary as a result of metastasis from primary sites in other parts of the body, especially in the latter stages of such malignant processes. A not in-

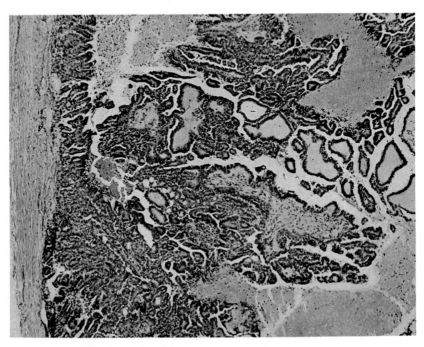

FIG. 24.16. Papillary serous cystadenocarcinoma

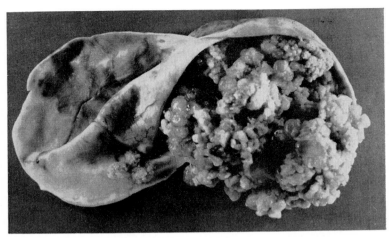

FIG. 24.17. Histologically malignant papillary vegetations lining interior of serous cystadenocarcinoma although capsule is smooth (6-year-old girl). (Courtesy of Dr. Don Walcott, San Jose, California.)

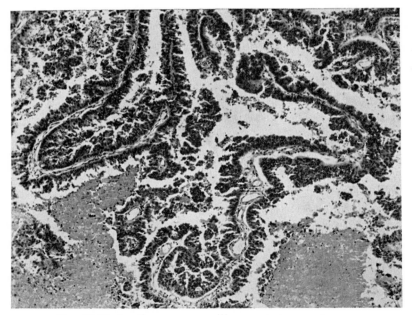

FIG. 24.18. Another serous papillary cystadenocarcinoma

frequent variety of secondary ovarian cancer is that seen in association with carcinoma of the gastrointestinal tract or of the secondary organs of digestion. This may present the same histological pattern in the ovary as in the primary tumor, this usually being adenocarcinoma.

Krukenberg Tumor. There is one particular variety of secondary ovarian carcinoma, however, which assumes special characteristics, and to which the designation of Krukenberg tumor is applied. This may be an accompaniment of primary carcinoma elsewhere, but especially in any portion of the gastrointestinal tract, most frequently the pylorus, but not infrequently the colon, rectum, small intestine, liver, or gall bladder. It should be emphasized that the term "Krukenberg tumor" should not be applied to any ovarian tumor secondary to a gastrointestinal lesion. The designation is purely on a histological basis.

Although it is generally believed that Krukenberg tumors are almost always metastatic, Woodruff and Novak have pointed out that about 20% *seem primary* in nature. An origin from teratoma, pseudomucinous cyst, or mucoid degeneration in a Brenner tumor would appear to furnish the proper ovarian environment for a Krukenberg pattern to evolve. Prolonged salvage without gastrointestinal signs or symptoms, or

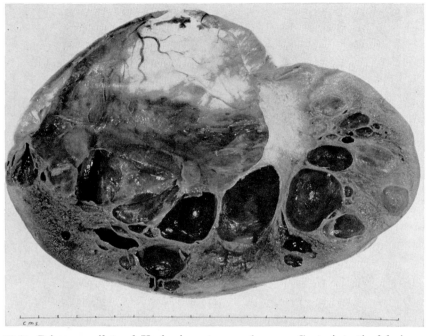

Fig. 24.19. Primary unilateral Krukenberg tumor of ovary. Gastrointestinal lesion well excluded; classic microscopic Krukenberg features. (Courtesy of Dr. Agnes Scott, Dumfries, Scotland.)

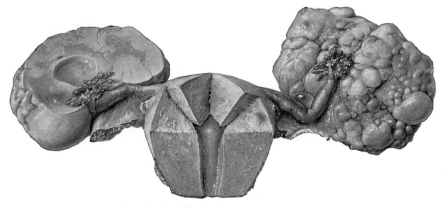

Fig. 24.20. Krukenberg tumor of ovary

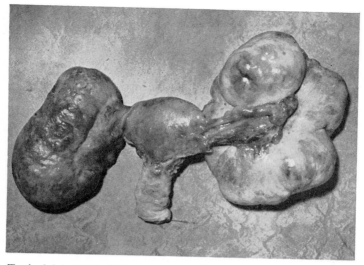

FIG. 24.21. Typical lobulated, kidney shaped Krukenberg tumors. (Courtesy of Dr. Albert Brown, Saskatchewan, Canada.)

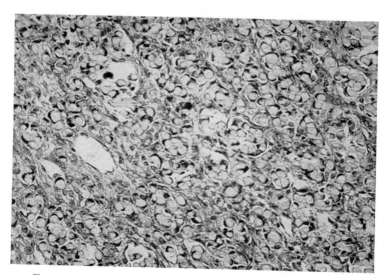

FIG. 24.22. Characteristic signet cells in a Krukenberg tumor

signet cells = "Cellule ad anello con castone" –

autopsy on women dead from other causes, would leave little doubt as to a not infrequent primary ovarian origin. One or two cases have occurred during pregnancy, as noted by Lawrence, Larson, and Hauge, and among the Ovarian Tumor Registry material utilized by Woodruff and Novak. The latter have found one 10-year salvage in a patient who had a characteristic unilateral primary Krukenberg tumor removed during pregnancy.

There has been considerable discussion as to the route by which carcinoma cells make their way to the ovary from such primary sites as the pylorus. Many believe that the cells after penetration of the stomach walls gravitate downward to the ovarian regions by way of the peritoneal fluid. There are many objections

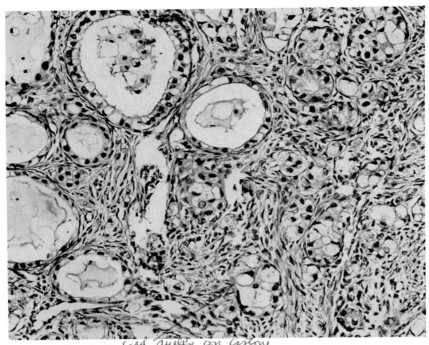

FIG. 24.23. Mucinous acini, *left*, with melting down to form signet-ring pattern on *lower right*

to this theory, and there is reason to believe that retrograde lymphatic transplantation is the important factor, while in some cases the hematogenous route plays the important role.

The tumors are generally bilateral (over 50%). They are solid and they have a tendency to retain the original ovarian contour, so that they are ovoid or kidney-shaped (Fig. 24.21). The surface is smooth, although often nodular, and the cut surface of variegated appearance, with frequently areas of gelatinous consistency.

Microscopically, the pattern of the Krukenberg tumor is quite distinctive, and the diagnosis is dependent only on the histological pattern, not on an associated or prior gastrointestinal lesion. Small nests or acini of epithelial cells are distributed throughout a fibrous or myomatous stroma, and especially characteristic are the so-called *signet cells*, in which the mucoid accumulation in the cytoplasm displaces the flattened nucleus to one side of the cell. A marked stromal hyperplasia mimicking sarcoma may be

present, and this stromal (thecal) reaction may lead to bleeding from a hyperplastic endometrium as noted by some authors. Although this type of estrogenic reaction is most commonly found in these tumors with a functioning stroma, Ober *et al.* report a Krukenberg tumor with androgenic effects. For a more complete discussion of this tumor type the reader may be referred to the paper of Woodruff and Novak.

EXTENSION OF OVARIAN CARCINOMA

The other ovary becomes involved in more than one-half of all cases of ovarian carcinoma, while the tube and the uterus are not infrequently the seat of metastatic extension, as one might expect from the richness of lymphatic intercommunication of these various organs. Even where the contralateral ovary appears grossly normal, cancer is found in the hilar lymphatics in 25 to 50% of cases. Especially frequent is extension to the peritoneum, occurring in over 75% of all cases. The lymphatic glands, especially those of the lumbar group, are involved in a very large proportion of the cases, especially in the later stages of the disease. Finally, metastases may occur to such distant organs as the liver, pancreas, lungs, pleura, and long bones.

CLINICAL CHARACTERISTICS OF OVARIAN CARCINOMA

The most important symptoms of ovarian carcinoma are unfortunately rather late ones, as the onset of this disease is almost always very insidious and "silent" in nature. The presence of a *mass* in the lower abdomen is the first indication of the disease in a considerable proportion of cases, and unfortunately by this time other organs are often involved. Moderate *heaviness* or occasional *pain* may be noted, but are more apt to be absent. The same statement may be made concerning *menstrual disorders*. If the patient is in the childbearing age there may be menorrhagia or even occasional slight metrorrhagia, but in the majority of cases no abnormality has been noted by the patient. In the postmenopausal cases, slight *bleeding* or a bloody discharge is noted in only a small proportion of the patients, and may be indicative of uterine metastasis. Thrombophlebitis, otherwise unexplained, may be due to silent tumor in proximity to the large veins. It has been amply demonstrated that the finding of tumor cells in the blood does not necessarily imply metastases.

Ascites is a relatively common accompaniment of ovarian cancer, especially of the papillary varieties. It is all too frequently indicative of peritoneal extension of the growth, but may be due merely to venous obstruction caused by partial torsion of the tumor, as in any other ovarian neoplasm. The ascites may be so extreme as to make palpation of the tumor impossible, and we have seen a number of instances in which only after paracentesis could the lower abdominal or pelvic masses be felt.

Ovarian Carcinoma in Pregnancy. This is a rather rare complication of pregnancy, albeit a rather serious one, for the symptoms and signs of pregnancy may mask those caused by the ovarian tumor. Jubb suggests certain suggestive

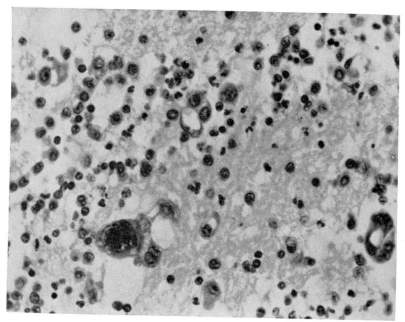

FIG. 24.24. Carcinoma cells in ascitic fluid in case of ovarian carcinoma

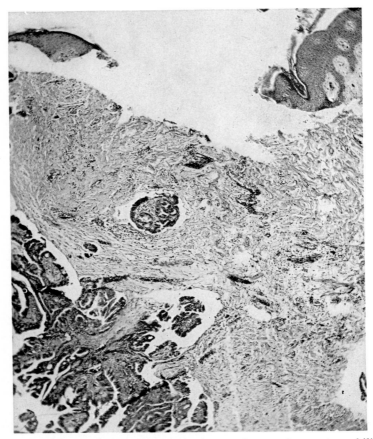

Fig. 24.25. Metastasis of papillary serous cystadenocarcinoma of ovary to umbilicus (see skin epithelium *above* and to the *right*). The histology is similar to that of primary ovarian growth.

features, as lower abdominal pain and discomfort or disproportionate enlargement of the abdomen (out of keeping with the degree of gestation). Less common are such surgical emergencies as rupture or torsion of the pedicle, and rarely obstruction to labor may occur. While the incidence of ovarian cancer in pregnancy is probably less than 0.5%, it is perhaps less commonly associated with the functioning ovarian tumors which Jubb has omitted from his case reports. Although his study would seem to support a conservative approach in the younger patient where the ovarian capsule is intact, this should depend upon the particular type and extent of the lesion. Conservative surgery can of course always be followed by more radical surgery whereas it is more difficult to replace removed organs.

Diagnosis. In a large proportion of cases the malignant nature of the tumors is not suspected before operation, and often not until the pathological examination is made. In many, however, a strongly presumptive diagnosis is possible, chiefly on palpatory findings. Vaginal smear rarely demonstrates exfoliated tumor cells, but Rubin and Frost note a frequent estrogenic effect in the maturation index (see Chapter 35). Preoperative culdocentesis may be helpful if the removed fluid is studied cytologically. This has been suggested as part of a routine "check-up" of even normal women, but we doubt if the usual patient would consent.

If pelvic examination reveals a mass occupying the position of the ovary, and if the mass is hard, fixed, and firm, ovarian carcinoma should be suspected, especially if the patient is in the cancer age. Benign solid tumors of the ovary, such as fibroma, give somewhat the same feeling, but they are less common. Benign cystic tumors, on the other hand, give a softer, elastic sensation to the examining hands, and are usually smoother in contour, as compared to the more nodular contour of most cancers. Many malignant tumors are partly cystic and partly nodular, and this very irregularity should be viewed with suspicion.

When such a tumor is associated with ascites, there can be little doubt as to its malignant nature. When the ascites is extreme, the tumor may be impalpable, and other causes of ascites, such as hepatic and cardiorenal disease or tuberculous peritonitis, may have to be eliminated. Occasionally paracentesis may be necessary to permit proper palpation of the pelvic organs, and a definite mass may then for the first time be felt. Microscopic examination of the centrifuged ascitic fluid may show typically malignant cells (Fig. 24.24).

Peritoneal washing at laparotomy has been suggested by some as being of prognostic value, if performed prior to operative manipulation and immediately after entry into the abdomen. We are not impressed with this method, however, because of the vagarious nature of ovarian tumors. Sometimes an apparently localized lesion is followed by massive recurrence. In other instances extensive disease seems compatible with longevity.

The symptoms themselves are rarely of much value in diagnosis. Postmenopausal bleeding, however, always calls for complete gynecological examination. While the form of malignancy producing this symptom is generally cervical or corporeal carcinoma, ovarian malignancy is not a rare finding. Culdoscopy is occasionally helpful in differentiating between a harmless uterine or tubal mass and a true ovarian neoplasm. When, however, there is any doubt as to whether a pelvic mass might be ovarian or not, exploration is indicated because of the very deadly nature of ovarian cancer.

Even at the time of surgery, the exact nature of an ovarian tumor may be uncertain, and in such instances a *frozen section* may be helpful. It is perhaps preferable to remove the whole adnexal mass, and allow the pathologist to select likely areas for section rather than blindly remove one or two areas for evaluation. While this may minimize errors, permanent sections will on occasion show malignancy that had not been noted on frozen section, so that the trained gynecologist will also strongly consider the gross appearance of the lesion at surgery.

Prognosis. The outlook for the patient with ovarian carcinoma is very grave, especially if one omits from consideration the dysontogenetic group (granulosatheca cell tumor, arrhenoblastoma, and dysgerminoma) in which the results are far better. There are few writers who report a 5-year survival rate of much more than 20 %, and indeed in some areas such as New York, ovarian cancer accounts for more deaths than cervical malignancy due to improved detection of the latter disease. Unfortunately cytopathological techniques rarely are useful in detecting cancer of the ovary.

Meigs reports only 9.7 % of 72 patients with solid ovarian carcinoma to have survived for 5 years, although 21.9 %, of 82 patients with cystic carcinoma were still living. The entire series of 154 cases gave a 5-year survival rate of 15.5 %. Munnell, Jacox, and Taylor in a recent study of 343 cases of ovarian cancers, reported 27 % of 5-year survivals, but if certain special types of relatively low malignancy, like granulosa cell and low grade cystic tumors, were excluded from the series the salvage is only 12 %. Kent and McKay record a surprisingly good salvage of 36.4 %, but their cases comprise a large number of favorable cystic tumors.

Treatment. The proper treatment of

ovarian carcinoma is *surgical*. Operation should be performed as early as possible, and should ideally comprise hysterectomy and bilateral salpingo-oophorectomy. Even when peritoneal involvement is disclosed, the primary lesions should be removed if this is safely possible, as there is rather general agreement that this retards the progress of the secondary extensions. Some degree of omentectomy decreases recurrent ascites, although it may predispose to intestinal obstruction.

Advanced Disease. Most gynecologists feel that ovarian carcinoma warrants exploration despite suggestive evidence of extrapelvic disease and even pulmonic or pleural spread. Admittedly the prognosis is poor but surgery is worthwhile (1) as a diagnostic measure, (2) in obviating incipient obstruction, and (3) as a palliative procedure by reducing tumor bulk, omental lesions, and ascites. Rarely there is profound regression following removal of the parent lesion, and modern methods of chemotherapy and irradiation often lead to prolonged remission although cure is minimal.

The postoperative employment of *irradiation therapy* has been almost universal, and is of undoubted value in prolonging life in many instances, with little regard as to tumor histology, as noted by Chu. There is scant evidence, however, of any curative effect. More recently, radioactive colloidal gold or phosphate has been placed into the peritoneal cavity and seems of considerable aid in preventing the recurrent ascites which is such a frequent problem in the implanting papillary tumors although damage to the intestinal tract has been an occasional complication. It is of no assistance where there are large masses and of course is rarely curative, merely palliative in increasing the life span. Details are available in the papers of Kron and of Elkins and Keettel.

The varied methods of chemotherapy are still uncertain and equivocal, but occasional patients have prolonged remissions of 1 or 2 years following drug therapy, despite advanced disease. On the other hand, certain tumors are not arrested, and just as there are varying degrees of radiosensitivity, we must anticipate differences in drug sensitivity and resistance. Chlorambucil, triethylenemalamine (TEM), and thiotriethylenephosphoramide (thio-TEPA), as reported by Navjoks, Crandall, and Treeter, are among the drugs utilized.

Parker and Singleton suggest increased longevity in certain drug-treated patients, and with this we would agree, although complete cure is unlikely. Severe bone marrow depression may ensue, but careful regulation of the drug may obviate this and other complications. We regard perfusion as a truly heroic and very dangerous procedure, to be utilized only when there is no alternative type of therapy.

SARCOMA OF OVARY

Sarcoma of the ovary is far less common than carcinoma, its *incidence* as compared with carcinoma being about 1:40. It *may occur at any age*. Most authors emphasize that it is frequent in children, but this is open to doubt, as so many ovarian tumors in children which were formerly diagnosed as sarcoma are now recognized as either granulosa cell carcinoma, dysgerminoma, or lymphomas.

Various types of sarcoma are found in the ovary, the spindle variety being more common than the round cell, although mixed forms often occur. The lymphomas, occasionally primary, and angiosarcoma are also described, but it appears that in the latter the perivascular arrangement of the cells is due to the fact that extensive degeneration has occurred except where the cells are near to their blood supply. Symptoms are identical to those of carcinoma.

TERATOMA

Teratoma of the ovary may be *cystic or solid*. The cystic form is represented by the benign dermoid, already described in the chapter on benign ovarian cysts. The *solid teratoma* differs from the simple dermoid not only in that it is a solid tumor, but also because it is malignant, and that it contains elements derived

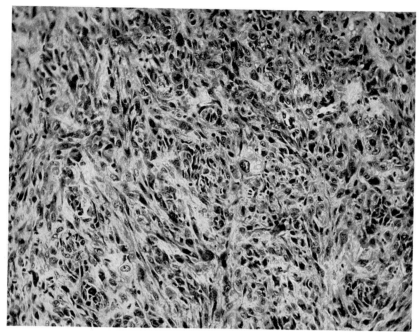

FIG. 24.26. Spindle cell sarcoma of ovary

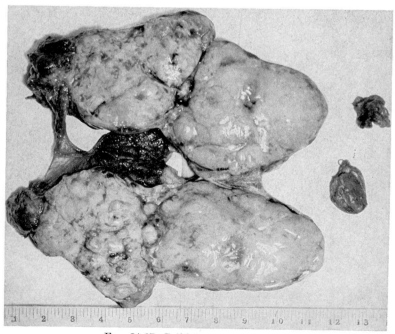

FIG. 24.27. Solid teratoma of ovary

from all three of the fetal layers. The term *embryonal carcinoma* is used by some for what we believe to be a typical teratoma; in other words, the lesion is the same despite the different terminology.

Within recent years we have been convinced that a third and somewhat intermediate form should be recognized, *a benign solid teratoma*, as noted by Peterson. We base this assertion on the fact that we have encountered a small group of dominantly solid teratomas, made up of tissues derived from all the fetal layers, but all very mature. Some of these have been extremely large, and some have occurred in children, so that one might at first suspect such tumors to be the malignant types of teratoma seen chiefly in children and usually fatal. The particular group we are describing, however, have all been benign clinically.

The *histogenesis* of teratoma is not clearly known, the two chief theories being: (1) an origin from segregated blastomeres, and (2) an origin from unfertilized sex cells. According to the first of these, blastomeres may be segregated in early stages of embryonic development, lying dormant until later life, when for some unknown reason they begin to differentiate into the tissues which they were originally designed to form. The weakness of this concept is that it does not explain why the ovary is such a seat of predilection for such teratomatous growths.

Perhaps somewhat more popular is the second theory. This is based on the fact that the ovary normally contains large numbers of germ cells, capable after certain preparatory changes of producing another human body if fertilized by the male element. Even without the latter, it is thought possible that a species of parthenogenetic development may occur because of certain stimulating if unknown factors which may arise, and that abortive and imperfect formation of various fetal tissues may thus occur.

According to this hypothesis, it will be seen that the histogenesis of teratoma is somewhat allied to the phenomenon of twinning. In this connection, it is worth noting that the chromosomal test for sex differentiation has been applied by Hunter, Lennox, and Durk to the study of a group of 21 teratomas, 12 occurring in females and 9 in males. All the teratomas borne by women were found to be

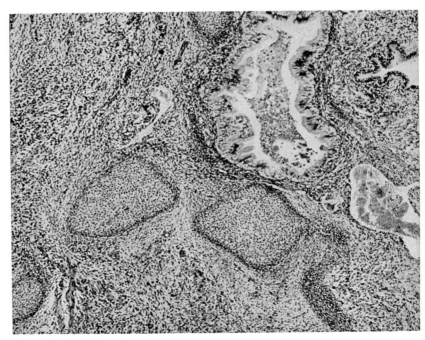

Fig. 24.28. Teratoma of ovary showing cartilage plates and a cavity lined by entodermic epithelium like that seen in pseudomucinous cystadenoma.

chemical methods of absolutely distinguishing between estrogen and androgen producing cells by virtue of enzyme response are not perfected.

DYSGERMINOMA (*neutra*)

Although Jakobovits notes occasional dysgerminomas that possess an estrogenic or androgenic effect, this is not regarded as an active tumor as far as endocrine effect is concerned. Since it is generally discussed with other functioning tumors which have been presumed to originate from some disorder in embryonic life (dysontogenetic), it seems logical to include it in this chapter.

Incidence. Morris and Scully note that dysgerminoma comprises 3 to 5% of all malignant ovarian tumors. Only about 540 cases have been reported, three-fourths of them occurring in the second or third decade of life.

Origin. This interesting tumor type is believed to arise from cells which date back to the early undifferentiated phase of gonadal development. In this phase the germ cells have not as yet acquired either male or female characteristics, so that, as might be expected, dysgerminoma has no effect on the sex characteristics of the patient. Such an origin, first suggested by Meyer, is given much support by the fact that an identical tumor occurs in the testicle, where it is commonly designated as seminoma or embryonal carcinoma. This is as one would expect with tumors which, as it were, lag behind the differentiating procession in gonads which later develop into either testes or ovaries.

The probable correctness of this theory of the origin of dysgerminoma is further indicated by the fact that in a considerable proportion of the reported cases the tumor has occurred in individuals showing some degree of gonadal deficiency, varying from minor degrees to actual pseudohermaphroditism. However, in such cases the tumor has no causal relation with the sex abnormality, which persists even when the tumor is removed. This is in contrast with certain other ovarian tumors which produce direct changes in sex characters, with return to normal after removal of the tumors.

Because a small proportion of dysgerminomas show various alien elements, there are some who look upon these tumors as of teratomatous origin, but the prevailing concept is that most cases of dysgerminoma originate as described above. However, the presence of teratoid elements impairs the prognosis. An origin from the mature oocyte, as suggested by Hughesdon, seems to us implausible.

Pathology. Grossly, these tumors are of solid type, although when large, they often show degeneration and cystic cavities. They may be very small, measuring only a few centimeters in diameter, or they may reach such large size as to fill most of the abdominal cavity. They are, when small, surrounded by a rather dense capsule, which, however, is often broken through as the tumor grows, with later infiltration of surrounding organs. The cut surface of the tumor is gray or grayish pink, but there are often areas of yellowish hue. The consistency is doughy but at times firm and rubbery. The growth is usually unilateral, although bilateral tumors have been noted in a few cases.

Microscopically, there are few tumors of the ovary which present such a distinctive picture, so that the diagnosis in most cases is easy, once one is familiar with this picture. The tumor is made up of rather large round or ovoid cells, arranged characteristically in alveoli separated by septa of partially hyalinized connective tissue which shows a characteristic infiltration with lymphocytes. The nuclei of the epithelial cells are large and rather deeply staining, and a varying number of mitoses are to be seen, although usually they are not numerous. Even in small tumors considerable areas of degeneration and hemorrhage are often present. Occasionally one finds large symplasmic giant cells, which have at times led to the mistaken diagnosis of associated

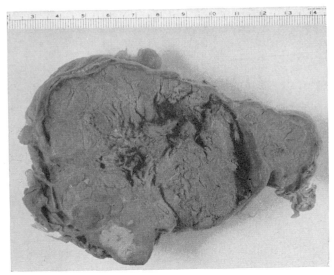

FIG. 25.1. Dysgerminoma—gross appearance

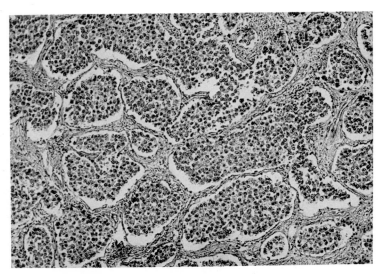

FIG. 25.2. Dysgerminoma—microscopic appearance

tuberculosis. Morris and Scully have described a *"gonadoblastoma,"* a combined dysgerminoma-sex cord tumor, which has only recently been accepted as a specific entity. Teter notes various androgenic and estrogenic combinations with these primarily germ cell tumors which he attributes to sex cord portions. He utilizes the term *gonocytoma* but notes several types according to the endocrine effect observed and the cell elements contained.

Malignancy. This tumor undoubtedly belongs in the malignant group, but there is much variation in this respect in individual cases. Certainly the degree of malignancy is not to be compared to that of the common types of primary ovarian cancer, and cure has in many cases followed simple removal of the

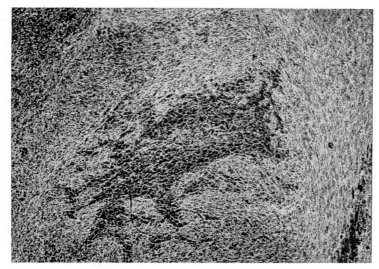

Fig. 25.15. Thecoma with lutein-like transformation in certain areas

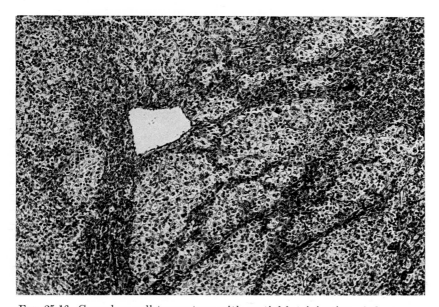

Fig. 25.16. Granulosa cell tumor type with partial luteinization of the tumor

phologically but not functionally like lutein cells, and that they are perhaps better to be spoken of as pseudolutein rather than lutein cells. In any case a feminizing effect is produced, rather than virilism which is so characteristic of the almost identical tumors of hilus cell origin. However, association of cell type and endocrine effect is inconstant.

PREGNANCY LUTEOMA

Sternberg describes a "pregnancy luteoma" as an ovarian enlargement (up to 12 cm.), which is generally solid, composed of eosinophilic, polyhedral cells, which are not a part of the corpus luteum of pregnancy, and may on occasion be bilateral. He is not certain whether this is a true neoplasm or merely a physio-

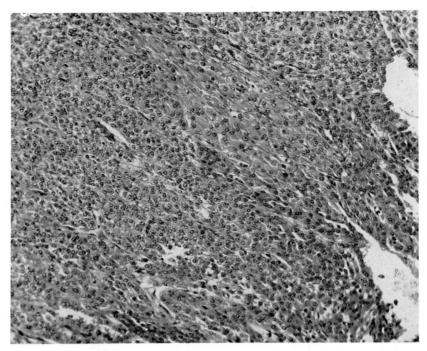

FIG. 25.17. Most areas show only a typical granulosa-thecal pattern with beginning luteinization in *right central area*.

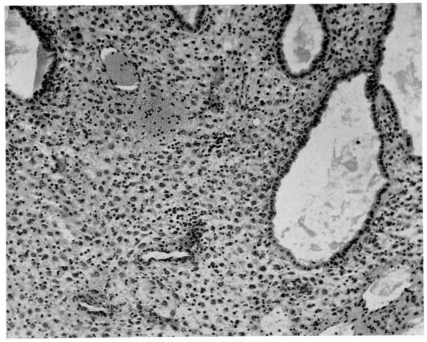

FIG. 25.18. Decidual transformation of endometrium in association with tumor shown in Figure 25.17.

logical response to pregnancy, similar to the theca lutein cysts so frequently seen in trophoblastic disease, and occasionally with normal pregnancy. Greene indicates that this particular picture should be regarded as a preexisting thecoma, which merely portrays the hormonal influences of pregnancy.

While we have seen a limited number of such ovarian enlargements, our own impression would be that it represents merely a profound exaggerated physiological response of the ovary to the increased endocrine stimulus of gestation. In the cases personally observed, it would be extremely difficult to exclude a hilus cell tumor on a purely morphological basis, although the concomitant pregnancy and absence of Reinke crystalloids is helpful. Histochemical determination of steroid 3β-ol dehydrogenase might be expected in a progesterone-secreting tumor as noted by Goldberg, Jones, and Woodruff.

Clinical Characteristics of Granulosa-theca Tumors. These neoplasms of the ovary may be considered a fairly common tumor, comprising probably nearly 10% of all solid malignant ovarian neoplasms. We have encountered more than 500 instances (including referred cases) of this neoplasm in our laboratory. The thecoma is much less common, although admixture is common. These tumors may occur at any age—before puberty, during the reproductive epoch, or after the menopause. While the larger tumors, like other ovarian neoplasms, may cause such symptoms as pain or discomfort, the more distinctive symptomatology is dependent upon the capability of the tumor cells to produce the estrogenic hormone. However, perforation of the tumor with intraperitoneal hemorrhage may lead to acute symptoms (French). Bilaterality is rare (approximately 5%).

When the tumor occurs *during reproductive life*, as it does in a large proportion of cases, the clinical syndrome is not so striking as when it occurs against the background of the prepuberal or postmenopausal phase, during which there is

normally little or no estrogenic hormone in the circulation. During the reproductive years, on the other hand, the tumor merely adds quantitatively to the cyclical hormonal content of the blood. No change would be expected in the secondary sex characters, for example, because these have long since been developed, while the effect upon menstruation would be merely a quantitative one, not unlike that which characterizes the relative hyperestrogenism which is associated with most cases of functional bleeding. Hyperestrogenism may be associated with normal menstruation, with hypermenorrhea, or with long periods of amenorrhea, as noted by Busby and Anderson, and these varying effects upon menstruation are noted with granulosa cell carcinoma. Nevertheless, pregnancy may concur with granulosa-theca cell tumors, and Diddle and O'Connor have noted this association in 37 of nearly 1200 reported cases of this type of lesion.

When, on the other hand, such tumors occur *in young children*, long before the inauguration of the normal estrogenic function of the ovary, the clinical manifestations of precocious puberty are evoked, *viz.*, precocious menstruation and the premature appearance of secondary sex characters, such as hypertrophy of the breasts, the appearance of axillary and pubic hair, puberal development of the external genitalia, and also hypertrophy of the uterus. With the removal of the tumor, these manifestations promptly regress, this constituting a crucial biological demonstration of the direct causal role of the tumor in the production of the symptoms. As a matter of fact, instances are recounted in which, after the removal of a unilateral tumor and disappearance of the abnormal symptoms, a recurrent tumor has developed in the remaining ovary, with again the production of precocious puberal symptoms and again their disappearance after the removal of the second tumor. It is of interest to note that the precocious menstruation of this syndrome is of the anovulatory, purely follicular type, in which respect it differs from certain other types of precocious

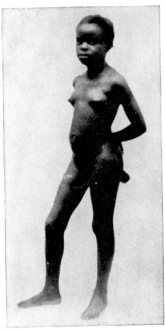

FIG. 25.19. Precocious puberty due to granulosa cell tumor in 7-year-old child.

puberty and menstruation in which both ovulation and menstruation occur. In the latter group, insemination might theoretically bring about fertilization at abnormally early ages.

In the *postmenopausal* group of cases, again, occurring at a life phase at which little or no estrogenic hormone is found in the blood, the tumors may produce a reestablishment of periodic menstruation-like bleeding, an estrogenic type of cytological specimen, and hypertrophy of the uterus with cases noted up to 84 years of age. No effect is seen upon secondary sex characters, presumably because of the higher threshold or unreceptivity of these at this phase of life. With the removal of tumors at this age, the abnormal menstruation of course ceases and, interestingly enough, the patient may experience a second menopause from the standpoint of the characteristic vasomotor phenomena.

It is generally accepted that estrogen is produced by associated theca cells. Our ideas in the past have always been that both granulosa and theca cells are capable of estrogenic production. More recently, however, Falck, utilizing intraocular transplants for study of various cell systems of granulosa and theca cells, has indicated that it is the *theca* interna cells that are actually responsible for the secretion of *estrogen*, but only where there is continuity with granulosa cells. Similarly his work would appear to indicate that the interstitial cells are capable of production of the estrogenic steroid if there is an association with granulosa or lutein cells. To further complicate this particular item we might simply mention the work of MacKinlay, whose review of granulosa cell tumors would seem to afford a strong suggestion that the granulosa and theca cells, normally estrogenic, may be converted into hilus or luteinized cells capable of androgen secretion. Such observations as the above would afford ample reason for accepting the possibility that any given endocrine-secreting tumor may excrete not a single but both types of sexual hormones. Our own feeling about the morphology of these tumors is well expressed in a recent study of the unclassified tumors of the Ovarian Tumor Registry. A number of pure thecomas have been observed with definite feminizing effects; however, Shippel, and Nokes, Claiborne, and Reingold report virilism as a sequel of thecomatous tumors.

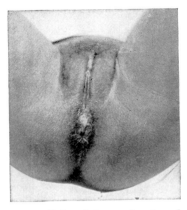

FIG. 25.20. Puberal type of external genitalia.

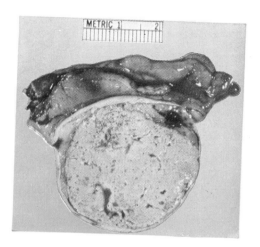

PLATE XXV. I. Arrhenoblastoma showing characteristic yellowish color with focal hemorrhage and smooth capsule. (From Novak, E. R., and Woodruff, J. D.: *Gynecologic and Obstetric Pathology*, Ed. 5 W.B. Saunders Company, Philadelphia, 1962.)

sions. A recent review by Novak and Mattingly has indicated that these (18) tumors were always small (less than 5 cm.), unilateral, benign, and virilizing (with one possible exception). An interesting if inexplicable association has been the presence of endometrial hyperplasia where uterine tissue was obtained.

A case report by Stewart and Woodard concerns the first malignant hilus cell tumor on record. Since the authors were kind enough to permit us to study their material, we can unanimously agree with their impressions of this clinically and histologically lethal tumor despite certain disagreement as noted in an addendum to the article by Boivin and Richart. In the material reviewed by us, Reinke crystalloids were plentiful. The concurrence of hilus cell tumors with gonadal dysgenesis (Turner's syndrome) has been summarized by Warren, Erkman, and Cheatum.

Tumors with Functioning Matrix (See also Chapter 23). It is becoming increasingly apparent to all pathologists that a certain number of ovarian tumors, not morphologically of the endocrinologically productive variety, possess hormonal activity. Indeed, these tumors may be of many types, both benign or malignant, and may produce either estrogenic or androgenic features.

It would appear that the ovarian stroma is capable of conversion into a steroid-secreting cell similar to a theca or Leydig cell. Consequently, a great many supposedly inert tumors such as Brenner, Krukenberg, and various carcinomas have appeared to exert a feminizing influence. Fewer androgenic tumors have been reported (Fig. 25.30), but a recent review by Scully notes 11 diverse tumors with virilizing tendencies.

From our own clinic Woodruff, Williams, and Goldberg have provided strong histochemical proof that certain tumors not usually recognized as endocrinologically active are capable of a hormonal

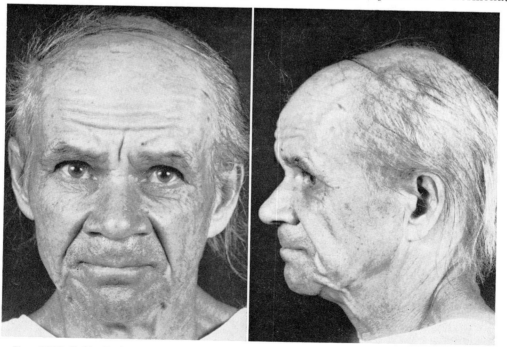

FIG. 25.30 (*left*). Patient with pseudomucinous tumor with marked hyperplasia of "stromal cells" showing profound virilism. "Stromal cells" histochemically resembled interstitial cells of the testis.

FIG. 25.31 (*right*). Lateral view of Figure 25.30

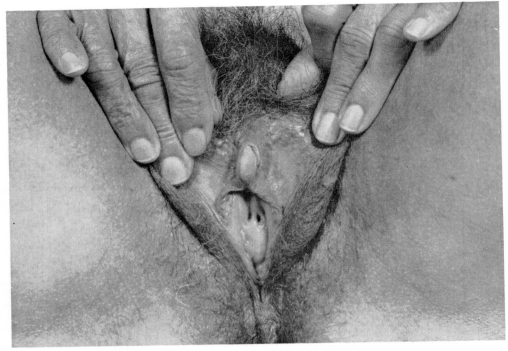

FIG. 25.32. External genitalia (same patient) with marked enlargement of clitoris

effect. It would seem likely that increasing knowledge of biosynthetic pathways will suggest that many tumors regarded as inert will show evidence of an endocrine effect even though on occasion any estrogenic trend may be nullified by an equal androgenic effect. Such is a premature impression of various ovarian neoplasms that have been studied by certain histochemical techniques in our own laboratory.

HOMOLOGY OF CERTAIN OVARIAN AND TESTICULAR TUMORS

A provocative approach to the study of the dysontogenetic group of tumors has been suggested by Teilum, whose studies have led him to believe in the homology of certain tumor groups occurring in the ovary and testis. This concept seems fundamentally sound, but it would be premature to completely accept the homologous group described by Teilum or to use his studies as a basis for revamping our present system of classification, inadequate as it admittedly is. Those interested in the details of Teilum's studies are referred to his various publications on the subject.

A recent study by Warner *et al.* describes the production of certain dysontogenetic tumors in various fowls and rodents by a variety of methods. They point out (and their photomicrographs suggest) many structural similarities. The authors are inclined to feel that the tumors arise from "reserve" cells capable of bipotential differentiation rather than from fetal rests, either androgenic or estrogenic. Although the "fetal rest" origin of various tumors is drawing more and more criticism in explaining tumorigenesis in general, and rightly so, we have always been lukewarm towards evoking a frequently undemonstrable "reserve cell" origin for certain tumors. The same authors suggest a generic name for the androgen and estrogen secreting tumors, namely "gynandroblastoma," with "androblastoma" and "gynoblastoma" proposed for the subtypes. These terms have the obvious disadvantage of confusion with what the terms used to mean. Indeed it is becoming increasingly apparent that

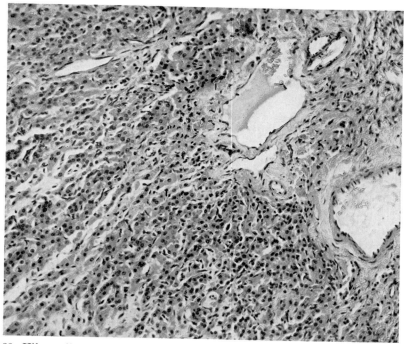

Fig. 25.33. Hilus cell tumor of ovary producing masculinization symptoms which regressed after removal of tumor.

any observed endocrine effect should be incorporated into the diagnosis even though a decisive hormone effect is not always apparent. For example, Shippel, Nokes *et al.*, and others report thecoma (usually regarded as estrogenic) as being associated with masculinization. Many other similar instances could be noted.

We might as well face the fact that certain tumors, classically of a certain type, may on occasion secrete the contrasexual hormone. Yet if one will recall the very close chemical structure of the steroids, why should this be unexpected from a neoplastic tumor? The mere shift of a keto or hydroxyl group from one to another area in the steroid would be all that would be necessary, and actual conversion of these steroids has been observed and made to occur in certain animals. MacKinlay speaks of the convertible nature of granulosa and theca cells which may become producers of androgen or androgen-like substances.

Whether the suggestion of Warner *et al.* be followed we doubt. The way of a re-

former in revising long accepted nomenclatures is always a difficult one. Yet any proposal that might in any way improve the tremendously confused status of the classification and nomenclature of this tumor group deserves serious consideration. At this writing our own preference is *gonadal stromal tumor*, feminizing, virilizing, or inert, as the case may be, and this has been discussed in the initial pages of this chapter.

Thyroid Tumors of the Ovary (Struma Ovarii). This group of tumors has been discussed in Chapter 24, "Malignant Tumors of the Ovary; Carcinoma of the Ovary."

REFERENCES

Amromin, G. D., and Haumeder, E. M.: Feminizing ovarian gynandroblastoma. Amer. J. Obstet. Gynec., 77: 645, 1959.

Ayerst, R. I., and Johnson, C. G.: Dysgerminoma; report of a case treated by surgery and x-ray therapy followed by term pregnancy. Obstet. Gynec., 14: 685, 1959.

Berger, L.: La glande sympathicotrope due hile de l'ovaire; ses homologies avec la gland interstitielle du testicule. Les rapports nerveuses des deux glandes. Arch. Anat., *2:* 255, 1923.

Berger, L.: Tumeur des celles sympathico-tropes de l'ovaire avec virilisation. Rev. Canad. Biol., *1:* 539, 1942.

Betson, J. R., and Eichen, P. M.: Isosexual precocity produced by an ovarian thecoma (in a 2½-year-old girl). Obstet. Gynec., *22:* 219, 1963.

Biskind, G. R., and Biskind, M. S.: Experimental ovarian tumors in rats. Amer. J. Clin. Path., *19:* 501, 1949.

Blocksma, R.: Bilateral dysgerminoma of ovary with pseudohermaphroditism. Amer. J. Obstet. Gynec., *69:* 879, 1955.

Boivin, Y., and Richart, R. M.: Hilus cell tumors of the ovary. Cancer, *18:* 231 1965.

Brody, S.: Clinical aspects of dysgerminoma of the ovary. Acta Radiol., *56:* 209, 1961.

Burslein, R. W., Langley, F. A., and Woodcock, A. S.: Clinicopathological study of estrogenic ovarian tumors. Cancer, *7:* 522, 1954.

Busby, T., and Anderson, G. W.: Feminizing mesenchymomas of ovary. Amer. J. Obstet. Gynec., *68:* 1391, 1954.

Diddle, A. W., and Devereux, W. P.: Ovarian mesenchymomas. Obstet. Gynec., *13:* 294, 1959.

Diddle, A. W., and O'Connor, K. A.: Feminizing ovarian tumors and pregnancy. Amer. J. Obstet. Gynec., *62:* 1071, 1951.

Dockerty, M. B., and Massey, E.: Malignant lesions of the uterus associated with estrogen-producing ovarian tumors. Amer. J. Obstet. Gynec., *61:* 147, 1951.

Dockerty, M. B., and McCartney, W. C.: Granulosa cell tumor, with the report of a 34-pound specimen and review. Amer. J. Obstet. Gynec., *38:* 698, 1939.

Dougherty, C. M., and Lund, C. J.: Solid ovarian tumors complicating pregnancy. Amer. J. Obstet. Gynec., *60:* 261, 1950.

Duckett, H. C., Davis, C. D., and Fetter, B. F.: Granulosa cell carcinom of the ovary. Obstet. Gynec., *2:* 611, 1953.

Dysgenminoma. Current opinions on clinical problems. Amer. J. Obstet. Gynec., *86:* 693, 1963.

Emig, O. R., Hertig, A. T., and Rowe, F. J.: Gynandroblastoma of the ovary. Obstet. Gynec., *13:* 135, 1959.

Falck, B.: Site of production of estrogen in rat ovary as studied in micro-transplants. Acta Physiol. Scand. (Suppl. 163), *47:* 5, 1959.

Falk, H. C., and Mason, V. C.: Arrhenoblastoma complicating pregnancy. Amer. J. Obstet. Gynec., *62:* 1160, 1951.

Flick, F. H., and Banfield, R. S. Jr.: Malignant theca cell tumors. Cancer, *9:* 731, 1956.

Flick, F. H., and Banfield, R. S., Jr.: Theca and granulosa cell tumors. Bull. Sloane Hosp. Wom., *2:* 31, 1956.

Francis, H. H.: Granulosa cell tumor of the ovary at the age of 85 years. J. Obstet. Gynaec. Brit. Comm., *64:* 274, 1957.

French, W. G.: Clinical behavior of granulosa-cell tumor of ovary. Amer. J. Obstet. Gynec., *62:* 75, 1951.

Ganem, K., Friedall, G. H., and Sommers, S. C.: A study of ovarian thecomatosis. Calif. Med., *96:* 254, 1962.

Geist, S. H., Gaines, J. A., and Pollock, A. D.: Experimental biologically active tumors in mice. Amer. J. Obstet. Gynec., *38:* 786, 1939.

Gershenfeld, O. B., Savel, L. E., and Diamond, E.: Ovarian dysgerminoma. J. Newark Beth Israel Hosp., *8:* 43, 1957.

Goldberg, B., Jones, S. E. S., and Woodruff, J. D.: A histochemical study of steroid 3β-ol dehydrogenase activity in some steroid-producing tumors. Amer. J. Obstet. Gynec., *86:* 1003, 1963.

Gordon, V. H., and Marvin, H. N.: Theca cell tumor of ovary in child one year of age. J. Pediat., *39:* 133, 1951.

Greenblatt, R. B., and Roy, S.: *The Hirsute Female,* edited by R. B. Greenblatt, p. 119. Charles C Thomas, Publisher, Springfield, Illinois, 1963.

Greene, R. R., Holzwarth, D., and Roddick, J. W., Jr.: "Luteomas of pregnancy." Amer. J. Obstet. Gynec., *88:* 1001, 1964.

Harris, H. R.: Granulosa cell tumor of the ovary (in a woman aged 82). J. Obstet. Gynaec. Brit. Comm., *64:* 272, 1955.

Hodgson, J. E., Dockerty, M. B., and Mussey, R. D.: Granulosa cell tumor of ovary; a clinical and pathologic review of 62 cases. Surg. Gynec. Obstet., *81:* 631, 1945.

Hughesdon, P. E.: The structure and origin of theca-granulosa tumors. J. Obstet. Gynaec. Brit. Comm., *65:* 540, 1958.

Hughesdon, P. E.: Thecal and allied reaction in epithelial tumors. J. Obstet. Gynaec. Brit. Comm., *65:* 702, 1958.

Hughesdon, P. E.: Structure, origin and histological relations of dysgerminoma. J. Obstet. Gynaec. Brit. Comm., *67:* 566, 1959.

Ingram, J. E., and Novak, E.: Endometrial carcinoma associated with feminizing ovarian tumors. Amer. J. Obstet. Gynec., *61:* 774, 1951.

Jakobovits, A.: Hormone production by miscellaneous ovarian tumors. Amer. J. Obstet. Gynec., *85:* 90, 1963.

Javert, C. T., and Finn, W. F.: Arrhenoblastoma; the incidence of malignancy and the relationship to pregnancy, to sterility, and to treatment. Cancer, *4:* 60, 1951.

Jones, E.: Dysgerminoma of the ovary; report of a case associated with teratoma of the ovary. Amer. J. Obstet. Gynec., *78:* 825, 1959.

Labotsky, J., Loewy, B. P., Lloyd, C. W., and

Rogers, W. F.: Studies of steroid-forming neoplasms. J. Clin. Endocr., *14:* 809, 1954.

Langley, F. A.: "Sertoli" and "Leydig" cells in relation to ovarian tumors. J. Clin. Path., *7:* 10, 1954.

Lees, D. H., and Paine, C. G.: Lipoid masculinizing tumors of the ovary. J. Obstet. Gynaec. Brit. Comm., *65:* 710, 1958.

Li, M. H., Gardner, W. W., and Kaplan, H. S.: Effects of x-ray radiation on development of ovarian tumors in intrasplenic grafts in castrated mice. J. Nat. Cancer Inst., *8:* 91, 1947.

Liebert, K. I., and Stent, L.: Dysgerminoma of the ovary with choriocarcinoma. J. Obstet. Gynaec. Brit. Comm., *67:* 627, 1960.

Mackinlay, C. J.: Male cells in granulosa cell ovarian tumors. J. Obstet. Gynaec. Brit. Comm., *64:* 512, 1957.

Mansell, H., and Hertig, A. T.: Granulosa and theca cell tumors and endometrial carcinoma; a study of their relationship and a survey of 80 cases. Obstet. Gynec., *6:* 385, 1955.

Maxwell, D. M. W.: Granulosa cell tumor producing symptoms 4 years following radium menopause. J. Obstet. Gynaec. Brit. Comm., *63:* 232, 1956.

McKay, D. G., Hertig, A. T., and Hickey, W. F.: Histogenesis of granulosa and theca cell tumors of human ovary. Obstet. Gynec., *1:* 125, 1953.

McKay, D. G., Robinson, D., and Hertig, A. T.: Histochemical observations on granuloma cell tumors, thecomas, and fibromas of ovary. Amer. J. Obstet. Gynec., *58:* 625, 1949.

Meyer, R.: Tubulläre (testikuläre) und solide Formen des Andreioblastoma ovarii. Beitr. Path. Anat., *84:* 485, 1930.

Meyer, R.: Pathology of some special ovarian tumors and their relation to sex characteristics. Amer. J. Obstet. Gynec., *26:* 505, 1933.

Morris, J. M.: Testicular feminization in male pseudohermaphroditism. Amer. J. Obstet. Gynec., *65:* 1192, 1953.

Morris, J. M., and Scully, R. E.: *Endocrine Pathology of the Ovary.* C. V. Mosby Company, St. Louis, 1958.

Morrison, C. W., and Woodruff, J. D.: Fibrothecoma and associated ovarian stromal neoplasia. Obstet. Gynec., *23:* 344, 1964.

Meuller, C. W., Topkins, P., and Laff, W. A.: Dysgerminoma of ovary; an analysis of 427 cases. Amer. J. Obstet. Gynec., *60:* 153, 1950.

Neigus, I.: Ovarian dysgerminoma with chorionepithelioma. Amer. J. Obstet. Gynec., *69:* 838, 1955.

Nokes, J. M., Claiborne, H. A., and Reingold, W. N.: Thecoma with associated virilization. Amer. J. Obstet. Gynec., *78:* 722, 1958.

Novak, E.: Dysgerminoma of ovary. Amer. J. Obstet. Gynec., *35:* 925, 1938.

Novak, E.: Masculinizing tumors of the ovary (arrhenoblastoma; adrenal ovarian tumors). Amer. J. Obstet. Gynec., *36:* 840, 1938.

Novak, E., and Brawner, J. N.: Granulosa cell tumors of the ovary; clinical and pathological study of 36 cases. Amer. J. Obstet. Gynec., *28:* 637, 1934.

Novak, E. R., and Long, J. H.: Arrhenoblastoma of the ovary. A review of the Ovarian Tumor Registry. Amer. J. Obstet. Gynec., in press.

Novak, E. R., and Mattingly, R. F.: Hilus cell tumors of the ovary (with a review of 18 cases). Obstet. Gynec., *15:* 425, 1960.

Novak, E. R., and Mattingly, R. F.: Functioning tumors of the ovary. Postgrad. Med., *30:* 438, 1961.

Novak, E. R., Woodruff, J. D., and Linthicum, J. M.: Evaluation of the unclassified tumors of the Ovarian Tumor Registry 1942–1962. Amer. J. Obstet. Gynec., *87:* 999, 1963.

Pedowitz, P., Felmus, L. B., and Grayzel, D. M.: Criteria for diagnosis of malignancy in theca cell tumors. Amer. J. Obstet. Gynec., *68:* 1519, 1954.

Pedowitz, P., Felmus, L. B., and Grayzel, D. M.: Dysgerminoma of the ovary; prognosis and treatment. Amer. J. Obstet. Gynec., *70:* 1284, 1955.

Pedowitz, P., and O'Brien, F. B.: Arrhenoblastoma of the ovary. Obstet. Gynec., *16:* 62, 1960.

Pick, L.: Über Adenome der männlichen und weiblichen Keimdrüse. Klin. Wschr., *42:* 502, 1905.

Plate, W. P.: Oestrogenic functie van de Tussencellen in de gonade. Nederl. T. Verlosk., *63:* 83, 1963.

Posner, A. C., Kushner, J. I., and Posner, L. B.: Ovarian dysgerminoma and pregnancy. Amer. J. Obstet. Gynec., *70:* 422, 1955.

Proctor, F. E., Greeley, J. P., and Rathmell, T. K.: Malignant thecoma of ovary. Amer. J. Obstet. Gynec., *62:* 185, 1951.

Rottino, A., and McGrath, J. F.: Masculinovoblastoma; primary masculinizing tumor of ovary (so-called large cell variety—hypernephroid—luteoma). Arch. Intern. Med. (Chicago), *63:* 686, 1939.

Sachs, B. A.: Leydig (sympathicotropic) cell tumor of ovary; report of case with virilism, including postmortem findings. J. Clin. Endocr., *11:* 878, 1951.

Sandberg, E. C.: The virilizing ovary. Obstet. Gynec. Survey, *17:* 165, 1962.

Saphir, W., and Parker, M. L.: Adrenal virilism. J. A. M. A., *107:* 1286, 1936.

Schiller, W.: *Pathologie und Klinik der Granulosazelltumoren.* Maudrich, Vienna, 1934.

Schneider, G. T.: "Functioning" ovarian tumors. Amer. J. Obstet. Gynec., *79:* 921, 1962.

Scully, R. E.: Androgenic lesions of the ovary. In *The Ovary*, International Academy of Pathology Monograph No. 3, edited by H. G. Grady and D. E. Smith, p. 143. The Williams & Wilkins Company, Baltimore, 1963.

Shippel, S.: Ovarian theca cell. J. Obstet. Gynaec. Brit. Comm., *57:* 362, 1950.

Sommers, S. C., Gates, O., and Goodof, I. I.: Late recurrence of granulosa cell tumors. Obstet. Gynec., *6:* 395, 1955.

Sternberg, W. H.: Morphology, androgenic function, hyperplasia and tumors of the human ovarian hilus cells. Amer. J. Path., *25:* 493, 1949.

Sternberg, W. H.: Nonfunctioning ovarian neoplasms. In *The Ovary*, International Academy of Pathologists Monograph No. 3, edited by H. G. Grady and D. E. Smith, p. 209. The Williams & Wilkins Company, Baltimore, 1963.

Sternberg, W. H., and Gaskill, C. J.: Theca-cell tumors; with a report of 12 new cases and observations on possible etiologic role of ovarian stromal hyperplasia. Amer. J. Obstet. Gynec., *59:* 575, 1950.

Stewart, R. S., and Woodard, D. E.: Malignant ovarian hilus cell tumor. Arch. Path., *73:* 91, 1962.

Teilum, G.: Homologous tumors in ovary and testis. Acta Obstet. Gynec. Scand., *24:* 480, 1944.

Teilum, G.: Arrhenoblastoma-androblastoma. Acta Path. Microbiol. Scand., *22:* 252, 1946.

Teilum. G.: Estrogen-producing Sertoli cell tumors (androblastoma tubulare lipoides) of the human testis and ovary; homologous ovarian and testicular tumors. J. Clin. Endocr., *9:* 301, 1949.

Teilum, G.: Ovarian neoplasms with endocrine significance. In *Progress in Gynecology*, edited by J. V. Meigs and S. H. Sturgis, Vol. 2, p. 48. Grune & Stratton, Inc., New York, 1950.

Teilum, G.: Endocrine varieties of "androblastoma" in ovary and testis. J. Obstet. Gynaec. Brit. Comm., *58:* 201, 1951.

Teilum, G.: Classification of ovarian tumors. Acta Obstet. Gynec. Scand., *30:* 292, 1952.

Teter, J.: A mixed form of feminizing germ cell tumor (gonocytoma II). Amer. J. Obstet. Gynec., *84:* 722, 1962.

Thoeny, R. H., Dockerty, M. B., Hunt, A. B., and Childs, D. S.: Study of ovarian dysgerminoma with emphasis on role of radiation therapy. Surg. Gynec. Obstet., *113:* 692, 1961.

Traut, H. F., and Butterworth, J. S.: The theca, granulosa, lutein cell tumors of the human ovary and similar tumors of the mouse's ovary. Amer. J. Obstet. Gynec., *34:* 987, 1937.

Tweeddale, D. N., Dockerty, M. B., Pratt, J. H., and Hranilovich, G. T.: Pregnancy with a recurrent granulosa cell tumor. Amer. J. Obstet. Gynec., *70:* 1039, 1955.

Vande Wiele, R. L.: Studies of the androgenic function of the ovaries. Bull. Sloane Hosp., *6:* 82, 1960.

von Kahlden, C.: Über eine eigentumliche Form des Ovarialkarzinoms. Zbl. Path., *6:* 257, 1895.

Warner, N. E., Friedman, N. B., Bomze, E. J., and Masin, F.: Comparative pathology of experimental and spontaneous androblastomas and gynoblastomas of the gonads. Amer. J. Obstet. Gynec., *79:* 971, 1960.

Warren, J. C., Erkman, B., and Cheatum, S.: Hilus-cell adenoma in a dysgenetic gonad with XX/XO mosaicism. Lancet, *1:* 141, 1964.

Watson, S. L.: Dysgerminoma complicating labor. Amer. J. Obstet. Gynec., *72:* 1177, 1956.

Waugh, D., Venning, E. H., and McEachern, D.: Sympathicotropic (Leydig) cell tumors of ovary with virilism. J. Clin. Endocr., *9:* 486, 1949.

Wilkins, L.: Feminizing adrenal tumor causing gynecomastia in boy of 5 contrasted with virilizing tumor in 5-year-old girl. J. Clin. Endocr., *8:* 111, 1948.

Woodruff, J. D., Williams, T. J., and Goldberg, B.: Hormone activity of the common ovarian neoplasm. Amer. J. Obstet. Gynec., *87:* 679, 1963.

transpulmonary cancer spread. Amer. J. Roentgenol., *72:* 409, 1954.

Ball, T. L., and Platt, M. A.: Urologic complications of endometriosis. Amer. J. Obstet. Gynec., *84:* 1516, 1962.

Barnes, J.: Endometriosis of the pleura and ovaries. J. Obstet. Gynaec. Brit. Comm., *60:* 823, 1953.

Bassis, M. L.: Pseudodeciduosis. Amer. J. Obstet. Gynec., *72:* 1029, 1956.

Beirne, M. F., and Berkheiser, S. W.: Umbilical endometriosis. Amer. J. Obstet. Gynec., *69:* 895, 1955.

Brosset, A.: Value of radiation therapy in treatment of endometriosis. Acta Obstet. Gynec. Scand., *36:* 209, 1957.

Carter, B.: Treatment of endometriosis (as part of a symposium). J. Obstet. Gynaec. Brit. Comm., *69:* 783, 1962.

Cavanagh, W. F.: Endometriosis. Bull. Sloane Hosp., *6:* 115, 1960.

Charles, O.: Endometriosis and hemorrhagic pleural effusion. Obstet. Gynec., *10:* 309, 1957.

Culver, G. J., Pereira, R. M., and Seibel, R.: Radiographic features of rectosigmoid endometriosis. Amer. J. Obstet. Gynec.[1] *76:* 1176, 1958.

Davis, C., Jr., and Truehart, R.: Surgical management of endometrioma of the colon. Amer. J. Obstet. Gynec., *89:* 453, 1964.

Duson, C. K., and Zelenik, J. S.: Vulvar endometriosis. Obstet. Gynec., *3:* 76, 1954.

Fallas, R.: Endometriosis. Amer. J. Obstet. Gynec., *72:* 557, 1956.

Fallon, J.: Endometriosis in youth. J. A. M. A., *131:* 1405, 1946.

Ferraro, L. R., Hetz, H., and Carter, H.: Polypoid endometriosis. Obstet. Gynec., *7:* 32, 1956.

Ferreira, H. P., and Clayton, S. G.: Three cases of malignant change in endometriosis, including two cases arising in rectovaginal septum. J. Obstet. Gynaec. Brit. Comm., *64:* 41, 1958.

Fertano, L. R., Hertz, H., and Carter, H.: Malignant endometriosis. Obstet. Gynec., *7:* 32, 1956.

Fredrikson, H.: Pregnancy after conservative surgery for ovarian endometriosis. Acta Obstet. Gynec. Scand., *36:* 468, 1957.

Frey, G. H.: Familial occurrence of endometriosis. Amer. J. Obstet. Gynec., *73:* 418, 1957.

Gardner, G. H.: Management of pelvic endometriosis. Obstet. Gynec., *5:* 538, 1955.

Gardner, G. H., Greene, R. R., and Ranney, B.: The histogenesis of endometriosis. Amer. J. Obstet. Gynec., *78:* 445, 1958.

Goldfarb, W. S.: A case of endometriosis in the episiotomy scar. Amer. J. Obstet. Gynec., *66:* 191, 1953.

Grayburn, R. W.: Ureteric obstruction due to endometriosis. J. Obstet. Gynaec. Brit. Comm., *67:* 74, 1960.

Greene, J. W., and Enterline, H. T.: Carcinoma arising in endometriosis. Obstet. Gynec., *9:*417, 1957.

Green, T. H., Jr., and Meigs, J. V.: Pseudomenstruation from posthysterectomy vaginal vault endometriosis. Obstet. Gynec., *4:* 622, 1954.

Hartz, P. H.: Occurrence of decidua-like tissue in the lung. Amer. J. Clin. Path., *26:* 48, 1956.

Hawthorne, H. R., Kimbrough, R. A., and Davis, H. C.: Concomitant endometriosis and carcinoma of the rectosigmoid. Amer. J. Obstet. Gynec., *62:* 681, 1951.

Hobbs, J. E., and Bortnick, A. R.: Endometriosis of lungs. Amer. J. Obstet. Gynec., *40:* 832, 1940.

Hughesdon, P. E.: Structure of endometrial cysts of the ovary. J. Obstet. Gynaec. Brit. Comm., *64:* 481, 1957.

Jacobsen, V. C.: The intraperitoneal transplantation of endometrial tissue. Arch. Path. Lab. Med., *1:* 169, 1926.

Javert, C. T.: Spread of benign and malignant endometrium in the lymphatic system with a note on co-existing vascular involvement. Amer. J. Obstet. Gynec., *64:* 780, 1952.

Kempers, R. D., Dockerty, M. B., Hunt, A. B., and Symmonds, R. E.: Postmenopausal endometriosis. Surg. Gynec. Obstet., *111:* 348, 1960.

Kimball, L. C., and Reeves, W.: Endometriosis following perforation of uterus. Amer. J. Obstet. Gynec., *73:* 422, 1957.

Kistner, R. W.: Newer progestins in treatment of endometriosis. Amer. J. Obstet. Gynec., *75:* 264, 1958.

Kistner, R. W.: Endometriosis. Fertil. Steril., *13:* 237, 1962.

Kistner, R. W., and Hertig, A. T.: Primary adenoacanthoma of the ovary. Cancer, *5:* 1134, 1952.

Koss, L. G.: Miniature adenoacanthoma arising in an endometriotic cyst in an obturation lymph node. Cancer, *16:* 1369, 1963.

Krohn, P. L.: Endometriosis and supernumerary ectopic ovarian tissue in a rhesus monkey. J. Obstet. Gynaec. Brit. Comm., *58:* 430, 1951.

Kunnar, D., Anderson, W., and Van Wyck, D.: Ovarian carcinoma arising in endometrial cyst. J. Obstet. Gynaec. Brit. Comm., *62:* 372, 1955.

Lane, R. E.: Endometriosis of the vermiform appendix. Amer. J. Obstet. Gynec., *79:* 372, 1960.

Lash, S. R., and Rubenstone, A. I.: Adenocarcinoma of the rectovaginal septum probably arising from endometriosis. Amer. J. Obstet. Gynec., *78:* 299, 1959.

Lattes, R.: A clinical and pathological study of

endometriosis of the lung. Surg. Gynec. Obstet., *103:* 552, 1956.

Meigs, J. V.: An interest in endometriosis and its consequences. Amer. J. Obstet. Gynec., *79:* 625, 1960.

Melody, G. F.: Endometriosis causing obstruction of the ileum. Obstet. Gynec., *8:* 468, 1956.

Meyer, R.: Adenomyosis, Adenofibrosis und Adenomyom. In *Handbuch der Gynakologie*, edited by W. Stoeckel. J. F. Bergmann, Munich, 1930.

Novak, E.: The significance of uterine mucosa in the fallopian tube, with a discussion of the origin of aberrant endometrium. Amer. J. Obstet. Gynec., *12:* 484, 1926.

Novak, E., and Alves de Lima, O.: Correlative study of adenomyosis and pelvic endometriosis. Amer. J. Obstet. Gynec., *56:* 634, 1948.

Novak, E. R.: Pathology of endometriosis. Clin. Obstet. Gynec., *3:* 413, 1960.

Novak, E. R., and Hoge, A. F.: Endometriosis of the lower genital tract. Obstet. Gynec., *12:* 687, 1958.

Nunn, L. L.: Endometrioma of thigh. Northw. Med., *48:*474, 1949.

Overton, O. H., Wilson, R. B., and Dockerty, M. B.: Primary endometriosis of the cervix. Amer. J. Obstet. Gynec., *79:* 768, 1960.

Park, W. W.: The occurrence of decidual tissue within the lung; report of a case. J. Path. Bact., *47:* 563, 1954.

Prince, L. N., and Abrams, J.: Endometriosis of perineum. Amer. J. Obstet. Gynec., *73:* 890, 1957.

Ridley, J. H., and Edwards, I. K.: Experimental endometriosis in the human. Amer. J. Obstet. Gynec., *76:* 783, 1958.

Russell, W. W.: Aberrant portions of the Müllerian duct found in an ovary. Bull. Johns Hopkins Hosp., *10:* 8, 1899.

Sampson, J. A.: Perforating haemorrhagic (chocolate) cysts of the ovary. Arch. Surg., *3:* 245, 1921.

Sampson, J. A.: Peritoneal endometriosis due to the menstrual dissemination of endometrial tissue into the peritoneal cavity. Amer. J. Obstet. Gynec., *14:* 422, 1927.

Sampson, J. A.: Postsalpingectomy endometriosis (endosalpingiosis). Amer. J. Obstet. Gynec., *20:* 443, 1930.

Sampson, J. A.: Pathogenesis of postsalping-

ectomy endometriosis in laparotomy scars. Amer. J. Obstet. Gynec., *50:* 597, 1945.

Scott, R. B., Novak, R. J., and Tindale, R.: Umbilical endometriosis and Cullen sign. Obstet. Gynec., *11:* 556, 1958.

Scott, R. B., and Wharton, L. R., Jr.: Effect of estrone and progesterone on growth of experimental endometriosis in rhesus monkeys. Amer. J. Obstet. Gynec., *74:* 852, 1957.

Scott, R. B., and Wharton, L. R., Jr.: The effect of testosterone on experimental endometriosis in rhesus monkeys. Amer. J. Obstet. Gynec., *78:* 1020, 1959.

Scott, R. B., and Wharton, L. R., Jr.: Effects of progesterone and norethindrone on experimental endometriosis in monkeys. Amer. J. Obstet. Gynec., *84:* 867, 1962.

Simon, H. B., Zimet, R. R., Schneider, E., and Morgenstern, L. L.: Bilateral ureteral obstruction due to endometriosis. J. A. M. A., *183:* 191, 1963.

Stevenson, C. S. (Editor): Symposium on endometriosis. Clin. Obstet. Gynec., *3:* 411, 1960.

Te Linde, R. W., and Scott, R. B.: Experimental endometriosis. Amer. J. Obstet. Gynec., *60:* 1147, 1950.

Thompson, J. D.: Primary ovarian adenoacanthoma. Obstet. Gynec., *9:* 403, 1957.

Wharton, L. R., Jr., and Scott, R. B.: Experimental production of genital lesions with norethindrone. Amer. J. Obstet. Gynec., *89:* 701, 1964.

White, R. J.: Simultaneous acute obstruction of the colon and terminal ileum from endometriosis. Surgery, *35:* 947, 1954.

Whitehouse, D. B., and Bates, A.: Endometriosis; results of conservative surgery. J. Obstet. Gynaec. Brit. Comm., *62:* 378, 1955.

Wietersen, F. K., and Balow, R. M.: Colonic endometriosis; roentgenologic aspects. Radiology, *69:* 839, 1957.

Williams, C., Jr.: Endometriosis of the colon in elderly women. Ann. Surg., *157:* 974, 1963.

Williams, G. A., and Richardson, A. C.: Endometriosis of cervix uteri. Obstet. Gynec., *6:* 309, 1955.

Williams, J. F., Williams, J. B., and Harper, J. W.: Thoracic endometriosis. Amer. J. Obstet. Gynec., *84:* 1512, 1962.

Zweibel, L.: Primary endometriosis of the cervix. Amer. J. Obstet. Gynec., *65:* 1350, 1953.

GRAVIDANZA ECTOPICA

È meglio parlare di gravidanza ectopica
che extrauterina. Infatti è ectopico qualunque
impianto dell'uovo al di fuori della mucosa
uterina: un uovo impiantato nel tratto
interstiziale della tuba non è uterino
né è extrauterino, si può ben dire però che è
ectopico —

27

ECTOPIC PREGNANCY

Definition. The term ectopic pregnancy is applied to pregnancy following implantation of the fertilized egg on any tissue other than the mucous membrane lining the uterine cavity. It is a better and more inclusive term than extrauterine pregnancy, as a pregnancy may be ectopic and yet be situated within the uterus, as in the case of interstitial or cornual pregnancy.

Under the heading of ectopic gestation may be included pregnancy in the tube, the uterine cornu, the interstitial portion of the tube, a rudimentary uterine horn, the cervix, the ovary, or the abdominal or pelvic peritoneum.

TUBAL PREGNANCY

Much of the most common type of ectopic pregnancy is that which occurs in the tube. The latter normally is concerned in the transportation of the fertilized egg to the uterus, but under certain conditions the egg may plant itself on the tube wall. The latter is ill adapted for either satisfactory nidation or later continuance of the gestation, so that with rare exceptions the embryo succumbs in an early stage.

Etiology. The causes ascribed for tubal pregnancy may be placed in two chief groups, *viz.*, (1) factors which delay or prevent the passage of the fertilized egg into the uterine cavity; and (2) factors which increase the receptiveness of the tubal mucosa to the fertilized egg.

(1) *Factors which Delay or Prevent Passage of Fertilized Egg into Uterine Cavity.* This is probably the more important of the two groups of causes. Partial obstruction of the tube by *chronic salpingitis* is most often concerned, not only because of the mechanical factor but also because of the impairment of ciliary activity and muscle peristalsis, both so important in the propulsion of the egg. Follicular salpingitis especially is believed to be a frequent cause, because of the formation of blind gutters into which a fertilized egg may stray.

Recent articles by Halbrecht and by Nokes *et al.* have pointed out that any pregnancy ensuing after chemotherapy for pelvic tuberculosis is very apt to be ectopic in nature. Halbrecht reports an astounding 66% incidence of extrauterine pregnancies in tuberculous patients, and he feels that a significant cause of ectopic pregnancy in general is spontaneous healing of unrecognized tubal tuberculosis, while the scarring and fibrosis may be a factor in the production of partial obstruction. This entity must be extremely less common in the United States than in Israel.

Congenital abnormalities of the tube, especially diverticula and accessory ostia, may likewise be concerned, as may also be *partial occlusion by adhesions or tumors* outside the tube. Finally, the occasional role of *transmigration of the ovum* is indi-

515

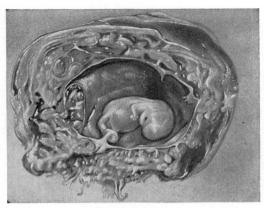

FIG. 27.1. Cut surface of tubal pregnancy sac at 2½ months showing embryo alive at time of operation.

cated by the fact that the pregnancy may occur in the tube opposite to the ovary containing the corpus luteum of pregnancy.

The egg does not implant itself until its burrowing apparatus, the trophoblast, has developed, and this normally takes place after the egg has reached the uterus. For this reason we believe the retardation of its progress is probably an important factor in tubal pregnancy, permitting the development of the trophoblast while the egg is still in the tube. It has been suggested that the increased use of penicillin in infections of the tube, through the prevention of complete occlusion of tubes which are otherwise damaged, may actually increase the incidence of tubal gestation, but the evidence on this point is not as yet convincing. Iffy has concluded that pregnancy may antedate the last menstrual period (LMP) and has provided a very persuasive correlation between the last menstrual period, the measurements of the early embryo, and any observations on the dates of coitus. His suggestion that menstruation may dislodge an early implantation with subsequent expulsion through the cornu and secondary tubal pregnancy is difficult to accept or deny. Since, however, pathological examination of tubes removed during the menstrual phenomenon only rarely reveal endometrium, we cannot help but

feel that Iffy's suggestion explains only a minority of cases of tubal gestation.

(2) *Factors Increasing Receptiveness of Tubal Mucosa to Fertilized Egg.* The second group of causes is less clearly demonstrable, although of undoubted importance in some cases. In some instances even areas of *typical endometrium may be found in the tube,* and in such cases it is easy to understand how a fertilized egg may implant itself. Again, in many cases of tubal pregnancy a greater or less degree of *decidual response* can be demonstrated histologically, indicating a responsiveness at least approaching that of the endometrium. Just what degree of importance is to be attributed to this factor of individual tubal responsiveness is still a matter of dispute, but it is certainly far less than that of retardation of the passage of the fertilized egg.

Incidence. Whereas it has been frequently quoted that 1 out of 300 pregnancies is ectopic, Fontanilla and Anderson, in an excellent statistical study, indicate that the occurrence is considerably more frequent. In Baltimore, ectopic gestation occurs once in 200 pregnancies among white women, once in 120 among Negroes, nearly a 50% difference. The authors feel strongly that the high incidence of inflammatory disease among Negroes is the responsible factor, and obviously consideration of any reported incidence should include the racial percentages.

The recent study by Bobrow and Bell from the Harlem Hospital in New York notes 1 ectopic pregnancy to every 64 live births, which would indicate (and we concur) the highest ratio ever recorded for any large American series, and approaches the figure of 1 ectopic in 28 pregnancies reported from Jamaica by Douglas. That repeat ectopic pregnancy may recur in the remaining tube in approximately 10% of cases (Schiffer) has been accepted by most gynecologists.

Pathology. Once the fertilized egg has implanted itself on the tubal mucosa, the early nidation changes are much like those seen in uterine pregnancy, except for

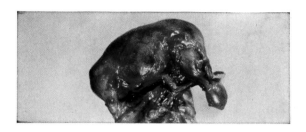

PLATE XXVII.I. Unruptured tubal pregnancy with extensive intratubal hemorrhage

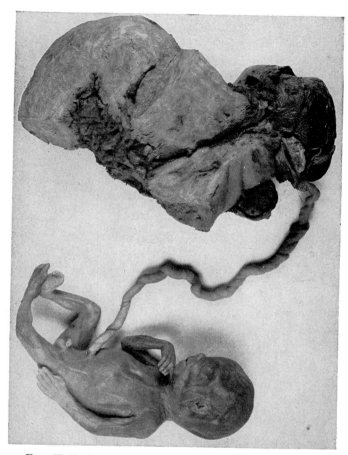

FIG. 27.15. Ruptured interstitial gestation with embryo

in Cavanagh's recent review. In Studdiford's case the implantation occurred in the posterior surface of the uterus about 1½ cm. medial to the insertion of the left tube. He suggests the following criteria on which proof of this type of pregnancy must rest: (1) that both tubes and ovaries are normal with no evidence of recent pregnancy; (2) the absence of any evidence of a uteroperitoneal fistula; and (3) the presence of a pregnancy related exclusively to the peritoneal surface and young enough to eliminate the possibility of secondary implantation following a primary nidation in the tube.

It may be well to mention that the surgeon, in dealing with an abdominal pregnancy, should generally not attempt to remove the placenta, which may be firmly fixed to mesentery and the abdominal viscera. Profuse hemorrhage can occur on manipulation, and the placenta, if left in situ, generally resorbs without sequelae. Removal of the fetus with ligation of the cord is usually the wise procedure.

Cervical Pregnancy. While exceedingly rare, the possibility of cervical pregnancy does exist. Just as, in placenta praevia, the egg may implant itself in the region of the internal os, so it may, in rare instances, implant on the cervical mucosa. As would be expected, this bizarre type of pregnancy produces profuse bleeding in the early months of pregnancy and necessitates surgical intervention, which may be of difficult and serious nature. In reporting a recent case Resnick notes only some 65 instances of a true

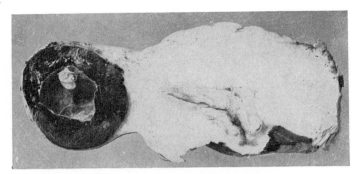

FIG. 27.16. Cut surface of uterus and cornual pregnancy. Note the thick decidua still in situ although evidences of its impending separation are already present.

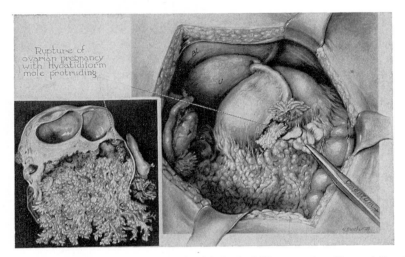

FIG. 27.17. Ovarian pregnancy associated with hydatidiform mole. (Case of Dr. Henry G. Bennett.)

cervical pregnancy in his exhaustive review of reported cases. He points out the difficulties in diagnosis and the mortality (20%), primarily due to hemorrhage, understandably due to repeated pelvic examinations in an effort to establish the diagnosis (Fig. 27.19).

Combined Pregnancy (Intra- and Extrauterine). There are now several hundred reported cases of combined pregnancy, one embryo being implanted normally within the uterus, the other ectopically in the tube. Interesting diagnostic problems may arise with such a combination. For example, rupture of the tubal pregnancy may cause serious intra-abdominal bleeding, with none from the vagina, since the integrity of the uterine decidua is maintained by the presence of

the lining intrauterine pregnancy. For a discussion of the clinical connotations of combined pregnancy, however, the reader must be referred to textbooks of obstetrics. Schaefer feels that the pathogenesis is a double-ovum twin pregnancy in which both ova are fertilized at a single coitus and separates this (combined) form from a compound pregnancy where an intrauterine is superimposed upon a preexisting resolving ectopic gestation. In any case diagnosis is seldom made because the slightly enlarged boggy uterus is felt to represent merely a decidual reaction. In adding an additional case, Brody and Stevens bring up to 506 the cases of combined pregnancy as well as providing an extensive review of the literature.

Posthysterectomy Ectopic Preg-

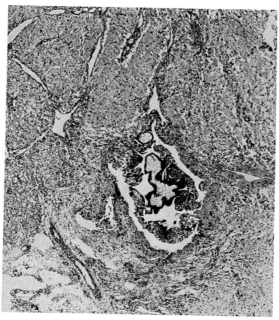

FIG. 27.18. Chorionic villi in ovarian pregnancy in which the implantation may have been in the corpus luteum which can be seen surrounding the villi in this section. (Courtesy of Dr. Herbert F. Traut, San Francisco, California.)

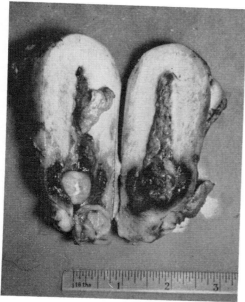

FIG. 27.19. Unusual cervical implantation. (Courtesy of Dr. L. Resnick, South Africa.)

nancy. Although we have seen a few cases of prolapsed fallopian tubes following hysterectomy, where the tubal fimbria protruded through the vaginal vault, it has been our impression that an ectopic pregnancy would be unlikely. The physiology of such a prolapsed tube without an intermediate uterus would seemingly be impaired so that the possibility of pregnancy would be minimal, and such would seem to be the rule.

While tubal pregnancy posthysterectomy is rare, the careful clinician cannot absolutely promise the woman patient that she will not become pregnant following removal of the uterus. Hanes has reported 11 cases of pregnancy following abdominal or vaginal hysterectomy. In 4 instances the pregnancy probably antedated the operative procedure, with conception occurring before and not recognizable at the time of surgery. Perhaps this occurs much more often than realized, with subsequent anemia and pelvic induration being construed as intraabdominal bleeding incurred by the surgery itself. Often this is self-limited, and does not require operative intervention.

In other instances years have occurred between the hysterectomy and the ectopic gestation so that we have no recourse but to assume that there is some tract whereby the sperm cell can ascend to fertilize an extruded ovum. We might also speculate that passage down the tube by the fertilized egg has been retarded, allowing the trophoblast and villi to undergo sufficient development to permit implantation in the tube or less commonly the abdomen. It might be considered mental cruelty to even remotely mention this remote possibility to the younger posthysterectomy woman.

REFERENCES

Angell, J. H., and Te Linde, R. W.: Further experiences in culdoscopy. Ann. Surg., 135: 690, 1952.

Armitage, G. L., and Armitage, H. V.: Combined intra- and extra-uterine pregnancy. Amer. J. Obstet. Gynec., 69: 885, 1955.

Bender, S.: Fertility after tubal pregnancy. J. Obstet. Gynaec. Brit. Comm., 63: 400, 1956.

Bisca, B. V., and Felder, M. E.: Coexistent interstitial and intrauterine pregnancy following homolateral salpingo-oophorectomy. Amer. J. Obstet. Gynec., 79: 263, 1960.

Bobeck, S. Endometrial reaction in ectopic pregnancy. Acta Obstet. Gynec. Scand., 36: 49, 1957.

Bobrow, M. L., and Bell, H. G.: Ectopic pregnancy: a 16-year survey of 905 cases. Obstet. Gynec., 20: 500, 1962.

Brody, S., and Stevens, F. L.: Combined intra- and extrauterine pregnancy. Obstet. Gynec., 21: 129, 1963.

Cavanagh, D.: Primary peritoneal pregnancy. Amer. J. Obstet. Gynec., 76: 523, 1958.

Charles, D.: The Arias-Stella reaction. J. Obstet. Gynaec. Brit. Comm., 69: 1006, 1962.

Clark, J. F. J., and Bourne, J.: Advanced ectopic pregnancy. Amer. J. Obstet. Gynec., 78: 340, 1959.

Crawford, J. R., and Ward, J. V.: Advanced abdominal pregnancy. Amer. J. Obstet. Gynec., 10, 549, 1957.

Cullen, T. S.: Bluish discoloration of umbilicus as diagnostic sign when ruptured extra-uterine pregnancy exists. In Contributions to Medical and Biological Research, edited by W. Osler, Vol. 1, p. 420, 1919.

de Brux, J., and Ancia, M.: Arias-Stella endometrial atypias. Amer. J. Obstet. Gynec., 89: 661, 1964.

Demick, P. E., and Cavanagh, D.: Unilateral tubal and intra-uterine pregnancy. Amer. J. Obstet. Gynec., 76: 533, 1958.

Donovan, W. H.: Ectopic pregnancy and maternal deaths. Obstet. Gynec., 7: 694, 1956.

Douglas, C. P.: Tubal ectopic pregnancy. Brit. Med. J., 2: 838, 1963.

Fontanilla, J., and Anderson, G. W.: Further studies on racial incidence and mortality of ectopic pregnancy. Amer. J. Obstet. Gynec., 70: 312, 1955.

Fulsher, R. W.: Tubal pregnancy following homolateral salpingectomy. Amer. J. Obstet. Gynec., 78: 355, 1959.

Grant, A.: The effect of ectopic pregnancy on fertility. J. Clin. Obstet. Gynec., 5: 861, 1962.

Grody, M. H., and Otis, R. D.: Ectopic pregnancy after total hysterectomy (report of a case). Obstet. Gynec., 17: 96, 1961.

Halbrecht, I.: Healed genital tuberculosis; new etiologic factor in ectopic pregnancy. Obstet. Gynec., 10: 73, 1957.

Hanes, M. V.: Ectopic pregnancy following total hysterectomy. Obstet. Gynec., 23: 882, 1964.

Hubbard, L. T.: Secondary abdominal pregnancy. Amer. J. Obstet. Gynec., 74: 431, 1957.

Iffy, L.: The role of premenstrual postmidcycle conception in the aetiology of ectopic gestation. J. Obstet. Gynaec. Brit. Comm., 70: 996, 1963.

Jarvinen, P. A., and Kinnunen, O.: Treatment of extra-uterine pregnancy and subsequent fertility. Int. J. Fertil., 2: 131, 1957.

Kistner, R. W., Hertig, A. T., and Rock, J.: Tubal pregnancy complicating tuberculous salpingitis. Amer. J. Obstet. Gynec., 62: 1157, 1951.

Kobak, A. J., Fields, C., and Pollack, S. L.: Intraligamentary pregnancy; extraperitoneal type of abdominal pregnancy. Amer. J. Obstet. Gynec., 70: 175, 1955.

Kroupa, W. E., and Bleicher, J. E.: Primary peritoneal implantation of ovum. Obstet. Gynec., 5: 165, 1955.

Laiuppa, M. A., and Cavanagh, D.: The endometrium in ectopic pregnancy. Obstet. Gynec., 21: 155, 1963.

Latto, D., and Norman, R.: Pregnancy in rudimentary horn of a bicornuate uterus. Brit. Med. J., 2: 926, 1950.

Malkasion, G. D., Hunter, J. S., and Remine, W. H.: Pregnancy in the tubal interstitium and tubal remnants. Amer. J. Obstet. Gynec., 77: 1301, 1959.

Mall, F. P.: On the Fate of the Human Embryo in Tubal Pregnancy. Contributions to Embryology Publication No. 221, Carnegie Institute of Washington, Washington, D. C., 1915.

Moyers, E. D., and Lack, A.: Primary ovarian pregnancy. Amer. J. Obstet. Gynec., 76: 518, 1958.

Murray, E.: Peritoneal factor in sterility. J. Clinic. Obstet. Gynec., 5: 836, 1962.

Nokes, J. M., Claiborne, H. A., Thornton, W. N., and Hsu, Y.: Extrauterine pregnancy associated with tuberculous sal-

tive the subsequent course has shown that rests of trophoblastic tissue have remained in the uterine wall, usually deep in the blood vessel spaces, so that they would be inaccessible to the curette, the so-called *syncytial endometritis.*

Nevertheless, Delfs has pointed out the extreme value of bioassays following evacuation of a mole. In 81 patients studied, 75% showed a normal chorionic gonadotrophin test (HCG) within 60 days, with a few more showing a slower decrease to average range. The residual cases, however, exhibit a high incidence of invasive mole or choriocarcinoma; therefore a persistently positive HCG of more than 2 months should be regarded as suggestive. If positive after hysterectomy, the prognosis is poor, for spread to other organs seems likely.

Brewer finds that after evacuation of a mole, HCG is elevated in 40% of patients as late as 60 days; of these 40%, one-half regress more slowly but the others progress into invasive mole or choriocarcinoma. We might regard *60 days* as the critical time where some decision must be made as to management of this still biologically active lesion.

Associated Ovarian Changes. In at least some cases of hydatidiform mole, as well as of its malignant prototype, chorionepithelioma, the ovaries exhibit an interesting change, in the form of a marked polycystic enlargement, with exaggerated luteinization of predominantly the theca cells. The incidence of these changes in hydatidiform mole would seem to vary between 10 and 25% according to different observers. The ovarian enlargement may be only moderate, or it may reach enormous proportions, the masses in some cases being described as of the size of a man's head. The time of appearance of such ovarian masses seems to be variable, and in some cases they have not appeared until after the evacuation of the mole.

These ovarian changes, including the characteristic *hyperreactio luteinalis,* represent an exaggerated response of the ovarian tissue to the abnormally great trophoblastic hormone production produced by the tumors, although the exact mechanism is not altogether clear. The multiple lutein ovarian cysts thus produced spontaneously disappear within a few months after removal of the mole, and no other treatment is indicated. Lynch, Kyle, and Raphael, as well as others, have indicated that this ovarian pattern is not pathognomonic of mole, or

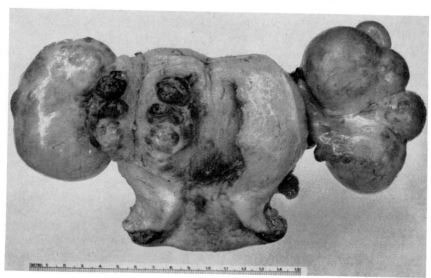

Fig. 28.10. Note bilateral ovarian cysts which may occur in conjunction with any type of trophoblastic disease. (Courtesy of Dr. Clayton Beecham, Philadelphia, Pennsylvania.)

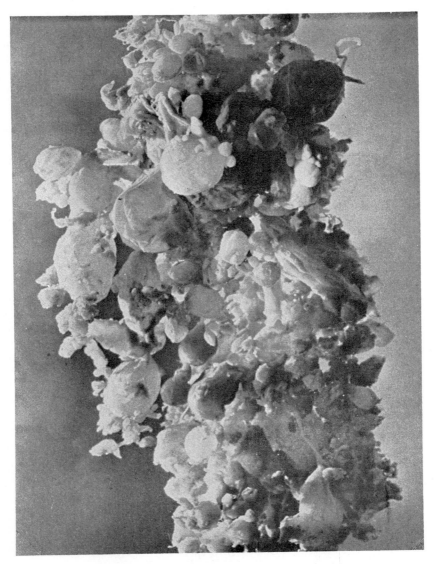

Fig. 28.11. Showing the grapelike gross pattern of hydatidiform mole

indeed, pregnancy, but may occur in un-related conditions. Shettles has recorded recurrent lutein cysts in successive preg-nancies. Girouard, Barclay, and Collins record 17 cases unassociated with mole or choriocarcinoma where these enlarged cystic ovaries occurred, presumably as a response to gonadotrophin stimulation.

Treatment. Once hydatidiform mole is diagnosed, the proper treatment is encouragement of evacuation of the uterus preferably by *Pitocin stimulation* but otherwise by surgery. This of course is followed by careful postoperative supervision with bioassays because of the possibility of later chorionepithelioma. While some put the *incidence of malig-nant change* as high as 10%, it is prob-ably less than this. Repeated moles are likewise rare, but have been reported by Posner, Kushner, and Posner. There are some gynecologists who resort to more

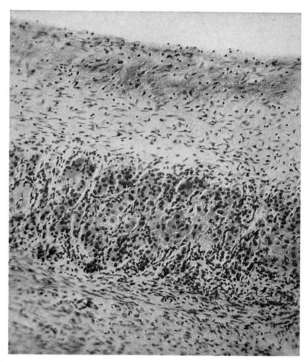

Fig. 28.12. Wall of one of multiple lutein cysts with hydatidiform mole, the lutein cells here being obviously of theca cell origin.

radical measures, such as hysterectomy, and this might seem justifiable where the patient has had all desired children and is elderly, for older women seem to show a considerably higher incidence of malignant degeneration.

Evacuation should be done with much care, to avoid penetration of the thinned-out uterine wall, but at the same time it should be done as thoroughly as possible. Retention of tissue, aside from malignant potentialities, may cause persistence of highly positive pregnancy tests for many weeks or even months, with the later unjustified assumption of chorionepithelioma. Whenever possible, the finger and ovum forceps should be used for the evacuation, although usually the cautious employment of the curette is also required. An injection of Pitocin during the procedure will harden the uterine wall and lessen the danger of perforation. Bleeding may be free, and a uterine pack may need to be inserted. If

the uterus is enlarged up to the umbilicus, hysterotomy is less bloody and permits more adequate evacuation of uterine contents.

Because diagnosis is rarely made early, this is the usual operative approach in this country; we have, however, been advised by Tow (Singapore) on the basis of personal experience, impossible for an American, that hysterotomy is rarely necessary. He states that initial bleeding during curettage may be extreme due to liberation of blood already trapped in the uterine cavity. Following initial hemorrhage, however, bleeding becomes much more moderate, and Tow advocates routine curettage with minimal complication. We frankly find it difficult to disagree with so experienced a clinician, and indeed American authors simply do not have the extensive personal experience of various Asian gynecologists in management of trophoblastic lesions.

The importance of after-supervision cannot be overemphasized, and monthly bioassay should be kept up for many months, until the tests at 6-month intervals are repeatedly negative. If the tests are persistently or increasingly positive, there will be no question as to the presence of actively functioning trophoblastic tissue in the uterus or elsewhere, and this may be due to malignancy. It is usually advisable, if there is any suspicion of the latter, to make x-ray examination of the lungs, which are frequent seats of metastasis in chorionepithelioma.

In the light of present knowledge, no conscientious gynecologist or obstetrician would fail to follow up such cases biologically. Sometimes the tests become negative within 2 weeks, but often they remain positive for months, indicating definitely the presence of functioning trophoblastic tissue. It is advisable that patients under study practice contraception, as an intercurrent new pregnancy could be very misleading.

If the test continues positive, and especially if the patient has bleeding and the uterus remains more or less subinvoluted, a second thorough curettage is indicated. This may reveal residual molar tissue or only necrotic portions of decidua. *If the test still remains positive and especially if the quantitative titer becomes higher*, more definitive therapy must be considered. There is increasing belief in the efficacy of such drugs as Methotrexate as the primary treatment of choriocarcinoma (see "Treatment").

On the other hand, hysterectomy should be considered in the older woman because of the greater frequency of malignant degeneration. In many instances it will afford considerable insight into the exact pathological nature of the trophoblastic disease. Otherwise we have only evidence of increased HCG which may be of diverse causes.

In a number of cases chorionepithelioma will not be revealed, but only residual trophoblastic tissue deep in the uterine wall and inaccessible to the curette. Occasionally, however, definite chorionepithelioma will be discovered.

In past years, a good many hysterectomies were done unnecessarily in the effort not to miss the occasional chorionepithelioma.

CHORIONEPITHELIOMA (CHORIOCARCINOMA)

This highly malignant neoplasm, for which both of the above names are used interchangeably, is derived from the chorionic epithelium. It may develop after full term delivery, miscarriage, or hydatidiform mole although previous pregnancy is not always recognized. In proportion to the relative frequency of these three antecedent conditions, the incidence after hydatidiform mole is disproportionately high. Fully 50% of all cases of chorionepithelioma are believed to follow vesicular mole. It should be repeated, however, that only in a very small proportion of cases, probably less than 5%, does malignancy develop, the benign mole being far more common than chorionepithelioma. The latter, indeed, is a very rare disease, and in many rather large clinics no case has been encountered. Furthermore, because of the frequent difficulty in microscopic diagnosis in this group of cases, it is quite certain that many cases reported as chorionepithelioma have really been highly proliferative but benign hydatidiform moles. It must be remembered that chorionepithelioma is a malignant tumor arising from the fetal trophoblast and not a tumor of the uterus, a curious condition of a tumor of one individual growing in and invading the tissues of another individual.

Pathology. The tumor appears as a dark, hemorrhagic grumous mass on the uterine wall, or in other cases in the substance of the latter, beneath the surface (intramural variety). Its surface soon shows extensive ulceration, with increasing spread on the surface or penetration of the musculature.

Microscopically it is characterized by a disorderly growth of trophoblastic tissue, usually in alveolar fashion, into the muscle, with destruction of the latter

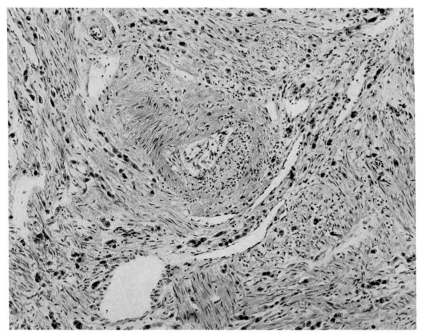

Fig. 28.20. Trophoblastic invasion of musculature beneath implantation area. This is a normal process, but has at times been wrongly diagnosed as syncytioma or chorionepithelioma.

persistently elevated HCG). Chemotherapy is begun if a positive titer persists more than 60 days after passage of a mole.

In previous years Methotrexate was considered in purely an adjuvant role to surgery, *i.e.*, where hysterectomy revealed choriocarcinoma and the level of HCG remained high with or without demonstrable evidence of residual or recurrent trophoblastic disease. The encouraging results stimulated Hertz, Ross, and Lipsett to a trial of primary chemotherapy without surgery. The astoundingly successful salvage has prompted optimism that there may be an adequate chemotherapeutic approach to at least a certain type of genital malignancy.

Although there have been many publications by these authors, the most recent and significant concerns 111 women with metastatic trophoblastic disease, of whom 75 were presumed to have choriocarcinoma, while the others had some form of metastatic trophoblastic disease. With Methotrexate, and occasionally such other agents as Vinblastine and actino-mycin D, an outstanding remission rate of 64% was produced, although not necessarily 5 years. With choriocarcinoma (75 patients), the remission rate was noted to be 60%; with mole and chorioadenoma this amounted to 75% in the 36 patients treated.

This is obviously a marked improvement on Brewer's compilation of women treated by surgery alone, for in 122 patients who had hysterectomy alone, the 5-year salvage was 41% where there were no metastases, but only 19% in the face of metastatic disease. Indeed, primary chemotherapy alone gives better results than when combined with surgery, and this has prompted Hertz to speculate about the danger of tumor emboli being disseminated by the manipulation of surgery.

A later study by Brewer on 28 cases, reaffirms the preferential role of chemotherapy, although pointing out, as do other authors, that hysterectomy may occasionally be necessary if there is failure of response of the HCG. Indeed, Lamb, Morton, and Byron indicate that chemotherapy alone should be reserved for the youthful patient desiring further pregnancy, and that combined chemotherapy and surgery should be the usual method of treatment. Such authors as Acosta-Sison and Manahan indicate that there is a place for hysterectomy, although acknowledging the tremendously beneficial results of chemotherapy.

Admittedly it is a great boon for the youthful patient to retain her uterus, and yet be assured a considerable chance of cure for what has previously been considered to be one of the most lethal forms of cancers. From the standpoint of the pathologist it is rather frustrating, because in the absence of hysterectomy, it is usually not possible to know what is being treated. Curettage alone is rarely diagnostic, and indeed hysterectomy is not always informative (as in those cases where no uterine tumor is present, although it probably arose in this organ, and was obliterated by the previously mentioned defense mechanism). Many cases then are probably treated only because of a persistently positive HCG, which may be due to many much less innocuous causes than choriocarcinoma. Indeed, we think it is remarkable that the diagnosis of choriocarcinoma has been made with assurance in so many cases in the absence of hysterectomy.

Perhaps primary chemotherapy might be the treatment of choice in the young woman desiring further pregnancy if there is a persistently positive or increasing titer after evacuation of a mole, even if curettage shows no evidence of choriocarcinoma. In the older woman, we might prefer hysterectomy with possibly adjuvant Methotrexate if there is evidence of true choriocarcinoma without invasive or metastatic tendencies.

Certainly, Methotrexate is a toxic drug, and must be administered cautiously because of such severe side effects as dermatitis, alopecia, bone marrow depression, stomatitis, and actual ulceration of the gastrointestinal tract. Deaths from this form of therapy are unfortunately not rare, and it would seem that such a toxic agent should be utilized only for treating a serious disease like choriocarcinoma. Chemically Methotrexate is 4-amino-n^{10}-methyl pteroylglutamic acid, a folic acid antagonist which may be given orally or intravenously in dosage varying according to the body weight, but generally up to 25 mgm. per day. A 5-day course followed by a week's resting stage is followed by repeated dosages, meanwhile measuring the response of the HCG. Failure of response after several courses might suggest trial of another drug, but if there is no decrease in the bioassay, hysterectomy deserves strong consideration. Indeed, Hertz has utilized this in cases where there was no demonstrable response of HCG following chemotherapy, and the titer showed no decline after repeated dosage of the different chemotherapeutic agents.

Retention of the uterus permits further pregnancy, and both Hertz and Brewer have noted this sequel after prolonged Methotrexate therapy. A negative bioassay for 1 year is considered a prerequisite for further attempts at pregnancy; during the year contraception should be practiced, and it would appear that oral pills in no way affect the level of HCG. The offspring of Methotrexate-treated mothers are normal; indeed one of the more interesting case reports is that of Freedman et al. A woman who had previously had an invasive mole was observed to have a rising titer of HCG, and was treated vigorously for 3 months by Methotrexate before it was appreciated that she had an intrauterine pregnancy, at which time chemotherapy was discontinued. Uneventful delivery of a term twin pregnancy subsequently occurred, despite the presumably toxic effects of chemotherapy. Spellacy, Meeker, and McKelvey record a patient with three pregnancies after a Methotrexate-treated choriocarcinoma (seemingly genuine), and they note 11 pregnancies in 7 patients.

The contributions by Hertz in the treatment of mole, invasive mole, and choriocarcinoma are monumental, for some regard this as a continuous disease spectrum. We might disagree with this tenet for only a few moles progress to

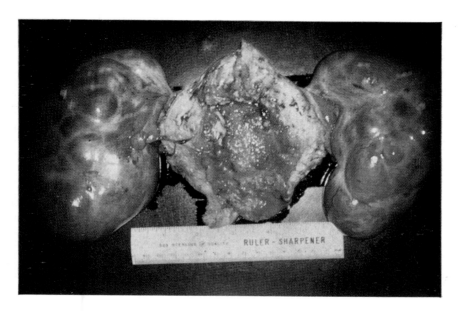

PLATE XXVIII.I. Huge theca lutein cysts with chorionepithelioma

choriocarcinoma, although many chorio-carcinomas are preceded by moles. While fervently agreeing with the work of Hertz, Ross, and Lipsett, it is difficult to quote exactly their latest statistics because of constantly increasing cases under treatment with different degrees of trophoblastic disease, often difficult to prove histologically, and some of which would almost certainly undergo spontaneous regression. This statement is in no sense meant to detract from the amazing results which have been obtained with drug therapy alone.

Our own feeling is that hysterectomy seems worthwhile where there is no evidence of extrauterine trophoblast in the older woman with a sustained titer following a mole. In the case with pulmonic or other metastatic tumor, we concur with the Roswell Park group (Hreshchyshyn *et al.*) that hysterectomy is of dubious value. The younger woman,

anxious for further pregnancy is the likely candidate for primary chemotherapy.

Pulmonary metastases are always difficult to evaluate unless lung surgery or biopsy has obtained tissue. X-ray reveals merely a shadow which may be metastasis, pneumonitis or other. If the shadow disappears, does it necessarily indicate regression of a metastatic lesion following treatment? X-ray changes should always be correlated with variations in the hormone titer. Above all, it should be noted that x-rays have cleared following hysterectomy alone. The use of chemotherapy has been discussed above.

Prognosis. There is wide divergence in reports as to the degree of malignancy of chorionepithelioma, although it had been felt to be one of the gravest of pelvic neoplasms. At one extreme one could find the gloomy and much-quoted statement of the late James R. Ewing that he had

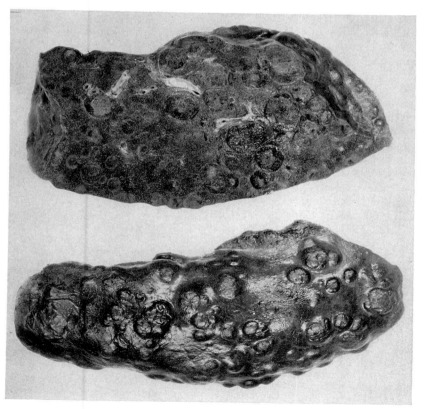

FIG. 28.21. Pulmonary metastasis in case shown in Figure 28.15.

never seen a patient with this disease survive. At the other extreme is the statement of Mathieu that only 5% of such cases end fatally. In view of the recent developments of chemotherapy, no one can be certain of the prognosis (see "Treatment"). It still seems desirable to mention some of the results obtained in the era prior to Methotrexate.

In a study of 74 cases of unquestioned chorionepithelioma from the Chorionepithelioma Registry, Novak and Seah found that 13 (17.5%) were living without recurrence after 1 year or more, an adequate follow-up period for this rapidly fatal disease which usually kills the patient within 6 months.

A later 5-year follow-up on these same Registry cases by Brewer reports a 15% salvage, so that it is apparent that if the patient lives 1 year her chances of a 5-year salvage are excellent. A more recent and more favorable report by the same author concerns 122 women (not the same group as above) treated by hysterectomy with a 32% 5-year survival, with a 41% salvage if no extrauterine disease, as compared to 19% if the disease had extended.

If this salvage seems much better than the earlier patients it should be noted that all of these women were treated by hysterectomy. In the early group with a 15% salvage, treatment was often minimal and indeed part of the figures include autopsy cases. It should be apparent that choriocarcinoma is justifiably regarded as a highly malignant tumor, but it should by no means be regarded as uniformly fatal. Indeed, the encouraging results with chemotherapy as noted by Hertz and Brewer might lead to such increasing salvage as became evident after various antibiotics were used to treat lobar pneumonia.

REFERENCES

Acosta-Sison, H.: Chorioadenoma destruens; a report of 41 cases. Amer. J. Obstet. Gynec., 80: 176, 1960.

Acosta-Sison, H.: Changing attitudes in management of hydatidiform mole (196 cases). Amer. J. Obstet. Gynec., 88: 634, 1964.

Adcock, L. L., and Hakanson, E. Y.: Vascular collapse complicating septic abortion. Amer. J. Obstet. Gynec., 79: 516, 1960.

Arias, R. E., and Bertoli, F.: Metastatic choriocarcinoma without primary lesion. Obstet. Gynec., 13: 737, 1959.

Attwood, H. D., and Park, W. W.: Embolism to the lungs by trophoblast. J. Obstet. Gynaec. Brit. Comm., 68: 611, 1961.

Bardawil, W. A., Hertig, A. T., and Velardo, J. T.: Regression of trophoblast. Obstet. Gynec., 10: 614, 1957.

Barr, F. G., and Okfay, A.: Primary ovarian hydatidiform mole. Amer. J. Obstet. Gynec., 79: 1088, 1960.

Barter, R. H., Dusbabek, J. A., Tyndol, C. M., and Erkenbeck, R. V.: Further experiences with the Shirodkar operation. J. Obstet. Gynec., 85: 792, 1963.

Beischer, N. A.: Hydatidiform mole with coexistent fetus. J. Obstet. Gynaec. Brit. Comm., 68: 231, 1961.

Bergman, P.: Bilateral multiple lutein cysts of the ovary complicating normal pregnancy. Obstet. Gynec., 21: 28, 1963.

Bobrow, M. L., and Friedman, S.: Hydatidiform mole in 12-year-old girl. Amer. J. Obstet. Gynec., 73: 448, 1957.

Bonnar, J., and Tennent, R. A.: Benign hydatidiform mole followed by later pulmonary choriocarcinoma. J. Obstet. Gynaec. Brit. Comm., 69: 999, 1962.

Borglin, N. E.: Missed abortion; analysis of 10-year series. Acta Obstet. Gynec. Scand., 36: 512, 1957.

Braungardt, C. D., Kaufman, R. H., and Franklin, R. R.: The outpatient management of incomplete abortion. Amer. J. Obstet. Gynec., 80: 151, 1963.

Brewer, J. I., Gerbie, A. B., Skom, I. H., Nagle, R. G., and Torok, E. E.: Chemotherapy in trophoblastic disease. Amer. J. Obstet. Gynec., 90: 566, 1964.

Brewer, J. I., Rhinehart, J. J., and Dunban, R. W.: Choriocarcinoma: report of five or more years survival from Albert Mathieu Chorionepithelioma Registry. Amer. J. Obstet. Gynec., 81: 574, 1961.

Brewer, J. I., Smith, R. T., and Pratt, G. B.: Choriocarcinoma. Amer. J. Obstet. Gynec., 85: 841, 1963.

Browne, F. J.: A case of chorionepithelioma of the uterus with pulmonary metastases cured by operation and x-rays. J. Obstet. Gynaec. Brit. Comm., 64: 852, 1957.

Buckell, E. W. C., and Owen, T. K.: Chorionepithelioma in mother and infant. J. Obstet. Gynaec. Brit. Comm., 61: 329, 1954.

Canlas, B. D.: Benign lesions of aberrant trophoblast in the lung. Obstet. Gynec., 20: 602, 1962.

Coppleson, M.: Hydatidiform mole and its complications. J. Obstet. Gynaec. Brit. Comm., 65: 238, 1958.

Corscaden, J. A., and Shettles, L. B.: Hydatidiform mole and choriocarcinoma. Bull. Sloane Hosp. Women, *5:* 41, 1959.

Cosgrove, R. A.: Missed abortion. Clin. Obstet. Gynec., *2:* 81, 1959.

Crisp, W. E.: Choriocarcinoma of the fallopian tube coincident with visible pregnancy. Amer. J. Obstet. Gynec., *71:* 442, 1956.

Daamen, C. B. F., Bloem, G. W. D., and Westerbeek, A. J.: Chorionepithelioma in mother and child. J. Obstet. Gynaec. Brit. Comm., *68:* 144, 1961.

Danforth, D. N.: Cervical incompetency as a cause of spontaneous abortion. Clin. Obstet. Gynec., *2:* 45, 1959.

Deane, R. M., and Russell, K. P.: Enterobacillary septicemia and bacterial shock in septic abortion. Amer. J. Obstet. Gynec., *79:* 528, 1960.

Delfs, E.: Quantitative chorionic gonadotrophin. Obstet. Gynec., *9:* 1, 1957.

D'Esposo, D. A.: Diagnosis and treatment of inevitable and incomplete abortions. Clin. Obstet. Gynec., *2:* 74, 1959.

Douglas, G. W.: Diagnosis and management of hydatidiform mole. Surg. Clin. N. Amer., *37:* 379, 1957.

Douglas, G. W.: Malignant change in trophoblastic tumors. Amer. J. Obstet. Gynec., *84:* 884, 1962.

Douglas, G. W., Thomas, L., Carr, M., Cullen, N. M., and Morris, R.: Trophoblast in the circulating blood during pregnancy. Amer. J. Obstet. Gynec., *78:* 960, 1959.

Driscoll, S. G.: Choriocarcinoma: An "incidental finding" within a term placenta. Obstet. Gynec., *21:* 96, 1962.

Editorial: Quantitative chorionic gonadotrophin. Maryland State J. Med., *11:* 611, 1962.

Freedman, H. L., Magagnini, A., and Glass, M.: Pregnancies following chemically treated choriocarcinoma. Amer. J. Obstet. Gynec., *83:* 1637, 1962.

Girouard, D. P., Barclay, D. L., and Collins, C. G.: Hyperreactio luteinalis. Obstet. Gynec., *23:* 513, 1964.

Green-Armytage, V. B.: Habitual abortion. Gynec. Prat., *9:* 7, 1958.

Greenhill, J. P. (Editor): *Yearbook of Obstetrics and Gynecology, 1957–1958.* p. 38. Year Book Publishers, Inc., Chicago, 1958.

Gutglass, M. F., and Adali, I.: Interstitial pregnancy. Amer. J. Obstet. Gynaec., *20:* 696, 1963.

Guttmacher, A. F.: Therapeutic abortion in a large general hospital. Surg. Clin. N. Amer., *37:* 459, 1957.

Haines, M.: Hydatidiform mole and vaginal nodules. J. Obstet. Gynaec. Brit. Comm., *62:* 6, 1955.

Haskell, J. G.: Diagnosis and treatment of threatening and habitual abortion. Clin. Obstet. Gynec., *2:* 64, 1959.

Hertig, A. T.: The placenta: some new knowledge about an old organ. Obstet. Gynec., *20:* 859, 1962.

Hertig, A. T., and Mansell, H.: *Hydatidiform Mole and Choriocarcinoma.* U. S. Armed Forces Institute of Pathology, Washington, D. C., 1956.

Hertig, A. T., and Sheldon, W. H.: Hydatidiform mole—a pathologico-clinical correlation of 200 cases. Amer. J. Obstet. Gynec., *53:* 1, 1947.

Hertz, R., Bergenstal, D. M., Lipsett, M. B., Price, E. B., and Hilbish, T. E.: Chemotherapy of choriocarcinoma and related trophoblastic tumors in women J. A. M. A., *168:* 845, 1958.

Hertz, R., Ross, G. T., and Lipsett, M. B.: Primary chemotherapy of nonmetastatic trophoblastic disease in women. Amer. J. Obstet. Gynec., *86:* 808, 1963.

Hertz, R., Ross, G. T., and Lipsett, M. B.: Chemotherapy in women with trophoblastic disease: choriocarcinoma, chorioadenoma destruens, and complicated hydatidiform mole. Ann. N. Y. Acad. Sci., *114:* 881, 1964.

Hobson, B. M.: The excretion of chorionic gonadotrophin by women with chorioadenoma and choriocarcinoma. J. Obstet. Gynaec. Brit. Comm., *66:* 282, 1959.

Hreshchyshyn, M. M., Graham, J. B., and Holland, J. F.: Treatment of malignant trophoblastic growth in women with special reference to amethopterin. Amer. J. Obstet. Gynec., *81:* 688, 1961.

Hsu, C., Huang, L., and Chen, T.: Metastases in benign hydatidiform mole and chorioadenoma destruens. Amer. J. Obstet. Gynec., *84:* 1412, 1962.

Hsu, C. T., Lai, C. H., Changchien, C. L., and Changchien, B. C.: Repeat hydatidiform mole. Amer. J. Obstet. Gynec., *87:* 543, 1963.

Hunter, J. S., Jr., and Dockerty, M. B.: Choriocarcinoma. Obstet. Gynec., *5:* 598, 1955.

Iffy, L., and Kenner, P.: The aetiology of early abortion. J. Obstet. Gynaec. Brit. Comm., *69:* 598, 1962.

Jackson, R. L.: Pure malignancy of the trophoblast following primary abdominal pregnancy. Amer. J. Obstet. Gynec., *79:* 1085, 1960.

Jacobson, F. J., and Enzer, N.: Hydatidiform mole with "benign" metastasis to lung. Amer. J. Obstet. Gynec., *7:* 868, 1959.

Javert, C. T.: Further follow-up on habitual abortion patients. Amer. J. Obstet. Gynec., *84:* 1149, 1962.

Jones, H. W., and Jones, G. E. S.: Double uterus as etiological factor in repeated abortion. Amer. J. Obstet. Gynec., *65:* 325, 1953.

Kadner, M. L., and Anderson, G. V.: Septic

abortion with hemoglobinuria and renal insufficiency with special reference to clostridium welchii infection. Obstet. Gynec., *21:* 86, 1962.

Kamm, M. L., and Beernink, H. E.: Uterine anomalies in habitual abortion and premature labor. Obstet. Gynec., *20:* 713, 1962.

Karen, Z., Zuckerman, H., and Brzezinski, A.: Pregnancy and delivery after forty. Obstet. Gynec., *21:* 165, 1963.

Kika, K., and Matruda, I.: Primary tubal hydatidiform mole. Obstet. Gynec., *9:* 224, 1957.

Kinch, R. A. H.: Management of prolonged retention of the dead fetus in utero. Canad. M. A. J., *85:* 932, 1961.

Kohl, G. C.: Hydatidiform mole and 4½-month fetus. Amer. J. Obstet. Gynec., *79:* 1091, 1960.

Lamb, E. J., Morton, D. G., and Byron, R. C.: Methotrexate therapy of choriocarcinoma and allied tumors. Amer. J. Obstet. Gynec., *90:* 317, 1964.

Lash, A. F.: Operations for habitual abortion. Clin. Obstet. Gynec., *2:* 1083, 1959.

Lash, A. F.: The incompetent internal os of the cervix; diagnosis and treatment. Amer. J. Obstet. Gynec., *79:* 552, 1960.

Logan, B. J.: Occurrence of a hydatidiform mole in twin pregnancy. Amer. J. Obstet. Gynec., *73:* 911, 1957.

Logan, B. J., and Motyloff, L.: Hydatidiform mole. Amer. J. Obstet. Gynec., *75:* 1134, 1958.

Lynch, M. J. G., Kyle, P. R., and Raphael, S. S.: Unusual ovarian changes (hyperthecosis) in pregnancy. Amer. J. Obstet. Gynec., *77:* 335, 1959.

MacLeod, J.: Role of spermatozoa in etiology of spontaneous abortion. Clin. Obstet. Gynec., *2:* 57, 1959.

MacRae, D. J.: Chorionepithelioma occurring during pregnancy. J. Obstet. Gynaec. Brit. Comm., *58:* 373, 1951.

Mall, F. P., and Meyer, A. W.: Studies on abortions; survey of pathological ova in Carnegie Embryologic Collection. Contrib. Embryol., *12:* 56, 1921.

Manahan, C. P., Manuel-Limson, G., and Abad, R.: Experience with choriocarcinoma in the Philippines. Ann. N. Y. Acad. Sci., *114:* 875, 1964.

Marikar, A. B., and Chandravadana, R.: Widespread skin secondaries in a case of chorionepithelioma. J. Obstet. Gynaec. Brit. Comm., *66:* 119, 1959.

Marquez-Monten, H., de la Vega, G. A., Robles, M., and Bolio, C. A.: Epidemiology and pathology of hydatidiform mole in the general hospital of Mexico. Amer. J. Obstet. Gynec., *85:* 856, 1963.

Marrubinia, G.: Primary choionepithelioma of the ovary. Acta Obstet. Gynec. Scand., *38:* 251, 1949.

McDonald, I. A.: Suture of the cervix for inevitable abortion. J. Obstet. Gynaec. Brit. Comm., *64:* 346, 1957.

Mercer, R. D., Lammert, A. C., Anderson, R., and Hazard, J. B.: Choriocarcinoma in mother and infant. J. A. M. A., *166:* 482, 1958.

Moore, J. H.: Hydatidiform mole in 53-year-old patient. Amer. J. Obstet. Gynec., *69:* 205, 1955.

Mule, J. G., and McCall, M. L.: The infected abortion. Clin. Obstet. Gynec., *2:* 87, 1959.

Nesbitt, R. E. L.: *Perinatal Loss in Modern Obstetrics.* p. 29. F. A. Davis Company, Philadelphia, 1957.

Nesbitt, R. E. L., Jr.: The outcome of pregnancy complicated by threatened abortion. Clin. Obstet. Gynec., *2:* 97, 1959.

Neuwirth, R. S., and Friedman, E. A.: Septic abortion. Amer. J. Obstet. Gynec., *85:* 24, 1963.

Nilson, L.: Hydatid form degeneration in aborted ova; histoipathological and clinical study. Acta Obstet. Gynec. Scand., *36:* 7, 1957.

Novak, E.: Pathological aspects of hydatidiform mole and chorionepithelioma. Amer. J. Obstet. Gynec., *59:* 1355, 1950.

Novak, E., and Koff, A. H.: Chorionepithelioma, with special reference to disappearance of primary tumor. Amer. J. Obstet. Gynec., *20:* 481, 1930.

Novak, E. R., and Mattingly, R. F.: Concept and management of hydatidiform mole and choriocarcinoma, Maryland Med. J., 1, 1961.

Novak, E., and Seah, C. S.: Choriocarcinoma of uterus. Amer. J. Obstet. Gynec., *67:* 993, 1954.

Novak, E., and Seah, C. S.: Benign lesions in Chorionepithelioma Registry. Amer. J. Obstet. Gynec., *68:* 376, 1954.

Overstreet, E. W. (Editor): Therapeutic abortion and sterilization. Clin. Obstet. Gynec., *7:* 14, 1964.

Park, W. W.: The occurrence of sex chromatin in chorionepitheliomas and hydatidiform moles. Brit. J. Path. Bact., *74:* 197, 1957.

Park, W. W.: Experimental trophoblastic embolism in the lungs. J. Path. Bact., *25:* 257, 1958.

Patterson, W. B.: Normal pregnancy after recovery from metastatic mole. Amer. J. Obstet. Gynec., *72:* 183, 1956.

Perlson, S. G., and Whitsitt, R. E.: Adjuvant therapy of choriocarcinoma with Methotrexate. Obstet. Gynec., *15:* 175, 1960.

Posner, A. C., Kushner, J. I., and Posner, L. B.: Repeated hydatidiform mole. Obstet. Gynec., *5:* 7€1, 1955.

Quigley, J. K.: Hydatidiform mole and toxemia of pregnancy. Amer. J. Obstet. Gynec., *74:* 1059, 1957.

Robinson, E., Shulman, J., Ben-Hur, N., Zuckerman, H., and Neuman, Z.: Immunity in chorioepithelioma. Lancet, *1:* 300, 1963.

Rock, J., and Hertig, A. T.: The human conceptus during the first two weeks of gestation. Amer. J. Obstet. Gynec., *55:* 6, 1948.

Schiffer, M. A.: A review of 268 ectopic pregnancies. Amer. J. Obstet. Gynec., *86:* 264, 264, 1963.

Schmorl, G.: Pathologisch-anatomische untersuching uber puerperal eclampsie. Leip. 319, p. 19.

Shettles, L. B.: Chorionepithelioma following full-term pregnancy. Amer. J. Obstet. Gynec., *69:* 869, 1955.

Shettles, L. B.: Recurrent theca lutein cysts. Obstet. Gynec., *21:* 339, 1963.

Shettles, L. B.: Ovulation: normal and abnormal. In *The Ovary*, International Academy of Pathology Monograph No. 3, edited by H. G. Grady and D. E. Smith, p. 135. The Williams & Wilkins Company, Baltimore, 1963.

Shirodkar, V. N.: A new method of operative treatment for habitual abortions in the second trimester of pregnancy. Antiseptic, *52:* 299, 1955.

Smalbraak, J.: *Trophoblastic Growths*. Elsevier Publishing Company, Amsterdam, 1957.

Southam, A. L., Sultzen, B. M., and Cohen, H.: Evaluation of a rapid immunological test for pregnancy. Amer. J. Obstet. Gynec., *85:* 495, 1963.

Speert, H., and Guttmacher, A. F.: Frequency and significance of bleeding in early pregnancy. J. A. M. A. *155:* 712, 1954.

Spellacy, W. N., Meeker, H. C., and McKelvey, J. L.: Three successful pregnancies in a patient treated for choriocarcinoma with Methotrexate. Obstet. Gynec., *25:* 607, 1965.

Spraitz, A. F., Welch, J. S., and Wilson, R. B.: Missed abortion. Amer. J. Obstet. Gynec., *87:* 877, 1963.

Stanton, E. F.: Pregnancy after forty-four. Amer. J. Obstet. Gynec. *71:* 270, 1956.

Stearns, H. C.: Choriocarcinoma and allied tumors. J. Clin. Obstet. Gynec., *5:* 747, 1962.

Stevenson, C. S.: Septic abortion with or without septic shock. J. Michigan State Med. Soc., *63:* 37, 1964.

Tedeschi, L. G., and Toy, B. L.: Experimental transpulmonary migration of trophoblast. Obstet. Gynec., *21:* 55, 1962.

Tenney, B., Little, A. B., and Wamsteker, E.: Septic abortion. New Engl. J. Med., *257:* 1022, 1957.

Thiele, R. A., and de Alvarez, R. R.: Metastasizing benign trophoblastic tumors. Amer. J. Obstet. Gynec., *84:* 1395, 1962.

Tietze, C.: In *Pregnancy Wastage*, edited by E. T. Engle (introduction). Charles C Thomas, Springfield, Ill., 1953.

Tow, S. H.: University of Singapore (Personal communication).

Wall, L. A.: Abortions; ten years' experience. Amer. J. Obstet. Gynec., *79:* 510, 1960.

Warburton, D., and Fraser, F. C.: Genetic aspects of abortion. Clin. Obstet. Gynec., *2:* 22, 1959.

White, T. G. E.: Chorionepithelioma of uterus in a postmenopausal woman. J. Obstet. Gynaec. Brit. Comm., *62:* 372, 1955.

Wilkins, L., Jones, H. W., Holman, G. H., and Stempfel, R. S.: Masculinization of female fetus associated with administration of oral and intramuscular progestins during gestation; nonadrenal female pseudohermaphroditism. J. Clin. Endocr., *18:* 559, 1958.

Wilson, R. B., Hunter, J. S., and Dockerty, M. B.: Chorioadenoma destruens. Amer. J. Obstet. Gynec., *81:* 546, 1961.

Wynn, R. M., and Davies, J.: Ultrastructure of transplanted choriocarcinoma and its endocrine implications. Amer. J. Obstet. Gynec., *88:* 618, 1964.

Zondek, B.: Importance of increased production and excretion of gonadotropic hormone for diagnosis of hydatidiform mole. J. Obstet. Gynaec. Brit. Comm., *49:* 397, 1942.

29

LEUKORRHEA

Leukorrhea is the term applied to any vaginal discharge other than blood. It is perhaps the most frequently encountered of gynecological symptoms, occurring in at least one-third of all gynecological patients. Certainly it has a greater nuisance value in its frequent recalcitrance to therapy. Rarely, however, is it of serious cause, and generally it is associated with simple infections of the cervix, vagina, or tube. Indeed the only justification for devoting a chapter to it is for the convenience of the medical student who is often asked the various causes of leukorrhea.

Leukorrhea, it need hardly be said, is a symptom and not a disease. Under normal conditions all parts of the genital mucous membrane are kept moistened, either by secretions of their own or by those having their source in a higher segment of the canal. Normally there is no escape of secretions to the outside, although there are comparatively few women who do not at some time or other in their lives have at least a slight external discharge. The discharge may consist of a mere excess of otherwise normal secretion, or it may consist partly or dominantly of abnormal exudates from pathological lesions at one point or another in the genital canal.

SOURCE AND CHARACTER OF GENITAL DISCHARGES

Vulva. Strictly speaking vulvar secretions do not come into the present discussion, as the vulva is an external structure. At times, however, vulvar secretions contribute to the leukorrhea complained of by the patient, who herself cannot know the source of the discharge.

In addition to the numerous sebaceous and sudoriferous glands found in the vulva, the vulvovaginal gland is to all intents and purposes a part of the vulva, and this gland plays the most important role in the lubrication of the vaginal introitus and the vulvar mucous membrane. It secretes a thick viscid mucus, which is greatly increased during sexual excitement. Finally, in the periurethral region of the vestibule are situated Skene's ducts and a considerable number of mucous crypts which likewise contribute to the lubrication of the vulvar structures. In infections of Bartholin's gland, there is often a profuse purulent discharge either from the duct or from a ruptured abscess. Such discharges are apt to be interpreted by the patient as of vaginal nature. The same statement may be made concerning discharges from the periurethral structures above mentioned, and may be extended even to the purulent exudate of actual acute urethritis.

Vagina. While the vagina is itself devoid of glands, its surface is normally kept moist by the secretion of the cervical glands, and to a much less extent by transudation from its own surface. Normally the secretion found in the vagina is acid in reaction, with a pH averaging 5%. This acidity is due to the acid-forming propensities of certain organisms normally found in the vagina, the chief being the large rod-shaped organism known as the bacillus of Döderlein.

The acid reaction is dependent upon the presence of the lactic acid produced by the action of these organisms upon the glycogen content of the vaginal epithelium. The latter undergoes constant desquamation, so that discharges of vaginal origin are characterized by the presence of many epithelial cells, giving the discharge a milky or curdy appearance. During pregnancy, vaginal desquamation is intensified, and a milky or curdy exudate is complained of by many women during the latter part of gestation. On the other hand, when actual inflammation and infection of the vagina occurs, as in trichomonas or monilial vaginitis, an exudate develops which is usually mucopurulent or purulent in character, extremely profuse, and associated with marked pruritus. There may be little or no odor to the discharge, or it may be very offensive.

Lang, Fritz, and Menduke have emphasized the frequency of associated trichomonal and candidal forms of vaginitis; even though only one type is apparent on wet smear, the other organism may be present on culture. There would appear relatively little difference in the bacteriological findings in pregnant and nonpregnant women although it is also stated that the gravid female is particularly prone to harbor these fungus type of infections.

Flagyl (metronidazole) is the new wonder drug for Trichomonas, but it is quite specific for this organism. The usual treatment is 250 mg. three times a day for 10 days for one or both sexual partners with vaginal therapy for the female on occasion. Concomitant antifungal therapy as with Mycostatin seems appropriate for a mixed infection. British authors who have a much more extended experience indicate that pregnancy is in no way complicated by use of this medication, the availability of which in this country was, until recently, markedly curtailed by the thalidomide tragedies. A recent double-blind study by Forster, Raminez, and Rapaport leaves little doubt as to the efficacy of the drug and the infrequency of complications.

Cervix. The mucous glands of the cervix are the chief source of the secretion normally found in the vagina, and it is not strange, therefore, that they are the chief source of leukorrheal discharge. The normal secretion is a clear, viscid, alkaline mucus, which varies in its amount and viscidity at different phases of the menstrual cycle. Recent investigations have shown, for example, that its permeability to the spermatozoa is greatest at about the time of ovulation. The secretion may be merely increased in amount without alteration in character, as a result of hyperactivity of the glands produced by hyperemic or endocrine factors.

The histological structure of the cervix, with its numerous gland invaginations, makes it peculiarly prone to persistent infections, characterized by increase and pathological alterations of the secretion. Invariably minor childbirth lacerations become secondarily infected, with resultant mucoid hypersecretion. Neoplasms of the cervix characteristically produce a discharge, and this is usually offensive and bloody.

Uterine Body. While the endometrium contains innumerable glands, these are inactive until the postovulatory phases of the cycle, and even then the secretion seems to be designed chiefly for local nutritional purposes in the event of pregnancy. At any rate it seems to add little to the secretory content of the lower genital canal. Aside from this, however, a certain amount of serous transudation undoubtedly occurs, and this may at times be increased in amount as a result of vascular or endocrine factors.

Even actual endometritis is commonly believed to be of little importance as a cause of leukorrhea. An exception to this is the occasional case of acute septic endometritis, in which a profuse purulent discharge may be given off from the uterine cavity. In cases associated with retention of placental tissue, this may be extremely odorous as a result of saprophytic invasion of the uterus. While not so easy to demonstrate, the histological appearance of chronic endometritis, sometimes showing considerable amounts of exudate in the gland lumina, makes it difficult to believe that this may not contribute to the vaginal discharge so often seen in such cases, and no doubt due chiefly to the associated cervical infection.

Finally, uterine polyps, submucous myomas, carcinomas, and other tumors are not infrequently the cause of uterine discharges, particularly when complicated by infection and necrotic changes.

Tubes. While certainly rare, leukorrhea of tubal origin may occur, the usually cited example being that of the so-called profluent salpingitis, in which a hydrosalpinx may periodically expel its content through a partially patent inner orifice into the uterus and thus cause gushes of watery fluid from the vagina. In most cases of hydrosalpinx, however, the uterine end of the tubal lumen is completely closed, so that the above mentioned mechanism must be extremely uncommon.

CAUSES

The chief causes of leukorrhea may be briefly summarized as follows.

Constitutional. These include such conditions as anemia, tuberculosis, chronic nephritis, and other diseases associated with general debility. In the same category may be included conditions which bring about circulatory disturbance, such as the chronic passive congestion of heart disease and cirrhosis of the liver.

Endocrine Disorders. Certain types of endocrine disorders may bring about leukorrhea, which is usually slight in amount and due to hypersecretion of the cervical glands. A good example of this is the moderate mucoid discharge not infrequently observed in patients suffering with functional uterine bleeding. In these the hypersecretion is due to the

excessive estrogen effect upon the cervical glands. An even simpler example is the premenstrual mucoid discharge seen in many normal women. The frequent leukorrhea of pregnancy is due partly to endocrine factors and partly to the hyperemia associated with gestation.

Inflammations of Any Part of the Genital Canal. These include (1) vulvitis or vulvovaginitis, (2) vaginitis, (3) cervicitis, (4) endometritis, and (5) salpingitis.

(*1*) *Vulvitis or Vulvovaginitis.* Numerous organisms may be concerned in the etiology of vulvitis, such as the *Micrococcus catarrhalis*, Streptococcus, Staphylococcus, *Hemophilus vaginalis*, tubercle bacillus, or the colon bacillus. Protozoal infections, especially with the trichomonas vagina, may occur, but these are far less important on the vulva than in the vagina. Fungus infection with the yeast organisms, especially the thrush fungus or the monilia, may likewise be encountered, and in children one may occasionally see inflammations produced by parasitic worms, especially the pinworm, or *Oxyuris vermicularis*. Gonococcal infection is relatively uncommon in this era.

(*2*) *Vaginitis.* The adult vagina is far more resistant to gonorrheal infection than that of the immature child, but inflammatory disease is not uncommonly produced by such organisms as the bacillus of Döderlein, the *Micrococcus catarrhalis*, Streptococcus, and the colon bacillus. The same organisms may be concerned in the vulvovaginitis of children, but the chief clinical type in this group was formerly produced by Gonococcus.

At the opposite end of the age scale may be put the fairly numerous cases of senile vaginitis and endometritis. As a result of the frequent cessation of ovarian function at the menopause, the lining of both the vagina and uterus becomes thin, atrophic, and prone to secondary infection. Not infrequently tiny areas of ulceration are produced, so that not only leukorrhea but also slight vaginal bleeding may be noted. Estrogen (stilbesterol) suppositories or creams are usually curative, and rarely lead to bleeding where the uterus is present.

(3) *Cervicitis*. This extremely common cause of leukorrhea is etiologically divisible into two groups, the gonorrheal and pyogenic. The latter, in which puerperal lacerations often play an important causative role, is the result of infection by various organisms, chiefly of Streptococcus and Staphylococcus groups (see Chapter 12 under "Cervicitis").

(4) *Endometritis*. Here again various organisms may be concerned, the gonococcus much less frequently than the pyogenic group, which so frequently, with saprophytes, are the secondary invaders in cases of retained pregnancy products and ulcerative or necrotic neoplasms.

(5) *Salpingitis*. In this rare source of leukorrhea, the causative organisms are almost always the Gonococcus, Streptococcus or Staphylococcus, or tubercle bacillus (see Chapter 20, "Chronic Pelvic Inflammatory Disease").

Other Local Pathological Conditions. These include a variety of conditions in almost any part of the genital canal. Among the most important are benign or malignant tumors, especially when infection and necrosis have occurred; uterine displacements; puerperal lacerations of the cervix; fistulas of one sort or another, especially frequent being the vesicovaginal and rectovaginal varieties; the retention of gestation products within the uterus; and the presence of foreign bodies such as neglected pessaries in the vagina or cervix, or bougies and other abortifacient implements in the uterus.

Diagnosis of Cause of Leukorrhea. The mere diagnosis of leukorrhea means nothing, being usually made by the patient herself. As already emphasized, leukorrhea is a symptom and not a disease, and the responsibility of the physician is to determine the cause if possible. This is simple in some cases, exceedingly difficult in others. The history of the case may be of great importance, as in the case of discharge developing after coitus with a partner in whom gonorrhea is known or suspected to exist. In all cases a complete appraisal of the patient's physical condition is indicated, with consideration of constitutional as well as local factors.

The routine of pelvic examination should be thorough, as outlined in Chapter 3, and this may readily reveal the source of the abnormal discharge, and often its probable nature. However, in a large proportion of cases, microscopic and bacteriological examinations are imperative. This is particularly true in the differentiation of cases in which a gonorrheal etiology is possible, and in the differentiation of vaginal leukorrhea, in which parasitic and fungus infections are so often concerned.

The character of the discharge is often suggestive, although never conclusive, of the source of the abnormal discharge. A thick, milky, or curdy discharge is suggestive of a vaginal source, a viscid mucopurulent one of a cervical source. The admixture of blood in leukorrheal discharges of women of middle life and beyond should always lead to the suspicion of malignancy, although similar discharges may be seen as a result of senile endometritis or ulcerative benign tumors. Such considerations, however, are merely of suggestive value, and cannot take the place of careful examination.

The examination of various special conditions characterized by leukorrhea, together with a discussion of examination techniques, is to be found in the appropriate chapters (on cervicitis and vaginitis).

TREATMENT

The treatment must obviously be based on removal of the cause, whatever this may be. Since the possible etiologic factors embrace such a large proportion of gynecological lesions, the reader is referred to the appropriate chapters for details of the treatment of the symptoms of leukorrhea. Similarly, most of the references will be so found with the individual chapters.

REFERENCES

Allen, E.: Diagnosis and treatment of leucorrhea. Med. Clin. N. Amer., *23:* 189, 1939.

Barringer, E. D.: Gonorrhea, syphilis and other infections of genital tract. In *Gynecology and Obstetrics*, edited by C. H. Davis, Vol. 2, Ch. 15, Section 2. W. F. Prior Company, Inc., Hagerstown, Maryland, 1940.

Barringer, E., Strauss, H., and Crowley, D. F.: Problem of clinical gonorrhea in the female. Amer. J. Obstet. Gynec., *25:* 538, 1933.

Bland, P. B., and Rakoff, A. E.: Clinical and therapeutic aspects of leucorrhea. J.A.M.A., *115:* 1013, 1940.

Brewer, J. I., Halpern, B., and Thomas, G.: *Hemophilus vaginalis* vaginitis. Amer. J. Obstet. Gynec., *74:* 834, 1957.

Forster, S. A., Raminez, O. G., and Rapaport, A. H.: Metronidazole and trichomonal vaginitis. Amer. J. Obstet. Gynec., *87:* 1013, 1963.

Gardner, H. L., Dampeer, T. K., and Dokes, C. D.: The prevalence of vaginitis. Amer. J. Obstet. Gynec., *73:* 1080, 1957.

Gray, M. S.: Trichomonas vaginalis in pregnancy: results of metronidazole therapy on mother and child. J. Obstet. Gynaec. Brit. Comm., *68:* 723, 1961.

Henricksen, E.: Pyometra associated with benign lesions of the cervix and corpus. Western J. Surg., *60:* 305, 1952.

Henricksen, E.: Pyometra associated with malignant lesions of the cervix and uterus. Amer. J. Obstet. Gynec., *72:* 884, 1956.

Hesseltine, H. C.: Vulval and vaginal mycosis and trichomoniasis. Amer. J. Obstet. Gynec., *40:* 641, 1940.

Holden, F. C.: Lesions of the cervix. In *Obstetrics and Gynecology*, edited by A. H. Curtis, Vol. 3, Ch. 85. W. B. Saunders Company, Philadelphia, 1933.

Hyams, M. N.: Chronic cervicitis. In *Progress in Gynecology*, Ed. 2, edited by J. V. Meigs and S. H. Sturgis, p. 410. Grune & Stratton, Inc., New York, 1950.

Johnson, D. G.: Infections of the cervix. Clin. Obstet. Gynec., *2:* 476, 1959.

Kleegman, S.: Office treatment of pathologic cervix. Amer. J. Surg., *38:* 294, 1940.

Lang, W. R.: Genital infections in female children. Clin. Obstet. Gynec., *2:* 428, 1959.

Lang, W. R.: Premenarchal vaginitis. Obstet. Gynec., *13:* 723, 1959.

Lang, W. R., Fritz, M. A., and Menduke, H.: The bacteriological diagnosis of trichomonal, candidal and combined infections. Obstet. Gynec., *20:* 788, 1962.

Liston, W. G., and Cruickshank, L. G.: Etiology and pathogenesis of leucorrhea in pregnancy; study of 200 cases. J. Obstet. Gynaec. Brit. Comm., *47:* 109, 1940.

McCoogan, L. S.: The treatment of vaginitis. Clin. Obstet. Gynec., *2:* 450, 1959.

Miller, N. F.: Nonspecific infections. In *Obstetrics and Gynecology*, edited by A. H. Curtis, Vol. 2, Ch. 57. W. B. Saunders Company, Philadelphia, 1933.

Reich, W. J., Nechtow, M. J., Zaworsky, B., and Adams, A. P.: Investigation and management of the patient with vaginal discharge. Clin. Obstet. Gynec., *2:* 441, 1959.

Symposium on clinical background of Flagyl. Research, *56:* 26, 1964.

Watt, L., and Jennison, R. F.: Metronidazole treatment of trichomoniasis in the female. Brit. Med. J., *1:* 276, 1962.

Wynne, H. M. N.: The vagina. In *Practice of Surgery*, edited by D. Lewis, Vol. 10, Ch. 12. W. F. Prior Company, Inc., Hagerstown, Maryland, 1940.

30

INFERTILITY

GENERAL CONSIDERATIONS

Definitions. *Sterility* is a term which can be correctly applied only to an individual who has some absolute factor preventing procreation. *Infertility*, however, is the inability to achieve pregnancy within a stipulated period of time, usually stated as 1 year. This view is adequately based on statistics. For example, Whitelaw found that 56.5 % of fertile couples achieve pregnancy within 1 month and 78.9 % within the first 6 months. *Primary infertility* is the term used to designate those patients who have never conceived, whereas *secondary infertility* indicates that the patient has had a pregnancy. This may be further qualified as secondary to term pregnancy, miscarriage, etc.

Occurrence. In the United States 12 % of all marriages are estimated to be involuntarily barren. Thus the problem is one of some magnitude.

Medical Considerations. Medically, infertility is a rather unique condition in that one must consider two individuals. As the husband or wife, or both, may have factors contributing to the condition, both must cooperate in the investigation. Although the woman is usually the most interested and aggressive in her desire for medical help, it is not satisfactory to initiate an infertility investigation without the cooperation of the husband. It is psychologically de-sirable to begin the evaluation of the husband and wife at the same time as this emphasizes for the couple the dual responsibility which they share in the condition.

Evaluation of the Problem. It has been adequately demonstrated that in formulating a prognosis the age of the wife and the duration of the marriage are major factors which must be taken into consideration along with the medical findings. Fertility in woman declines after the age of 35 years. Guttmacher has shown that marriages of women between the ages of 16 and 20 years have only a 4.5 % infertility rate; the incidence has risen to 31.3 % for women married between the ages of 35 and 40 years, and after the age of 40 the infertility rate approaches 70 %. This is further substantiated by the relative infrequency of pregnancy after the age of 45 years. This so-called "aging factor" is, however, a difficult one to assess. A routine infertility investigation in older women may fail to reveal any abnormality. In a preliminary study of ovaries removed in the over 50-year-old woman we have found evidence of recent ovulation in 15 % despite almost uniform absence of pregnancy beyond the age of 48. Indeed we have found histological proof (corpus luteum) of ovulation in a few women past the age of 55.

It may therefore be assumed that the

571

infertility is caused by a defect in the ovum itself, making it unfertilizable. The increased incidence of congenital anomalies and miscarriages in pregnancy among older women might seem to substantiate this theory. The duration of the infertility, which has long been recognized as a reliable yardstick for prognosis, obviously serves as an indication of the seriousness of the condition.

According to statistics from various clinics, 20 to 50% of patients investigated for infertility can be helped. It is estimated that with our present investigative techniques between 10 and 30% of the patients will be found to have no discernible etiological factors responsible for the infertility.

There is no evidence for fertility differentials of racial origin. Guttmacher estimates the average number of children per couple married before the age of 20 years, without the use of contraception, to be approximately 9.5, and this figure is the same for five different nationality groups.

INVESTIGATION

Although it was once thought unjustifiable to initiate an infertility investigation short of 3 years of barren marriage, it now appears that no couple who seeks medical aid for infertility should be turned away without some consideration of their problem, be it real or fancied. This is scientifically justifiable on the basis of the statistics just cited and psychologically desirable, as often the fears of the overanxious couple can be allayed by a few explanations and suggestions from a sympathetic and well informed physician. Such a discussion may, perhaps, prevent the development of major psychological problems which aggravate or cause infertility.

The Initial Interview. The investigation of the infertile couple begins with a careful history and physical examination which will exclude major medical or gynecological conditions. A proper history must include the age of the patient and her husband, the duration of the marriage, previous marital histories of both parties, and other efforts to obtain medical aid, as well as a medical and social history. Physical examination includes a vaginal smear with maturation index and an examination of the cervical mucus in addition to the usual general examinations of urine for sugar and protein, a hematocrit, and white count. It is generally impossible to make an etiological diagnosis at the first visit. However, it is well to make a tentative diagnosis if there are suggestive factors in the history or physical examination, as these observations are valuable signposts in focusing our attention on important details during the subsequent examinations and tests.

At the first visit it is wise to discuss with the patient and her husband, if possible, the need for a complete investigation, as well as the time and expense involved, the statistical probabilities of help, and the value of the investigation from a prognostic point of view. The couple should be advised that if treatment seems indicated, it is usually necessary to allow at least 1 year before evaluation of therapy is possible. At this time it is well to set up a subsequent appointment with both the husband and wife to discuss the investigational findings and recommendations.

Fundamental Tests. Pertinent investigations must include tests of the five major factors concerned with fertilization and implantation of an ovum: (1) the occurrence of ovulation, (2) the production of normal sperm, (3) the presence of adequate cervical mucus which can act as a transport medium for sperm and as a sperm repository, (4) the patency of tubes for transport of sperm up and ovum down, and (5) the development of the endometrial implantation site which depends upon both ovarian endocrine function and end organ response.

If no abnormalities are found in the above studies, certain ancillary factors must be checked. A protein-bound iodine, a basal metabolic rate, a glucose tolerance

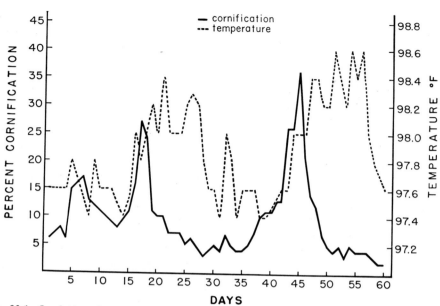

Fig. 30.1. Ovulation determined by cornification pattern of urinary sediment smears. The vaginal smear pattern parallels that of the urinary cells. Ovulation can be seen to coincide with the cornification peak. (From Vincze, L. O., Taft, P. D., and McArthur, J. W.: J. Clin. Endocr., 19: 281, 1959.)

test, and a 17-ketosteroid assay will detect metabolic disease processes which are associated with infertility problems. However, it is our experience that when there is no evidence of ovarian insufficiency, these diseases are usually not the cause of the infertility. A psychiatric evaluation or a psychological test may be advisable. The blood grouping of husband and wife may also have some significance, as there is statistical evidence to indicate that blood incompatibilities may occasionally be the cause of infertility.

If, at the end of the complete examination, no cause is found for the infertility, and after 1 year no pregnancy has occurred, a culdoscopic examination should be performed. This may reveal unsuspected endometriosis or peritubal or periovarian adhesions. If no cause for infertility is found, no treatment should be given. It is likewise inadvisable to repeat tests after one has satisfactorily established a diagnosis, as such unnecessary procedures or therapy can prove harmful, interfering with the process of fertility rather than improving it. The

one possible exception to this rule for patients with no discernible infertility factors is the use of synthetic progestational compounds. As suggested by Garcia, Pincus, and Rock, progestational drugs may be used in an effort to put the ovary at rest, with the hope that at the end of the treatment period a rebound phenomenon will occur allowing for improved ovarian function and pregnancy.

OVULATION

Of the many methods advocated for the detection of ovulation, four are currently outstanding as clinically proved and applicable: (1) the cornification of the daily vaginal smear pattern or urinary sediment followed by a progestational smear (Fig. 30.1); (2) increased amount and fluidity of the cervical mucus followed by a decreased amount of mucus and absence of the fern formation (Fig. 30.2); (3) the biphasic basal body temperature graph (Fig. 30.3); (4) secretory changes observed in the endometrium (Figs. 30.4 and 30.5).

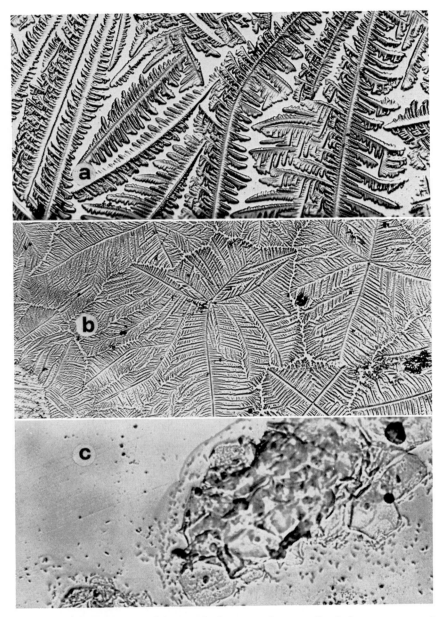

Fig. 30.2. Ovulation determined by cervical mucus changes. Ovulation occurs at the time when fern formation is strongly positive (*a* and *b*); when progesterone is present the mucus shows a negative reaction or only a slightly positive reaction (*c*).

Of these the first two are most useful in predicting the probable occurrence of ovulation, as the changes take place within the 24-hour period preceding ovulation. However, such findings can be associated with follicular maturation without ovulation and therefore must be interpreted absolutely in the light of knowledge of the entire cycle. The latter two tests are not useful in predic-

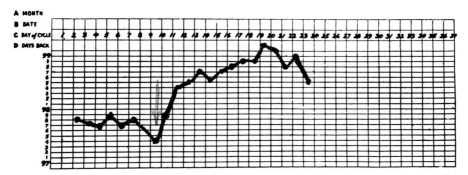

FIG. 30.3. Typical ovulatory basal temperature record in a 24-day cycle. Ovulation probably occurs at the low point prior to the continuous rise. In this case it would be on Day 10.

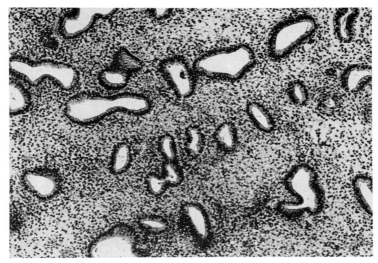

FIG. 30.4. Proliferative type of endometrium with no suggestion of secretory activity and indicating nonoccurrence of ovulation.

tion of ovulation but are perhaps more reliable in the retrospective evaluation of the cycle, as they are a function of progesterone and therefore imply ovulation by determination of an active corpus luteum.

As far back as 1904 van de Velde reported that the normal basal body temperature throughout the menstrual cycle is biphasic. The temperature is taken orally as soon as the patient awakens each morning, and before she moves about, eats, drinks, or smokes. This low point occurs at or about the time of ovulation, although there is still some uncertainty as to the precise chronological relationships involved.

Other clinical tests are currently available but as yet are either unsatisfactorily tested or perfected. The presence of glucose in the cervical secretions as measured by glucose oxidase was reported almost simultaneously by Birnberg *et al.* and by Doyle and has been further assayed by Cohen; the detection of urinary gonadotrophins by the Farris test depends upon the evaluation of an ovarian hyperemia reaction in the mouse ovary and, although readily reproducible by the originator, is either too subjec-

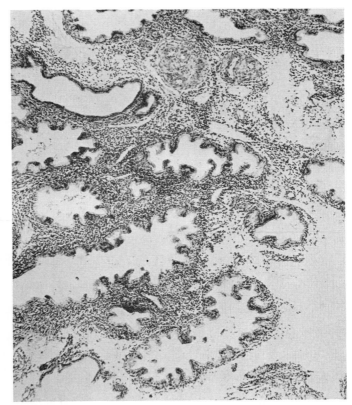

FIG. 30.5. Normal progestational endometrium removed by suction curette on the 27th day of cycle.

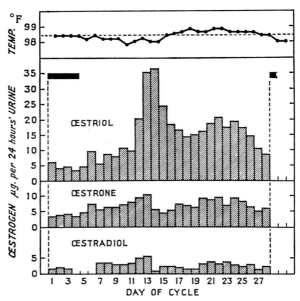

FIG. 30.6. Urinary estrogen excretion during a normal 28-day cycle correlated with the basal temperature record. The estrogen peak occurs just prior to ovulation. (From Brown, J. B.: Lancet, *1:* 320, 1955.)

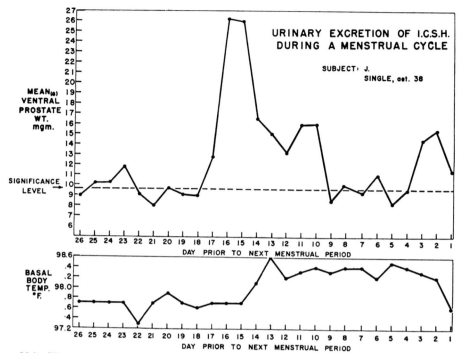

FIG. 30.7. Illustrating the pituitary gonadotrophin peak which occurs just prior to ovulation. Interstitial cell-stimulating hormone (*I.C.S.H.*) assay by the McArthur technique. (From Ingersoll, F. M., and McArthur, J. W.: Amer. J. Obstet. Gynec., *77*: 795, 1959.)

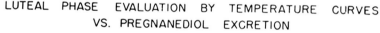

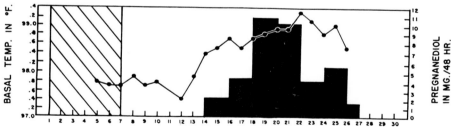

FIG. 30.8. The basal body temperature charted with the urinary pregnanediol excretion (Astwood gravimetric method). The pregnanediol is plotted in *black blocks*, indicating the amount in milligrams per 48-hour periods. The base line represents the days of the menstrual cycle, counting Day 1 as the first day of menstruation. Pregnanediol excretion begins at the 14th day.

tive or too dependent upon specific animal strains to be practical.

Methods which depend upon complicated hormone analyses are too expensive and too time-consuming to be clinically applicable; these are the detection of urinary estrogenic peaks which occur about 24 hours before ovulation (Fig. 30.6); measurement of total urinary gonadotrophins which exhibit a peak just prior to ovulation (Fig. 30.7); and urinary pregnanediol excretion (Fig. 30.8), which is a retrospective test for ovulation in that it measures progesterone production by the corpus luteum.

For a summary of recent attempts at

timing ovulation, the reader is referred to a review by Speck.

Ovulation Defects. The etiology of ovulation defects has been discussed in detail in Chapter 31, "Amenorrhea," and will be simply itemized here. Generalized major factors are: (1) nutrition; (2) metabolic disease, *e.g.*, pituitary insufficiency, hyper- or hypothyroidism, diabetes, the adrenogenital syndrome and related diseases, and Cushing's disease; (3) chronic illness; (4) psychogenic disturbance; (5) neurogenic disturbances; and (6) specific ovarian factors. These latter comprise ovarian tumors, polycystic ovaries of Stein, and congenitally defective ovaries, such as those in Turner's syndrome which lead to ovarian failure.

The treatment of anovulation depends upon the etiology, and any specific factor found must be specifically treated as indicated, by diet, thyroid, or adrenal hormone. Pituitary insufficiencies or neurogenic disturbances leading to inadequate pituitary excitation and secondarily to inadequate ovarian stimulation should theoretically be best treated by substitution therapy with pituitary hormones. Gemzell and others have demonstrated that this therapy is satisfactory. The use of cyclic steroid hormones, estrogens followed by progestogens, in an effort to stimulate pituitary function, although less expensive and less complicated, is usually unsuccessful. Clomiphene is also useful in patients with an intact pituitary gland. These therapeutic agents will be discussed in detail under the treatment of amenorrhea. Ovarian tumors must be surgically removed; the Stein-Leventhal ovary must be wedge-resected or treated with clomiphene. Unfortunately there is no treatment for ovarian failure at this writing, since attempted application of the newer grafting techniques has been unsatisfactory.

SPERM

Evaluation. As least two semen analyses should be performed for proper evaluation of the male factor. If these do not show a satisfactory agreement, samples should be taken until a reasonable assessment of fertility capacity has been reached. Samples should not be collected after a specific abstinence period but in accord with the usual intercourse habits of the couple. A clean, wide-mouthed container should be used for collecting the specimen, which may be procured either by induced ejaculation or by intercourse with withdrawal. A total ejaculate must be obtained, as any loss may seriously influence the sperm count. The sample should be collected and brought to the laboratory within 1 hour, if possible, marked with the hour of collection and the date of the previous intercourse. Liquefaction of seminal fluid may be expected to occur at room temperature within 20 minutes. Failure of liquefaction indicates a lack of proteolytic enzyme and makes the evaluation of the sample difficult. The quality of the semen is judged by the motility of the sperm, the numbers per milliliter, and the presence of abnormal forms. The total volume is also recorded and is of some importance as the normality of the sample frequently varies inversely, within limits, with the amount of the semen. Thus a large volume is often indicative that the sperm is of poor quality. The total sperm count is not of too great importance. The number of epithelial cells and leukocytes present is obviously significant.

Although absolute criteria of male fertility cannot be obtained with the present rather crude methods of evaluation, the following standards may be considered as representative of the usual fertile male. *Count per milliliter:* normally fertile, above 60,000,000 per ml.; subfertile, between 20,000,000 and 60,000,000 per ml.; sterile, less than 20,000,000 per ml. *Volume:* 2.5 ml. *Motility:* 60% (motility within 4 hours). *Differential:* less than 25% abnormal forms (Fig. 30.9).

The occurrence of an abnormal differential with an otherwise normal semen analysis is rare. The studies of Leuchten-

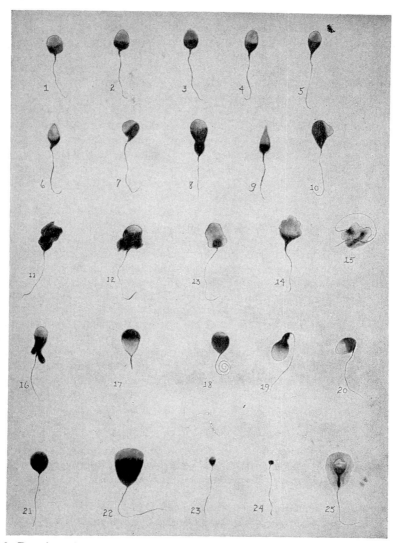

FIG. 30.9. Drawing of spermatozoa as seen under oil immersion, approximately, ×1200. *1–5*, normal variation; *6–10*, common abnormalities of the shape of the head; *11–15* and *25*, immature forms; *16–20*, abnormalities of the size of the head; normal semen contains a maximum of 20% of abnormal forms. (From Israel, S. L.: *Mazer and Israel's Diagnosis and Treatment of Menstrual Disorders and Sterility*, Ed. 4. Paul. B. Hoeber, Inc., New York, 1959.)

berger *et al.* have suggested the deoxy-ribonucleic acid (DNA) content of spermatozoa might be used as a fertility index. These authors' investigations indicate that the DNA value will detect deficiencies in otherwise apparently normal semen. From a theoretical point of view this would be attractive, as the DNA is a measure of chromosomal mate-rial and thus would be an accurate measure of genetic abnormalities. Studies by Knudsen in animal husbandry indicate that certain forms of nondysfunction of chromosomes which would give rise to increased or decreased DNA measurements, are incompatible with reproductive capacity.

The survival time of sperm in the

human female genital tract is still debatable but, at the proper time in the cycle, motile sperm can normally be seen in the cervical mucus 48 hours after intercourse and it is not unusual to find adequate numbers of motile sperm after 76 hours. It is also apparent in certain types of experimental animals that sperm require a 24-hour period in the female genital tract in order to acquire fertilizing ability. This property has been called *capacitation* and has been extensively studied in the rabbit by Chang. This interesting phenomenon is reviewed by Noyes.

Seminal Insufficiency. Seminal insufficiency can be attributed to constitutional factors such as nutritional problems, acute or chronic illness, general metabolic disease, specific poisonings or occupational hazards, central defects occurring in the pituitary or hypothalamic areas, specific diseases within the genital tract such as infections causing blockage to the vas and scarring of the tubular elements, or congenital defects of testicular development such as the Klinefelter syndrome. Diagnosis can be facilitated by a 17-ketosteroid determination, a urinary gonadotrophin assay, and a testicular biopsy. Testicular failure is indicated by a low 17-ketosteroid and a high urinary gonadotrophin excretion and confirmed by the microscopic appearance of the testicles.

For detailed and specific treatment the reader is referred to urological texts. For the treatment of many constitutional factors general hygiene is important: limitation of smoking and elimination of excessive alcohol, attention to diet and adequate rest, relief of emotional tension states, treatment of any chronic illness or metabolic disease. Specific hormone therapy has been occasionally successful; this involves the administration of testosterone, first described by Heckel, until the sperm count is reduced to zero, at which time the drug is withdrawn and the pituitary, which has been suppressed, is allowed to resume its function. This pituitary rebound phenomenon sometimes produces a much improved sperm count which may or may not be permanent. Unfortunately, there is no method for detecting which group of patients will respond to the testosterone rebound phenomenon and it is estimated that approximately only 20% of men showing low sperm counts, presumably due to inadequate pituitary stimulation, will show improvement on this form of therapy. Human pituitary gonadotrophin therapy has also been successful in restoring spermatogenesis and fertility (MacLeod).

For those men having blockage of the vas deferens, surgical therapy may help on occasion. For those having destruction of the testis or congenitally defective spermatogenic elements, no therapy is available, and adoption or donor insemination must be considered. In the unusual case in which hypospadias is present so that deposition of spermatozoa on the cervix is inadequate, or in which a neurological cord lesion occurs, semen may be obtained mechanically and artifical insemination attempted.

A more concentrated semen sample can be obtained by collection of a split ejaculate since the first portion of the ejaculate often contains the majority of sperm. In men whose counts are between 20,000,000 and 60,000,000 sperm per ml., this method of concentration, followed by cervical insemination, may on occasion be justifiable. Other means of mechanical concentration are centrifugation of the ejaculate and the use of a millipore filter, as described by Perloff.

Artificial Insemination. The procedure of artificial insemination or, as we prefer to call it, semiadoption, is still a highly controversial one. It is a medical problem which also involves moral issues. These issues must be resolved by each physician according to his own conscience. The entire subject of artificial insemination in the human is very adequately treated in the book by Schellen.

Any physician who takes it upon himself to perform this service should remember that he accepts a grave responsibility.

He is, in effect, placing an adopted child in a home and in so doing must be sure that this home is worthy and capable of contributing happiness and security to the child. It has been our practice to interview couples over a 3- to 6-month period before instituting therapy or to request a psychiatric interview in an effort to evaluate the stability of the individuals and their compatibility as a couple. A child, be it natural, adopted, or semiadopted, cannot be regarded as cementing material for a marriage. If there is dissension, the rearing of a baby offers one more matter for disagreement.

In addition to repeated interviews with the couple, there are several rules of thumb which should be followed. First, the husband must have been aware of his inadequacy for at least a year prior to the first serious consideration of the planning of insemination. Second, the physician must be convinced that the husband is taking the initiative and not being pushed by an overaggressive and overanxious wife. Third, there must be no religious background in either partner which would suggest that either might harbor moral scruples about the procedure. Fourth, every possible medical investigation and aid must have been employed to diagnose and treat the cause of the male infertility. Fifth, a basal temperature chart, Rubin's test, and endometrial biopsy must indicate normal fertility in the female.

In the first interview it is explained to the couple that they must count on at least 3 months, with the possibility of 6 months, of insemination prior to anticipating success. The figures given by Behrman *et al.* for the occurrence of conception in 50% of the women within 3 months and in 90% within 6 months are strikingly similar to those quoted for normal fertile couples by Tietze, Guttmacher, and Rubin, again confirming the rationale for instituting infertility investigations after 1 year of barren marriage if the couple so desires.

The problem of mixing semen is complicated by the occurrence of sperm agglutination in some specimens. It is therefore practical to request that intercourse be practiced prior to insemination; or, if the couple prefers, the husband's semen is concentrated and used intercervically while the donor's is used in a cervical cap. Intrauterine insemination should probably never be performed. In women with regular menstrual cycles, our figures indicate that a single insemination is as satisfactory as repeated inseminations and this observation is substantiated by Kleegman.

The selection of a donor is of course of utmost importance. He should be physically fit, emotionally stable, intelligent, and free of any history of congenital hereditary defects. In addition his semen analysis must be in the normally fertile range. Every effort should be made to match his blood group and type with that of the patient to be inseminated.

CERVICAL MUCUS

The examination of the cervical mucus with reference to the amount, quality, and presence or absence of infection should be made at the first office visit. The quality of mucus is judged by the viscosity and *spinbarkeit* (ability to spin a thread) as well as the number of epithelial cells and bacteria and the crystallization patterns. A good estrogenic mucus is watery and clear, has excellent *spinbarkeit* (5 cm. or longer) and few, if any cells. When the mucus is dry, fern patterns may be seen. These are characteristic of the mucus in the preovulatory and ovulatory phase. In the pre- and postmenstrual phase, when estrogen influence is either low or dominated by progesterone, the mucus is scanty, thick, cloudy, and contains numerous cellular elements, and the dried sample does not exhibit ferning. The changes in the mucus throughout the cycle have been described by LaMarr, Shettles, and Delfs (Fig. 30.10) and elaborated upon by Pommerenke and his associates.

A postcoital examination (the Sims-Huhner test) should be scheduled at approximately ovulation time. The patient is requested to have intercourse

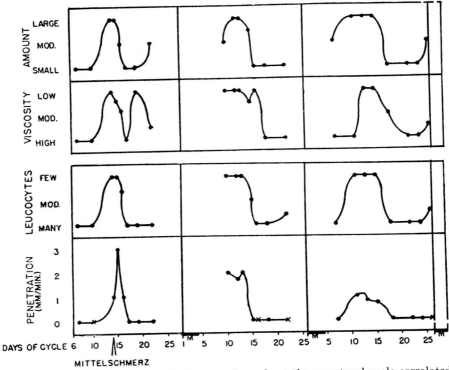

FIG. 30.10. Characteristics of cervical mucus throughout the menstrual cycle correlated with sperm penetrability. *Curves* are a composite from three cycles of a single individual. (From data reported by LaMarr, J. K., Shettles, L. B., and Delfs, E.: Amer. J. Physiol., *129:* 234, 1940.)

within 12 to 24 hours of her visit. It is often well not to make an issue of this as many husbands do not do well with command performances and the patient may be allowed to call for her appointment the day on which she is prepared. In order to make this test as uniform as possible, recordings should be standardized in certain broad aspects. The last menstrual period, the date of the previous intercourse, the hour of the last intercourse, and the hour of the examination must be recorded. The cervix should be wiped free of all vaginal contaminants and the mucus aspirated from the cervix by a pipette with a fine tip attached to a good suction ball. The removal of the mucus is further facilitated by clipping it off with a long clamp. The amount of mucus is estimated as poor, fair, or abundant. The quality and presence or absence of infection are recorded, and the number of actively progressive sperm per high power field as well as those wtih poor or no activity. A successful test is one in which there are 5 or more actively motile sperm per high power field.

A successful Sims-Huhner test implies (1) satisfactory intercourse techniques, (2) normal mucus for the transport and preservation of sperm, and (3) adequate ovarian estrogenic function, as well as (4) at least the possibility of a normal male fertility. This test, however, does not substitute for a semen analysis but merely complements it. An unsuccessful Sims-Huhner test may result from a variety of causes. Faulty intercourse techniques, oligo- or azoospermia, or poor timing of the test are among the more usual causes since sperm consistently survive and penetrate mucus only in the preovulatory and ovulatory mucus. An inadequate ovarian estrogenic function, cervical infection, or in rare instances, a specific vaginitis due to *Candida krusei* are other causes. There remains a small residue of cases of unexplained etiology. These are the patients who show no evidence of infection, no evidence of ovarian insufficiency, and whose husbands have a normal semen analysis.

The treatment of the so-called "hostile mucus" depends upon the etiology of the condition. Those patients showing an inadequate estrogenic mucus at the ovulatory time of the cycle can be treated by the daily administration of 0.1 mg. of stilbestrol, or its equivalent, or 0.5 mg. of stilbestrol suppositories every night. If suppositories are used they should be discontinued at the 12th day of a 28-day cycle or approximately 2 days prior to the ovulation date. In the majority of patients the dosage of 0.1 mg. of stilbestrol daily is too small to interfere with the menstrual rhythm, and therefore can be administered continuously. If cervical infection is present, this may not always be amenable to cauterization. Chemotherapy should be tried; a broad spectrum antibiotic four times a day for 10 days, as advocated by Horne and Rock, has proved successful in the majority of cases. However, as recurrences are frequent it is wise to give medication at the onset of the menstrual period in order to insure a normal mucus at the time of ovulation. If a vaginal infection of *C. krusei* exists, this can usually be eradicated by scrubbing the vagina with green soap and painting with a 2% aqueous solution of gentian violet every other day for three times. No treatment is known for the normal type of estrogenic-appearing mucus with no evidence of infection which, nevertheless, fails to support sperm activity. Fortunately these cases are extremely rare.

TUBAL FUNCTION

Tubal tests serve not only as diagnostic procedures but also as therapeutic ones in that they tend to overcome minor obstructions. There are three accepted methods for establishing the patency of fallopian tubes. The first is gas insufflation described by Rubin in 1920 and known by his name, Rubin's test. This procedure is the least likely to be associated with any complication and is, therefore, preferable as a first test unless the history or pelvic findings suggest an abnormality which indicates some pelvic pathology. In this case another form of tubal test may be preferable. The Rubin's test is best performed by using a mercury manometer, and tubal patency is estimated to exist if gas is heard to pass through the tubes at pressures below 180 mm. of mercury. Partial occlusion is probably present if pressures above 180 and below 200 are obtained, and tubes are completely obstructed for practical purposes if pressures of 200 or over are unsuccessful. By using a mechanical system, Rubin found that tubes requiring 200 mm. of mercury for passage of gas were too small to transport a particle the size of an ovum.

The second method of tubal evaluation is by means of a hysterosalpingogram. This examination is indicated when the Rubin's test is unsuccessful and especially when operative procedures are contemplated. Because of the high amount of radiation to the ovaries which this procedure entails, it should be limited to carefully selected cases. A water-soluble, opaque medium is preferable to an oil-soluble medium (Fig. 30.11) which carries a greater potential for serious complications such as oil emboli and granulomata. Protagonists of oil-soluble media believe that there is a greater therapeutic value in these media but the facts substantiating these claims are tenuous, and such nebulous evidence does not seem to warrant the additional risks.

The third method of assessing tubal function is by means of culdoscopy. The Decker culdoscopic procedure (Fig. 30.12), performed simultaneously with the insertion into the cervix of a No. 14 Foley catheter with a 5-cc. bulb (to be inflated to not over 2 ml.), allows the instillation of indigo carmine into the tubes and any blockage may be demonstrated under direct vision. This method is the treatment of choice if there is some

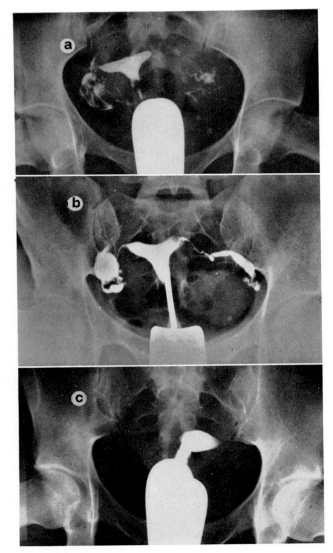

FIG. 30.11. *a*, normal hysterosalpingogram showing outline of delicate tube and spill into peritoneum on left. The right tube is obscured by massive peritoneal spill on the right. The sweeping, smeared appearance is characteristic when water-soluble media are used. *b*, obstruction at the fimbriated ends of tubes with bilateral hydrosalpinx. There is an arcuate uterus. *c*, bilateral tubal occlusion at the cornu. The uterine cavity has been distorted by overdistention with radiopaque medium.

question about the accuracy of the Rubin's test or a discrepancy between two tests. It is also useful when extratubal or periovarian adhesions are suspected. Because of the preponderance of tubal factors responsible for infertility in the female, a culdoscopic examination should be offered when the infertility investigation has failed to demonstrate any etiological factor and no pregnancy has resulted within 1 year after completion of the total investigation.

As a word of warning it must be remembered that neither a Rubin's test nor

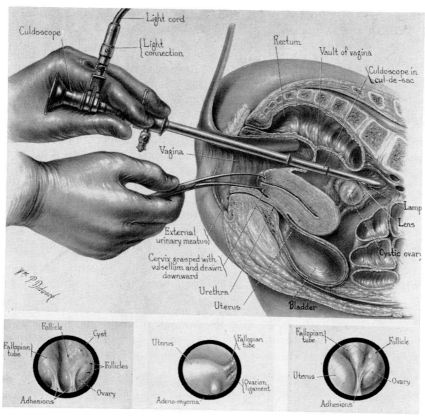

FIG. 30.12. Culdoscope in place. The culdoscope can be seen passing through the trochar sheath. The trochar is introduced into the cul-de-sac through the posterior vagina, which has been "tented" by pushing the cervix forward and downward. The trochar is then withdrawn and the culdoscope inserted. (From Decker, A.: *Culdoscopy*, W. B. Saunders Company, Philadelphia, 1952.)

hysterosalpingogram is infallible. Each can be technically unsatisfactory, giving false results of either a positive or a negative nature. Therefore three tests, preferably of different types, must be performed before a diagnosis of tubal occlusion can be made and certainly before considering a tubal plastic procedure. On the other hand, it is not justifiable to perform repeated tubal studies if a normal test has been obtained. As previously stated, if real doubt exists a culdoscopic examination should be made. No tubal procedures should be repeated before a 3-month interval, as any such intrauterine manipulation produces some tissue damage.

Tubal occlusion may be the result of adhesions from pelvic inflammatory dis-ease due to gonorrhea, tuberculosis, or postabortal or postpartum infections. Adhesions may be due to endometriosis or other more unusual causes of blood in the peritoneal cavity, such as an unrecognized ectopic pregnancy, a ruptured corpus luteum cyst, or a bleeding follicle at ovulation. Extrapelvic inflammatory processes such as an appendiceal abscess may also occasionally cause tubal adhesions with occlusions.

The treatment of tubal occlusion must usually be surgical in the final analysis. However, as indicated, at least three tubal patency tests should be performed in an effort to rupture adhesions. Pelvic diathermy may be used, and recently corticosteroids have been advocated for pelvic inflammatory disease, as noted in the review by Kurland and Loughran.

All of these medical procedures should be given an adequate trial prior to the discussion of surgery. A tubal plastic procedure in our opinion should be undertaken only as a last resort since the chances of success are slight.

The data on 2285 operations collected by Siegler and Hellman from questionnaires to 734 gynecologists showed an over-all livebirth rate of 16.5%. The breakdown according to the tubal location indicated that tubal lysis, as might be expected, is most successful—29% pregnancies in 930 operations. For operations upon the tubal fimbriae, there was a 20% pregnancy rate among 891 operations. The worst results were with tubal implantation for obstruction at the cornua. Here the pregnancy rate was but 16% and the livebirth rate was but 9% of 272 operations. A report from the Mayo Clinic, in 1964, on results in 75 tubal plastic procedures, interestingly enough gives almost the same over-all statistics, e.g., 16% livebirths and 24% pregnancies. However, the intertubal implantation procedure was the most successful in this series, resulting in 10 livebirths out of 22 implantations. For a complete discussion of techniques the reader is referred to a monograph by Shirodkar.

The patient should wait until the last opportunity at which the operative procedure may be performed with any reasonable expectation of success. The age of 30 years is our arbitrary standard. She should then be adequately informed concerning the poor prognosis of the operation. A thorough investigation for other factors which might be contributing to the infertility is mandatory.

THE ENDOMETRIUM

A study of the premenstrual endometrium gives information about the implantation site for the fertilized ovum and the ovarian luteal function as well as presumptive evidence concerning ovulation. This, therefore, is an extremely important test.

An endometrial biopsy can be obtained by a Novak curette (Fig. 30.13). The biopsy should be timed according to the basal temperature chart to be approximately 2 days prior to menstruation, as this time is the most satisfactory for accurate endometrial dating by criteria of Noyes, Hertig, and Rock.

If the presumptive diagnosis of a luteal phase defect is made, it is well to recheck the endometrial dating by using a thorough curettage. The diagnosis of a luteal phase defect is substantiated if the histological pattern is 2 days behind the expected date. An inadequate endometrium may reflect (1) an inability of the endometrium to respond to hormone stimulation which, in our experience, is unusual, or (2) an insufficiency of progesterone production by the ovary.

The cause of this condition may be due either to factors discussed under the sections on ovarian failure in Chapter 31—that is, nutritional insufficiencies, metabolic disease processes, chronic illnesses, or deficient pituitary stimulation (neurogenic)—or to specific inherent ovarian defects. The inadequate luteal phase is more apt to be associated with early repeated miscarriages but can occasionally be severe enough to cause primary infertility.

The treatment of the inadequate luteal phase is dependent upon the etiology. However, if the specific factors have been corrected as well as possible or if no specific factors are found, progesterone substitution therapy must be instituted. Usually the most satisfactory substitution therapy is the administration of 12.5 mg. of progesterone intramuscularly daily, given within 2 days after ovulation and continued until the menstrual period begins. This amount of progesterone is adequate for the repair of the average luteal defect but is not enough to override a normal menstrual period. A repeat biopsy while the patient is on therapy will tell whether or not the defect has been repaired. If this amount of progesterone is inadequate, 25 mg. of progesterone can be given daily until approximately 2 or 3

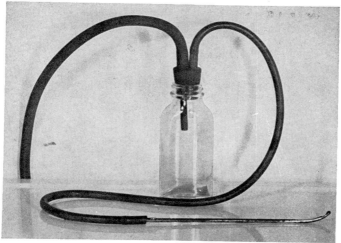

FIG. 30.13. Novak suction curette. This is attached either to an electric suction apparatus or to a simple water pump although tissue for biopsy may be obtained without either.

days before the period is expected, at which time the dosage may be reduced to 12.5 mg. or its equivalent. In this fashion one can prevent a pseudopregnancy reaction.

Synthetic progestogens are not advised since the effect upon the endometrium is often not equivalent to that of progesterone. Chorionic gonadotrophin from human pregnancy urine can also be used as a luteotrophic agent. A daily dose of 2500 IU given 2 days after ovulation has occurred will produce an adequate stimulation of corpus luteum function and is usually insufficient to cause pseudopregnancy. If in addition to the luteal phase defect, there is an estrogenic deficiency, as judged by an inadequate cervical mucus, 0.1 mg. of stilbestrol daily throughout the menstrual cycle will, as eported by Hughes and Van Ness, sometimes be sufficient to produce a proper endometrial build-up for a progestational response.

If infection is present, proper antibiotic therapy must be instituted. If there is endometrial scarring, as in Asherman's disease, repeated gentle curettage may suffice. Tuberculous endometritis as a factor in infertility is discussed in Chapter 21, "Tuberculosis of Female Generative Organs."

REFERENCES

Adams, C. E., and Chang, M. C.: Capacitation of rabbit spermatozoa in the Fallopian tube and in the uterus. J. Exp. Zool., *151:* 159, 1962.

Behrman, S. J., Buettner, J. J., Heglar, R., Gershowitz, H., and Tew, W. L.: ABO (H) blood incompatibility as a cause of infertility; a new concept. Amer. J. Obstet. Gynec., *79:* 847, 1960.

Brown, J. B.: Urinary excretion of estrogens during the menstrual cycle. Lancet, *1:* 320, 1955.

Campos Da Paz, A.: Crystallization phenomena of cervical mucus in the human being and in animals. Proc. Int. Fertil. Assn., *1:* 595, 1953.

Cohen, M. R.: Glucose reagent stick test compared with other criteria for detection of ovulation. Fertil. Steril., *10:* 340, 1959.

Cooper, G., Jr., and Williams, R.: Radiation dosage to female gonads during diagnostic roentgenographic proceedings. J.A.M.A., *170:* 766, 1959.

Corner, G. W., Farris, E. J., and Corner, G. W., Jr.: Dating of ovulation and other ovarian crises by histological examination in comparison with the Farris test. Amer. J. Obstet. Gynec., *59:* 514, 1950.

Decker, A.: *Culdoscopy.* W. B. Saunders Company, Philadelphia, 1952.

Farris, E. G.: A test for determining the time of ovulation and conception in women. Amer. J. Obstet. Gynec., *52:* 14, 1946.

Garcia, C. R., Pincus, G., and Rock, J.: Effects of three 19-*nor*-steroids on human ovulation and menstruation. Amer. J. Obstet. Gynec., *75:* 82, 1958.

Gemzell, C. A., Diczfalusy, E., and Tellinger, G.: Clinical effect of human pituitary follicle-stimulating hormone (FSH). J. Clin. Endocr., 18: 1333, 1958.

Guttmacher, A. F.: Fertility of man. Fertil. Steril., 3: 281, 1952.

Hanton, E. M., Pratt, J. H., and Banner, E. A.: Tubal plastic surgery at the Mayo Clinic. Amer. J. Obstet. Gynec., 89: 934, 1964.

Heckel, N. J.: Production of oligospermia in man by the use of testosterone propionate. Proc. Soc. Exp. Biol. Med., 40: 658, 1939.

Heckel, N. J., and MacDonald, J. H.: Rebound phenomena of spermatogenic activity of human testis following administration of testosterone propionate; further observations. Fertil. Steril., 3: 49, 1952.

Higdon, A. L.: Pregnancy in women over 40. Amer. J. Obstet. Gynec., 80: 38, 1960.

Horne, H. W., Jr., and Rock, J.: Oral Terramycin therapy for chronic endocervicitis in infertile women. Fertil. Steril., 3: 321, 1952.

Hotchkiss, R. S., Pinto, A. B., and Kleegman, S.: Artificial insemination with semen recovered from the bladder. Fertil. Steril., 6: 37, 1955.

Hughes, E. C., and Van Ness, A. W.: In Progress in Gynecology, edited by J. V. Meigs and S. H. Sturgis, Vol. 2. Grune & Stratton, Inc., New York, 1950.

Ingersoll, F. M., and McArthur, J. W.: Longitudinal studies of gonadotrophin excretion in the Stein-Leventhal syndrome. Amer. J. Obstet. Gynec., 77: 795, 1959.

Israel, S. L.: Mazer and Israel's Diagnosis and Treatment of Menstrual Disorders and Sterility. Ed. 4. Paul B. Hoeber, Inc., New York, 1959.

Jones, G. E. S., and Pourmand, K.: An evaluation of etiologic factors and therapy in 555 private patients with primary infertility. Fertil. Steril., 13: 398, 1962.

Jones, G. E. S., Wood, J., Bishop, D., and Donoho, R.: Vaginal fungi and their relation to sperm survival. Amer. J. Obstet. Gynec., 70: 1271, 1955.

Kleegman, S. J.: Therapeutic donor insemination. Fertil. Steril., 5: 7, 1954.

Klinefelter, H. J., Jr., Reifenstein, E. C., Jr., and Albright, F.: Syndrome characterized by gynecomastia, aspermatogenesis without A-leydigism and increased excretion of FSH. J. Clin. Endocr., 2: 615, 1942.

Knudsen, O.: Studies on spermiocytogenesis in the bull. Int. J. Fertil., 5: 389, 1958.

Kurland, I. I., and Loughran, C. H.: Corticosteroids in the treatment of nonpatent fallopian tubes. Amer. J. Obstet. Gynec., 81: 243, 1961.

LaMarr, J. K., Shettles, L. B., and Delfs, E.: Cyclic penetrability of human cervical mucus to spermatozoa in vitro. Amer. J. Physiol., 129: 234, 1940.

Leuchtenberger, C., Leuchtenberger, R.,

Schrader, F., and Weir, D. R.: Reduced amounts of desoxyribose nucleic acid in testicular germ cells of infertile men with active spermatogenesis. Lab. Invest., 5: 422, 1956.

Lorimer, F.: Culture and Human Fertility. Columbia University Press, New York, 1954.

MacLeod, J.: Human semen. Fertil. Steril., 7: 368, 1956.

MacLeod, J., Artemis, P., and Ray, B. S.: Restoration of human spermatogenesis by menopausal gonadotrophins. Lancet, 1: 1196, 1964.

MacLeod, J., and Gold, R. Z.: The male factor in fertility and infertility. V. Effect of continence on semen quality. Fertil. Steril., 3: 297, 1952.

Marcus, S. L., and Marcus, C. C.: Cervical mucus and its relation to infertility. Obstet. Gynec. Survey, 18: 749, 1963.

Moszkowski, E., Woodruff, J. D., and Jones, G. E. S.: The inadequate luteal phase. Amer. J. Obstet. Gynec., 83: 363, 1962.

Novak, E.: Suction-curet apparatus for endometrial biopsy. J.A.M.A., 104: 1497, 1935.

Noyes, R. W., Hertig, A. T., and Rock, J.: Dating the endometrial biopsy. Fertil. Steril., 1: 1, 1950.

Parker, A. S., Jr.: Management of sterility. Surg. Clin. N. Amer., 25: 566, 1945.

Perloff, W. H.: A simplified technic for the concentration of seminal fluid. Fertil. Steril., 11: 262, 1960.

Pommerenke, W. T.: Cyclic changes in the physical and chemical properties of cervical mucus. Amer. J. Obstet. Gynec., 52: 1023, 1946.

Rubin, I.: Non-operative determination of patency of fallopian tubes in sterility; intrauterine inflation with oxygen and production of a subphrenic pneumoperitoneum. J.A.M.A., 74: 1017, 1920.

Schellen, A.: Artificial Insemination in the Human. Elsevier Publishing Company, Amsterdam, 1957.

Shirodkar, V. N.: Contributions to Obstetrics and Gynecology, p. 65. The Williams and Wilkins Company, Baltimore, 1960.

Siegler, A.: Tubal plastic surgery, the past, present, and future. Obstet. Gynec. Survey, 15: 680, 1960.

Siegler, A., and Hellman, L.: Tubal plastic surgery. A retrospective study of 50 cases. Amer. J. Obstet. Gynec., 86: 448, 1963.

Sobrero, A. J., Silberman, C. J., Post, A., and Ciner, L.: Tubal insufflation and hysterosalpingography. Obstet. Gynec., 18: 91, 1961.

Southam, A., and Buxton, L.: Factors influencing reproductive potential. Fertil. Steril., 8: 25, 1957.

Speck, G.: Determination of time of ovulation. Obstet. Gynec. Survey, 14: 798, 1959.

Stone, A., and Ward, M. E.: Factors responsible for pregnancy in 500 infertility cases. Fertil. Steril., 7: 1, 1956.

Tietze, C.: Statistical contributions to the study of human fertility. Fertil. Steril., 5: 88, 1956.

Tietze, C., Gutmacher, A. F., and Rubin, S.: Time required for conception in 1727 planned pregnancies. Fertil. Steril., 1: 338, 1950.

Vara, P.: Results and experience in the surgical treatment of sterility. Gynaecologia (Basel), 147: 445, 1959.

Vincze, L. O., Taft, P. D., and McArthur, J. W.: A study of cornification in vaginal, buccal, and urinary sediment smears. J. Clin. Endocr., 19: 281, 1959.

Whitelaw, M. G.: Statistical evaluation of female fertility. Fertil. Steril., 11: 428, 1960.

31

AMENORRHEA

GENERAL CONSIDERATIONS

Definitions

Amenorrhea is not a disease but a symptom and may be arbitrarily defined as the absence of menses for 3 months or longer. *Primary amenorrhea* is defined as the failure of menses to appear initially and should not be diagnosed before the patient has reached the age of 18 years. *Secondary amenorrhea* implies the cessation of menses after an initial menarche. *Physiological amenorrhea* is the normal absence of menses before puberty, during pregnancy and lactation, and after the menopause. *Cryptomenorrhea* signifies that menstruation actually occurs but does not appear externally because of obstruction of the lower genital canal. *Oligomenorrhea* is defined as a reduction in the frequency of menses; the interval must be longer than 38 days but less than 3 months. This must not be confused with the term *hypomenorrhea*, which is used to designate the reduction in the number of days or the amount of menstrual flow.

Incidence

It is difficult to arrive at a statistical evaluation of the occurrence of amenorrhea and oligomenorrhea in a general gynecological practice but it probably comprises less than 5% of patients. This figure will, of course, vary with the socioeconomic status of the patients as well as the geographical location. Kaeser finds the incidence of primary amenorrhea among 15,000 gynecological patients, over a 10-year period, to be 0.65%.

Classification

As indicated, amenorrhea and oligomenorrhea are symptoms which may be caused by a variety of etiological factors. A single individual with a constant etiological background may show at various times any or all of the pathological manifestations of menstruation, including dysfunctional uterine bleeding, oligomenorrhea, amenorrhea, infertility, and habitual abortion. It is most satisfactory, therefore, whenever possible, to make the classification of these symptom complexes on the basis of the underlying etiological disturbance. The following outline shows the etiological classification of amenorrhea to be used in the discussion.

Etiological Classification of Amenorrhea

I. Lesions of central origin
   A. Neurogenic
     1. Organic
     2. Idiopathic hypothalamic dysfunction — Stein syndrome
     3. Inhibition of the prolactin inhibition factor—Chiari-Frommel
   B. Pituitary disturbances
     1. Insufficiency
       a. Destructive processes (Shee-

trophins it is especially important that the urinary gonadotrophin assay be below 6.6 mµ/24 hours. If the patient has a detectable pituitary function of her own this will invalidate the dosage calculation and complications due to overdosage, which are multiple cysts and multiple pregnancies, will arise. The Stein-Leventhal syndrome is also specifically excluded as the polycystic ovary is peculiarly sensitive to gonadotrophin stimulation.

The dosage schedule which has been found satisfactory is 1500 to 2000 mg. equivalents of FSH, standardized against the European Standard menopausal urine preparation (IRP-HMG) given daily for approximately 10 to 14 days. When a rapid urinary estrogen assay is not available, the clinical evaluation suggested by Igarashi and Matsumoto can satisfactorily be used. A daily vaginal smear for a maturation index, and observation for the occurrence of cervical dilatation and estrogenic mucus, will indicate when a full estrogenic response has been obtained. This usually occurs between 10 and 14 days and, if no response has been obtained by 14 days, treatment should be discontinued. At the full estrogen response, following a 1-day rest period, 2500 IU of HCG are given for 4 days. In our experience this has been an adequate dose schedule to induce ovulation in the hypogonadotrophic, amenorrheic patient, and still low enough to obviate the complications of overdosage.

The major complications of gonadotrophin therapy are superovulations with multiple cyst formation and subsequent multiple pregnancies. These complications have led to death through rupture of the cysts, or rupture of the uterus during pregnancy. Therefore, it cannot be emphasized too strongly that, prior to treatment, an etiologic diagnosis must be established and a proper selection of patients must be made to insure that they do not have endogenous gonadotrophic function. A proper exogenous dosage must be employed and frequent pelvic examinations made; the maximum ovarian size is reached between 7 and 10 days after the initiation of the chorionic gonadotrophin which triggers the ovulation.

Pituitary suppression therapy in the production of ovulation as suggested by Garcia, Pincus, and Rock is usually as disappointing as cyclic steroid therapy. A synthetic progesterone with estrogen added is the most efficient therapy, and, beginning on the 5th-cycle day, 5 mg. daily are given for 24 days each month during a 3- to 6-month period. Treatment is not infrequently complicated by irregular bleeding during the first cycle. Following suppression, the gonadotrophic rebound may, on occasion, induce an improved ovarian function. As there is evidence that, at least, some progestational agents also have a direct effect upon the ovary caution must be used in the selection of the progestogen.

Although low dosage irradiation of the ovaries for the correction of menstrual abnormalities has been repeatedly demonstrated to be therapeutically effective, the radiation biologist and geneticist have been so emphatic in their caution against the use of therapeutic x-rays that most gynecologists have abandoned this form of treatment. The viewpoint is summarized by Glass in his review on radiation hazards.

Clomiphene

A number of years ago, a weak synthetic estrogen, tri-para-anisylchloroethylene (Tace) was developed as an antiestrogenic, and possibly an antifertility, drug. Many derivatives were synthesized in an effort to derive an antiestrogenic compound which would block gonadotrophin secretion. Experimental evidence indicated that clomiphene (Fig. 31.3) was satisfactory in the rat as it produced pituitary inhibition, blocked estrogen activity, and inhibited pregnancy. Subsequent clinical trials proved that in the human the reverse effect was produced; gonadotrophin secretion was increased and stimulation of ovarian function and excessive estrogen production ensued.

Although clomiphene is still classified as an experimental drug there have been

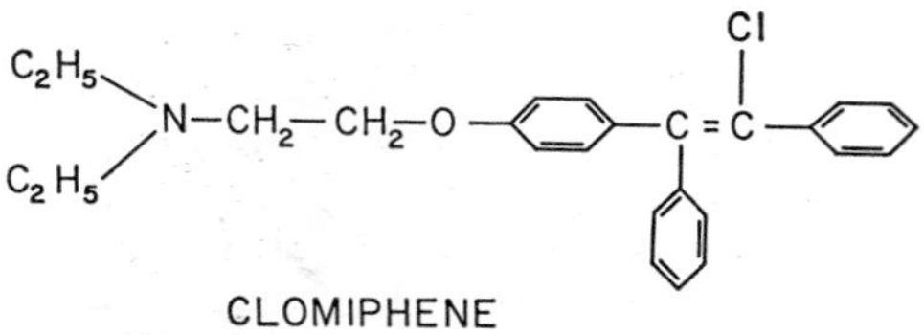

CLOMIPHENE

FIG. 31.3. Formula of clomiphene, 2 [p-(2-chloro-1,2-diphenylvinyl)phenoxy]triethyl-amine.

so many successful clinical trials, with so few and such relatively mild complications, that it is reasonable to believe the drug will soon be commercially available. Its mode of action is apparently to block estrogen at the hypothalamic level, thus removing the inhibition to pituitary gonadotrophin production and allowing a gonadotrophic flood. The increased gonadotrophic secretion causes excessive ovarian stimulation with excretion of urinary estrogen, ovulation, and normal corpus luteum function.

The success rate of such therapy, as with any drug, depends upon the care and skill used in making an etiologic diagnosis when selecting patients suitable for therapy. The classic indication for clomiphene treatment is hypothalamic hypogonadotrophism. The inclusion of the Stein-Leventhal syndrome as a hypothalamic disease can be justified on the basis of experimental evidence and analogy with other endocrine metabolic disease states (p. 598).

The most serious complications reported are the occurrence of multiple ovarian cysts with rupture, and multiple pregnancies. As the pathologic picture is similar to that seen with pituitary gonadotrophin administration, it seems clear that these effects are the results of a pituitary stimulation.

Transitory blurring of vision and hot flushes are not infrequent symptoms and an occasional patient notices some loss of scalp hair. This alopecia, however, has not been severe and regression occurs rapidly after cessation of treatment. If care is taken in using an initial low dosage over a short period and the patient is observed for evidence of ovarian stimulation and not retreated until the initial reaction has subsided, these complications of over stimulation can usually be avoided. Liver function studies should be made if there is a history of any liver disease, since clomiphene is excreted by way of the bile ducts.

Although many dosage schedules have been reported, it would seem that 50 mg. daily for 5 to 10 days, repeated after 30 days if necessary, is a good standard procedure to start with. The lowest dosage should be used in patients with the Stein-Leventhal syndrome. If no effect is observed after 3 cycles, the dosage can be increased to 100 mg. daily for 5 days. It is recommended that the total dosage in any single case not exceed 600 mg. in 1 month.

Although no adverse effects on the fetus have been reported in humans treated during early pregnancy, clomiphene has produced fetal anomalies in experimental animals. It is therefore recommended that treatment be avoided during pregnancy.

Thyroid

Thyroid has long been advocated as of therapeutic value in the correction of menstrual disorders; however, its empiric and indiscriminate use should not be encouraged. It will prove useful only when there is evidence of a low thyroid function as reflected in the basal metabolic rate, blood cholesterol, protein-bound iodine, or ^{131}I uptake. When such evidence exists adequate thyroid dosage must be used and overdosage avoided; 0.2 to 0.3 mg. of sodium levothyroxine daily is usually sufficient and 3 months is the shortest possible therapeutic trial period. A repeat basal metabolic rate should show some improvement at this time. If there is none, however, this is not necessarily an indication for increased dosage, and reevaluation is advisable. There is no evidence that triiodothyronine is more efficient in hypothyroidism than are thyroid hormones; however, a therapeutic effect can be obtained more rapidly. If this drug is used it must be remembered that one cannot rely upon the protein-bound iodine as a standard for judging adequate replacement. The protein-bound iodine will be suppressed as a result of depression of pituitary production of thyrotrophic hormones and resultant thyroid inactivity. Under these circumstances a basal metabolic rate serves as a guide. Triiodothyronine is indicated when the hypometabolic state exists; this condition is characterized by a normal protein-bound iodine and lowered basal metabolic rate.

Nutrition

A good nutritional status is mandatory for the ultimate success of any treatment and must not be overlooked in our zeal for less mundane therapy.

LESIONS OF CENTRAL ORIGIN

Lesions of central origin can be subdivided into three major groups: (1) neurogenic, (2) psychogenic, and (3) pituitary. Neurogenic amenorrhea may be further subdivided into organic brain disease and idiopathic hypothalamic failure; psychosomatic amenorrhea into major and minor psychosis, emotional shock, anorexia nervosa, and pseudocyesis; and pituitary amenorrhea into pituitary insufficiency, tumors and congenital deficiency of gonadotrophic hormone production.

Neurogenic Lesions and Organic Brain Disease

Organic. The diagnosis of organic brain disease is made with the help of the physical examination and history of encephalitis (Fig. 31.4) or related infections, accidents, injuries, or exposure to toxic substances such as lead or carbon monoxide. Laboratory findings are characterized by a low, or low normal, urinary gonadotrophin excretion, lowered urinary estrogen excretion and a moderately atrophic vaginal smear. Depending upon the severity, or the position, of the neurological lesion, there may be associated abnormalities of laboratory findings related to thyroid, adrenal, or pancreatic functions. The electroencephalogram is a valuable diagnostic aid.

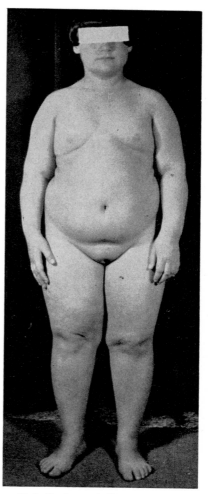

FIG. 31.4. Postencephalic obesity and absence of sexual development. (From Sevringhaus, E. L.: *Endocrine Therapy in General Practice.* Year Book Publishers, Inc., Chicago, 1938.)

Kinnunen and Kauppinen, in a survey of 78 patients who had amenorrhea following brain injury, indicate that the duration of unconsciousness is a fairly good index of the possibility of amenorrhea. The prognosis in patients with neurogenic amenorrhea is poor except for those following acute trauma. Under these circumstances recovery may occur. Adequate pituitary hormone therapy should be successful in bypassing the neurological lesions. In our series of 352 patients with amenorrhea, 9 had organic brain disease; 3 were related to central nervous system syphilis, 3 to traumatic epilepsy (probably from birth injuries), and 2 to cerebral accident; in 1 case there was a history of carbon monoxide poisoning and in the other a motor accident; 1 patient had multiple sclerosis.

Idiopathic Hypothalamic Insufficiency. In hypothalamic failure either the hypothalamic cells are defective in their secretory ability or they are excessively sensitive to inhibitory stimulation. In either case there is a lack of stimulation to the pituitary gonadotrophic cells.

The cardinal symptom of idiopathic hypothalamic failure is infrequent, but usually ovulatory, menstruations; the menstrual irregularity dates from the menarche and is often associated with a family history of menstrual irregularities. On physical examination there are no detectable neurogenic or psychogenic factors, and despite a normal encephalogram the laboratory findings are similar to those in patients with organic brain disease.

There is usually no indication for therapy among this group of patients, as pregnancy frequently occurs without difficulty. However, if infertility is a problem, regular menstruation with a reasonable expectation of ensuing pregnancy can usually be initiated with clomiphene. As this drug is still quite new patients should be followed carefully, with frequent repeated pelvic examinations, to be sure that ovarian cysts have not been induced. Dosage should not be over 600 mg. total per month to avoid possible complications of alopecia, flushes, and visual symptoms mentioned in the preceding section on clomiphene.

Among our 352 amenorrhea patients, 9 were diagnosed as having idiopathic hypothalamic failure. The prognosis in the group of patients is good and 4 of 6 patients adequately followed became pregnant.

The STEIN-LEVENTHAL SYNDROME. The Stein-Leventhal syndrome is characterized by bilateral polycystic ovaries in association with infertility and anovulatory menstrual irregularities. These are manifest as either amenorrhea, oligomenorrhea, or functional uterine bleeding. A mild or marked degree of hirsutism is usually present (Fig. 31.5). The one single criterion which must always be present to substantiate the diagnosis is bilaterally enlarged ovaries. Therefore the diagnosis cannot be made without some form of visualization of the ovaries. Stein has for many years advocated gynecography; however, culdoscopy is another method of visual diagnosis.

The differential diagnosis must often be made between the Stein syndrome and mild adrenal hyperplasia. A prolonged cortisone suppression test is sometimes helpful in this regard. A sufficient amount of adrenal hormone is given to maintain a suppression of 17-ketosteroid secretion to 6 mg. per 24 hours, or below, over a 6-month period; 25 to 50 mg. of cortisone acetate or its equivalent daily is usually satisfactory. The classic response in a patient with the Stein-Leventhal syndrome is a single ovulation usually within the first 6 weeks of treatment followed thereafter by a reversion to her previous state of anovulation. If continued ovulatory menses do not ensue or suppression cannot be sustained, a Stein syndrome is suspect. An adrenal tumor, however, may also be associated with these laboratory findings, and if the ketosteroid excretion is remarkably elevated, especially if there is also a high dehydroepiandrosterone excretion, this is most likely.

As described in Chapter 23, the ovaries of a patient with the Stein-Leventhal syndrome should be $1\frac{1}{2}$ to 2 times enlarged. They are often the size of the uterus which is frequently small, allowing one to feel three structures of equal size in the pelvis. Macroscopically, the ovaries are pearly white in appearance with multiple cysts beneath the capsule. Microscopically, they are characterized by a capsule formed by hyalinization of the interstitial tissue of the cortex directly beneath the germinal epithelium. This

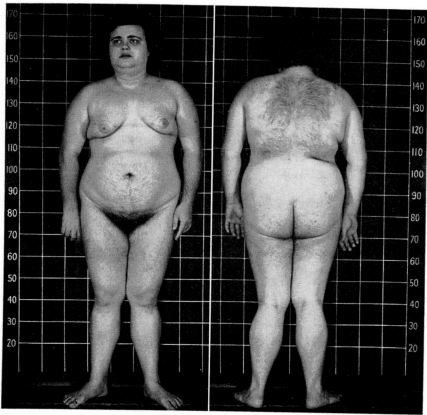

FIG. 31.5. Patient with a Stein syndrome illustrating the difficulty which may be encountered in differentiating the condition from Cushing's syndrome by the physical appearance of the patient.

hyalinization may engulf the primordial follicles. There are numerous follicular cysts which characteristically have a thin granulosal lining and a marked luteinization of the theca interna. There are no corpora lutea present, although there may be evidences of old corpora albicantia (occasionally, however, even in a typical Stein-Leventhal syndrome a sporadic ovulation can occur). As all of these elements are present at times in the normal ovary and the findings represent simply an exaggeration of the normal, there is no diagnostic pathologic picture. Comparison of the "Stein-Leventhal ovary" and the ovary removed with hysterectomy performed for recurrent anovulatory bleeding would suggest that

histological differentiation is impossible except for the marked bilateral enlargement of the "S.L." ovary; in other words, the difference is merely quantitative.

Therefore, the diagnosis cannot be made as a pathologic entity and one can only report the ovarian findings as "compatible with" those seen with the Stein-Leventhal syndrome. Contrariwise, however, although a positive finding is not diagnostic, a negative correlation, e.g., "not compatible with," is good evidence that one is *not* dealing with a Stein-Leventhal syndrome.

The excessive follicle maturation and hyperluteinization are indications of excessive gonadotrophic stimulation and excessive steroid production. Laboratory investigations indicate that this is indeed the case. Ingersoll and McArthur demonstrated that total urinary gonadotrophins are elevated, and, if a fractionation study is carried out, it is the ICSH which is responsible for the elevation. In patients who show endometrial hyperplasia and hyperestrogenism (25% of all cases), the urinary estrogen excretion is above normal while in patients who show hirsutism, the 17-ketosteroid excretion is usually slightly elevated or in the high normal range indicating excessive androgen secretion. This has been proved by the demonstration that in the polycystic ovary the ovarian vein blood contains excessive amounts of testosterone, as well as by *in vitro* experiments of Sandor and Lanthier. These authors have shown that slices from ovaries of patients with the androgenic form of the Stein-Leventhal syndrome transform Δ_4-androstene-3,17-dione into testosterone at a more rapid rate than do slices from ovaries of normal women.

Other laboratory tests such as the vaginal maturation index, and the endometrial biopsy vary depending upon whether or not the ovary is producing excessive androgen or excessive estrogen. In the variety associated with excessive androgen production, the maturation index shows a complete shift to the left or a midzone shift with atrophic endometrium, while in the estrogenic variety, the maturation index may be completely shifted to the right and the endometrium may show marked adenomatous hyperplasia (see Chapter 15).

Stein recognized many years ago that it was impossible to treat the syndrome with suppressive doses of steroids. Keettel, Bradbury, and Stoddard reported apparent hypersensitivity of the Stein-Leventhal ovary to pituitary gonadotrophins and described a remarkable ovarian enlargement which occurred following the use of these substances. Crooke *et al.* extended this work and indicated that under gonadotrophic stimulation polycystic ovaries could be made to produce excessive amounts of estrogen and to ovulate with the production of normal or high amounts of progesterone. In our own experience it was found that

ovarian cyst formation was produced only if pituitary gonadotrophins (predominantly FSH) were given and not if human chorionic gonadotrophin was given alone.

In resumé then, the whole picture represents a patient with the paradoxical finding of *excessive gonadotrophin production* and ICSH predominance over FSH, in association with *excessive ovarian steroid formation* either androgen or estrogen. Additional *estrogens do not suppress* the *excessive gonadotrophin* production and stimulation with pituitary *gonadotrophins causes a hyperresponse* with multiple cyst formation.

Although the exact pathogenesis of the Stein-Leventhal syndrome is still not completely documented, the existing evidence establishes it as a disease of the neuroendocrine homeostatic control mechanism and places it in the same category as Cushing's syndrome and perhaps Graves' disease, hyperthyroidism. These diseases are characterized by excessive pituitary activity in the paradoxical presence of excessive target organ hormone formation, hyperresponsiveness to pituitary stimulation and lack of response to pituitary suppression in the absence of a pituitary tumor. The explanation for these aberrations of physiology is a block in the hypothalamic center or centers which control the pituitary secretion and release of trophic hormones.

The exact nature of the agents which block the hypothalamic centers in the case of the Stein-Leventhal syndrome is unknown but it would seem, from a review of case histories, that this may be of varied origin. Experiments in the rat by Barraclough indicate that gonadotrophic centers can be blocked by androgen given within 3 days of birth. That some stimulation early in life may often be responsible for the condition in the human, is indicated by the fact that many patients exhibit their symptoms from the onset of the menstrual function. In addition to the possible effect of steroids as blocking agents for the hypothalamic nuclei, one would have to consider emotional stress and other factors in the external environment such as drugs and illnesses. These stimuli, through their effect upon the hypothalamus, alter the secretion and release of the pituitary gonadotrophins, changing the ratio of FSH:ICSH. It is probably the changing ratio which determines the enzymic mechanism of the ovarian theca cells and sets the equilibrium in favor of either estrogen or androgen production. The high ICSH in relation to FSH also inhibits ovulation and corpus luteum formation. By using human pituitary gonadotrophins in amenorrhoeic, hypogonadotrophin patients, Diczfalucy has shown that if the ICSH value is too high in relation to the FSH value, ovulation does not occur. When additional FSH is given, as in our experiments and those of Crooke et al., ovulation does occur in Stein-ovaries, further substantiating the theory.

Although the pathogenesis is uncertain, the treatment is well documented. A bilateral wedge resection operation will cure the menstrual irregularities in 85% of the patients and pregnancy can be expected in 75% of the married women. The rate of recurrence is low if patients are carefully selected. The explanation for the success of the wedge resection is problematical. Reports in the current literature seem to substantiate the fact that clomiphene is also a successful therapeutic agent in the Stein-Leventhal syndrome. The therapy was first suggested by Kistner with MRL-25, an early analogue of the drug. At the present time, the optimum dosage is still uncertain but is in the range of 50 mg. daily for 5 days, given at monthly intervals. A small dosage is preferable as with larger dosage it is possible to produce ovarian cyst formation. It is also wise to preclude a pregnancy until the cycle has been satisfactorily regulated.

One would have to surmise that with both methods of therapy, surgical and clomiphene, one is shifting the gonadotrophic ratio in favor of FSH against ICSH. It is easy to explain this syndrome if one accepts the *hypothesis* that there is an ICSH inhibitory center in the hypothalamus (Chapter 2). If this center is blocked (and it is this one that controls the cyclic release of ICSH), then the tonic center, which is constantly stimulating ICSH production, predominates and a constant high ICSH prevails with relatively normal FSH values. This abnormal ratio inhibits ovulation. Therapy, by some neurohumoral mechanism, unblocks the ICSH inhibitory center.

The indications for treatment in Stein-Leventhal syndrome are infertility, functional uterine bleeding, and, in the rare instance, hirsutism. Functional uterine bleeding is an important indication for therapy; as mentioned in the chapter on carcinoma of the fundus, there is certain evidence that this condition may precede endometrial carcinoma. Hirsutism would constitute an indication in a young girl who was rapidly developing an extreme amount of hair. Under these circumstances, operation would be done *only* with the full knowledge of the patient that the hirsutism already present may not regress and with the hope that progression will be forestalled. In the absence of functional uterine bleeding or marked hirsutism, it is wise to postpone surgical treatment until such a time when fertility is of importance. Medical treatment can, of course, be used with fewer reservations. In our series of amenorrheic women there were 23 with bilateral polycystic ovaries. Nine of these patients had a wedge resection operation and all 9 were cured of menstrual irregularities; 4 of 5 married women became pregnant.

Inhibition of the Prolactin Inhibiting Factor (PIF). Occasionally, after a pregnancy one observes persistent lactation and failure of menses to reappear. These symptoms are characteristic of the *Chiari-Frommel* syndrome and are associated with an atrophic vagina and uterus and a low urinary gonadotrophin excretion. Theoretically, the condition represents an inhibition of the prolactin-inhibiting factor of the hypothalamus. Although usually due to physiologic causes, it may be associated with a tumor causing destruction of the center or tracts involved. The results of treatment are often unsatisfactory; however, continuous high dosage of progestene and clomiphene citrate have both been reported as occasionally successful.

Pituitary Amenorrhea

Pituitary Insufficiency (Sheehan's Disease). The most common cause of pituitary insufficiency is necrosis of the anterior lobe due to a traumatic labor or delivery, as classically described by Sheehan. Nassar has inferred from experimental work that the use of ergot may predispose to pituitary thrombosis. However, the pituitary is normally enlarged during pregnancy and may, on occasion, thrombose spontaneously. Depending upon the severity of the thrombosis, there is postpartum collapse and hyperpyrexia. After an immediate recovery there is an absence of lactation and amenorrhea. The initial physical signs are uterine and vaginal atrophy with a slight, or occasionally marked, gain in weight (Fig. 31.6). Signs characteristic of the late stages are loss of axillary and pubic hair, lowered blood pressure, and loss of weight. Thus the final stage is that initially described by Simmonds for pituitary cachexia (Fig. 31.7). Such patients are susceptible to infections and other forms of stress and thus live in a precarious state. Sheehan describes acquisition of pigment due to intermedin, and although theoretically this is possible since the intermediate and posterior lobe of the pituitary are supposedly unaffected by the venous thrombosis, in our experience this finding is certainly unusual.

It is reported that some patients, over a period of years, tend to have an amelioration of the disease probably due to a compensatory hypertrophy of the remaining pituitary cells. If satisfactory temporary replacement therapy can be obtained, patients have been reported to have become pregnant, and Murdoch and Govan say this is the best treatment of the condition as, under the pregnancy stimulation, the pituitary gland hypertrophies. On the other hand, Israel and Constan warn that this can be an ex-

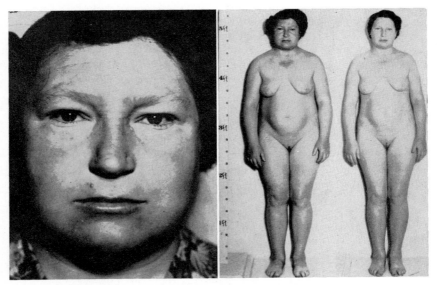

Fig. 31.6. Late stage of Sheehan's syndrome. *Left,* patient at the age of 35 years. This patient had amenorrhea of 16-years duration. Her last pregnancy, at 19 years of age, was associated with severe postpartum hemorrhage. *Center,* before treatment. Notice mild obesity, puffiness of face (myxedema), and loss of pubic hair. *Right,* after 8 months of treatment with 2 grains of thyroid daily.

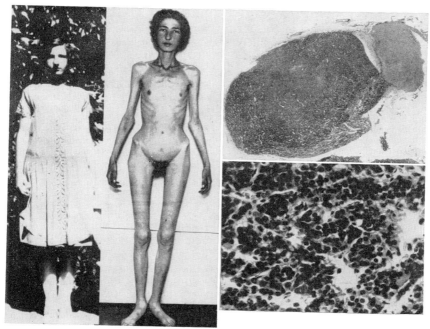

FIG. 31.7. Cachectic state, resembling Simmonds' disease, caused by pituitary destruction due to chromophobe adenoma. *Left,* patient at 11 years of age, just prior to onset of illness. *Center,* at the age of 17 years. This patient had amenorrhea of 6-years duration and a 65-pound weight loss. Notice extreme emaciation and lack of breast development; but pubic hair is still present. *Right,* low and high power photomicrographs of the pituitary chromophobe adenoma. (From Lisser, H., and Escamilla, R. F.: *Atlas of Clinical Endocrinology.* C. V. Mosby Company, St. Louis, 1957.)

tremely dangerous situation for, as a result of the stress of labor and delivery, collapse and death may occur.

The laboratory findings are characteristic of panhypopituitarism: a lowered or absent gonadotrophin excretion, a low 17-ketosteroid and 11-corticosteroid excretion, a low protein-bound iodine and basal metabolic rate, a flat glucose tolerance test, and anemia.

The treatment is replacement therapy, with 25 mg. of cortisone acetate, or its equivalent, daily. On occasion it may be necessary to use in addition 96 mg. of desiccated thyroid a day to give these patients a general feeling of well-being. Although replacement steroid therapy will induce menstruation, it is certainly not indicated except for psychological reasons. When sterility is a problem, pituitary gonadotrophin therapy is the treatment of choice if one has the temerity

to care for the pregnancy which may ensue under such precarious conditions. In the last decade we have seen an even dozen patients fulfilling the criteria for Sheehan's disease.

Pituitary Tumors. Although pituitary tumors are uncommon in any series of amenorrhea patients, the reverse is not true, in that amenorrhea is an extremely common symptom among women with pituitary tumors. In a series of 15 young women who had pituitary tumors, all had amenorrhea as one of the presenting symptoms (Jagiello). Thus it is most important to keep this etiological factor in mind and to make the diagnosis when it does occur.

A history of headache and visual disturbances with amenorrhea is suggestive of an intracranial difficulty. However, these may be late symptoms and a slow growing lesion can exist for years prior to their onset. The specific laboratory diagnostic aids are (1) an x-ray of the sella turcica, and (2) a color visual field examination, as the first diagnostic sign may be the encroachment of the tumor on the optic tracts with an ensuing defect in red perception.

Any type of pituitary tumor can produce amenorrhea. The most common type, the *chromophobe adenoma*, usually has no specific endocrine symptoms and produces amenorrhea through gross destruction of pituitary tissue. However, prolactin-producing chromophobe adenomas which are associated with the *Ahumada-del Castillio syndrome*. This is characterized by persistent lactation in the absence of a previous pregnancy, extreme atrophy of the uterus and vaginal mucosa, small ovaries, and a copious milky secretion from the breasts bilaterally. Breast secretion may, on occasion, be enough to cause the patient annoyance and embarrassment, whereas in other instances it may be noticed only by the physician during the breast examination. When an associated defect in the sella turcica is present, the diagnosis is assured. However, in our experience, only about a quarter of the patients show this defect. A case has been reported by Bricaire *et al.* with complete laboratory data including a prolactin assay which was reported as high, 20 pigeon units per 100 ml. of serum.

Two patients in the series reviewed showed a chromophobe adenoma without associated endocrine symptoms. One was cured of the adenoma surgically and the other died postoperatively. If the pituitary has been destroyed, amenorrhea, of course, persists following operative therapy, and the only curative treatment would be substitution gonadotrophic therapy.

The *basophilic adenoma* is associated with *Cushing's syndrome* which will be discussed in the section on adrenal, under "Lesions of Intermediate Origin." The *acidophilic adenoma* is associated with the signs and symptoms of *acromegaly*, and 85% of young women with acromegaly are said to have menstrual disturbances. The physical appearance of the patient with this condition is usually the best diagnostic aid. There is excessive growth of hands and feet and an increase in coarseness of all of the features. This is associated with an increase in the size of the nose and prognathous of the lower jaw. There may be unusual muscular weakness, polyuria, and polydipsia in the later stages. The laboratory findings are characterized by the absence of urinary gonadotrophins and the presence of a diabetic type of glucose tolerance curve and an increased metabolic rate or protein-bound iodine. It is important to recognize these tumors prior to the occurrence of severe visual field defects as pressure on the optic nerves may cause blindness. These adenomas are ordinarily radiosensitive, and some form of radiation therapy should be employed. When the condition is arrested, amenorrhea is usually corrected. However, if pressure necrosis of the pituitary has occurred, the amenorrhea may be permanent.

Congenital Deficiency of Gonadotrophic Hormones (Hypogonadotrophic Eunuchoidism). This condition is extremely rare. It is theoretically due to a specific failure of the pituitary to produce gonadotrophic hormones. However, there is no pathology available on the pituitaries of any of these individuals to date.

The diagnosis is made when primary amenorrhea occurs with a eunuchoid stature in the absence of urinary gonadotrophins. A familial occurrence is reported. The pathology of the ovary shows follicles in all stages of evolution but no evidence of ovulation or corpus luteum formation. Again, the treatment of choice in these cases is substitution gonadotrophin therapy. Because of the familial occurrence a chromosomal defect might be suspected.

Psychogenic Amenorrhea

Psychogenic amenorrhea can be further subdivided into (1) major and minor psychosis, (2) emotional shock, (3) pseudocyesis, and (4) anorexia nervosa.

DD → between Ah. del Castillo S. and C. Frommell

Major and Minor Psychosis. The diagnosis is made on the basis of the patient's psychiatric symptoms. The endocrine assays have been reviewed by Ray, Nicholson-Vailey, and Grappl and are found to show low normal values within the range seen in patients having neurogenic disturbances. This would indicate, as one might expect, that the final common pathway for the production of the amenorrhea is through a depressed pituitary function. The most common major psychosis associated with amenorrhea is a depressive state. However, according to Kroger and Freed, amenorrhea may also occur in the less profound psychiatric disturbances and may be a manifestation of emotional immaturity, overtly expressing the patient's subconscious attitude of a distaste for intercourse, a fear of pregnancy, or of promiscuity.

Some of these conditions are relatively easy to diagnose, as the amenorrhea immediately follows an unfortunate emotional experience. In other patients the diagnosis is made on an exclusion basis in that no other etiological factor can be found and the patient is emotionally unstable.

The treatment consists of psychiatric care, and, with the present psychiatric approach, the prognosis is poor. It is unusual to be able to induce ovulation with cyclic steroid therapy, but gonadotrophic therapy is usually successful. However, it is questionable whether such patients should be treated in this substitution fashion until psychiatric care has been administered.

There were 7 patients among our series with this diagnosis and the course of the amenorrhea seemed to parallel the course of the psychiatric disturbance. Two were improved psychiatrically and these were cured of their amenorrhea.

Emotional Shock. Any traumatic experience may be followed by amenorrhea and the history is the diagnostic criterion. Amenorrhea is usually temporary, and menses may be expected to resume within 6 months. The laboratory investigation, according to Faierman, indicates lowered pituitary function. Bass reported that amenorrhea occurred in 50% of women interned in concentration camps during World War II; the onset was within 4 weeks of internment and spontaneous remission occurred in 94% of the women in spite of deteriorating food supplies. A nutritional basis would therefore seem to be excluded. A number of such reports have been reviewed by Randall and McElin.

The experience with shock treatments for various psychiatric disturbances has been interesting in this regard; Liepelt reports that 84.7% of 300 patients receiving such therapy have some period of amenorrhea, ranging from 6 weeks to 13 months. The treatment of amenorrhea secondary to emotional shock or trauma is largely reassurance followed by gonadotrophin substitution therapy if necessary.

Pseudocyesis. This condition is characterized by (1) an obsession of pregnancy, (2) weight gain, (3) normal secondary sexual characteristics and pelvic organs, (4) lactation, and (5) an impaired ovulatory mechanism. Since secondary sexual characteristics and pelvic organs are normal, it may be assumed that the estrogenic function is maintained at least to some degree. The lesion would therefore seem to be localized to a disturbance of the FSH:ICSH ratio. A corpus luteum cyst or ectopic pregnancy may be associated with similar symptoms and these diagnoses, as well as the possibility of a missed abortion, must be excluded.

The laboratory findings are characterized by a low normal gonadotrophin excretion, estrogens within the normal range and a midzone shift in the vaginal smear pattern. A negative serum chorionic gonadotrophin assay will also assist in the differential diagnosis. Endometrial biopsy or curettage should be considered only if an intrauterine pregnancy can be excluded.

As the basis of this disturbance is often due to the patient's desire to become pregnant and inability to do so, the problem can frequently be handled by a gynecologist without psychiatric help. A discussion .and explanation of her problems, together with the initiation of an infertility investigation, will often suffice.

There were 4 patients with this diagnosis in our series. None received psychiatric care but were handled entirely by a gynecologist and all have had a return of regular menstrual periods. There have been 3 subsequent pregnancies. As cited by Rakoff, the prognosis among this group of patients is apparently good.

Anorexia Nervosa. Anorexia nervosa is characterized by severe malnutrition with no associated lethargy or inanition. This persistent feeling of well-being, in spite of profound weight loss, distinguishes the condition from the pituitary cachexia seen with Simmonds' disease. The other characteristic of the syndrome is that the patient is unable to give an accurate account of her food intake and, either willfully or compulsively, falsifies the record. This preoccupation with weight and the inability to eat is the overt manifestation of a severe psychological disturbance. The associated loss of weight is secondarily responsibe for the amenorrhea. The physical examination is characterized by emaciation, a fine lanugo type of hirsutism, normal axillary and pubic hair, and atrophy of internal and external genitalia (Fig. 31.8).

The laboratory findings in our experience are compatible with a low or absent total pituitary function. This is in accordance with Emanuel's findings, although Bliss and Migeon report only a lowered gonadotrophic function. The differential diagnosis between anorexia nervosa and panhypopituitarism of Simmonds' disease is made on the appearance of the patient in conjunction with the history.

As the etiology is psychogenic the treatment is psychiatric rather than endocrine. However, because of the very cleverly concealed personality problems, it is often difficult to persuade the family that psychiatric care is necessary, or desirable. If the patient accepts advice and weight gain is accomplished, menses recur within 3 months after a minimal ideal weight is regained. Dally and Sargeant have advocated a hospital regimen of combined chlorpromazine and insulin. Chlorpromazine is given in massive dosage increasing from 150 mg. a day to as much as 1000 mg. a day. Insulin is started with 5 units and progressively increased to drowsiness, the average morning dose in the reported series being 60 units. The courses are interrupted for three large meals a day. This regimen serves to restore the patient's nutritional status to such an extent that she is able to accept treatment for her psychological problems. The condition is not to be taken lightly, as 10 to 20% of patients with anorexia nervosa develop irreversible, fatal malnutrition.

There were 12 women in our series with this disturbance, 6 of whom have been adequately followed. Only 1 patient accepted treatment and gained weight. Her menses returned promptly and she has since become pregnant.

LESIONS OF INTERMEDIATE ORIGIN

Intermediate problems concerned with the production of amenorrhea are those factors which exert their effect somewhere between the central stimulatory and pituitary gonadotrophic functions and the ovarian or end organ levels. These may be divided into chronic illness, metabolic disease, nutritional factors, and disease of organs concerned with the excretion and metabolism of the steroid hormones.

Chronic Disease

Although any chronic disease process associated with inanition can be associated with amenorrhea, by far the most common one is tuberculosis. Tuberculosis may exert its influence through constitutional factors or specifically by destruction of the ovary or endometrium. These latter causes have been discussed under the organs involved. Diagnosis of a chronic disease process is made on the basis of an increased sedimentation rate, elevation of white count, and the presence of a low grade fever. Normal menses re-

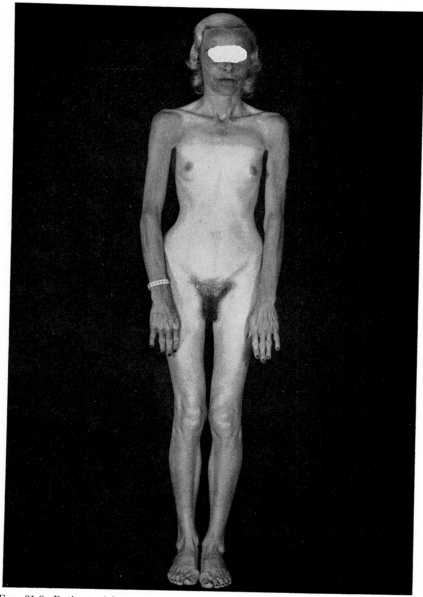

FIG. 31.8. Patient with anorexia nervosa. Note the normal amount of pubic hair

appear when the disease process is arrested or cured. Only 2 patients in the reported series had amenorrhea associated with tuberculosis.

Metabolic Disease

Disturbances of the pituitary and ovarian function are discussed under these specific headings and metabolic disease is herein divided into three categories: disturbances of the thyroid, the pancreas, and the adrenal.

Thyroid. Both *hypo-* and *hyperthyroid* states may be associated with menstrual irregularities and amenorrhea. These diagnoses must be made by some specific test for thyroid function such as the basal metabolic rate, the protein-bound iodine, or an ^{131}I uptake. To confirm the diagnosis of hypothyroidism the basal metabolic rate should be −10 or below, and the protein-bound iodine under 4 μg. per 100 ml. of serum; two or more tests should be made. It must also be remembered that the diagnosis of hypothyroidism cannot be made in the presence of malnutrition, as lowered thyroid function invariably exists under these conditions. The diagnosis of hyperthyroidism cannot be made unless the basal metabolic rate is consistently +20 or above and the protein-bound iodine is 8 μg. per 100 ml. of serum or above. In either case some clinical signs and symptoms of hypo- or hyperthyroidism should be present. The classic signs of hypothyroidism are sensitivity to heat and cold, a tendency to constipation, dryness of the skin and hair, and slow reaction time. Hyperthyroidism is characterized by an elevation of the pulse rate, a fine tremor, some loss of weight, excessive perspiration, a lid lag, and occasionally exophthalmos.

The treatment of hypothyroidism is the administration of desiccated thyroid. The usual dosage is between 96 and 128 mg. daily. Therapy must be continued for at least 3 months and as long thereafter as necessary to maintain the basal metabolic rate or the protein-bound iodine at normal levels or both. Therapy should be interrupted periodically and patients checked for remissions. There is usually no indication for the use of tri-iodothyronine in patients with simple hypothyroidism. If or when it is given it must be remembered that the protein-bound iodine is no longer of value as a guide to therapy, and a basal metabolic rate must be used. Either severe hypothyroidism to the point of myxedema or hyperthyroidism warrant medical consultation. In the treatment of hyperthyroidism antithyroid drug therapy is usually to be desired, and some form of propylthiouracil, administered over long periods of time, will usually result in a

euthyroid state. Unless there is a suspicion of malignancy, or unless there is resistance to antithyroid drug therapy, thyroidectomy is usually not advisable. Radioactive iodine treatment carries the theoretical possibility of late carcinogenic effects and in addition may produce permanent amenorrhea, perhaps through its effect upon the ovary. Therefore, especially in women of the childbearing age, this type of therapy is not recommended.

In our own series of amenorrheic patients there were 34 with hypothyroidism and 2 with hyperthyroidism. The prognosis is relatively good; of 30 patients adequately treated and followed 28 were improved and 8 became pregnant.

When a euthyroid state is achieved in Graves' disease, the menstrual abnormalities are usually promptly corrected and fertility is restored. Among our own patients, however, the 2 women with this condition who were treated with radioactive iodine have remained amenorrheic despite apparently normal thyroid function.

Pancreas. Although *diabetes mellitus* is more apt to be associated with functional bleeding, amenorrhea is occasionally present. There are at least three theoretical causes for the menstrual disturbance. First, the difficulty may be due to the diabetes *per se*, resulting from the insulin deficiency; second, it can be caused by associated nutritional deficiencies; or third, it can be caused by the emotional disturbances which occur so frequently with this disease, especially if the diabetic control is poor.

The classic signs and symptoms are obesity followed by weight loss, polyuria, polydipsia, and nocturia. Often it is the monilial vulvovaginitis, commonly associated with diabetes, which brings the patient to the doctor; therefore the gynecologist may be the first who has the opportunity of making the diagnosis. It should be unnecessary to state that in the presence of these symptoms a determination for urinary sugar must be obtained.

The important laboratory finding is an

elevated fasting blood sugar. It has been our experience that when the diabetes is satisfactorily controlled, the menstrual periods become regulated. Although some observers have advocated the use of estrogen therapy in the menopausal type of diabetes, this rather unorthodox form of treatment is certainly not applicable to most patients, and the interesting observations of Houssay tend to shed light on the physiological defects of the disease rather than to serve as a practical aid to therapy.

An interesting experimental approach to the problem led Foglia *et al.* to conclude that the pancreatectomized rat exhibits alterations of the estrous cycle and disturbances of fertility prior to the development of frank diabetes. As there is some evidence that anatomical changes can be detected in the prediabetic human, these findings are of additional importance.

There were 6 women with amenorrhea and diabetes in the series reported by us and although there were no pregnancies, 4 were symptomatically improved with good diabetic control only.

Adrenal. The two outstanding adrenal syndromes associated with menstrual abnormalities are the *adrenogenital syndrome* and *Cushing's disease.* Addison's disease is occasionally associated with amenorrhea in its late stages and under these circumstances it is impossible to say that the cachexia is not the major factor rather than the adrenal insufficiency.

CONGENITAL ADRENAL HYPERPLASIA. Probably the most dramatic form of the adrenogenital syndrome has been classically described by Glynn as female pseudohermaphroditism, and the laboratory aspects have been elaborated upon by Wilkins. The characteristic features are the deformity of the external genitalia, precocious virilism, short stature, deep skin pigmentation, and an absence of menses. There are all transitions between marked congenital adrenal hyperplasia and postpubertal virilization.

The disease is a heritable one, caused by a specific enzyme deficiency which prevents the adrenal from synthesizing cortisol (Chapter 8). Depending upon the specific enzyme deficiency which the patient has inherited certain specific urinary metabolites will be increased. In the classic form the urinary ketosteroid excretion is markedly elevated, usually being in the range of 50 mg. per 24 hours. An elevated pregnanetriol excretion indicates an insufficiency of the 21-hydroxylase enzyme and blockage of adrenal production of cortisol at the 17-hydroxyprogesterone step. The hypertensive form of congenital adrenal hyperplasia has an increased urinary excretion of pregnan-3α,17α,21-triol-20-one (THS) indicating defective 11-β-hydroxylation. This form of the disease may be unassociated with an increased 17-ketosteroid excretion (Fig. 31.9).

The adrenal pathology is characterized by a hyperplasia of the zona reticularis and either anatomical absence, or a failure of fat accumulation in, the zona fasciculata.

In the severe forms of congenital hyperplasia the deficiency of cortisone causes excessive pituitary adrenocorticotrophin (ACTH) production, which in turn produces the abnormally stimulated adrenal. The steroids which are secreted by the adrenal, in lieu of cortisone, suppress the pituitary gonadotrophins, and ovarian insufficiency and amenorrhea ensue.

There is reason to believe that certain patients with postpubertal virilization also have the same, or a related, problem but to a milder degree. This is evidenced by the course of the disease and the clinical and laboratory findings, and substantiated by the adrenal histology. There are, however, a majority of hirsute patients with many similar clinical findings who apparently do not have a true enzymic insufficiency, as in the congenital form of adrenal hyperplasia, but rather are suffering from a physiologic insufficiency induced by stress. There is some evidence that in a predominately Mediterranean population, where hirsutism is relatively common, the rate of adrenal *androgen* to *corti-*

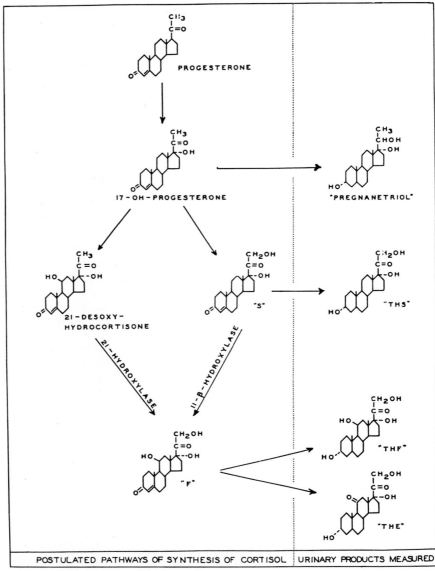

POSTULATED PATHWAYS OF SYNTHESIS OF CORTISOL | URINARY PRODUCTS MEASURED

Fig. 31.9. Urinary corticoids in the adrenogenital syndrome showing the possible theoretical implications in relation to precursor steroids. S, 17α-hydroxydeoxycortisone; THS, pregnan-3α,17α-21-triol-20-one; F, 17α-hydroxycorticosterone (cortisol); THF, pregnan-3α,11β,17α,21-tetrol-20-one; THE, pregnan-3α,17α,21-triol-11-20-dione.

sol production is increased. Blackman, in a morphological study of the adrenal of hirsute women, noted an increase in the size of the *zona reticulata* regardless of the cause of the hirsutism. Both observations substantiate the belief that in women with a hirsute tendency there is a "variation" of normal adrenal function.

Dorfman *et al.* have demonstrated that Δ_4-androstenedione inhibits 11β-hydroxylase activity in the adrenal. If a patient has a tendency to synthesize adrenal androgens excessively, under *stress* the increased rate of synthesis of andro-stenedione might be sufficient to start a vicious circle.

Bush and Mahesh have published a fascinating case report of twins, one of whom developed hirsutism under particularly stressful circumstances. Both twins exhibited a high androgen:cortisol ratio following ACTH stimulation. The authors postulate that chronic stress constituted a prolonged ACTH test for the one twin who thereby produced enough androgen to initiate the hirsutism. There may be many such women in the general population who have either a very slight congenitally defective adrenal cortex or simply represent the extreme of the normal variation in the rate of adrenal androgen production. If the adrenal secretion rate is accelerated by stress, symptoms such as hirsutism, acne, oligomenorrhea and infertility appear.

The treatment for congenital adrenal hyperplasia, postpubertal virilization and related disturbances is cortisone substitution therapy; 50 mg. of cortisone acetate or its equivalent, daily by mouth, is usually adequate to maintain a ketosteroid excretion suppression of about 5 mg. per 24 hours, which is the desirable level. If it is impossible to maintain the suppression, one must suspect a tumor of the adrenal or ovarian pathology as discussed in this chapter under "The Stein-Leventhal Syndrome."

In the relatively mild forms it is often possible to maintain a suppression with as little as 25 mg. of cortisone acetate daily (or its equivalent) after the initial suppression has been well established. In the congenital form, which is due to a genetic deficiency of a specific adrenal enzyme, therapy will need to be continued throughout life. However, in the form induced by stress, once the vicious circle has been interrupted, steroid therapy can be discontinued until the next stressful situation develops.

There were 46 women in this category in our series of amenorrheic patients. Four had severe forms of congenital adrenal hyperplasia and 42 were cases of related dysfunctions. Of 27 patients adequately treated and followed, 23 were improved and 8 of 13 married patients achieved a pregnancy.

CUSHING'S DISEASE. In contrast to congenital adrenal hyperplasia, Cushing's disease represents a hyperfunction of the entire adrenal cortex including the cortisone-secreting zona fasciculata. The pituitary-adrenal homeostatic mechanisms are out of control as there is excessive ACTH production in the presence of excessive cortisol. Cushing in his initial publication believed that the syndrome was always the result of a pituitary tumor or pituitary basophilism. Since the initial paper, however, it has become clear that bilateral adrenal hyperplasia may occur without a demonstrable pituitary lesion and adrenal tumors are not infrequently responsible for the condition. In addition to these possibilities, Heinbecker has implicated the hypothalamus as the primary disease site. Thus, when Cushing's disease exists, the differential diagnosis must be made among a pituitary tumor, bilateral hyperplasia of the adrenals, or adrenal tumor.

In addition to the three principle primary sites of origin for the syndrome, there is a fourth unusual one. Two reports have appeared in the literature of Cushing's disease resulting from an adrenal rest tumor in the ovary (Kepler et al. and Rottino and McGrath). In this era of corticosteroid therapy for many diseases, the physician should also be alerted to the possibility of an iatrogenic factor in the production of a Cushing-like picture.

The subject of etiology has been extensively reviewed by Plotz, and according to autopsy findings in 97 cases, carcinoma of the adrenal occurred 16 times, adenoma 11 times, benign hyperplasia 58 times. A pituitary adenoma was associated with adenomatous hyperplasia 40 times and with carcinoma and benign adrenal adenoma once. There were changes in the paraventricular nucleus in 8 instances, and these 8 instances were distributed evenly among the adrenal carcinomas, hyperplasias, and pituitary adenomas.

Cushing's disease is characterized by obesity, amenorrhea, moon face, hirsutism, hypertension, purple striae, erythemic acne, and easy bruisability. The pelvic organs are usually normal and there is no enlargement of the clitoris or marked vaginal atrophy. When the full-blown picture exists the syndrome is so striking that the diagnosis is blatant; however, in the early stages it may be extremely difficult (Fig. 31.10). The laboratory findings are characterized by an elevation of the urinary and blood corticoids. The urinary 17-ketosteroid assay is usually normal or only moderately elevated; if an adrenal tumor is present it may be markedly elevated. There is a polycythemia, diabetic glucose tolerance curve, and x-ray evidence of osteoporosis. The typical response to ACTH stimulation is an over-reaction with at least a 3-fold increase of the urinary and blood corticoids. It is usually impossible to suppress the urinary corticoids below 10 mg./24 hours by cortisone. When an adrenal tumor is present there is usually no response to ACTH stimulation or cortisol suppression. Unfortunately, however, not all tumors are autonomous and some do show a response.

The treatment of the disease depends upon its etiology. Sosman recommends irradiation of the pituitary for those patients without adrenal tumors. Certainly this is the method of choice if a pituitary tumor can be demonstrated. However, most authorities have recommended adrenal extirpation for bilateral adrenal hyperplasia. The decision between pituitary irradiation and adrenalectomy is further complicated by the difficulty in excluding the possibility of an adrenal tumor. This may be attempted by perirenal carbon dioxide insufflation, by laminography, by simple intravenous pyelograms with attention to the adrenal shadow, or by adrenal angiogram. In our experience none of these is completely satisfactory.

It is often possible to decide at operation, by the appearance of one adrenal, whether or not there is a tumor in the other. If at operation the exposed gland is atrophied, it should be left in situ with a presumptive diagnosis of a contralateral tumor. If, however, the exposed adrenal is hypertrophied it is removed with all or 90% of the opposite gland. When the partial operation is performed there is always a possibility that a second operation will be necessary; however, this seems like a worthwhile risk to take in an effort to prevent lifelong invalidism with dependence upon prolonged, expensive replacement therapy.

Stress Obesity. A borderline clinical picture with moderately elevated urinary corticoids occurs more frequently than true Cushing's disease. It is thought that this picture represents the response of certain individuals to the "*stress of obesity.*" There were 7 such patients in our series of amenorrheic women, and the treatment was simple weight reduction. The one patient who cooperated and reduced to a normal figure had a remission of all her symptoms.

Nutritional Amenorrhea

One of the basic influences which determines how any endocrine gland may act, or indeed any substitution therapy, is the diet. Richter has ably demonstrated this clinical factor in a laboratory animal, by using self-selective diets in rats. Adrenalectomized, parathyroidectomized, and pancreatectomized animals can all adjust to their deficiencies if allowed a sufficient choice of diet.

In the human the importance of malnutrition in reproductive function has been demonstrated. Disturbances of reproductive functions can be caused in animal experimentation by specific caloric deficiencies, protein deficiencies, or vitamin deficiencies with special reference to vitamins A, B, and C. Whether one or all of these factors operate in nutritional amenorrhea of the human is undetermined. There is a relatively large literature by European authors on the occur-

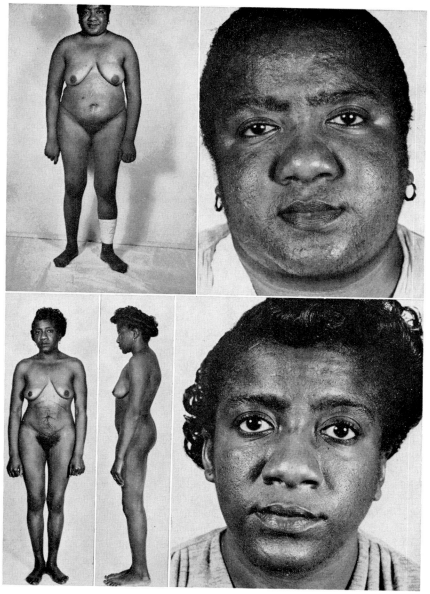

FIG. 31.10. Patient with Cushing's disease due to benign hyperplasia of the adrenal glands. *Upper,* before adrenalectomy the characteristic obesity, moon face, and hirsutism can be seen. Although the purple abdominal striae are not apparent the acniform rash can be seen on the chest. *Lower,* after operation the patient has regained her normal appearance. Some hirsutism persists. (From Jones, H. W., Jr., and Scott, W. W.: *Hermaphroditism, Genital Anomalies and Related Endocrine Disorders.* The Williams & Wilkins Company, 1958.)

rence of nutritional amenorrhea during World Wars I and II but it is generally difficult for the authors to separate nutritional from psychogenic factors. Heyne-mann was of the opinion that nutrition played an important part in war amenorrhea, as he observed an increase in the incidence in Germany after 1944 when the deterioration of food supplies occurred. Plotz believed that the protein deficiency aspects were most important and reported that 17 of 19 women with nutritional amenorrhea of over 1 year's duration responded to an amino acid preparation. The first vaginal bleeding occurred after an average of 31 days of therapy and permanent success was achieved in almost every case.

It is the general opinion, quoted by Seitz, that nutritional amenorrhea is usually reversible; 80% of the patients reviewed recovered with improved nutrition. However, the prognosis is graver when the nutritional damage occurs at or just prior to puberty. This is in keeping with the experience in animal experimentation, reviewed by Asdell, which indicates that the younger the animal when nutritional damage occurs the more difficult it is to repair. There is also some evidence that residual damage may result; Klebarow reports a 75% incidence of infertility among concentration camp victims of World War II who suffered severe malnutritions, in contrast to a 25% incidence of infertility in the general population. He further states that this may be attributable to damage of the germinal cells, as impaired spermatogenesis, under similar circumstances, was found among males. Stafko, in an examination of ovaries of 120 women who died of starvation, found an absence of primordial follicles and replacement of the cortical layer with scar tissue indicating that the amenorrhea might be primarily due to ovarian damage. The occurrence of amenorrhea in patients with exogenous obesity is somewhat more difficult to explain but may be based on some relative dietary imbalance associated with the abnormal caloric intake.

The treatment of both malnutrition and obesity is directed toward general dietary habits—either weight gain or weight reduction, with a well balanced high protein diet. Of 16 recent patients with exogenous obesity and amenorrhea, only 9 were adequately treated and followed. Seven were improved with regular menses when a normal weight was acquired, and

1 became pregnant. Two were unimproved. There were 9 patients with malnutrition and 6 were followed. Only 3 showed a satisfactory weight gain and all 3 responded with regular menses.

Disturbances of Steroid Excretion and Metabolism

Liver Cirrhosis. The conjugation and metabolism of estrogens and progesterone takes place in the liver; the excretion is accomplished to a large extent through the bile and hepatic portal system to the bowel. In cirrhosis of the liver, impairment of conjugation of estrogen leads to an excess of circulating active estrogens. This may result in functional bleeding interspersed with periods of amenorrhea. Although this is certainly the most common menstrual cycle aberration associated with cirrhosis, Green and Rubin report 18 patients having amenorrhea as the menstrual symptom. The diagnosis is made on the basis of the physical findings and liver function tests.

The treatment is medical and the prognosis is poor.

LESIONS OF PERIPHERAL ORIGIN

Ovarian

Ovarian causes for amenorrhea can be classified as follows.

(1) *Ovarian insufficiency:* (a) congenital defects, gonadal dysgenesis, and related conditions; (b) the premature menopause, congenital and acquired.

(2) *Ovarian dysfunction:* Stein-Leventhal syndrome (possibly hypothalamic in origin).

(3) *Ovarian tumors:* (a) arrhenoblastoma, hilus cell tumor, and adrenal rest tumor; (b) granulosa cell tumor; (c) dysgerminoma.

All of these conditions, with the exception of the ovarian tumors, are characterized by the laboratory finding of an elevated urinary gonadotrophin assay. Although the values in the patients with the Stein-Leventhal syndrome may be lower and more variable than those found in other types, they also tend to be moderately elevated.

Congenitally Defective Gonads.
GONADAL AGENESIS (TURNER'S SYN-
DROME). In 1938 Turner described a
syndrome of "infantilism," congenital
webbed neck, and decubitus valgus.
Albright, Smith, and Fraser, in 1942,
demonstrated the association of this
syndrome with an elevated urinary gonadotrophin titer, and Wilkins and Fleischmann in 1944 described the pathology
which was characterized by absence
of gonads and the presence of normally
developed but immature Müllerian ducts.
The gonads are represented grossly by a
primitive streak of white or yellow, and
microscopically by stroma only or by
stroma and Leydig cells. In 1954 a
number of investigators independently
reported that a majority of these patients
had a negative or male type chromatin
pattern, and in 1959 Ford and Jones
reported that at least some of these patients with negative chromatin patterns
represented not an XY but an XO
configuration of sex chromosomes. These
contributions provided the building stones
for a satisfactory explanation of the
syndrome. Those patients who show an
OX or a fragmented XX chromosomal
configuration can be explained on the
basis of nondysjunction of the sex
chromosomes associated apparently with
other chromosomal abnormalities to
account for the concomitant congenital
defects. Patients who have a normal XX
chromosome pattern may represent the
result of embryonic gonadal damage
prior to the 8th week of development.
Under these circumstances, in the absence
of the embryonic gonadal organizers, the
Müllerian ducts are retained and the
external genitalia develop in a female
manner, according to the experimental
embryological investigations of Jost.

Every stage of developmental anomaly
can be seen in the negative chromatin
patients—from gonads with a few Leydig
cells associated with female genitalia and
hypertrophy of the clitoris only (first
described by Pich in 1937), to almost
normal testicular development and male
external genitalia except for hypospadia.
For a complete summary of this abnormal
development see the text by Jones and
Scott.

The clinical features of a typical Turner's syndrome are so characteristic that
one can recognize such a patient as she
walks into the consultation room. There
is shortness of stature, webbing of the
neck, deformity of the carrying angle, a
shield type chest with nipples placed far
laterally, no breast development, and
scanty or absent axillary and pubic hair.
From this typical picture of Turner's
syndrome and dwarf stature there are all
gradations through the normal stature
with eunuchoid proportions (Fig. 31.11)
to gigantism with or without other stig-
mata. In addition a number of other
associated congenital defects have been
described, the most important one being
coarctation of the aorta.

The laboratory findings are characteristic in that there must be an elevated
urinary gonadotrophin level, and most of
the patients exhibit a negative chromatin
pattern; the buccal smear, therefore, is
often the most rapid and least expensive
way to make a diagnosis. Thyroid studies
are normal. The urinary 17-ketosteroid
excretion is normal or low.

Until such a time when transplantation
of organs is feasible, the treatment of this
condition will remain as substitution
therapy only. Estrogen is given in interrupted dosage, depending upon the
amount of drug necessary to induce vaginal bleeding: 0.5 to 2 mg. of stilbestrol, or
its equivalent, daily through the 25th
day of each month, discontinued and
resumed the 1st day of the following
month.

In cases of dwarfism, if the patient is
pubertal and epiphyseal fusion has not
occurred, smaller dosages of estrogen over
longer periods of time should be tried in
an effort to induce a maximal growth
spurt prior to epiphyseal closure which
will occur with estrogen stimulation.
Whitelaw et al. report a growth of 9.5
cm. in a year in a patient treated with
an anabolic steroid and suggest that this
form of therapy should be given until
epiphyseal closure or failed response

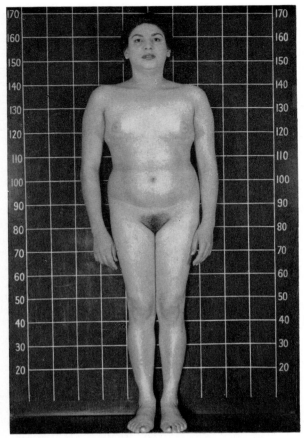

FIG. 31.11. Gonadal dysgenesis with normal height. Notice typical shield chest with nipples placed far laterally. Buccal smear showed a negative chromatin pattern and the gonadotrophin hormone (FSH) level was elevated.

occur. They advise liver function tests and observation for androgenicity.

Therapy may be expected to induce normal breast development, vaginal cornification, and menstruation. The induction of menstruation is usually desirable for psychological reasons. Pregnancy, of course, cannot be expected to occur, and axillary and pubic hair will usually remain scanty or absent unless an androgenic stimulus is supplied. This is possibly due to an associated adrenal insufficiency but might also be indirect evidence for the normal occurrence of an ovarian androgen. If coarctation of the aorta is present surgical correction wherever possible should be advised, and if webbing of the neck is deforming, plastic surgery can offer excellent cosmetic results. It is

well to have a psychological evaluation, and therapeutic consultations if necessary, to insure that the patient is adjusted to her limitations and will thus be able to live a completely normal life except for ability to bear children.

There were 20 patients with gonadal agenesis among our series of 352 women with amenorrhea.

TRUE HERMAPHRODITISM. True hermaphroditism is extremely rare. A summary of the 58 cases reported in the literature up to 1955 can be found in the textbook on this subject by Jones and Scott. Most true hermaphrodites are raised as men and this was the case in 39 of the 58 patients reported. This indicates, of course, that in a majority of instances the external genitalia are masculine rather than feminine in appearance. The condition should be suspected in patients who show some ambiguity of the external genitalia, associated with breast development. Minimal hirsutism may occur but has been absent in the majority of the reported cases.

These cases are interesting from the point of view of experimental embryology, as they indicate that the male gonad exerts a strong influence on the development of external genitalia. Thus, even in the 16 patients in the literature who showed an ovary on one side and an ovotestis on the other, only 8 had been raised as females. The Müllerian duct must be more positively influenced by the ovarian organizer, since a normal uterus was present in about half of the patients. Almost all of these individuals menstruated; thus, in contrast to gonadal dysgenesis, the ovarian tissue present in true hermaphrodites is functioning.

The diagnosis can be suspected by the physical findings, and the laboratory data are of very little assistance. The chromatin pattern can be positive or negative and the 17-ketosteroid and gonadotrophin assays are within normal range. The diagnosis therefore is made by the pathologist at the time of operation, and the treatment is surgical correction.

MALE HERMAPHRODITISM. Male hermaphrodites show ambiguous external genitalia, no breast development, minimal hirsutism, and a negative chromatin pattern. This condition has been discussed in Chapter 8 in detail. There was 1 such congenital abnormality among our series of patients.

TESTICULAR FEMINIZATION. This interesting form of hermaphroditism is characterized by a normal female appearance with excellent breast development and completely normal female external genitalia. However, in about a third of the cases there is either no axillary or pubic hair, or the axillary and pubic hair is extremely scanty. There is a short or absent vagina and no cervix. The differential diagnosis must be made between this condition and that of congenital absence of the Müllerian ducts. A negative chromatin pattern is confirmatory of a diagnosis of testicular feminization.

The laboratory findings are bizarre and can vary widely. Some patients show an elevated urinary gonadotrophin. Others show urinary gonadotrophins in the normal range. Most patients have a 17-ketosteroid excretion compatible with a normal male, and estrogen excretion compatible with a normal female. Morris has recently reported a comprehensive survey of his experience with this condition. The findings in the testis have been described in detail in Chapter 8. The assumption is that this is a heritable developmental enzymatic defect of the testosterone target organs.

The treatment is operative removal of the testes after the age of puberty and vaginal plastic procedure if indicated. One patient among the 252 with amenorrhea was found to have this condition.

Ovarian Insufficiency. PREMATURE MENOPAUSE, CONGENITAL. The idiopathic premature menopause can be familial or sporadic. The description, in 1959 by Jacobs and Baikie, of a patient with a premature menopause who showed a triplo-X chromosomal pattern associated with multichromocenters in cells from a buccal smear, indicates that this condition may also be associated with nondysjunction of chromosomes or a disturbance related to gonadal dysgenesis. The ovaries of such individuals may appear small and deformed or almost normal grossly. Microscopically, the appearance is indistinguishable from that of a normal ovary.

ACQUIRED DEFECTS. In addition to the congenital types of ovarian defects, ovarian destruction can occur in association with (1) tuberculous pelvic inflammatory disease, (2) irradiation, or (3) operative procedures. Very occasionally, primary amenorrhea results when pelvic tuberculosis occurs in a prepubertal child. Such a case has been described by Reiss. Under these circumstances, of course, eunuchoid proportions and gigantism are associated.

The diagnosis of a premature menopause can be suspected when the patient gives a history of hot flushes; but the laboratory finding of an elevated urinary gonadotrophin is the absolute criterion. There is no cure for a premature menopause, and therapy must be substitutional only. This is discussed in Chapter 34. There were 24 patients, among the series reported, who had a premature menopause.

Ovarian Tumors. Amenorrhea related to ovarian tumors has been discussed in Chapter 25.

End Organs: Uterine and Vaginal Cryptomenorrhea

The conditions embraced under this heading are: traumatic occlusion of the vagina; the imperforate hymen; congenital absence or atresia of the vagina; vaginal septa; congenital absence of the Müllerian ducts; traumatic occlusion of the cervix; and destruction of the endometrium.

Occlusion of the Vagina and Cervix. The term *gynatresia* is applied to occlusion of any part of the genital canal. It may be of congenital or acquired origin.

CAUSES. The congenital causes embrace any of the forms of congenital occlusion which have been discussed in Chapter 7, "Congenital Anomalies of the Female Generative Organs." The most important is imperforate hymen, although occasionally the congenital block involves the cervical or vaginal segment of the canal.

SYMPTOMS. When atresia of the cervix or any part of the vagina is present, or when the hymen is imperforate, the menstrual discharge, if it occurs, is retained behind the obstruction. Of these causes, imperforate hymen is much the most common. The retained blood distends the vagina (*hematocolpos*) while with succeeding periods there is distention of the cervix (*hematotrachelos*), uterine cavity (*hematometra*), and finally even of the tubes (*hematosalpinx*).

With each succeeding period there is increasing pain and discomfort. When the uterine distention becomes marked, a bulging enlargement of the lower abdomen develops, and the patient's discomfort may be extreme, especially at the time of the periods. Difficulty in voiding is a common symptom.

DIAGNOSIS. The diagnosis in such cases is usually easy, especially in the case of imperforate hymen. The distended hymen actually bulges forward from the pressure of the retained blood (see Plates VII.I and VII.II), and fluctuation can be felt both through the hymen and on rectal examination. In the less frequent cases in which the obstruction is higher up, the diagnosis is not always so obvious, but a history of regularly recurring menstrual molimina, with increasing menstrual discomfort without external menstrual flow, together with the finding of a fluctuating mass on bimanual abdominorectal palpation, will leave little doubt as to the nature of the condition.

TREATMENT. The treatment in the case of imperforate hymen is simple, consisting simply in slow evacuation of the blood through a crucial incision in the hymen. Strict asepsis must of course be observed, and most writers, whether justifiably or not, warn of the especial proneness of such patients to infection. After evacuation of the blood, the hymen may be excised, or as some prefer, gently but widely divulsed, to avoid agglutination and secondary closure.

In the case of obstruction higher up, the problem is not so simple. If the lower vagina is involved, and the septum thin, somewhat the same plan may be followed as with imperforate hymen. But if the obstruction is higher and the intervening mass of tissue thick, much care is necessary in evacuating the blood, and the later treatment may involve some form of plastic operation for what is essentially absence of the vagina.

Acquired Gynatresia. Gynatresia is by no means always due to congenital factors, and as a matter of fact the acquired variety is more frequent. The portions of the genital canal which by their occlusion may cause retention of the genital discharge are the cervix and the vagina. Especially frequent is the cervix, the canal of which is normally much the narrowest portion of the uterovaginal tract.

CAUSES. The most important causes of acquired gynatresia are the following.

Senile Contraction. Although atrophy of the genital canal, including its mucosa, occurs normally after the menopause, it may in some women be so extreme as to cause blockage of the cervix and occasionally of the vagina. This is especially true because of the proneness of the thin, senile mucous membrane to secondary infection and ulceration. As a result of complete occlusion of the cervical canal in the woman who is no longer menstruating, the retained discharge consists of pus rather than blood, although there may be a bloody admixture because of the presence of granulation tissue in the wall of the retention cavity. Such retention of pus in the uterine cavity is called *pyometra.* It is very gradual in development, with often no symptoms for many months. Attention is called to the condition in many cases by the seepage of slight amounts of blood from the granulation tissue in the cervical canal, whereas in other cases there may be pelvic discomfort or even the development of a mass.

Malignant Disease. One of the most common of all causes of gynatresia is malignant disease, usually of the cervix. Either epidermoid or adenocarcinoma may be responsible, and in most cases there has been an antecedent history of bleeding from the cancer. A not uncommon occurrence, especially in older women, is to encounter the pyometra in the course of diagnostic curettage performed because of postmenopausal bleeding. In other cases the pyometra develops in the late stages of carcinoma whose existence has long been known.

Radiotherapy and Cauterization. As a result of the radiotherapy universally employed for carcinoma of the cervix, stricture or complete atresia of the cervical canal may occur, with pyometra as the usual result. Such postradiation strictures may not develop until a long time, even several years, after the application of radium. The widely prevalent and sometimes injudicious or improper use of the cautery in the treatment of cervicitis has left in its wake a definite incidence of strictures of the cervix and even complete atresia of the canal. The same result may follow the use of chemical caustics, such as strong solutions of nitrate of silver, within the cervix.

Surgical Operations. An occasional result of operations upon the cervix is the occurrence of stricture or atresia. This may follow even simple dilatation when this is associated with laceration of the tissue, but is more likely to occur after cervical cauterization, conization, or such plastic operations as the Sturmdorf tracheloplasty or cervical amputation.

SYMPTOMS. When a previously normal woman ceases to menstruate, but suffers severe colicky pain at the time of the expected period, the possibility of gynatresia should be suspected, especially if there is a history of one of the causative factors enumerated above. The pain recurs at each menstrual date, and pelvic examination will usually, within a month or two, reveal evidence of distention of the uterus, if, as is most common, the obstruction is in the cervix. The latter becomes large and broad, and develops a peculiar elastic feel, with sometimes distinct fluctuation. Later the body of the uterus likewise becomes large and fluctuant.

When the gynatresia occurs in postmenopausal women, its development is much more insidious and its recognition more difficult, because the retained genital secretion is far less in amount than the normal menstrual flow. In a large proportion of cases pyometra is found accidentally, as already mentioned. The retained secretion commonly undergoes secondary infection, and there may be fever or chills, in addition to increasing pelvic discomfort and slight bleeding.

DIAGNOSIS. When such symptoms as have been described lead to the suspicion of cervical occlusion, the diagnosis can be made reasonably certain by direct exploration of the cervical canal by the uterine sound, always under strict aseptic precautions. When the occlusion is light, the probe itself may be followed by a telltale trickle of blood or pus. When the blockage is tight even a very fine probe will fail to enter the uterus. In such cases the diagnosis can be made by passing a large caliber aspirating needle through the cervical wall into the distended cavity.

TREATMENT. The treatment of the common forms of acquired gynatresia consists of dilatation followed by drainage. The dilatation may be a comparatively simple office procedure, although it must be repeated from time to time, as most strictures of the cervix have a tendency to contract down. Small olive-pointed metal dilators are ordinarily most useful.

Congenital Absence of the Müllerian Ducts. This condition is characterized by a normal development and normal endocrine findings, with absence of the uterus and upper third of the vagina. As mentioned previously, it must be differentiated from testicular feminization and this can be done by the buccal smear which is positive, or feminine, in type. Once the diagnosis is made it must be determined as accurately as possible whether there is absence of the uterus as well as a congenital absence of the upper third of the vagina. In rare instances there is simply a vaginal constriction band and a normal uterus is present above. In this case, of course, a surgical procedure will assure normal reproductive function, whereas, if the uterus is absent, the only procedure required is either a vaginal plastic operation or the use of a Frank tube to produce a vagina by pressure, as described in 1928. One patient in the present series had a transverse vaginal septum and was cured by simple incision.

Destruction of the Endometrium and Traumatic Strictures of the Cervix. This condition has been classically described by Asherman. Although usually associated with secondary amenorrhea, the condition can, very occasion-

ally, be the cause of primary amenorrhea, as when pelvic tuberculosis has involved the endometrium extensively prepubertally. Aside from tuberculosis, cervical stenosis and endometrial sclerosis are almost always secondary to a dilatation and curettage or some other intracervical or intrauterine procedure which has been unduly traumatic or associated with an inflammatory process. A postpartum or postabortion curettage, as well as procedures associated with criminal abortions, classically predispose to this type of scarring.

Diagnosis of amenorrhea associated with destructive or congenital lesions of the end organs is made on the basis of an examination and curettage which demonstrate a vaginal or cervical obstruction or scarring of the endometrium. The basal temperature chart indicates ovulation in the absence of menstruation, and after the administration of adequate amounts of estrogen withdrawal fails to induce menstruation. Although frequently advocated as a diagnostic aid in this condition, the hysterogram is usually unsatisfactory.

The treatment of the condition is repeated dilatation of the cervix and curettage. Although this seems paradoxical, the therapeutic effect is probably due to the "freshening up" of the scar tissue, allowing the remains of the basalis layer of the endometrium to regrow. Various operative procedures, originating with that of Strassman, have been advocated for the correction of the condition. These differ mainly only in the use of different materials to substitute for the endometrial lining. The success obtained with any of these procedures can probably be attributed to the regenerative powers of the endometrium when the cervix is patent.

There were 6 patients with cryptomenorrhea in our series of amenorrheic women, and 2 have become pregnant after repeated curettages.

PHYSIOLOGICAL AMENORRHEA

Physiological types of amenorrhea need only be mentioned briefly as associated with puberty, pregnancy, and the menopause.

Delayed Puberty

The diagnosis of delayed puberty might be best included under lesions of the nervous system, as it is now our concept that puberty is initiated by maturation of the hypothalamus rather than of the pituitary.

Statistically speaking, the diagnosis cannot be made until after the age of 17 years, although any delay of menstruation after 14 years is considered delayed over the average age. The diagnosis is made when the history, physical findings, and laboratory data are all within normal limits, and it is facilitated if there is a family history of a delayed menarche. The causes are numerous, the most important being poor general health, nutrition, or hygiene.

A careful follow-up examination should be made yearly until one is sure that the correct diagnosis has been established. There were 3 patients among our group with this diagnosis and all 3 are menstruating regularly at the present time.

Pregnancy and Postpartum Amenorrhea

Any patient presenting with amenorrhea is presumed to be pregnant until proved otherwise. If the physical examination is equivocal, a pregnancy test can be performed to exclude the diagnosis. Postpartum amenorrhea is usual, especially if the patient nurses her baby. The normal duration of this amenorrhea is between 6 weeks and 3 months if the patient does not lactate. If the patient has nursed, menses usually return within 6 months of delivery, or 6 weeks after cessation of lactation; any period of amenorrhea longer than this can be considered as prolonged, lactation amenorrhea. A differential diagnosis must be made between this physiological condition and true Sheehan's disease, pituitary necrosis caused by the destruction of the gland at the time of the traumatic delivery. If there is a history of a postpartum dilatation and curettage, the possibility of endometrial sclerosis must also be entertained. The diagnosis of postpartum amenorrhea is made on the basis of a history of an uncomplicated delivery and normal laboratory findings. However, this differential diagnosis is not to be made didactically for, if destruction of the pituitary (Sheehan's disease) has not been complete, the findings may be identical with those of postpartum lactation amenorrhea. The Chiari-Frommel syndrome is another variant.

Time will usually suffice to cure the condition but cyclic steroid therapy will often suppress the pituitary prolactin and predispose to a more rapid resumption of regular menses.

In the series of amenorrheic women reported there were 16 with prolonged postpartum amenorrhea. Fourteen patients were followed adequately and 8 have had subsequent pregnancies; an additional 3 have menstruated regularly and 3 remain amenorrheic.

SUMMARY

In summary, amenorrhea and oligomenorrhea must always be regarded as symptoms, not a disease. The decision as to whether or not these symptoms require investigation or treatment must be made on the basis of the individual case. Investigation is usually indicated if infertility is a complaint, if the patient is anxious or disturbed about the absence of menstruation, or if there are associated signs and symptoms suggestive of a serious physical problem. When primary amenorrhea exists it is always important to determine if an anatomical abnormality of the genitalia exists. No intelligent approach can be made to treatment until a proper etiological diagnosis has been attained. With the addition of human pituitary gonadotrophins and clomiphene to our therapeutic armamentaria, the results of therapy are more encouraging.

REFERENCES

Ahumada, J. C., and Del Castillo, E. B.: Amenorrea y galactorrea. Bol. Soc. Obstit. Ginec., *11:* 64, 1932.

Albright, F., Smith, P. H., and Fraser, R.: A syndrome characterized by primary ovarian insufficiency and decreased stature; report of 11 cases with digression on hormonal control of axillary and pubic hair. Amer. J. Med. Sci., *204:* 625, 1942.

Allen, W. M., and Woolf, R. B.: Medullary resection of the ovaries in the Stein-Leventhal syndrome. Amer. J. Obstet. Gynec., *77:* 826, 1959.

Asdell, S. A.: Reproduction. Ann. Rev. Physiol., *12:* 537, 1950.

Asherman, J. G.: Traumatic intra-uterine adhesions. J. Obstet. Gynaec. Brit. Comm., *57:* 892, 1950.

Barraclough, C. A.: Production of anovulatory, sterile rats by single injections of testosterone proprionate. Endocrinology, *68:* 62, 1961.

Bass, F.: L'amenorrhée au camp de concentration de Terezin (Theresienstadt). Gynaecologia (Basel), *123:* 211, 1947.

Bergman, P.: Clinical treatment of anovulation. Int. J. Fertil., *3:* 27, 1958.

Bickers, W.: Amenorrhea and oligomenorrhea; etiology and treatment. Amer. J. Obstet. Gynec., *56:* 893, 1948.

Blackman, S.: Concerning the function and origin of a reticular zone of the adrenal cortex; hyperplasia in the adrenogenital syndrome. Bull. Hopkins Hosp., *78:* 180, 1946.

Bliss, E. L., and Migeon, C. J.: Endocrinology of anorexia nervosa. J. Clin. Endocr., *17:* 766, 1957.

Bricaire, H., Moreau, L., Elissade, B., and Bouvier, J. M.: Amenorrhoea and galactorrhoea syndrome in connection with a nonmalignant chromophalic tumor of the hypophysis. Ann. Endocr. (Paris), *19:* 719, 1958.

Burns, R. K., Jr.: The effects of male hormone on differentiation of the urogenital sinus in young opposums. Contrib. Embryol., *31:* 163, 1945.

Bush, I. E., and Mohesh, V. B.: Adrenocortical hyperfunction with sudden onset of hirsutism. J. Endocr., *18:* 1, 1959.

Crooke, A. C., Butt, W. R., Palmer, R., Morris, R., Edwards, R. L., Gaylor, G. W., and Short, R. B.: The effect of human pituitary follicle-stimulating hormone and chorionic gonadotrophic in Stein-Leventhal syndrome. Brit. Med. J., *1:* 1119, 1963.

Cushing, H.: The basophil adenomas of the pituitary body and their clinical manifestations (pituitary basophilism). Bull. Hopkins Hosp., *50:* 137, 1932.

Dally, P. I., and Sargeant, W.: A new treatment for anorexia nervosa. Brit. Med. J., *1:* 1770, 1960.

Decourt, J., and Michard, J.: Les amenorrhees psychogenes. Sem. Hop. Paris, *25:* 3352, 1949.

di Paola, G., and Lelio, M.: Respuesta inusitada de los ovarios a la gonadotrofinas. Obstet. Ginec. Lat. Amer., *12:* 490, 1954.

Drill, V. A., and Pfeiffer, C. A.: Effect of vitamin B-complex deficiency, controlled inanition, and methionine on inactivation of estrogen by the liver. Endocrinology, *38:* 300, 1946.

Emanuel, R. W.: Endocrine findings in anorexia nervosa. J. Clin. Endocr., *16:* 801, 1956.

Engle, E. T.: Luteinization of ovary of monkey by means of combined use of anterior pituitary extract and extract of pregnancy urine. Endocrinology, *18:* 513, 1934.

Everson, C., Williams, E., Wheeler, E., Swenson, P., Spivey, M., and Eppright, M.: The occurrence of five B-vitamins in the tissues of pregnant rats fed rations satisfactory and unsatisfactory for reproduction. J. Nutr., *36:* 463, 1948.

Forbes, A. P., Henneman, P. H., Griswold, G. C., and Albright, F.: Syndrome characterized by galactorrhea, amenorrhea and low urinary FSH; comparison with acromegaly and normal lactation. J. Clin. Endocr., *14:* 265, 1954.

Ford, C. E., and Jones, K. W.: Sex chromosome anomaly in a case of gonadal dysgenesis (Turner's syndrome). Lancet, *1:* 711, 1959.

Garcia, R., Pincus, G., and Rock, J.: Effect of three 19-*nor*-steroids on human ovulation and menstruation. Amer. J. Obstet. Gynec., *75:* 82, 1958.

Geist, S. H.: Reaction of mature human ovary to Antiuitrin-S. Amer. J. Obstet. Gynec., *26:* 588, 1933.

Gitlow, S., and Kurschner, D. M.: Estrogen, diabetes and menopause. Arch. Intern. Med. (Chicago), *72:* 250, 1943.

Glass, B.: Hazards of atomic radiation to man; British and American report. J. Hered., *47:* 260, 1956.

Green, P., and Rubin, L.: Amenorrhea as a manifestation of chronic liver disease. Amer. J. Obstet. Gynec., *78:* 141, 1959.

Greene, O., Migeon, C., and Wilkins, L.: Urinary steroids in the hypertensive form of congenital adrenal hyperplasia. J. Clin. Endocr., *20:* 929, 1960.

Guinet, P., and Mornex, R.: L'eunuchisme hypogonadotrophique chez la femme. Rev. Lyon. Med., *6:* 39, 1957.

Hamblen, E. C.: Results of preoperative administration of extract of pregnancy urine; study of ovaries and endometria in hyperplasia of endometrium following such administration. Endocrinology, *19:* 169, 1935.

Hartman, C. G.: Use of gonadotropic hormone in adult rhesus monkey. Bull. Hopkins Hosp., *63:* 351, 1938.

Heinbecker, P.: Pathogenesis of Cushing's syndrome. Medicine, *23:* 225, 1944.

Heynemann, T.: Die Nachkriegsamenorrhoe. Klin. Wschr., *26:* 129, 1948.

Igarashi, M., and Matsumoto, S.: Induction of human ovulation by individualized gonadotrophin therapy. Amer. J. Obstet. Gynec., 73: 1294, 1957.

Ingersoll, F. M., and McArthur, J. W.: Longitudinal studies of gonadotrophin excretion in Stein-Leventhal syndrome. Amer. J. Obstet. Gynec., 77: 801, 1959.

Israel, S. L.: Empiric usage of low-dosage irradiation in amenorrhea. Amer. J. Obstet. Gynec., 64: 971, 1952.

Israel, S. L., and Constan, A. S.: Unrecognized pituitary necrosis (Sheehan's syndrome); a cause of sudden death. J. A. M. A., 148: 189, 1952.

Jacobs, P. A., and Baikie, A. G.: Evidence for the existence of the human super female. Lancet, 2: 423, 1959.

Jones, H. W., and Jones, G. E. S.: Gynecological aspects of adrenal hyperplasia and allied disorders. Amer. J. Obstet. Gynec., 68: 1330, 1954.

Jones, H. W., Jr., and Scott, W. W.: Hermaphroditism, Genital Anomalies and Related Endocrine Disorders. The Williams & Wilkins Company, Baltimore, 1958.

Jost, A.: Hormonal factors in the development of the fetus. Cold Spring Harbor Symposia Quant. Biol., 19: 167, 1954.

Jungck, E. C., and Brown, W. E.: Human pituitary gonadotropin for clinical use; preparation and lack of antihormone formation. Fertil. Steril., 3: 224, 1952.

Kaeser, O.: Zur Aetiologie der primaren Amenorrhoe. Gynaecologia, 127: 220, 1949.

Keettel, W. C., Bradbury, J. T., and Stoddard, F. J.: Observations on the polycystic ovary syndrome. Amer. J. Obstet. Gynec., 73: 954, 1957.

Kepler, E. J., Dockerty, M. V., and Priestley, J. T.: Adrenal-like ovarian tumor associated with Cushing's syndrome (so-called masculinovoblastoma, luteoma, hypernephroma, adrenal cortical carcinoma of the ovary). Amer. J. Obstet. Gynec., 47: 43, 1944.

Kinnunen, O., and Kauppinen, M.: The effect of brain injury on the menstrual cycle. Acta Endocr. (Kobenhavn), 6: 183, 1951.

Klebarow, D.: Fertilitatsstorungen als spatfolge chronischen hungers und schwerer seelischer Traumen. Geburtsh. Frauenheilk., 9: 420, 1949.

Knobil, E., Kostyo, J. L., and Greep, R. O.: Production of ovulation in the hypophysectomized rhesus monkey. Endocrinology, 65: 487, 1959.

Knobil, E., Morse, A., Wolf, R. C., and Greep, R. O.: Action of bovine, porcine and simian growth hormone preparations on the costochondral junction in the hypophysectomized rhesus monkey. Endocrinology, 62: 348, 1958.

Kroger, W. S., and Freed, S. C.: Psychosomatic aspects of sterility. Amer. J. Obstet. Gynec., 59: 867, 1950.

Leathem, J. H.: Anti-hormone problem in endocrine therapy. Recent Progr. Hormone Res., 4: 115, 1949.

Liepelt, A.: Die Auswirkungen der Elektroshockbehandlung auf den Menstrationszyklus bei psychiatrischen Erkrankungen. Z. Geburtsh. Gynaek., 132: 65, 1950.

Loeser, A. A.: Effect of emotional shock on hormone release and endometrial development. Lancet, 1: 518, 1943.

Martin, E.: Die hemmende Wirkung des prolan. Deutsch. Med. Wschr., 56: 580, 1930.

Mattingly, D., Mills, I. H., and Prunty, F. T. G.: Postpubertal adrenal virilism with biochemical disturbances of the congenital type of adrenal hyperplasia. Brit. Med. J., 1: 1294, 1960.

Mischell, D. R., and Molyoff, L.: Practical value of endometrial biopsies in amenorrhea. New York J. Med., 40: 928, 1940.

Morris, J. M., and Mahesh, V. B.: Further observations on the syndrome "testicular feminization." Amer. J. Obstet. Gynec., 87: 731, 1963.

Murdoch, R., and Govan, A. D. T.: Therapeutic effect of subsequent pregnancy in Simmonds' disease. J. Obstet. Gynaec. Brit. Comm., 58: 18, 1951.

Mussey, R. D., and Haines, S. F.: Amenorrhea and oligomenorrhea associated with low basal metabolic rates. Amer. J. Obstet. Gynec., 27: 404, 1934.

Nassar, G., Greenwood, M., Djanian, A., and Shanklin, W.: The etiological significance of ergot in the incidence of postpartum necrosis of the anterior pituitary; a preliminary report. Amer. J. Obstet. Gynec., 60: 140, 1950.

Novak, E., and Hurd, G. B.: Use of anterior pituitary luteinizing substance in treatment of functional uterine bleeding. Amer. J. Obstet. Gynec., 22: 501, 1931.

Pich, G.: Über den angeborenen Eierstockmangel. Beitr. Path. Anat., 98: 218, 1937.

Plotz, C., Knowlton, A., and Ragan, C.: Natural history of Cushing's syndrome. Amer. J. Med., 13: 597, 1952.

Plotz, J.: Die Bedeutung der Aminosauren fur die Ebstehung und Behandlung der Nechkriegsamenorrhoe. Z. Geburtsh. Gynaek., 132: 13, 1950.

Rakoff, A. E.: Hormonal changes following low dosage irradiation of pituitary and ovaries in anovulatory women. Fertil. Steril., 4: 263, 1953.

Randall, L. M., and McElin, T. W.: Amenorrhea. Charles C Thomas, Springfield, Ill., 1951.

Ray, J. H., Nicholson-Vailey, U., and Grappl, A.: Endocrine activity in psychiatric patients with menstrual disorder. Brit. Med. J., 2: 843, 1957.

Reifenstein, E. C.: Psychogenic or "hypo-
thalamic" amenorrhea. Med. Clin. N.
Amer., *1252:* 1103, 1946.
Reiss, H. E.: Primary amenorrhoea as a mani-
festation of tuberculosis. J. Obstet. Gy-
naec. Brit. Comm., *65:* 735, 1958.
Robertson, J. D.: Glinski and aetiology of
Simmonds' disease (hypopituitarism).
Brit. Med. J., *1:* 921, 1951.
Rydberg, E., and Pedersen-Bjergaard, K.:
Effect of serum gonadotropin and chorionic
gonadotropin on human ovary. J. A. M. A.,
121: 1117, 1943.
Seitz, L.: Die sekundare Amenorrhoe in ihrer
Abhangigkeit von Stoffwechsel und
Psyche. Geburtsh. Frauenheilk., *10:* 165,
1950.
Sheehan, H. L.: Post-partum necrosis of anterior pituitary. J. Path. Bact., *45:* 189,
1937.
Sherman, H. C., Campbell, H. L., and Ragan,
M. S.: Analytical and experimental study
of the effects of increased protein with
liberal calcium and riboflavin intakes;
complete life cycles. J. Nutr., *37:* 317,
1949.
Simmonds, M.: Über embolische prozesse in
der Hypophysis. Arch. Path. Anat., *217:*
226, 1914.
Solomon, D. H., Beck, J. C., Vander Laan,
W. P., and Astwood, E. B.: Prognosis of
hyperthyroidism treated by anti-thyroid
drugs. J. A. M. A., *152:* 201, 1953.
Sosman, M. C.: Cushing's disease—pituitary
basophilism; Caldwell Lecture. Amer. J.
Roentgen., *62:* 1, 1949.
Staemler, H. J.: Der Einfluss gonadotroper
Hormone auf ovarielle Fehlbildungen.
Arch. Gynaek., *187:* 711, 1956.
Stein, J. F.: Diagnosis and treatment of bi-
lateral polycystic ovaries in the Stein-
Leventhal syndrome. Int. J. Fertil., *3:*
20, 1958.
Stein, J. F., and Leventhal, M. L.: Amenor-
rhea associated with bilateral polycystic

ovaries. Amer. J. Obstet. Gynec., *29:* 181,
1935.
Strassman, E. O.: Surgical reconstruction of
a functional uterine cavity in 6 patients
having complete atresia. Southern Med.
J., *49:* 458, 1956.
Tompkins, P.: Treatment of imperforate
hymen with hematocolpos; a review of
113 cases in the literature and a report
of 5 additional cases. J. A. M. A., *113:*
913, 1933.
Turner, H. H.: A syndrome of infantilism,
congenital webbed neck, and cubitus
svalgu. Endocrinology, *23:* 566, 1938.
Van Wagenen, G., and Simpson, M. E.: Induction of multiple ovulation in the
(*Macaca mulatta*) rhesus monkey. Endocrinology, *61:* 316, 1957.
Westman, A.: Untersuchungen uber die
Wirkung des gonadotropin hypophysen-
vorderlappenhormones Antex (Leo) auf
die Ovarien der Frau. Acta Obstet. Gynec.
Scand., *17:* 392, 1937.
Whitacre, F. E., and Barrera, B.: War amenorrhea. J. A. M. A., *124:* 399, 1944.
Whitelaw, M. J., Thomas, S. F., Graham, W.,
Foster, T. M., and Brock, C.: Growth
response in gonadal dysgenesis to the
anabolic steroid Norethandrolone. Amer.
J. Obstet. Gynec., *84:* 501, 1962.
Wilkins, L.: *The Diagnosis and Treatment of
Endocrine Disorders in Childhood and
Adolescence.* Charles C Thomas, Spring-
field, Ill., 1950.
Wilkins, L., and Fleischmann, W.: Ovarian
agenesis; pathology, associated clinical
symptoms and bearing on theories of
sex differentiation. J. Clin. Endocr., *4:*
257, 1944.
Wilson, J. G., and Warkany, J.: Malformations
in the genito-urinary tract induced by
maternal vitamin A deficiency in the rat.
Amer. J. Anat., *83:* 357, 1948.
Zondek, B.: Hypophysenvorderhappen. Arch.
Gynaek., *144:* 133, 1930.

32

ABNORMAL UTERINE BLEEDING

Abnormal uterine bleeding can be classified under two major etiological headings, (1) anatomical and (2) functional. Bleeding is *anatomical* in origin if it is caused by a lesion in some part of the genital tract. The characteristic history is menometrorrhagia. Although bleeding episodes may appear at irregular and unpredictable times, the patient is often able to identify regular menstrual intervals in addition to the abnormal bleeding phases. This is because there is no interference with the ovarian ovulatory phenomena.

Functional uterine bleeding (or dysfunctional) is abnormal bleeding unassociated with tumor, inflammation, or pregnancy. As the condition is usually associated with an ovarian dysfunction and anovulation, the characteristic history is one of complete irregularity of the menstrual interval, prolonged menses frequently alternating with episodes of amenorrhea.

ANATOMICAL FACTORS

This group embraces lesions of the uterus, tubes, or ovaries (Fig. 32.1). Among the more important anatomical causes of abnormal uterine bleeding are the following.

Cervical Polyps. The bleeding with cervical polyps is characteristically slight and intermenstrual, being provoked by muscular exertion, such as defecation, and especially by coitus (*contact bleeding*).

Many polyps cause no bleeding at all, being discovered only accidentally. The slight intermenstrual or postcoital bleeding which often occurs is like that seen in the early stages of cervical carcinoma, and the gynecologist breathes a sigh of relief when, in a patient with such suspicious symptoms, he finds instead of carcinoma one or more cervical polyps protruding from the canal.

Cervical Erosions or Ectropion. With either erosion or ectropion the cervical mucosa may be reddish, granular, and vascular, producing slight bleeding of the type described for cervical polyp. When the tissues are very vascular, bleeding on slight touch, there should always be a suspicion of carcinoma, and biopsy is indicated.

Carcinoma of Cervix. By far the *most important cause of uterine bleeding*, from the standpoint of its life-and-death significance to the patient, is that due to uterine cancer, especially of the cervix. Characteristically this, in the early stages, is of the spotting, intermenstrual type, and is frequently noted especially after coitus. Such bleeding is always suspicious of a cervical lesion, such as cancer or polyp, and always demands careful examination of the cervix. Such an examination, moreover, must always include a speculum examination under the best possible light, a Papanicolaou smear, and where a

625

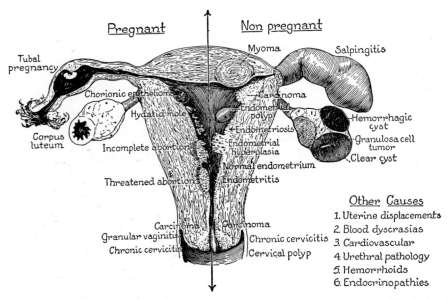

Fig. 32.1. Composite diagrammatic drawing showing chief causes of uterine bleeding. (From Henriksen, E.: Amer. J. Obstet. Gynec., *41:* 179, 1941.)

suspicious but doubtful lesion is found, biopsy must be taken to determine whether or not cancer is present. The bleeding in cancer is the result of the surface ulceration seen even in the early stages of malignancy.

Endometrial Polyps. These are much less likely to cause bleeding than cervical polyps, because of their protected position within the uterine cavity. As a matter of fact, the smaller endometrial polyps ordinarily cause no symptoms at all, being found accidentally on curettage or hysterectomy for other indications. In the larger polyps, and especially those which develop pedicles sufficiently long to allow obtrusion of the polyp into the cervical or even the vaginal canal, bleeding is a common symptom. It is the result of ulcerative changes in the dependent portion of the polyp, and at times of necrosis due to interference with the blood supply.

Retention of Gestation Products. This is *one of the most common of all causes of uterine bleeding,* chiefly because of the frequency of abortion, both spontaneous and induced, although placental tissue is not infrequently retained after full term delivery as well. The bleeding may be slight or it may be exceedingly profuse.

The continuance of bleeding after abortion usually indicates retention of gestational products (Fig. 32.2). In some cases considerable masses of placenta may be retained for long periods of time with little or no bleeding, while in others only small particles may be associated with prolonged and profuse bleeding. Occasionally such retained tissue becomes firmly incorporated with the uterine wall, and may form large or small *placental polyps* (Fig. 32.3). The bleeding is sometimes due to failure or inability of the uterine muscle to contract, but in other cases is due to the opening up of large venous sinuses when the uterus tries to expel portions of placental tissue still attached to the uterine wall.

Chronic Endometritis. Endometritis is not a common cause of uterine bleeding and, when the association occurs, it is probable that the factor responsible for the bleeding is the chronic metritis which, as Schwarz has shown, is not infrequently associated with the endometritis, and which interferes with uterine contractility.

Subinvolution of the Uterus. This condition is seen most frequently in association with marked retroflexion and

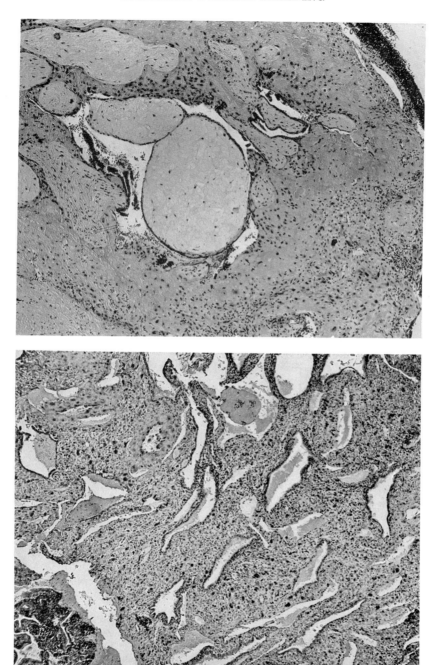

Fig. 32.2. *Top*, old degenerated "shadow" villi in postabortal curetting. *Bottom*, decidual and trophoblastic cells in curettings following recent abortion.

retroversion of the acquired type. The incompleteness of the normal involution of the puerperal uterus leaves it large, boggy, and congested, and menstrual excess is not uncommon as a result of the uterine hyperemia.

Carcinoma of the Corpus Uteri. Adenocarcinoma of the uterine body is a

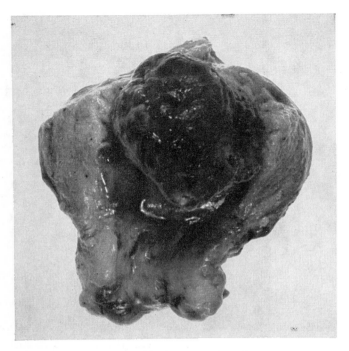

FIG. 32.3. Large placental polyp of uterus

common cause of uterine bleeding, especially of the postmenopausal type. In about one-fourth of the cases this disease develops during reproductive life, when the abnormal bleeding may be both menstrual and intermenstrual, the latter being the more significant. In early stages it is only slight and occasional, appearing often as a blood-tinged watery discharge. In those patients who develop adenocarcinoma after the menopause, the early bleeding is of the same slight degree, but later it becomes increasingly persistent and more profuse.

Sarcoma of the Uterus. Sarcoma of either the cervix or corpus uteri is far less common than carcinoma, and it produces bleeding of the same type as the latter.

Myoma of Uterus. This exceedingly common cause of uterine bleeding is most likely to occur when the tumors are of the submucous or interstitial variety, the subperitoneal growths having no tendency to cause hemorrhage. Even when a myoma is present, the *bleeding is often*

due to associated ovarian dysfunction. Furthermore, it should be remembered that the finding of myomas in a patient who is bleeding does not justify the conclusion that the tumors cause the bleeding, which may be due to some very different intrauterine condition, such as cancer or retained placental tissue.

Hydatidiform Mole and Chorionepithelioma. These lesions are occasionally encountered by the gynecologist, although the latter is exceedingly rare. The bleeding of hydatidiform mole appears in the early months of pregnancy, usually the third to the fifth, and is often associated with a disproportionately large uterus as compared with the duration of the pregnancy. *Quantitative serum chorionic gonadotrophin assays* are often of value in arriving at a diagnosis. Chorionepithelioma manifests itself by persistence of bleeding after the evacuation of a hydatidiform mole, or after miscarriage or full term delivery. Here again quantitative chorionic gonadotrophin tests may be helpful, although the diagnosis is often not made until later stages, and sometimes not until metastases have appeared (Chapter 28).

Ectopic Pregnancy. In few other conditions is the menstrual history as suggestive as with ectopic pregnancy. Menstruation is usually delayed for a few days or several weeks, followed by uterine bleeding which is typically of a spotting character, accompanied by pain in one side of the pelvis. Such a history, together with the finding of a unilateral adnexal mass, should always lead to the suspicion of tubal gestation. While a definite anatomical lesion is present in such cases, the mechanism of the bleeding is at least partly due to hormonal factors, as discussed in Chapter 27, "Ectopic Pregnancy."

Tuberculosis of the Genital Tract. The usual primary seat of genital tuberculosis is in the tubes, but the endometrium is secondarily involved in the majority of cases. Bleeding is frequent but not invariable, and amenorrhea or hypomenorrhea may be noted in some cases, espically in very late stages.

Adnexitis. Inflammatory disease of the tubes and ovary may cause not only uterine bleeding, but also disturbances of menstrual rhythm, especially in the form of shortened intervals (polymenorrhea). In many cases, the probable immediate factor is ovarian dysfunction rather than pelvic hyperemia.

Tumors of the Ovary. While any type of ovarian neoplasm may at times cause uterine bleeding, the proportionate incidence of this symptom is greater with those tumors characterized by the production of estrogen. This group includes especially granulosa cell carcinoma and thecoma although other tumors not of the "endocrine variety" may likewise exert a hormonal influence, in most instances by virtue of hyperactive stromal cells. Even large growths of other types, malignant or benign, are most frequently accompanied by no external bleeding.

Tumors of the Tube. These are extremely rare, but the most important of them, carcinoma, is not infrequently associated with bleeding. The blood undoubtedly finds its way into the uterus from the ulcerating intratubal neoplasm giving a serosanguinous discharge referred to as hydrosalpinx.

Treatment. The treatment of uterine bleeding due to any of the anatomical causes enumerated above must obviously be directed toward removal or correction of these various etiological factors. Each is discussed under the appropriate chapter heads.

DYSFUNCTIONAL UTERINE BLEEDING

Definition. Dysfunctional uterine bleeding may be defined as abnormal bleeding from the uterus unassociated with tumor inflammation or pregnancy. Although apt to occur at the extremes of the menstrual life, such bleeding may occur at any age and is one of the most common gynecological complaints.

Pathology. Schröder, in 1915, by a correlated histological study of the uterus and ovaries, concluded that the bleeding disorder to which he gave the name of metropathia hemorrhagica, is produced by abnormal persistence of unruptured follicles, with consequent absence of functioning corpora lutea and with the production of hyperplasia of the endometrium as a result of the abnormally persistent and excessive estrogenic stimulation. This is still the accepted explanation for perhaps the largest number of cases of functional bleeding.

Pathological studies have shown that although functional uterine bleeding can be associated with any type of endometrial pathology, the most common finding is a nonsecretory pattern. In a recent survey of 158 patients with this diagnosis, 85 were found to have endometrial hyperplasia, 38 a nonsecretory pattern including atrophic endometrium, and 35 a secretory pattern. The division of patients into those with nonsecretory and secretory patterns is important as it distinguishes *anovulatory* from *ovulatory* types of bleeding. The classification is of clinical significance, as these two types of functional uterine bleeding have different etiological

BASAL TEMPERATURE RECORD

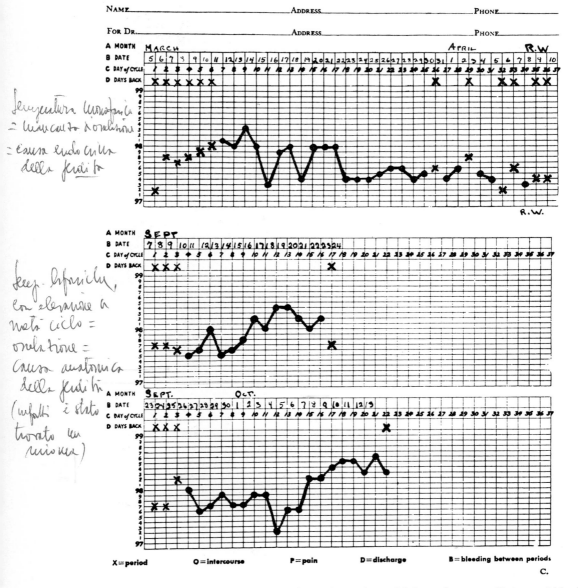

X=period   O=intercourse   P=pain   D=discharge   B=bleeding between periods

C.

FIG. 32.4. *Upper,* basal temperature chart of a patient with irregular, sporadic type of bleeding. The temperature graph is monophasic, indicating an anovulatory pattern. *Middle and lower,* basal temperature charts of a patient with profuse vaginal bleeding at irregular intervals, from 17 to 27 days. The charts are biphasic, indicating ovulatory bleeding with an occasional excessively short menstrual interval. At curettage a submucous myoma was diagnosed.

backgrounds and respond to different forms of therapy.

Bleeding associated with a secretory pattern must be regarded as anatomical until proved otherwise. If all anatomical factors can be excluded, the functional disturbance is usually of neuromuscular, vasomotor, or hematological origin, not

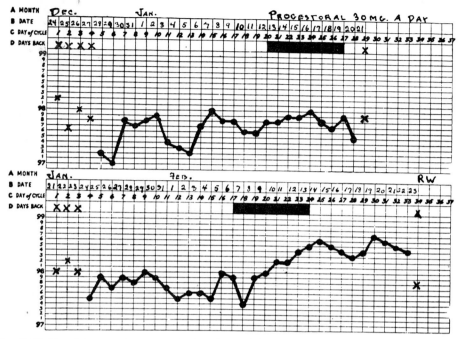

FIG. 32.6. Basal temperature record of patient with anovulatory type of functional bleeding. The *top chart* is monophasic. The *black area* indicates the time during which 30 mg. of oral ethisterone were given daily. This dosage is insufficient to produce any thermogenic effect. Withdrawal bleeding occurred 2 days after cessation of therapy. The *lower chart* is ovulatory. Bleeding does not occur until 10 days after cessation of therapy, indicating a "breakthrough" or escape.

Therefore, if the patient is bleeding at the time therapy is instituted, bleeding will not be controlled until 6 or 8 days after cessation of therapy. If the patient is not bleeding when treatment is begun, her menstrual period usually begins within 2 to 4 days after cessation of therapy. In the 2% of patients who require adjunctive estrogen, 1 mg. of stilbestrol, or its equivalent, may be given immediately with the progesterone and for 17 consecutive days preceeding the next cycle of progesterone therapy.

Progestational Drugs. When progestational-like compounds (19-*nor*-methyltestosterone and its analogues) are used to control dysfunctional bleeding these are employed either cyclically as progestogens in small doses (5.0 mg. daily for 5 days) or continuously in large doses (10 to 30 mg. daily for 2 to 3 weeks) as pituitary suppressants. The larger dose is said to have the advantage of suppressing bleed-

ing within 24 to 48 hours. Suppression is usually maintained throughout the course of therapy but occasionally there is some breakthrough bleeding.

During the last decade a number of steroids have been synthesized which have some progestational activity orally or intramuscularly. The majority of these, however, also have certain androgenic properties and some even show inherent estrogenic characteristics. It is therefore extremely important that one should not think of such drugs as interchangeable with "progesterone." It is necessary to know the specific effect of the specific type of steroid one is using.

Although it was initially thought that ovulation was inhibited by progestational agents, and this certainly has been demonstrated under some circumstances, other experiments indicate that additional mechanisms may be of some importance.

TABLE 32.1

Progestational therapy for anovulatory dysfunctional bleeding

Method of Administration	Clinical Name	Trade Name	Dosage
Intramuscular	Progesterone		5 mg./d. 3–5 d. q. 28 da. × 3 mo.
	17α-Hydroxyproges- terone caproate	Delalutin	125 mg. stat. & q. 28 da. × 3 mo.
Oral	Δ⁶-Dehydroretro- progesterone	Duphaston	15 mg./d. 3–5 d. q. 28 da. × 3 mo.
	Ethistherone	Lutocylol Ora-lutin Pranone Progestoral	30 mg./d. 3–5 d. q. 28 da. × 3 mo.
	6α-Methyl-17α-hy- droxyprogesterone acetate	Provera *FARLUTAL*	10 mg./d. 3–5 d. q. 28 d. × 3 mo.
	Norethynodrel (with estrogen added)	Enovid	5 mg./d. 3–5 d. q. 28 da. × 3 mo.
	Norethistherone	Norlutin	5 mg./d. 3–5 d. q. 28 da. × 3 mo.
Suppositories	Progesterone	Colposterone	25 mg. vaginally q. n. × 5 n. q. 28 da. × 3 mo.

Lunenfeld was unable to induce ovulation with human gonadotrophins in a patient under the influence of 6α-methyl-17α-acetoxyprogesterone and ethinyl estradiol, indicating that the ovary was refractory to gonadotrophin stimulation. Goisis, working with the baboon, was also able to find suggestive evidence that this compound specifically inhibited ovarian function. His observations indicated divergent effects of different synthetic progestogens on the pituitary and ovary.

A list of the more frequently used progestogens with the trade names and dosages used for the treatment of anovulatory dysfunctional bleeding is given in Table 32.1.

Chorionic Gonadotrophin. Although the use of chorionic gonadotrophin seemed theoretically promising and initially practical, most subsequent reports have been disappointing. Bergman, however, reports a series of 361 patients with excellent clinical results using 4500 IU of chorionic gonadotrophin, given in 3 doses of 1500 IU each, on 3 consecutive days each month. With this regimen ovulation was apparently induced.

Estrogens. The use of high dosages of oral estrogens (25 mg. or more of stilbestrol daily), or of intravenous estrogen as a hemostatic agent, is undesirable, as a vicious circle is established. Although intravenous estrogens have been reported as having hemostatic properties, Kudish and Rapaport were unable to demonstrate that they affected the plasma clotting time in humans. Kelly has recently reviewed the evidence for the rationale of the use of intravenous estrogen and concludes that "there is no concrete experimental evidence to justify the endorsement of estrogen given by the intravenous route for any therapeutic indication."

The great individual variation in response to estrogens makes it extremely difficult to establish a satisfactory routine dosage and withdrawal schedule. The rationale of estrogen therapy in dysfunctional bleeding was initially based on the theory that the abnormal bleeding resulted from a drop in the estrogen level. Estrogen was therefore given in an effort to maintain a uniform estrogen milieu. The metabolic studies of Brown, Kellar, and Matthew have failed to substantiate

ing or breast symptoms warrant additional examinations.

For the woman under 40 who needs castration, it is sometimes desirable to insert one or two 25-mg. estradiol pellets into the incision, and, at the 6-week postoperative examination, to prescribe estrogen suppositories (stilbestrol, 0.5 mg.) during the first 3 to 7 days each month, depending upon symptoms and vaginal cytology. Such a regimen usually prevents flushes from developing and maintains vaginal pliability and lubrication.

Therapy in all cases should be maintained until the age of 45 or 50 years and then should be discontinued slowly over a year's time. Again, no rule of thumb will prove successful for all women and each must be individualized according to her needs.

SENILE VAGINITIS AND URETHRITIS. The predominating symptoms of senile vaginitis are discharge, itching, burning, and dyspareunia. The symptoms of senile urethritis are urinary frequency and nocturia unassociated with infection. The most effective therapy for these local symptoms is by the vaginal route as described in the preceding paragraph. If constriction of the vaginal lumen has occurred, this is an additional factor causing dyspareunia and some form of manual dilatation will also be necessary to reestablish normal function and painless intercourse. Pyrex test tubes in graduated sizes make the most satisfactory dilators.

The response of senile urethritis to estrogen suppositories is frequently dramatic.

OSTEOPOROSIS. Osteoporosis is characterized by the x-ray evidence of decalcification of bone, decrease in stature, kyphosis, and eventually severe joint pain and debility associated with multiple fractures. The role played by steroid hormones in maintenance of calcium in bone has not been completely elucidated by the biochemists but is clearly demonstrated clinically in the occurrence of epiphysial closure at puberty and osteoporosis associated with conditions causing gonadal hypoplasia, for example, Cushing's disease and acromegaly. The incidence of symptomatic menopausal osteoporosis among the general population is difficult to estimate, as is the frequency of its occurrence after a premature menopause, but it is certainly not an uncommon finding 10 years or more after cessation of ovarian function.

An instructive report by Caldwell on the experimental production and treatment of osteoporosis in the rat, indicates that after removal of gonads and adrenal glands all animals developed osteoporosis within 100 days (perhaps the equivalent of 20 years in the human life span). Recovery was most rapid and complete with estradiol treatment alone. Lesser degrees of recovery occurred with combinations of estradiol and testosterone and virtually no improvement was obtained with testosterone only.

The experimental results are in accord with the clinical findings, for although testosterone, cortisone, and the synthetic anabolic steroids have been advocated in the treatment of this condition, it is our experience that none, either alone or in combination with estrogens, has proved more effective than estrogens alone. The most satisfactory, and least expensive, schedule used for the treatment of menopausal osteoporosis is 1 mg. of stilbestrol daily for 25 days each month, ending with a single monthly injection of 25 mg. of progesterone or a 3-day course of an oral progestogen, 30 mg. of ethisterone or its equivalent daily. This schedule will usually produce monthly bleeding which, although troublesome, is warranted by the remarkable relief from painful bone symptoms which ensues. Relief from pain can be expected within the first month and it is not unusual to have a return of function concomitantly.

Initial investigators were surprised and disappointed not to see evidence of x-ray changes associated with the dramatic clinical improvement. It is now thought that the production of such x-ray evidence takes a protracted period of time probably amounting to 10 years or so.

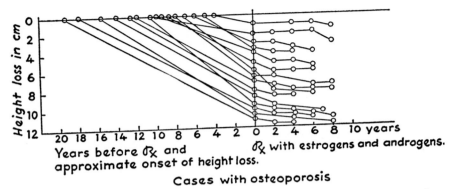

Cases with osteoporosis

FIG. 33.1. Treatment of patient with postmenopausal osteoporosis. In most cases there was a cessation of height loss within 2 years after institution of therapy. (From Hernberg, C. A.: Acta Endocr. (Kobenhavn.), *34:* 51, 1960.)

Albright suggested using the height as a standard of improvement, because all patients show a progressive loss of height with the passage of time. As improvement occurs and osteoporosis is arrested, the height becomes stationary. Hernberg has demonstrated the value of this criterion and the arrest of height loss by the prophylactic use of estrogens (Fig. 33.1). (For a complete review see the article by Handelsman.)

CARDIOVASCULAR HYPERTENSIVE AND ARTERIOSCLERIC DISEASE

Treatment and Prophylaxis

The clinical observation that vascular disease is less common among young women than among men in a similar age group is complicated by a multiplicity of factors and it cannot be assumed that estrogen is the most important one. To cite only two major causes which are also undoubtedly involved, *stress* from the strenuous competitive activities of man concerned with making a place of social and economic security for himself and family is far greater than the stress to which the average woman is exposed. *Excessive smoking*, which has also been seriously implicated by Hammond and Horn in the production of arteriosclerosis, has, until quite recently, been practiced largely by men.

The two major pieces of evidence which

link estrogens with cardiovascular disease are first the statistical studies on the differential occurrence of the disease in normal young men and women, and in menopausal and castrate women with and without estrogen replacement therapy, and second the effect of estrogens on the serum cholesterol to phospholipid ratio. Of still controversial nature is the relationship between these blood changes and arteriosclerosis. Experimental work has demonstrated in the rat that a high cholesterol to phospholipid ratio predisposes to cardiac arteriosclerosis and hypertension. The cardiac but not thoracic artery changes can be prevented by estrogen administration. In the rabbit, serum lipids do not change with estrogen administration and estrogens have no effect upon the occurrence of arteriosclerosis in this species. Findings in the human are interestingly similar to those in the rat in that Wuest, Dry, and Edwards found increased coronary atherosclerosis and hypertensive disease in women who had oophorectomies 10 years or more prior to death, when compared to normal women of similar ages. Novak and Williams, in a parallel study, investigating atherosclerosis of the coronary arteries and the aorta, found no difference in the amount of atheromatous disease between castrate and normal women in comparable age groups. Davis demonstrated increased electrocardiogram changes and hyper-

34

MISCELLANEOUS PROBLEMS OF GYNECOLOGY

DYSMENORRHEA

Dysmenorrhea, or menstrual pain, is probably the most common of all symptoms of gynecological disorders, and is the greatest cause of lost work hours among women. In spite of its great frequency, and despite the fact that it has been the subject of extensive discussion and study for more than a hundred years, it remains one of the unsolved problems of gynecology.

Definition

Primary dysmenorrhea is menstrual pain observed in the absence of any noteworthy pelvic lesion and due to factors intrinsic in the uterus itself. Characteristically the pain begins with the onset of menstruation and lasts over a few hours, although in some cases it may continue throughout several days. Although it is most frequently of a colicky, labor-like nature, the pain is sometimes described as of severe aching character. It may be severe enough to require bed rest of one to several days each month, and may be accompanied by diarrhea, nausea, and vomiting. In the so-called *secondary variety*, demonstrable pelvic disease of one sort or another is present and is the ostensible cause of the menstrual pain. Although dysmenorrhea may appear with the very first period, in a surprisingly large proportion of patients menstrual pain is not complained of until many months or even several years after initiation of the function. One explanation for this is that the inaugural cycles of many girls are of the anovulatory type, and these are characteristically painless. When ovulation begins, primary dysmenorrhea not infrequently develops.

Causative Factors and Their Management

Many theories have been advanced to explain the causation of primary dysmenorrhea, and it seems clear that a number of factors may be concerned. Chief among them are those enumerated below, with a discussion of the management of these various factors.

Psychogenic. Although many women suffer no discomfort whatsoever during menstruation, a moderate amount of pelvic heaviness and even an occasional cramp may be considered as within normal limits. Indeed, the line between this normal discomfort and real dysmenorrhea is a very shadowy one, and the distinction is commonly made subjectively by the patient herself, on the basis of the incapacity produced. It is this subjective nature of the disorder which has made its study so difficult. It needs no more than a knowledge of human nature to justify the statement that the same degree of peripheral stimulus which in the well balanced, phlegmatic individual will be expressed as a moderate discomfort will manifest itself in the high-strung, supersensitive girl by severe and perhaps incapacitating pain.

The psychogenic element, therefore, is one which can never be lost sight of in the management of cases of dysmenorrhea, and a comprehensive study includes a consideration of factors which may accentuate the subjective element in the particular case. Among these are a congenitally unstable and high-strung nervous system, psychic trauma, especially when related to the menstrual periods, and wrong ideas as to the significance and normality of the menstrual function. Many times a young girl, at the beginning of her menstrual life, is coddled by an overly anxious mother into the belief that menstruation is a time when she should really consider herself "unwell." To such a girl, especially if reared in a household where one or more members of the female contingent suffer from dysmenorrhea, the transition to menstrual invalidism is an easy one.

So important are these factors that there are some authorities who assert that the cause of primary dysmenorrhea is invariably psychogenic, a view which we do not share. On the other hand, we are convinced of the prime role of the psychogenic factor in many cases. To unearth such etiological factors as these, it is not necessary to submit the patient to a pyschoanalytical examination, but it is important that the physician possess common sense and understanding. He must take the trouble to review the history of the disorder, especially in its inceptional phases, and to set before the patient the fact that menstruation should not normally interfere materially with the usual work or activities of the normal girl. The physician can soon learn the probable importance or unimportance of the psychogenic factor in the individual case, and thus determine the importance or the futility of intensifying the psychotherapeutic approach. In at least a small proportion of cases, we believe it possible literally to talk a girl out of her dysmenorrhea through a policy of sympathetic understanding, reassurance, and education.

Constitutional. Closely and often indistinguishably linked with the purely subjective group of causes is the factor of constitutional debility of one sort or another, as observed in patients who because of anemia, tuberculosis, diabetes, overwork or many other possible causes, suffer a lowering of the threshold of pain, primarily because of physical factors, but often with a strong admixture of nervous and psychic factors as well. Certainly a part of the treatment of every case of dysmenorrhea should be to outline a regimen calculated to raise the patient's general health level in every possible way, and these measures alone will in some cases cause disappearance or marked amelioration of the dysmenorrhea.

Obstructive. One of the first theories for the explanation of dysmenorrhea was that it was due to obstructive cervical lesions, acute anteflexion of the uterus, or cervical stenosis. Although it is probably true that mechanical obstruction plays a part in the etiology of a small proportion of cases, no one now believes it to play the essential role in dysmenorrhea which was formerly attributed to it. In many dysmenorrheic women the uterus shows no flexion and the cervix is not stenosed, whereas in women who experience no pain whatsoever there may be a sharp anteflexion or retroflexion and the canal may be of pinpiont variety.

Hypoplasia of the Uterus. The fact that underdevelopment of the uterus is noted in many cases of dysmenorrhea has led many to stress its etiological importance, although here again the evidence is unconvincing. Various theories have been suggested to explain how hypoplasia can cause dysmenorrhea, but none has obtained acceptance. Even when hypoplasia exists one must think of a more fundamental underlying defect.

Endocrine Factors. This brings us to the last category of etiological factors, represented by endocrine aberrations of one sort or another. On clinical rather than scientifically demonstrable grounds, the frequently crampy character of primary dysmenorrhea has been rather generally, although not unanimously, accepted as due to *exaggerated uterine contractility*, and we have learned a good deal as to the endocrine factors which govern the contractility of the uterine musculature. Novak and Reynolds reported studies upon the rabbit uterus which seemed to indicate very clearly that the *normal stimulant of uterine contractility is the estrogenic hormone*, while *progesterone is the normal inhibitor* of this contractility. Csapo's work in vitro substantiates these views.

If the estrogenic hormone is responsible for the heightened uterine contractility which appears to characterize primary dysmenorrhea, there are two clinical observations which seem perplexing and paradoxical. The first of these is the fact that in cases of dysfunctional bleeding, associated usually with a relative excess of estrogen and a deficiency or complete absence of progesterone, menstrual pain is characteristically absent. The second is the fact that primary dysmenorrhea so often does not date from the inauguration of menstruation at puberty, but makes its appearance at a later period, varying from a few months to perhaps 2 years after puberty.

These observations would indicate that dysmenorrhea is apparently not due to mere dominance of estrogenic hormones but rather to some sort of imbalance between the estrogen and the progesterone. This view, which has been suggested on circumstantial grounds, was given considerable support by the classic studies of Sturgis and Albright, who were able to prevent dysmenorrhea by inhibiting ovulation. We are still as far as ever from the solution of the underlying mechanism of the pain. Whatever the underlying mechanism of dysmenorrhea may be, it has seemed rational as a part of the treatment of this disorder to attempt to inhibit contraction of the uterine musculature. This plan is based on the still unproved assumption, improbable though it may seem, that the immediate factor of the production of dysmenorrhea lies in exaggerated and painful labor-like contractions of the muscles.

Treatment

Endocrine Therapy. There are several endocrine approaches to the therapy of dysmenorrhea and these may be briefly summarized.

ESTROGENS. From the studies of Sturgis and Albright, to which reference has already been made, it seems possible to convert an ovulatory cycle into an anovulatory one by administering estrogens in adequate dosage in the early part of the cycle; and often such inhibition of ovulation brings about relief from pain with the next flow. Stilbestrol, 1 mg., given for 12 days beginning shortly after the onset of the period, usually on the first or second day, will often abolish ovulation quite effectively, although much larger doses, 5 mg. daily, are probably necessary to bring about this effect consistently. Unfortunately the use of this dosage is often associated with severe nausea. Although effective in the treatment cycle, the benefits do not usually extend beyond the month of therapy. Furthermore, minor disturbances of menstrual rhythm or flow may be noted. In many patients it is also difficult to repeat the inhibition month after month as the patient's own cycle tends to break through. Even a temporary relief, however, is a boon to the patient who has come to dread the advent of menstruation because of the severe suffering it entails; and those in whom the dysmenorrhea is severe would prefer to have a short course of therapy repeated from time to time rather than to suffer menstrual pain constantly. Aside from this the psychic lift given by the treatment is important in interrupting the pain habit pattern, and the beneficial effects of the estrogenic substance when used in promoting uterine development are not unimportant considerations. Because of the inhibition of ovulation, upon which the effectiveness of this treatment depends, one would not wish to resort to it with any persistence in the case of women anxious for pregnancy.

PROGESTERONE. There are two major uses of progesterone for the control of dysmenorrhea. The first is the older method that was used in the membranous type of dysmenorrhea in an effort to restore the estrogen-progesterone balance. This therapy consisted of the administration of 60 to 80 mg. of ethisterone daily, beginning about 4 days prior to the period and continuing through the first 2 days of the period. An alternative method is the injection of 250 mg. of a long acting progestational substance (17-hydroxy-progesterone caproate) 1 week prior to the onset of menses. The rationale of this therapy was that there was a sudden withdrawal of progesterone causing profound ischemia and a muscle imbalance. It was postulated that by giving additional progesterone throughout the withdrawal period the rapid withdrawal could be cushioned.

The most recent and most successful form of therapy for dysmenorrhea involves the use of the synthetic progestogens for the inhibition of ovulation. These substances are potent pituitary inhibitors in relatively small dosages and are generally unassociated with the unpleasant side effects of stilbestrol. Unlike estrogens, they can be used in the same dosage month after month with a similar suppression of ovulation and beneficial effects. As little as 2.5 mg. of 19-*nor*-(methyl or ethyl)testosterone, given daily during the first 25 days of each cycle, is a sufficient dose to suppress ovulation. Although side effects are minimal with this small dosage, occasionally one incurs gastrointestinal symptoms, abdominal cramps, irregular bleeding, or amenorrhea. The same theoretical considerations, of course, apply to the use of these substances in the suppression of ovulation as to the use of estrogens, and again the treatment is effective only in the cycle of therapy and no permanent relief is attained. However, as everyone's experience demonstrates that dysmenorrhea is invariably provoked by general psychic tension, sometimes a course of 3 to 6 months of treatment will carry a patient through an unusually difficult time and it will then be possible to control her symptoms with more general measures for several months, after which treatment can be reinitiated if necessary.

TESTOSTERONE. Testosterone is of value in the treatment of dysmenorrhea only when endometriosis is the etiological factor (Chapter 26). Methyltestosterone, 5 mg. daily over a 6-month period, is usually adequate to control symptoms. This dosage is not associated with any evidence of virilization and will not interfere with ovulation and normal menstruation. An occasional patient who has an acne tendency, however, may find that the acne is exaggerated. It would be important, therefore, to use progestogens if this skin condition exists.

Presacral Neurectomy. The operation of presacral neurectomy or sympathectomy is a rational and frequently effective procedure in an occasional patient with unusually severe dysmenorrhea which has proved intractable to more conservative procedures. It gives complete or almost complete relief from pain in perhaps 60 to 70% of the cases. Although only occasionally indicated in primary dysmenorrhea *per se*, a more frequent application, at least in our hands, has been as a supplementary procedure in conservative operations performed for such conditions as endometriosis when associated with severe dysmenorrhea.

Treatment during Dysmenorrhea Attack. Very little new information can be added to a discussion of the treatment of the dysmenorrhea attack. Once the pain has been initiated, it is apt to run its course. The local use of heat and analgesics such as acetylsalicylic acid and sodium Amytal to induce sleep will suffice for all except the occasional case. When nausea is an associated finding, rectal suppositories must be employed. Too much stress cannot be laid on the risk of resorting to the two drugs which will always relieve the pain, morphine and alcohol. It should be unnecessary to emphasize that no habit-producing drug should ever be used, as the condition must be regarded as a chronic illness and under these circumstances the possibility of addiction is too great a hazard. Every attempt should be made to prevent the condition, as it is easier to stop the pain before its inception than after it is well established. This can frequently be done by the use of analgesics, and these in combination with other types of drugs such as psychic energizers and tranquilizers. A few of the most effective ones are Edrisal, Equagesic, Zactirin, and Daprisal. Medication should be given at the first sign of menstruation and repeated every 3 hours through the first or second day if necessary. Some patients respond better to an anticholinergic drug such as Trasentine. A smooth muscle relaxant, isoxsuprine hydrochloride (Vasodilan), 10 to 20 mg. 3 or 4 times a day is more effective for others.

Summary of Management. No therapy of such a subjective pain disorder as primary dysmenorrhea can be based purely on endocrine considerations, for cognizance must also be taken of constitutional and psychogenic factors as a basis for the management of these patients. Although endocrine factors alone may be responsible in some cases and the same is true of constitutional or psychogenic factors, in most cases more than one of these three chief etiological factors may exist. As a part of the treatment of primary dysmenorrhea, endocrine therapy or surgery may properly be employed, but the physician who depends upon these entirely and who takes no cognizance of other possible factors is sure to meet with failure in a large proportion of cases. In addition to the general and constitutional measures, psychotherapy and reassurance with advice to try to remain up and about rather than going to bed during the pain of the attack seem preferable to the uncertainties and inconvenience of endocrine therapy. A few doses of aspirin or some antispasmodic will usually tide the girl over the worst of her trouble. When the dysmenorrhea is more protracted and severe, however, endocrine therapy should be tried before resorting to more radical measures such as presacral neurectomy. The evidence now clearly indicates what has long been suspected, that primary dysmenorrhea is a disorder of ovulating women and that it is probably relievable by preventing ovulation. This can apparently be done for any one particular cycle by progestogen therapy or estrogens given in the early phase of the cycle.

PREMENSTRUAL TENSION AND EDEMA

Premenstrual tension in minor degrees is relatively common; extreme degrees are rare and may be very distressing. The milder forms of the condition are characterized by nervousness and restlessness, but, in the severe types, the condition of the patient closely approaches a psychotic state with striking personality changes and emotional outbursts which make her difficult both for the family and physician. On the other hand, the most characteristic complaint may be incapacitating headaches which may on occasion be associated with sensory or motor symptoms of cerebral vascular spasms. The condition appears to be closely related to premenstrual edema and the two frequently coexist.

Premenstrual edema was described by Thomas in 1933 and a number of reports have since appeared. It must be remembered that many normal women show a slight gain of weight during the premenstrual period. Sweeney, for example, found that 30% of a group of normal women studied by him showed a gain of 3 or more pounds. This agrees with our observations. In the occasional patient, however, the weight gain may be far greater and is obviously due to retention of fluid. There is often marked edema with puffiness of the face and eyes, swelling of the feet and ankles. In one such patient there was a weight gain of as much as 15 pounds during the cycle; the eyes were almost closed by the edematous eyelids, and there was swelling and pitting of the feet and ankles. The edema usually begins a few days before the onset of menstruation, but may also appear at ovulation time. Toward the beginning of menstruation, or sometime immediately after its cessation, marked polyuria occurs with rapid disappearances of edema. The condition may be noted at any age during the menstrual era, but in our experience it is most common during the 4th decade.

The earliest studies on the problem were made by Frank, who related the symptoms to estrogen retention produced by a high renal threshold of excretion. Early metabolic studies by Thorn, in the human, and Krohn and Zuckerman, in the baboon, confirmed the role of estrogen in fluid retention. However, although some patients do show both preovulatory and premenstrual edema paralleling the ovarian estrogen secretion pattern, as with dysmenorrhea, premenstrual tension usually occurs in the ovulatory cycle, linking it at least circumstantially to progesterone secretion. As with dysmenorrhea also, no abnormality of the ovarian hormone production or metabolism has been demonstrated and the normal hormonal balance is attested by the ability of most patients to retain a normal reproductive function. Because of the associated edema, it has been suggested that the condition may also represent a disturbance of adrenal aldosterone function. Reich has demonstrated an increased aldosterone secretion in normally menstruating women premenstrually. However, if any hormonal imbalance exists, it must certainly be superimposed on a very specific type of sympathetic nervous system and is influenced by external environmental factors, everyday stress and strain, and dietary indiscretions such as inadequate or infrequent meals, excessive coffee, alcohol, or nicotine. A recent study by Copper has produced some substantiation for this conclusion. His results indicate that there is a definite association of premenstrual tension with a psychotic personality type while there is no such correlation with dysmenorrhea.

Thus, it seems that we may consider the condition of premenstrual tension and edema as due to secondary aldosteronism with three major components which contribute to the pathogenesis. First, and certainly fundamental, is the psychotic personality; second, the environmental stress; and third, the shifting ovarian physiology which is, so to speak, the "straw that breaks the camels back," in producing a secondary aldosteronism. For a better understanding of the physiology a paragraph on aldosteronism seems appropriate.

Aldosteronism. Aldosteronism due to a tumor or hyperplasia of the adrenal *zona glomerulosa* was first described by Krohn and is characterized by hypertension, muscular weakness, polyuria, polydypsia, and high sodium and low serum potassium, but no edema. The absence of edema is explained by Bartter in the following manner. The aldosterone or sodium-retaining factor causes increased sodium resorption by the renal tubules; the expansion of volume of extracellular fluids causes increased cellular filtration rate and thereby an increased sodium secretion. Thus, there is relatively little sodium retention and therefore no edema.

In contrast, secondary aldosteronism described as hypersecretion due to factors outside of the adrenal glomerulosa zone, is usually associated with the state of edema. Some factors known to produce secondary aldosteronism are: corticotropin, potassium, progesterone, and changes in body fluid volume. In addition to these, surgical trauma and anxiety states have been implicated. It seems apparent that the edema is dependent upon the increased aldosterone secretion, since under experimental conditions in animals, adrenalectomy will usually eliminate the edema.

We can then reconstruct the picture of a harassed housewife, endowed with a psychotic personality who by her 4th decade is burdened with more anxiety than she is able to handle. Having ovulated, she is now producing progesterone and increased amounts of estrogen which lead to mild fluid retention. These two factors, the progesterone and the fluid retention, stimulate increased aldosterone production, which then causes more fluid retention, thus creating the vicious circle which produces symptoms of headache, irritability, depression, and swelling (Frank). The intercellular edema itself then causes increased tension, headache, and anxiety. The anxiety further stimulates aldosterone production, and thus the syndrome grows in proportion. It is often difficult to know where the chain begins and how to interrupt it.

It is interesting that the older patients reported by Reich showed more pronounced increases of aldosterone in the premenstrual phase and this may be related to the increased frequency of the condition during the late 30's and early 40's. We have been inclined to attribute this to the additional stress which most patients undergo in association with the greater responsibilities of age.

Treatment. The clinical management of the *premenstrual tension* syndrome is a reminder that medicine is still an art and not an exact science. This statement indicates that the therapy is by no means a standardized one.

In the milder cases and in the younger group of patients, especially when edema is the predominating symptom, ammonium chloride, 0.6 gm. 3 times daily during the last 2 weeks of the menstrual cycle, associated with a salt-poor diet and 3 regular high protein meals a day, may suffice, if the initial point of attack has been made simultaneously on adjusting the stress and strain of everyday living. Within the past few years a number of commercial preparations have been available which are based on this general diuretic plan of therapy. Combined with dietary salt limitations, these are often effective in the treatment of both premenstrual tension and premenstrual edema (Premens, Neobromth, etc.). For more severe edema problems Diuril, 500 mg. can be given once or twice a day for 2 or 3 days during the onset of swelling. Prolonged, continuous therapy is inadvisable, as marked edema will occur on withdrawal of medication. When severe emotional disturbances exist these should be treated only in conjunction with a psychiatrist.

When headache is the major symptom, it has been our experience that 25 mg. of methyltestosterone daily for 2 or 3 days premenstrually and, if necessary, at the time of ovulation, will often prove a great help. When the symptoms are seen in women approaching middle life, especially if headaches are severe and associated with vascular spasms causing unilateral parasthesias, irradiation induction of the menopause may be indicated. Although this specifically does not apply to patients with edema or tension, when done after careful study and consideration with the full understanding and desire of the patient, it has been our experience that this method of treatment is highly satisfactory for the relief of premenstrual headaches. Contrary to the fears of most physicians concerned in handling such patients, they do not have excessive hot flushes or other adverse symptoms of the menopause.

In recapitulation, although one can alleviate the symptoms of premenstrual tension and edema by salt restriction and diuretics, by inducing anovulatory cycles, or by giving 25 mg. of methyltestosterone daily for not over a 10-day period each month, little of permanent value can be expected from any therapeutic regimen without concomitant psychotherapy. Let us not resort to operative procedures as a desperate therapeutic attempt. It has been our experience that, especially in those patients with edema, the symptoms will remain even following a bilateral oophorectomy and hysterectomy. A psychiatrist is a much better recourse.

VICARIOUS MENSTRUATION

This is of historical interest mainly and is the designation applied to certain rare cases in which extragenital hemorrhages of one source or another take place at periodical intervals corresponding to the menstrual cycle. The most frequent site of the bleeding is from the nasal mucous membrane in the form of epistaxis. This variety, according to Roth, makes up about 30% of all cases. It has long been known that a biological relation exists between the nasal mucous membrane and the female generative organs. Investigations by Mortimer *et al.* have demonstrated the responsiveness of certain areas in the nasal mucous membrane to estrogen stimulation. The local hyperemia and other vascular changes produced by the ovarian hormones would seem to offer a satisfactory explanation of this type of vicarious bleeding.

Vicarious menstruation has been described as occurring from a great variety of other sources: the stomach, intestines, lungs, mammary glands, skin, and various skin lesions such as ulcers or navi, kidneys, abdominal fistulas, umbilicus, external auditory meatus, eyes, and eyelids. Many of the cases in older literature, for example those of fistulas or of umbilical origin, are no doubt explainable by the existence of endometriosis or fistulas communicating with the uterus or tubal lumen.

Treatment. The treatment of the condition depends upon the exact diagnosis as well as the source of the bleeding. In the nasal type of vicarious menstruation, cauterization of the nasal spur responsible for the bleeding is usually recommended. When bleeding occurs elsewhere an investigation for endometriosis should be made and, if confirmed, excision of the area when possible is most expedient. Either methyltestosterone, 5 mg. daily, can be used as described for the treatment of endometriosis, or 20 mg. of a synthetic progestogen in combination with estrogens, as in the commercial preparation Enovid. An alternate therapy is a combination of long acting estrogen and progestational steroids, given by intramuscular injection.

INTERMENSTRUAL PAIN (*MITTEL-SCHMERZ*) AND BLEEDING

These two conditions may be discussed together, in spite of the fact that the pain often occurs without the bleeding, and *vice versa*. They are apparently both linked in some manner with the phenomenon of ovulation, although little is known as to the exact mechanism.

Intermenstrual pain, occurring usually at approximately the midinterval period, with many individual variations as to the exact day of the cycle, was described by Priestley as far back as 1872. Such pain may be slight, or it may be as severe as the more intense forms of dysmenorrhea. The duration may be only a few hours, but in some cases 2 or 3 days. There may or may not be associated *bleeding*, sometimes so slight as to cause only a brownish discharge, in other cases sufficiently free and prolonged as to mimic a menstrual flow. To such scanty flows, regularly interpolated between the periods, the Germans have applied the term *kleine Regel* (little period). In the occasional case this interval type of bleeding is so free that the patient states that she menstruates twice a month. Even when there is no macroscopic bleeding with *Mittelschmerz*, blood corpuscles may often be found in microscopic examination of the vaginal discharge.

Etiology. The chronological relation between intermenstrual pain and bleeding on the one hand, and ovulation on the other, has led to general agreement that there is some sort of causal relation between them. The bleeding would seem logically explainable by the *temporary drop in estrogen* immediately following ovulation, but there is greater difficulty in explaining the pain. As Reynolds states, "one can only speculate upon whether the occurrence of *Mittelschmerz* betokens impending ovulation, the act of ovulation or recent ovulation." Only a few studies of actual *operative findings* in such cases have been reported, the most complete being that of Wharton and Henriksen. In 9 of their 21 patients some evidence of bleeding from the ovary was found; in others the findings were negative. Some have suggested that the pain may be most logically explained on the basis of slight intraabdominal hemorrhage.

Treatment. When intermenstrual bleeding is very slight, and has been known to occur with such periodicity that there is little reason to doubt its functional nature, no treatment is necessary except reassurance and perhaps simple analgesics. Where there is doubt on this point, diagnostic curettage may be necessary to

35

CLINICAL CYTOLOGY

Cytopathology studies health and disease through *micro*biopsies, cellular samples. As extremely small as these specimens are, they at times hold more information than larger tissue samples removed by surgery. While usually coming from the surface of organs, these samples reflect the deeper processes accurately, cover a wider surface area for examination than the usual biopsies, do not remove viable tissue and, thus, afford unequaled opportunity not only to detect and diagnose disease but to study the biologic behavior of disease processes *unaltered* by surgical intervention or surgical removal.

Successfully introduced into clinical medicine by Papanicolaou and Traut in 1943, it has been accepted into our armamentarium after extensive use and proof of reliability. In the United States, great clinical emphasis has been placed upon its unequaled ability to detect *early cancer*. This has speeded its development and acceptance, but has overshadowed its other potentials. In Europe, Latin America and, more recently, the United States its great assistance in the understanding of *endocrine* status is being developed and exploited. Further, it has proved very useful in filling out the assessment of patients' sensitivity or resistance to irradiation, and the understanding of the whole problem of *host response* to infections, neoplasias, and therapy. By provid-

ing a rapid and accurate method of determining X sex chromosomal make-up, it has opened many new vistas in cytogenetics and the understanding of the complex and compound problems of *sex determination*, intersexuality, and hermaphroditism.

The clinical simplicity and rapidity with which each specimen is obtained, has placed its consultation at the fingertips of every practicing physician regardless of specialty, training, or experience. *Techniques* for the clinical preparation of these cytopathology specimens are depicted at the *end* of this chapter.

Both the clinician and the consulting pathologist must have a clear, accurate picture of each other's problems and perspective in order for cytopathology not to mislead but to guide securely. Together these physicians must strive for a complete understanding of the patient as a whole.

SEX DETERMINATION AND CYTOGENETICS

Not too long ago it would have seemed that the determination of a patient's sex as female would have to be a prerequisite before consideration in gynecological and obstetrical cytology. This paradox has arisen from mushrooming evidence in the field of cytogenetics which is shedding much light on many clinical problems but, as with any new knowledge, is raising a host of others.

Basis for Determination

In the mitotic cell at metaphase, "squash" preparations or air dried preparations of properly incubated blood, bone marrow, and other cell cultures allow morphological study of individual chromosomes. In this fashion counting and identification of all 44 autosomes and two sex chromosomes is possible. In the resting (metabolic) nucleus, chromosomes are threadlike and not individually identifiable; yet, the XX chromosome pair can be determined by the presence of a female sex chromocenter or Barr body. Following the work of Barr, many investigators have confirmed the fact that epidermal cells of human females contain a peripheral clump of chromatin on the nuclear membrane, which is absent in the male. This sex chromocenter is present in exfoliated cell nuclei in the easily obtainable clinical specimens of both vaginal and buccal smears (Fig. 35.1). In the neutrophilic polymorphonuclear leukocyte, this sex difference manifests itself by a small lobe or nuclear "drumstick" appendage in a female's nucleus, which is absent in a male's nucleus. The two methods appear to be in agreement, but because of its greater clinical ease of preparation and its more objectively reproducible results, only the *exfoliated squamous epithelial cell* method and results will be considered in detail.

The Clinical Method

The buccal mucus membrane is scraped (see Fig. 35.30, "Clinical Preparation of Specimen"); the milky cellular fluid so obtained is spread on a glass microscopic slide and immediately dropped in fixative (95% ethyl alcohol). A good hematoxylin nuclear chromatin stain will usually suffice, such as the routine Papanicolaou or hematoxylin and eosin (H & E) stains. More satisfactory, however, are certain stains which preferentially demonstrate deoxyribonucleic acid (DNA) while de-emphasizing the bacteria and granular artifacts which can obscure a clear cut

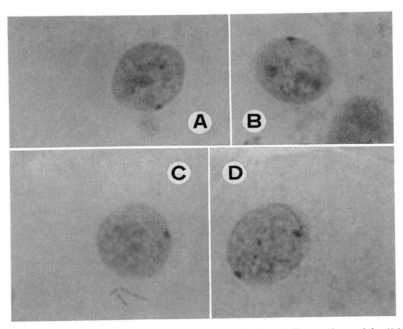

Fig. 35.1. Normal female sex chromocenter or Barr body in "chromatin-positive" intermediate cells. The chromocenter measures around 1.0 μ in diameter, fusing with the nuclear membrane at any point around the rim of a well preserved resting (metabolic) nucleus. *A, B,* and *C* are from buccal smears; *D* is from a Fast smear (single slide, vaginocervical) ($\times$2000).

finding with hematoxylin. These include aceto-orcein, cresyl violet, Biebrich scarlet, thionine, and Feulgen. Of this group, the former has proved so reliable and valuable that a permanent aceto-orcein mount (various aceto-orcein staining methods have been modified into a permanent mount, and incorporated into the present routine technique) is routinely prepared on all of our buccal smear preparations, with a Papanicoloau stain on a duplicate slide if one is available.

Procedure. Allow cell spread to fix in 95% ethyl alcohol (EOH) 15 minutes or longer. Refilter aceto-orcein stain immediately before use. Hydrate slide through 50% EOH and water (distilled). Stain in aceto-orcein stain for 5 minutes. Wash for 10 seconds in gentle stream of distilled water (wash bottle) and dehydrate rapidly (five dips each) through 50% EOH, 70% EOH, 80% EOH, and 95% EOH. Stain in fast green stain for 1 minute and rapidly (five dips each) pass through 95% EOH, 100% EOH, and 100% EOH-xylol. Clear in xylol for 5 minutes, permanently mount, and examine.

Stain Preparations (Stock and Working). ACETO-ORCEIN STAIN. To 45 ml. glacial acetic acid (80° to 85° C.) add 1.0 gm. of orcein with rapid agitation. Gradually add this solution to 55 ml. of distilled water (room temperature), stirring constantly. Cool in running water bath and filter (No. 1 paper). Store in brown screw cap jar. Improving with age, stain must be refiltered just before each use.

FAST GREEN STAIN. To 100 ml. of 95% ethyl alcohol add 0.03 gm. of fast green, with agitation to dissolve. Store in screw cap jar.

"Chromatin-positive" is a useful clinical term for individuals with chromatin accumulations on the nuclear rim of approximately 1-μ diameter which *blends in* with the membranes of over 15% of well preserved nuclei; those with its absence, one termed as "chromatin-negative." This reduces the possibility of psychological trauma of emotionally undesirable information reaching the patient.

Normal childbearing *females* are chromatin-*positive*, whereas normal *males* are chromatin-*negative*. Study of "squash" preparations of metaphase cells reveals 46 chromosomes. Formally thought to total 48, the human chromosomal endowment has been shown, by these more sensitive cytogenetic methods, to be 46. These consist of 22 pairs of autosomes (non-sex chromosomes) and one pair of sex chromosomes. In the normal female, the latter are XX; in the male, they are XY. On present evidence, it appears that any cell requires one X sex chromosome to be in the metabolic phase. Thus, a second X sex chromosome may be found in the clumped, presumably non-metabolic phase clump. This resulting chromatin is responsible for the nuclear membrane chromocenter of chromatin-positive individuals (Fig. 35.1).

Nondisjunction

Chromosomal aberrations are rapidly being discovered and shown clinically to be linked to certain sexual and developmental abnormalities. In the development of the ovum or sperm, failure of a pair of chromosomes to separate during miotic division is referred to as nondisjunction. When this occurs, both (or neither) chromosomes enter the gamete, while the complement (neither or both) is lost to heredity into a polar body. In lower forms of life nondisjunction occurs with increased frequency in older individuals. This aging tendency likewise appears to apply to man, at least in mongolism and Klinefelter's syndrome. Mental status, physical make-up, and endocrine balance are frequently affected in the clinical entities produced from nondisjunction.

Nondisjunction of Sex Chromosomes. Most individuals with *Turner's syndrome* (XO) or gonadal-agenesis have an endowment of only 45 chromosomes. The 22 autosomal pairs appear to be intact, but only one sex chromosome is present (XO). Although these patients are physically female, they are chromatin-*negative*.

Persons with *Klinefelter's symdrome* (XXY) or testicular dysgenesis are chromatin-*positive* even though of male habi-

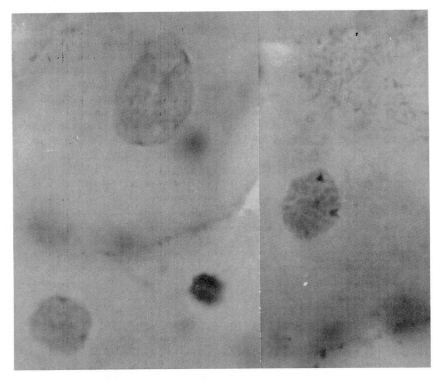

Fig. 35.2. "Superfemale" (XXX) with two sex chromocenters, or Barr bodies in intermediate cells of a buccal smear. *Left*, two cells, each having two diagnostic sex chromocenters widely separated on the nuclear membrane. *Right*, the same patient with two chromocenters. One, being on the nuclear membrane in profile, is diagnostic; however, the other one, being on a superior or inferior membrane, is not diagnostic as it does not blend in with the membrane in profile. The diagnostic one is forked; at times it appeared paired in this individual (aceto-orcein, permanent stain, ×2000).

tus. Their total chromosomal count is usually 47. Again the 22 autosomal pairs appear to be intact but there are three sex chromosomes, two X and one Y. Some have four sex chromosomes, three X and one Y giving *double* chromocenters.

In lower forms of life, "*superfemales*" (XXX) are well known to geneticists. Only recently have they been documented in man. Cytogenetically, these individuals possess 22 apparently intact autosomal pairs; however, as with the usual Klinefelter's syndrome, they have three sex chromosomes, but differ from it in that all are alike (XXX). They are not only chromatin-*positive*, but have *double* chromocenters widely separated on the nuclear membrane (Fig. 35.2). At times each of these chromocenters appears to be paired or forked.

Extremely rare variants occur such as XXXY (with Klinefelter's, two Barr bodies) and XXXXY (three Barr bodies), and other forms appearing in mosaic. Many miscellaneous forms of nondisjunction of the sex chromosomes have not been clinically demonstrated. It is very probable that, as with lower species, some of these produce "lethals," such as OY, with death of the fetuses in utero or perinatally.

Nondisjunction of Autosomes. LeJeune found that mongolian idiocy is associated with an extra chromosome in one of the smallest of the autosome sets (trisomy), with 47 chromosomes resulting. At times, the extra chromosome attaches to another one, which results in a total of 46 but with one abnormally large. Trisomy in other non-sex chromosomes is being discovered with increased frequency. They usually produce no evident change in the metabolic (resting) nuclear pattern, showing the single sex chromocenter (Barr body) only in females.

Developments in cytogenetics have been so rapid recently that many of our fundamental concepts are being basically altered; not only our concepts of genetics, but also of our approaches to many clinical problems. Physiological and biochemical genetics is playing an ever increasing role in our recognition, appreciation, and handling of these clinical entities.

Thus, normal females (XX) have positive nuclear sex chromatin ($♀$), whereas normal males (XY) have negative sex chromatin ($♂$) or lack of the Barr body. Male pseudohermaphrodites (XY with female external genitalia) have negative chromatin ($♂$), whereas female pseudohermaphrodites (XX with male external genitalia) have positive chromatin ($♀$). Turner's syndrome patients (XO with female habitus) have negative sex chromatin ($♂$). Klinefelter's syndrome patients (XXY with male habitus) have positive sex chromatin ($♀$). "Superfemales" (XXX with female habitus) and some Klinefelter's (XXXY with male habitus) have "double positive" sex chromatin. Many of the patients reported with nondisjunction of the sex chromosomes have been sterile and mentally deficient.

ENDOCRINE EVALUATION BY CYTOHORMONAL STUDIES

Endocrinopathies detected for therapy in today's medical practice are rarely overt. Most are subtle and obscured by structural and functional changes seeming to have other, nonendocrine bases. In addition, a wide variety of diseases are associated with endocrine abnormalities or produce them as by-prodcts. Prompt determination of the patient's hormonal status, with accurate recognition of its variance from normal, is a key to detection of the underlying cause and to its proper management.

Cytohormonal determination is a readily available tool which has been made easily accessible to the clinician by rapid and simple methods for obtaining specimens. With proper interpretation it can offer valuable assistance which is either detective and directive to more elaborate procedures, or is definitive and diagnostic.

The Cytological Basis for Hormonal Evaluation. As with other systemic states in medical practice, determination of status is made from an aliquot with extrapolation to the whole. Because of this, aliquot samples must be picked with care and with full knowledge of limitations, and interpreted wisely. To be complete, knowledge of endocrine status should be gained from all possible sources, including accurate clinical observations, biochemical assay of blood and urine, and cytohormonal evaluation.

As with clinical observation, cytohormonal evaluation must recognize the complex endocrine interplay which is mirrored in the cellular spread. One is not dealing with a single compound evaluation, as with biochemical determination.

Individual sensitivity to compounds vary. Further, the presence of undetermined substances may be overlooked by focusing one's attention solely upon the few for which objective determinations can be made by biochemical assay. Cytologically adjudging patient endocrine response is a physiological test of the actual reaction in that individual patient.

Specifically, cytohormonal evaluation is based upon the reactions of certain cells (while *in situ*) to the complex endocrine milieu. It is dependent upon the *types* of hormonally active compounds present at that time, their *dose level* of activity and the patient's ability for *tissue response*. Fortunately, the latter is somewhat constant and predictable from patient to patient; it is dependent, however, upon other endocrine-enzymatic systems active at that time, e.g., thyroid status, previous injury to the tissue (for example, radiation), and differences in response inherited by the tissues of the end organ. In certain clinical situations, cytopathological endocrine determinations yield detective, diagnostic, or therapeutic information unobtainable by other methods.

All living tissues respond to their endocrine-enzymatic milieu. Some, however, recognizably change their morphological and physiological states with great sensitivity, to reflect accurately the delicate hormonal balance present throughout the body at that time. Such a systemic mirror for the interplay of certain clinically important substances is the vaginal epithelium (Kahn). Extremely sensitive to the sexually active compounds (estrogens, progestogens, androgens), it is also sensitive in varying degrees to others (corticoids, thyroxines, vitamins, cyclic antibiotics, digitoxins, etc.). The buccal mucous membrane, the external skin (Fell and Mellanby), and the urinary tract epithelium show similar responses which are weaker and less dependable.

No tissue is as sensitive an indicator (of hormonal status) as is the epithelium of the upper vagina in quality, quantity, and rapidity of response. Regardless of the controversy over its embryological origin, vaginal epithelium faithfully mirrors the status of the Müllerian and associated tissues.

The Specimen. The *vaginal pool specimen*, with its spontaneously exfoliated vaginal epithelial cells, is a very satisfactory specimen for hormonal evaluation. The lateral vaginal wall responds to hormones with somewhat greater sensitivity than the whole vault and its direct scraping gives an evaluation relatively free from uterine contamination or from cells exfoliated into the pool hours or days before. However, there is individual variation in response and site of such sensitive areas; further, and of more importance, among clinicians there is variation in the area selected and in the pressure of scraping, so that the artificially exfoliated cells represent varying depths of cellular layers.

Cytohormonal evaluation depends upon the state of the epithelial cells lying at the surface; natural exfoliation therefrom yields a reproducibility and reliability which cannot be achieved when specimen depth artificially varies. The vaginal pool specimen is a part of the routine Fast smear (single slide, vaginocervical).

When *daily serial* cytohormonal evaluation is of importance, the patient herself can easily take vaginal pool smears which are completely comparable, reproducible, and reliable. Posterior vaginal pool material can be relied upon for reproducible cytohormonal evaluation.

The specimen of mucus is obtained from the pool in the posterior vaginal fornix by aspiration, by gentle removal with a a wooden blade or nonabsorbent swab without scraping the epithelium, or even from the posterior blade of the speculum (see Fig. 35.28, "Clinical Preparation of Specimens"). It is then spread on a slide, fixed, and stained as in the classical Papanicolaou-Traut method for an accurate evaluation and permanent record; or, for an immediate clinical impression, it can be stained fresh by Rakoff's rapid stain and microscopically examined directly. A combination of both is valuable. The latter temporary preparation allows for immediate recognition of overt abnormalities for prompt institution of therapy, but does not allow for future reference. The permanent preparation allows a complete evaluation of subtle endocrine changes and comparison with previous and subsequent preparations.

In *children* and the *aged*, great care must be exercised to obtain the specimen only from the vaginal vault. It must not be contaminated by touching either the labia, the vestibule, or the ungloved examiner's fingers. A nonabsorbent cotton swab, moistened with saline and introduced through a nasal speculum, gives an adequate vaginal pool specimen for cytohormonal evaluation of a child.

General Pattern Response. The vaginal epithelium is capable of producing carbohydrates, proteins, and crystalloids in varying aqueous concentrations. Additional quantities come from higher up the tract in the endometrium, endosalpinx, and peritoneum. Many of these are under endocrine influence, but other factors also effect them. Nervous and psychic stimuli alter their production; irritation, inflammation, and bleeding change or obscure them. Neutrophils appear and disappear under hormonal influences, but slight infections invalidate and obscure their significance.

As the significance of these elements is unpredictable, they are usually of dubious assistance and for most endocrine determinations are best disregarded, routinely. Occasionally they will clarify an obscure problem.

Cellular Morphology Response. Cellular morphology yields the most dependably valuable information. Both the relationships of one cell to another and their individual state of cellular maturation are evaluated. The former includes their sticky behavior with clumping *versus* a tendency to remain separate as individual cells, and a cytoplasmic crinkling and folding upon itself *versus* a tendency to be flat.

By far the most informative and reliable is the state of maturation which the cells of the vaginal epithelium attain at their time of exfoliation. Thus, natural exfoliation is of basic importance to hormonal evaluation; artifacts of scraping can be disastrous. The endocrine-enzymatic milieu in which the squamous cells are bathed has the greatest influence upon the length of time they remain attached as part of the epithelium and upon the state of maturation they develop. Compounds reach the cells with effectiveness either from the vessels below the basement membrane or from the vaginal lumen above the epithelial surface—both systemic and suppository therapy produce the characteristic effects.

Clinical endocrine cytology produces predictable and reproducible results. Its pattern parallels the pattern of tissues taken simultaneously at biopsy. The most objective, reproducible, and generally valuable methods for determining endocrine status cytologically are based upon assessing the state of maturation attained by the cells of the squamous epithelium at their time of exfoliation. The percentage of cells with nuclear pyknosis is referred to as the karyopyknotic index (K.I.). The percentage of cells showing cytoplasmic acidophilia is termed the cornification index (C.I.). These and the important parabasal type cell exfoliation are evaluated in the total maturation index (M.I.).

Maturation Index (M.I.). A concise and objective method for accomplishing endocrine evaluation is the maturation index. This cytohormonal evaluation expresses conveniently the level of cellular maturation attained at the time of exfoliation, as a delicately changing ratio. A differential of the three major types of cells shed from the stratified squamous epithelium is performed on vaginal pool material or lateral vaginal wall material; *viz.:* parabasal cells, intermediate cells, and superficial cells (Fig. 35.3). (The nomenclature used for these three major types of cells shed from squamous epithelium is the International Nomenclature which was informally agreed upon in 1958. Nomenclature used previously differs from this.

Thus, 10/55/35 represents the M.I. of a patient exfoliating 10% parabasal cells, 55% intermediate cells, and 35% superficial cells, and reflects their ratio on the surface of her vaginal epithelium. This is analogous to the Arneth index, in which nuclear morphology reflects the level of neutrophilic maturation at the time of their exfoliation from marrow into circulating peripheral blood; likewise, a shift to the left denotes less mature cells being released (exfoliated), whereas a shift to the right indicates more mature cells.

The three normal cells shed from the noncornified, stratified, squamous vaginal epithelium are usually easily told apart. First, one determines the cytoplasmic thickness (Fig. 35.3). If it is *thick*, the cell is a *parabasal*. If the cytoplasm is "wafer-thin" the cell is a squame of either intermediate or superficial type, and one then determines the nuclear size and chromatin pattern. If the nucleus of this squame is plump and vesicular, with an intact chromatin pattern, the cell is termed an *intermediate;* if it is pyknotic, shrunken, and hyperchromatic and lacks chromatin pattern, the cell is a *superficial.*

A sharp distinction is usually obvious with a good nuclear stain, such as the Papanicolaou stain, on properly fixed

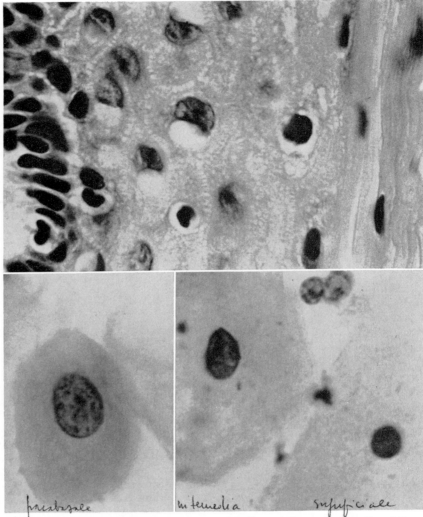

parabasale *intermedia* *superficiale*

Fig. 35.3. Noncornified, stratified, squamous epithelium of the vaginal vault and its exfoliated cells. *Upper section from left to right:* basement membrane, true basal cells, parabasal cells, intermediate cells, superficial cells (×1100). *Lower left,* parabasal cell (exfoliated, in vaginal smear); cytoplasm is *thick* from nucleus to cell border (×1500). *Lower right,* intermediate cell (*left*) and superficial cell (exfoliated, in vaginal smear); cytoplasm of both is uniformly "wafer-thin" from nucleus to cell border. The intermediate cell nucleus is vesicular and retains chromatin pattern. The nucleus of the superficial cell is pyknotic and has lost chromatin pattern. A neutrophil is in upper midfield (×1500).

material. In poor nuclear stains and in dried or poorly fixed cell preparations a sharp differentiation may be difficult. Under phase contrast, pyknosis is accompanied by a very characteristic red sheen to the nucleus. Cytoplasmic color is not of assistance in separating a parabasal from a squame; between an intermediate and a

superficial cell, however, there is some rough correlation. With a Papanicolaou stain, Shorr stain, and Rakoff stain, intermediate cells tend to have green, blue, or gray cytoplasm, whereas superficial cells usually are termed acidophilic, with an affinity for yellow, orange, or red. There is not an absolute correlation, as cytoplasmic color is affected by more artifacts than is nuclear pyknosis, for example, mild infections, drying, fixative, pH, and stain. It does give a rapid albeit rough impression.

Strict cellular morphology, *i.e.*, cytoplasmic maturation (thick *versus* thin) and nuclear maturation (viable *versus* pyknotic), gives the most consistently reproducible endocrine evaluation for clinical purposes. These two are the only factors utilized for determining the M.I.

One must be very careful not to include metaplastic or dysplastic cells in the M.I. Contaminating cells from endocervical dysplasia or from vaginal dermatological conditions must be recognized as not belonging in the normal squamous series, and therefore not counted in the M.I. The cells of the dysplastic series have larger than normal nuclei, with a nuclear membrane frequently wrinkled as if it had somewhat shriveled. In addition, the chromatin is not in the fine reticular pattern of a normal squamous cell, but tends to be coarser with granular clumping. With severe dysplasia the cytoplasm may be scanty, and the cell would approach the appearance of a parabasal cell if it were not for the enlarged, coarse nucleus. Dyskaryotic cells must *not* be included in the M.I.

Under certain conditions superficial cells can become more mature (hypermature) by losing their nuclei (see Fig. 35.13). As normal vaginal epithelium is nonkeratinizing squamous, these cells are not present in normal vaginal smears. These anucleate superficial cells are usually shed from keratotic epithelium of irritation, reaction, neoplasia, or dermatosis, which usually appears clinically as a leukoplakia; at times they will appear with extremely high levels of estrogen or tissue sensitivity to the drug, as with excessive therapy, tumors, etc. It is a normal occurrence in rhesus monkeys at menarche, but not in humans with a normal cycle.

Under certain conditions parabasal cells can produce orangophilic cytoplasm which may, on rare occasions, be truly keratinized. In addition, some parabasal cell nuclei may occasionally become pyknotic. The true identity of both of these cells as being parabasal is evident from the thickness of their cytoplasm, with failure to show the thin squamification of intermediate and superficial cells. Such abnormal parabasal cells can be found in severe atrophy, in inflammation, and in an androgen "spread" pattern.

Other forms of expressing cellular maturation include the karyopyknotic index (K.I.), which expresses the percentage of squamous epithelial cells having pyknotic nuclei, and the cornification index (C.I.), expressing the percentage of cells having yellow, orange, or red cytoplasm. It is obvious from the foregoing that these two indices usually will approximate closely the right hand figure of the maturation index; at times, however, they will significantly differ. More complicated methods of expression are in use by some, but they appear to offer no more clinical assistance than those mentioned.

Recently a term, maturation count, has been introduced. This greatly confuses the clinician by expressing the *same* cell-types in *reverse* order to the maturation index and offers nothing in addition. The two must not be confused.

Cytohormonal Patterns

The *normal patterns* and their *great variations* must be thoroughly understood before attempting to interpret abnormalities. Therefore, for better comprehension and clinical correlation it is valuable to consider the normal female life span in *five* periods (Plate XXXV.I). Three of these are clinically well defined—*childhood, reproductive, postmenopausal*—separated by the objective occurrences: *birth, menarche, menopause,* and *death.* Because of the endocrine turbulence occurring at menarche and menopause, even though clinically they might appear to be fairly sharply defined in most individuals, there is great value in considering the *perimenarchal* and *perimenopausal* periods in great detail; these, of course, overlap the three major periods.

From the endocrine point of view, therefore, the normal female life span is conveniently considered in five periods: *childhood, perimenarchal, reproductive, perimenopausal, and postmenopausal.* To understand the endocrine cellular patterns, one should first consider the basic modes in which the vaginal epithelium and its exfoliated cells have to react to individual hormones.

Normal Cytohormonal Patterns of the Basic Stimulating Agents. ESTROGENS. All layers of the epithelium become thickened and proliferated. This is marked in the squames, where intermediate and superficial cells become most numerous on the surface. A great many of these mature to superficial cells with a resultant shift to the right of the M.I. Thus, when a patient with a completely atrophic pattern of 100/0/0 is given increasing doses of estrogens, either systemically or by suppository, there will be a progressive shift of the M.I. to the right, with the degree of shift proportional to the amount of estrogens administered. A moderate dose will produce an M.I. of 0/50/50, a large dose will approach 0/0/100. At the same time that clinical

and cytological inflammation due to atrophy decreases, cellular degeneration is strikingly reduced, the smear appears "clean," and the cells tend to be distributed singly without curling.

PROGESTOGENS. Proliferation of the squames is also a major feature of progesterone, but maturation progresses only through the intermediate cell stage when exfoliation occurs. The M.I. shifts toward the midzone, to 0/100/0 if dosage is sufficient. Superficial cells are not produced on pure progesterone, estrogen being needed to mature the cells to superficial type. In tissue, the intermediate cells have plump and delicate cytoplasm, which completely collapses on cell spread to a characteristically thin wafer. The cytoplasm curls and cells stick together in masses. Mucus is abundant if the systemic hormonal pattern background is proper; if the epithelium has been "primed" with estrogens, cytolysis occurs. The background of the cell spread is "messy" with mucus, neutrophils, and cellular debris.

ANDROGENS. Androgens do not perfectly oppose estrogen proliferation. In fact, proliferation is the rule under

---

PLATE XXXV.I. Cytohormonal evaluation; maturation index (M.I.) of a woman's lifetime. The endocrine periods of the female—a composite based upon cytohormonal determinations of individual patients. This schematically represents the fluctuations of the three levels of epithelial surface cell maturation (parabasal, intermediate, superficial) which occur under the influence, mainly, of various hormones. Estrogen produces superficial cell maturation (M.I. to right, toward 0/0/100). A moderate degree of this effect is noted at ovulation (M.I., c. 0/40/60). Progesterone and cortisone cause intermediate cell maturation (M.I. to midzone, toward 0/100/0). A moderate degree of this effect is noted at menstruation (M.I., c. 0/70/30), and extreme effect at birth and pregnancy (M.I., 0/95/5) and estratrophy (M.I., 0/100/0). Lack of all maturing factors, or repression of their effect, causes no maturation beyond parabasal cells at exfoliation (M.I. to left, toward 100/0/0). A moderate degree of this effect is noted during childhood (M.I., c, 80/20/0), and extreme effect at postpartum and teleatrophy (M.I., 100/0/0). The period of childhood is relatively constant and predictable. The reproductive period is constant from cycle to cycle. Atrophy in the postmenopausal period is of two main types: estratrophy (M.I., 0/100/0) with complete lack of estrogen effect, and teleatrophy (M.I., 100/0/0) with complete lack of effect of all maturing substances. Conversely the perimenarchal and the perimenopausal periods are extremely difficult to evaluate because of the wide range of normal possibilities serving as an unpredictable base line. In all cytohormonal evaluations it is thus essential to know everything possible about the patient endocrinologically, such as age, date of last menstrual period (LMP), date of previous menstrual period (PMP), drug therapy, radiotherapy, surgery, etc.

androgens, but the cells on the surface mature to all three types. Thus, one finds parabasal cells lying on the surface alongside of superficial and intermediate cells. The M.I. is a "spread" pattern, approaching in some a flat 33/34/33 but tending to shift more to the left. In other patients, more intermediate cells or parabasal cells are present, even approaching 100/0/0; however, the trend remains for the index to "spread," as androgens do not typically produce 100% of one cell type. A clue that one may be dealing with androgens can be found in a "spread" pattern with abnormally small superficial cells (*wafer-thin* polygonal cytoplasm) and small parabasal cells having *thick* orangophilic cytoplasm with nuclear pyknosis. Mucus may be present. Inflammation also causes "spreading" of the M.I. and, as an androgen pattern may appear inflammatory and obscuring, these two conditions can be easily confused. Androgen, therefore, does not produce a diagnostic pattern, but at times comes very close to it.

CORTISONE. Drugs having the cortisone effect produce proliferation similar to progesterone, with the surface cells maturing to intermediate type. The M.I. approaches 0/100/0, according to the dosage, but the cells do not tend to curl or stick to the degree that one finds with progesterone. Mucus is usually scanty or lacking, and the smear may appear strikingly "clean." One must bear in mind that the adrenal cortex also produces estrogenic, progestogenic, and androgenic compounds which affect the vaginal epithelium characteristically if in sufficient dosage.

MISCELLANEOUS SUBSTANCES. Various other compounds may affect the hormonal pattern of the vaginal epithelium. Digitalis produces an intermediate cell maturation, with a midzone shift in the M.I. Likewise, some of the cyclic broad spectrum antibiotics cause an M.I. shift. Absence or severe reduction of some compounds will change the cellular response. Avitaminosis A causes an M.I. shift to the right, whereas extreme hypothyroidism causes an M.I. shift to the left.

COMPOUNDING EFFECT. It is important to realize that effects of substances acting in succession or simultaneously may be simply additive or may qualitatively change each other's response. The effect of progesterone upon an unstimulated atrophic vaginal epithelium, for instance, differs markedly from one "primed" with estrogens.

INFLAMMATORY EFFECT. In addition to bringing forth leukocytes and other inflammatory elements, inflammation alters the level of maturation attained by the surface cells and makes cytohormonal evaluation unsatisfactory. The general effect is to increase the cell types in the minority, at the expense of the cell types in the majority. This "spread" of the M.I. (*e.g.*, 0/30/70, 70/30/0, and 0/95/5 all tending to become 33/34/33) is roughly proportional to the severity of the inflammation, and is dependent upon its etiology. When severe, inflammation may result in hypermaturity of the superficial cell sufficient to cause it to lose its nucleus, forming areas of leukoplakia which exfoliate this abnormal, anucleate superficial cell. When severity is restricted to an extremely small area of the epithelium (such as in chronic irritation from a pessary or in a localized dermatosis), such extreme cellular artifacts exfoliated from this area into otherwise healthy vaginal secretions may appear paradoxical. In addition to this alteration of cellular maturation, severe inflammation can be so obscuring and so destructive of cells that the preparation is useless. Clearing inflammation in any effective way which does not employ agents altering the epithelial maturation, allows true hormonal pattern to be evaluated.

Normal Cytohormonal Patterns of the Endocrine Periods. CHILDHOOD PERIOD. This period produces one of the most dependable and constant patterns, except for the very beginning and end of the period (Plate XXXV.I). *At birth* the vaginal epithelium of the female infant

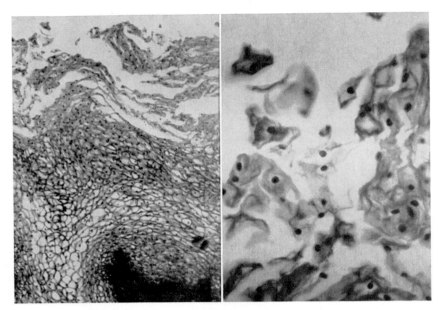

FIG. 35.4. Vaginal epithelium, female fetus, 6 months gestation. *Left,* the lush epithelium so typical of both a female fetus *en utero* and a pregnant woman (H & E stain, ×40). *Right,* intermediate cells exfoliating from the surface of the same epitheli um. Maturation index, 0/95/5 (see Fig. 35.6) (H & E, ×160).

is thick and lush in response to circulating maternal hormones, including massive progesterones, estrogens, and adrenocortical compounds (Fig. 35.4). The surface cells are mainly of intermediate type, so that the M.I. of the cell spread is characteristic of pregnancy, 0/95/5 (Fig. 35.6). Desquamation rapidly takes place and within a few weeks it becomes the thin atrophic epithelium so characteristic of *childhood,* with the M.I. markedly shifted to the left (*c.* 100/0/0 or 70/30/0). The surface cell matures to the parabasal level at exfoliation, with only a few intermediates and with *no* superficials. In the absence of inflammation or irritation and with the certainty that the vaginal smear has not been contaminated with introitus cells, the superficial cell is normally absent until the onset of the perimenarchal period. An appearance of this cell in the childhood period is significant.

PERIMENARCHAL PERIOD. Around the age of 8 years (Rakoff), and with great individual variation, there begins a gradual increase of noticeable sex steroid activity until the reproductive level is reached at menarche, about the age of 14 (Plate XXXV.I). This gradual increase is evidenced in the vaginal epithelium by thickening and proliferation, with increasing numbers of surface cells maturing to the intermediate and superficial types as sex hormone production increases. The vaginal smear mirrors this, with an increasing shift to the right of the M.I., until the appearance of menses and the full-blown cellular endocrine pattern of the reproductive age. Therefore, as this perimenarchal period is a continuing transition from childhood atrophy (M.I., *c.* 100/0/0 to 70/30/0) to the lush epithelium of the reproductive period, (M.I., *c.* 0/70/30 to 0/40/60), great variation can be encountered. Age is the major factor in evaluating endocrine status of this period. When the menarche appears, there is still adjustment for many. Some have not yet reached a full reproductive M.I., whereas others for a

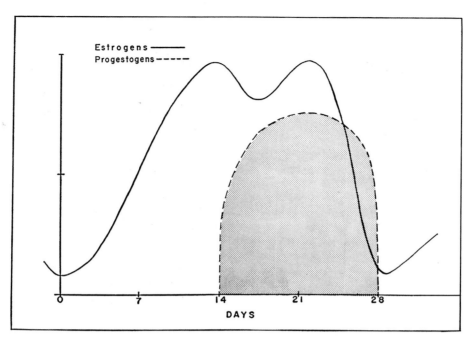

Fig. 35.5. Menstrual cycle. A diagrammatic composite of the interplay in levels of systemic estrogens and progestogens which occurs during the menstrual cycle of a woman in her reproductive period of life.

period of time exceed normalcy and have an M.I. with an extreme shift to the right.

REPRODUCTIVE PERIOD. From onset to cessation of menses the endocrine milieu shows great cyclic fluctuation. Following the initial period of endocrine adjustment in the establishment of menses and extending into the disruption of endocrine interplay of the perimenopausal period, the pattern is a series of lunar cycles. Although the hormonal patterns vary widely within each cycle, they are usually mirrored in repetition for a given individual. Their constancy is broken normally only by childbearing, so that the cellular patterns of the *menstrual cycle*, of *pregnancy*, and of the *postpartum period*, are characteristic.

Throughout the *menstrual cycle* with a normal ovulatory pattern (Plate XXXV.II), superficial cells and intermediate cells vary in exfoliation from 30 to 70% (M.I. from *c.* 0/40/60 to *c.* 0/70/30) in response to estrogen and

progesterone levels. At the time of ovulation, high estrogen is present (Fig. 35.5), with a moderate shift of M.I. to the right (*c.* 0/40/60) (Plate XXXV.II). With ovulation, circulating estrogen drops rapidly. Shortly thereafter estrogen rises with the development of the corpus luteum during the secretory phase, but at this time accompanied by progestogens (Fig. 35.5). Just before menstruation the progestogen opposition is at its highest and produces a moderate M.I. shift to the midzone (M.I., *c.* 0/70/30). During menstruation both estrogen and progestogen sharply drop. Soon, from the developing new follicle, estrogen again rises alone during the proliferative phase, shifting the M.I. to the right until the ovulatory pattern (M.I., *c.* 0/40/60) is once more reached, 2 weeks before menses. Except postpartum, the parabasal type cell does not exfoliate normally until the later years of the reproductive period, or the perimenopausal period; in some patients

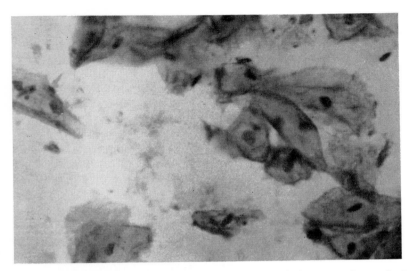

Fig. 35.6. Gestation. This Fast smear of a 23-year-old woman in her seventh month of gestation shows the "midzone" shift in the maturation index, 0/95/5, so typical of pregnancy. It is also found during fetal life and at birth (see Fig. 35.4). The intermediate cells fold into "navicular" forms and tend to adhere together (×160).

(estratrophy) it may not exfoliate at any time during the reproductive and post-menopausal periods (Plate XXXV.I). As with a single basal body temperature determination, a *single* vaginal smear evaluation gives only limited endocrine information. This is not only because of the great endocrine variations encountered during the menstrual cycle, but also because of the fact that many combinations of various factors can produce similar static cytohormonal patterns. *Daily* vaginal pool aspiration smears obtained and prepared by the patient, with her basal body temperature, are invaluable in detecting ovulation, anovulation, time in cycle, endocrinopathies, etc. Such complete cytohormonal evaluation yields valuable dynamic endocrine information.

In *pregnancy*, the cytohormonal pattern is characteristic. With conception the normal luteal phase M.I. shift toward the midzone proceeds just as in the nonpregnant menstrual cycle; however, when the pattern reaches the menstrual M.I. (*c.* 0/70/30), it does not recede but continues its midzone climb. Within a few weeks it has reached the pattern so characteristic of pregnancy (Fig. 35.6),

with the extreme M.I. midzone shift (0/95/5) maintain throughout gestation. The levels of estrogens, progestogens, and cortical steroids are so massive in the normal pregnancy (Fig. 35.7), that this M.I. is not altered by usual doses of hormones. This forms the basis for Wied's test for menopausal amenorrhea *versus* pregnancy (see p. 684). Direct effect of infection upon the vaginal epithelium, however, will artificially alter even the hormonal pattern of pregnancy, with a characteristic inflammatory "spread" of the M.I. (*e.g.,* from 0/95/5 toward *c.* 33/34/33). Thus, when the usual pregnancy M.I. of 0/95/5 varies markedly either to the right or to the left in the *absence* of inflammation, it is significant; hormonal change must be great indeed, to effect such an alteration in a pattern normally held to by massive levels of hormones. Abortions having an endocrine basis are heralded by a bizarre M.I. usually to the right but at times either "spread" or to the left. If this threatened or impending abortion then leads to fetal death, it is signaled by a drastic shift of

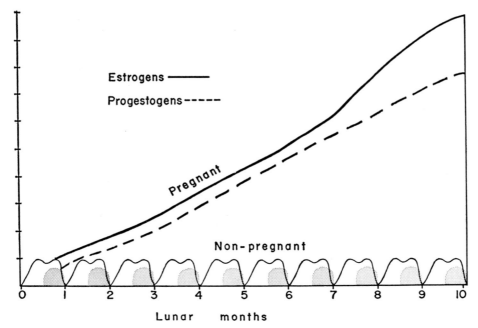

Lunar months

FIG. 35.7. Gestation. A diagrammatic composite of the systemic estrogens and progestogens of a pregnant patient, superimposed upon those expected if she were not pregnant.

the M.I. to the left, similar to the postpartum pattern.

The *postpartum* pattern is striking. Around the time of delivery another mammoth hormonal change takes place. The M.I., heavily shifted to the midzone throughout pregnancy, apparently briefly shifts to the right (Pundel) and then suddenly plunges completely to the left (0/95/5 to 100/0/0) (Plate XXXV.I). This teleatrophic postpartum or lactational pattern (Fig. 35.8) is striking in a young woman. It can be altered by hormones administered for suppression of lactation. After varying lengths of time it gradually returns to the normal menstrual cyclic pattern. Of great interest is Pundel's report of a significant change in cytohormonal pattern a few days *before* normal termination of pregnancy, with a slight shift to the right and then the significant shift to the left of the M.I. He has used this to indicate extreme postmaturity in a few cases, with successful saving of some of the infants. Others have been unable to entirely confirm the findings in much smaller series, but the work

is recent and remains clinically a very important finding to exploit. Determination of fetal sex from alterations of maternal cytohormonal pattern by fetal endocrine production has proved fruitless in spite of earlier encouraging reports. The maternal hormonal level which establishes the normal pregnancy pattern is massive relative to the minute alteration which any fetal production might play.

PERIMENOPAUSAL PERIOD. For years, both before and after the actual cessation of menses, there are gradually progessive alterations in the orderly cyclic endocrine patterns of the reproductive period. These are mirrored in the vaginal epithelium and its cytohormonal pattern (Plate XXXV.I). This process of alteration begins in the latter part of the reproductive period and continues through the menopause and for years thereafter, with the cyclic hormonal variations decreasing in intensity and frequency. The onset of this perimenopausal period is gradual and varies greatly among individuals; if cessation of cycles does occur

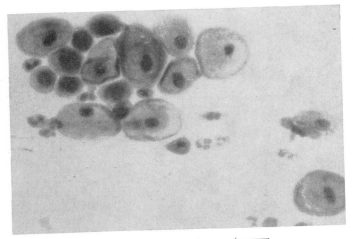

FIG. 35.8. Postpartum or lactation; maturation index, 100/0/0. This peculiarly teleatrophic pattern contains only parabasal cells. It occurs abruptly at the end of gestation and is a marked change from the lush intermediate cell exfoliation of pregnancy (see Fig. 35.6) (×160).

before death, it is likewise insidious and without clinical fanfare.

Cytohormonally, patients appear to fall into two well defined categories, those developing *estratrophy* (M.I., 0/100/0) with complete lack of estrogen effect (Fig. 35.9) and those developing *tele-atrophy* (M.I., 100/0/0) with total absence of evidence of any effect of vaginal maturation (Fig. 35.10). The reasons for the difference are not clear. Adrenal cortical function undoubtedly plays a larger role than generally appreciated, and probably accounts for the M.I. "midzone" shift of estratrophy; but why all do not follow this pattern is not clear. Variations in hypophysial response to feedback may underlie these patterns, and at times adrenal androgens are suspected of playing a role.

In the development of *estratrophy* throughout the perimenopausal period, there is an increasing number of intermediate cells exfoliated at the expense of superficials, without significant production of parabasals. This shift toward the midzone of the M.I. (0/100/0) is gradual, and estratrophy is eventually reached years after actual cessation of menses. This is not an atrophic vaginal epithelium,

clinically, but is lush and resistant; however, of great importance is the absence of superficial cells. This total lack of apparent estrogen stimulation may reflect relatively high or unopposed cortisone levels.

In the development of the second frequent pattern, that of *teleatrophy* (Fig. 35.10), there is a gradual increase in exfoliation of parabasal cells at the expense of superficial cells, and later of the intermediate cells. Finally complete atrophy, or teleatrophy, appears with total shift of the M.I. to the left (100/0/0). Clinically, vaginal atrophy is present and the epithelial resistance is low. Senile vaginitis is frequent in this group.

There is no "normal" or typical pattern of a woman at the time of her last menses, the range of normalcy being extremely wide. Some pass through the menopause with a "young" pattern, whereas others are more atrophic. The established pattern is more one of default than of strong endocrine levels, and is thus labile and sensitive to small doses of hormones or inflammation. Wied (1957) has taken advantage of this in differentiating between a menopausal missed period and pregnancy. The strong endo-

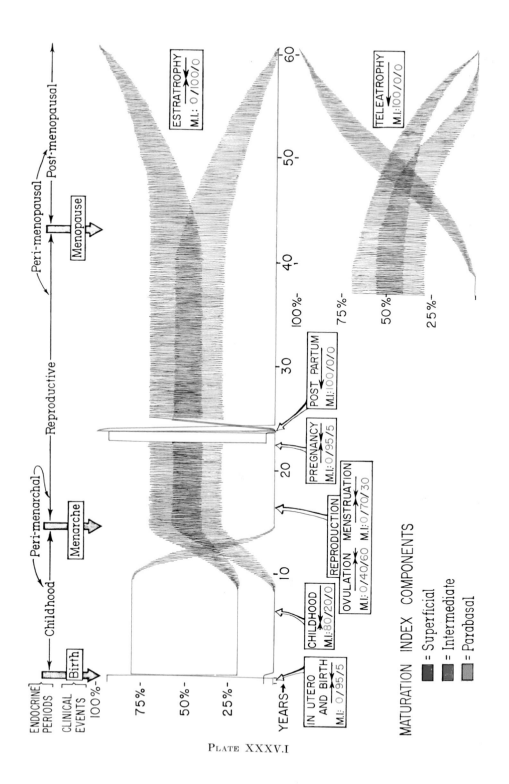

PLATE XXXV.I

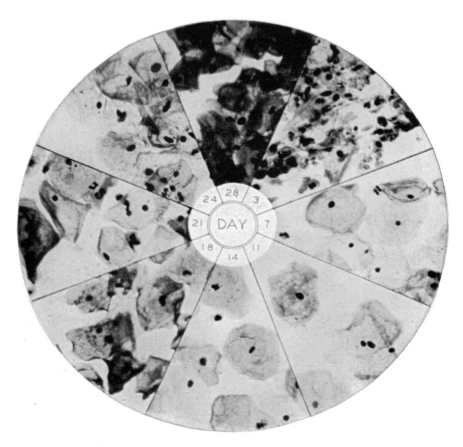

PLATE XXXV.II. The cytohormonal menstrual cycle. Vaginal smears were taken at 3- to 4-day intervals; normal 28-day cycle; menstruation commenced on the 1st and 29th days; age 21. At ovulation (Day 14) the maturation index (M.I.) is 0/40/60, the cells lie singly and flat, and the background is "clean." Immediately before menstruation (Day 28) the M.I. is 0/70/30, cells clump and curl, and the background is "dirty." Note endometrial cells on Day 3 (×70).

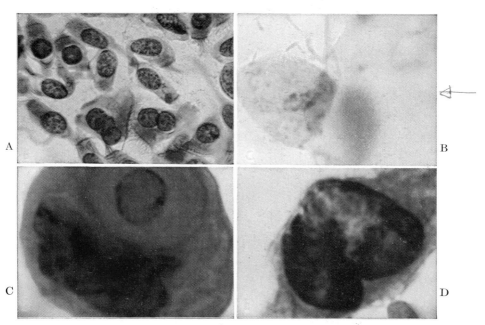

PLATE XXXV.III. *A*, ciliated endocervical cells in a Fast smear (×520). *B*, *Trichomonas vaginalis, left*, lying on the edge of the cytoplasm of a superficial cell. Döderlein bacilli above. Note the pale nucleus of the Trichomonas, with green cytoplasm containing red granules (Fast smear, ×1378). *C*, malignant "pearl" exfoliated from invasive squamous cell carcinoma of the cervix. These two cells have extremely hyalinized and keratinized cytoplasm. An unusual hyper-maturation for cervical carcinomas. The lower nucleus has many malignant criteria (Fast smear, ×1378). *D*, undifferentiated cell from invasive carcinoma (Fast smear, ×1378).

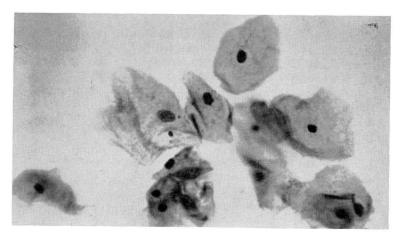

FIG. 35.12. A Fast smear of a 20-year-old patient with testicular feminization demonstrated at subsequent operation. A normal appearing girl with good breast development and normal external genitalia, she had never menstruated. The nuclei contain no Barr bodies ("chromatin-negative"), and the cytohormonal pattern shows good estrogen production with a normal maturation index of 0/62/38 (×160).

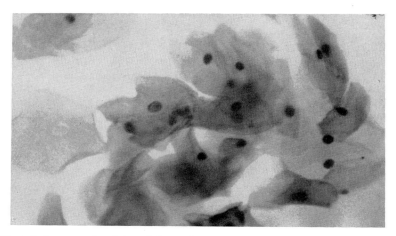

FIG. 35.13. A fast smear of a sister of the patient shown in Figure 35.12. This 17-year-old girl also has testicular feminization, demonstrated at subsequent operation, with negative sex chromatin; however, her cytohormonal pattern shows a more extreme estrogen response, with numerous anucleate superficial cells produced (*left*). The maturation index is 0/32/68, with 18 of the 68 superficials being anucleate (×160).

usually present in the vaginal smear cytohormonal pattern. Male pseudo-hermaphrodites may have evidence of androgen in their cytohormonal pattern, but may approach estratrophy or teleatrophy according to their age.

SECONDARY AMENORRHEA OR OLIGO-MENORRHEA (see Chapter 31). In evaluating unexplained secondary amenorrhea or oligomenorrhea, one should consider the cytohormonal status, the possibility of anovulation, and the cytogenetic status (*i.e.*, XXX). In determining the presence or absence of ovulation in these patients, daily smears should be extended past the usual 30 days in order to detect the extremely long periods encountered with many irregular menses (see "Clinical Techniques," p. 809). The cytohormonal levels of Stein-Leventhal syndrome patients is constant without the cyclic ovulatory shift. Patients with persistent follicular cysts also show anovulation, but their constant daily pattern approximates that found normally at the time of ovulation, estrogen without progesterone. Some patients with Sheehan's syndrome who retain appreciable partial pituitary function have a cytohormonal pattern falling within normal range but without the cyclic ovulatory shift. Mild or moderate hypothyroidism produces cytohormonal patterns within normal range, but without ovulation if the disorder is severe enough. In extreme hypothyroidism the M.I. is shifted to the left toward teleatrophy.

Cytohormonal pattern falling within normal range is also found in systemic illnesses, emotional disturbances, simple physical blockage, or endocrinopathies of borderline severity.

Secondary amenorrhea or oligomenorrhea with *abnormal cytohormonal pattern* bespeaks severe systemic illness, endocrinopathy, or emotional disturbances. Three major cytohormonal patterns should be sought, either in pure form or combinations, a shift in the M.I. to the right, to the midzone, or to the left.

The extreme *M.I. shift to the right* (approaching $\overrightarrow{0/0/100}$) is that of high estrogen effect. This is found in persisting follicle cysts, certain ovarian and adrenal tumors, some endometrial hyperplasias, and adenocarcinomas. In rare instances various miscellaneous hormonally associated states are found with this pattern, such as endometriosis, myomas, and mammary disease (adenofibromas, chronic cystic mastitis, carcinoma); these are not, however, found in any consistent pattern. One must always be alert for exogenous estrogens in its many and frequently overt forms of administration.

The extreme *M.I. shift to the midzone* (approaching estratrophy $\overrightarrow{0/100/0}\overleftarrow{}$) bespeaks lack of estrogen effect in the presence of nonestrogenic maturing stimula-

tion. The most frequent situation is ovarian failure with adequate adrenal cortical function remaining. Oophorectomy, either from surgery or adequate irradiation, removes ovarian estrogen and progestogen production, leaving adrenal cortical function. During the reproductive age the latter normally is overwhelmingly of cortisone type compounds, which produce exfoliation at the intermediate cell level of maturation $\overrightarrow{0/100/0}\overleftarrow{}$. The small amounts of estrogen and progestogen compounds produced by the adrenal cortex are normally insufficient to alter this cytohormonal pattern in the face of overwhelming cortisone effect. Hypopituitary function from tumors, Simmonds' disease, anorexia nervosa, and radiation ablation may be partial with a spread M.I. pattern simulating inflammation. The usual mild or moderate Sheehan's syndrome appears to result from a selective lack of gonadotrophins resulting in a cytohormonal shift to the midzone (M.I., $\overrightarrow{0/100/0}\overleftarrow{}$) typical of ovarian ablation with continuing adrenal cortisone production. When pituitary injury has been more severe and widespread in its trophic effects, Sheehan's syndrome will also produce a spread cytohormonal pattern and even, in very severe ablation, complete teleatrophy. Other menstrual disturbances associated with a M.I. midzone shift include functioning ovarian mesenchymal tumors producing progestogens, functional adrenal tumors, and certain drug administrations. The most frequent cause for secondary amennorrhea with an approximate estratrophy pattern $\overrightarrow{0/95/5}\overleftarrow{}$ is, of course, pregnancy. This is due not to lack of estrogens, as in true estratrophy $\overrightarrow{0/100/0}\overleftarrow{}$, but to its overwhelming opposition by progestogens and adrenal corticoids.

The extreme *M.I. shift to the left* (approaching teleatrophy, $\overleftarrow{100/0/0}$) is found with secondary amenorrhea or oligomenorrhea when there has been no maturation of the vaginal epithelium past the immature parabasal cell. At times the vaginal epithelium is at fault, but usually the maturing stimuli are absent. In the first instance the vaginal epithelium is incapable of reacting to maturing substances in normal fashion owing to inherent inadequacies following injury (*e.g.*, extensive irradiation for cervical carcinoma) or from lack of elements basic to fundamental cellular metabolism (*e.g.*, thyroid deprivation in cretins or extreme hypothyroidism). In the second instance, and most frequently, a normal vaginal epithelium capable of full maturation may be deprived of sufficient amounts of specific maturing substances such as estrogens, progestogens, corticoids, etc. This is responsible for the teleatrophy of extreme panhypopituitary function found in severe Simmonds' disease, anorexia nervosa, Sheehan's syndrome, and ablation. One must remain aware of the peculiar lactational teleatrophy and amenorrhea normally present postpartum, which persist for varying lengths of time (Plate XXXV. I and Fig. 35.8).

MAMMARY LESIONS. Some lesions of the breast are associated with bizarre cytohormonal patterns. They are neither consistent nor diagnostic. Adenofibromas are the most frequent mammary lesions of youth associated with an M.I. shift to the right, at times beyond normal limits. Chronic cystic mastitis, usually with a normal pattern, can also be associated with an M.I. shift to the right, or a spread pattern. Adenocarcinoma is associated with virtually any pattern, either extremely abnormal or normal.

Cytology can be of assistance in clinically evaluating the endocrine status of a patient with *advanced* or metastatic adenocarcinoma of the breast who is within the perimenopausal period. The 5-year postmenopausal clinical rule-of-thumb for endocrine supplemental or ablative therapy, can be augmented by cytohormonal evaluation. In the absence of inflammation, this can qualitate and roughly quantitate remaining endocrine activity to evaluate estrogenic stimulation, androgenic effect, or teleatrophy (Frost *et al.*; Masukawa *et al.*) and may assist in choosing therapy. In following such patients cytohormonally, an unexplained change in pattern often heralds, by a few months, a clinical relapse.

COMPOUNDING STATES. It is no rarity for multiple lesions in the above categories to present together. It is well documented that there is an increased frequency of the association and either simultaneous or subsequent occurrence of ovarian tumors, endometrial hyperplasias or carcinomas, myomas, endometriosis, and mammary lesions. Some bizarre cytohormonal patterns persist for years after the removal of a lesion, such as an extreme M.I. shift to the right in an 80-year-old patient, living and well without evident recurrence or related disease, 16 years after hysterectomy for endometrial adenocarcinoma.

ARTIFICIAL VAGINA. It is interesting to note that vaginal grafts from the thigh may show varying degrees of endocrine response after becoming well established. This coincides with their secretory ability, as demonstrated by Masters. Their cytohormonal pattern is not entirely normal, however, as they retain some true cornification with an extreme M.I. shift to the right and exfoliation of numbers of anucleate superficial cells.

Childhood Abnormal Cytohormonal Patterns. The cytohormonal pattern of childhood is so constantly predictable, at or near teleatrophy with no superficial cells (Plate XXXV. I), that abnormalities are usually obvious. Adrenogenital syndrome with adrenocortical hyperplasia, is associated with an abnormal cytohormonal pattern varying according to the amounts of estrogens, progestogens, and androgens being produced. As the effect of the latter usually predominates, the corresponding androgenic M.I. spread pattern is the most frequent cytohormonal finding. An M.I. shift to the right during childhood, especially before perimenarche, is distinctly abnormal and bespeaks estrogens. Ovarian granulosa-theca cell tumors produce significant M.I. shifts to the right, as does systemic estrogen therapy for childhood atrophic vaginitis.

INFLAMMATION

General Inflammation. Many agents including trauma, chemicals, radiation, infections, and tumors, bring forth a nonspecific inflammatory host response. This heavy leukocytic, hemorrhagic, or necrotic exudate often obscures diagnostic elements. The maturation index is "spread," so that cytohormonal evaluation becomes invalid. Neoplastic elements are rendered unrecognizable from obscuring and degeneration, whereas, at times, non-neoplastic cells are sufficiently altered morphologically to tempt a false cancer diagnosis by the unwary.

CHRONIC TRAUMA

Irritation from a long standing pessary, prolapse, or foreign body produces a M.I. shift to the right in addition to the general inflammatory exudate. Anucleate superficial cells are exfoliated from leukoplakic areas. While multinucleated giant cell histiocytes are most frequently associated with Trichomonas infection, some foreign bodies (*e.g.*, iodinated fats used to determine tubal patency and embedded sutures) may bring them forth.

INFECTIONS

Viral Infections. The usual background pattern in viral infection is a great leukocytic outpouring with cellular destruction, especially of epithelial cells. Some viruses produce inclusion bodies in either the nucleus, the cytoplasm, or both, the former yielding the most diagnostic information. Intranuclear inclusion bodies usually have cleared "halo" areas about them (Figs. 35.14 and 35.15) in contradistinction to giant nucleoli or chromocenters. As nuclei with viral inclusions are degenerating, their chromatin is smudged and is both plastered onto the outer edge of the inclusion as well as margined onto the inner surface of the nuclear membrane, leaving a clearing between which forms the "halo." Cytoplasmic inclusion bodies are much less helpful, diagnostically, as they are diffi-

cult to distinguish from debris of phagocytosis or degeneration, as well as from cellular organelles or inclusions of metabolism. Various viruses have been identified in the urogenital tract but these undoubtedly represent merely a small fraction of those present either locally or as part of a systemic involvement. Salivary gland viral infection during pregnancy can produce congenital infection in the infant with resultant cytomegalic inclusion disease of the newborn. While this is a generalized infection of the infant, it produces characteristic cells in the renal tubular epithelium which exfoliate into the urine to yield a clinical diagnosis (Fig. 35.14).

Other viral or possible viral-associated diseases have been associated with inclusions in the vaginal smear (Varga and Browell). Two types of cells with intranuclear inclusions which have many features in common and may well represent the same condition, are the bizarre cells associated with condyloma acuminata (Naib and Merckling) (Fig. 35.15) and those identified serologically (Stern) with herpes simplex infection. These inclusions tend to be irregular and are found in extremely multinucleated cells superficially resembling syncytiotrophoblasts from which they are to be differentiated.

Bacterial Infections. Acute neisserial, streptococcal, staphylococcal, hemophilic, and pleuropneumonic infections are associated with exudation of neutrophils and serum. Blood is not infrequent. There is marked cellular destruction and obscuring of both cytohormonal pattern and evidence of cancer. Usually these acute infections are vaginal whereas the subacute and chronic infections reside up in the paraurethral glands, the vulvovaginal glands, and, especially, the endocervical canal and glands. Chronic infections involving the endocervix, including tuberculosis, are usually associated with various stages of metaplasia and varying degrees of dysplasia. The latter sheds cells of the dyskaryotic series (Fig. 35.21) corresponding to the degree of atypia or dysplasia (see p. 701). While most bacteria can be morphologically classified in

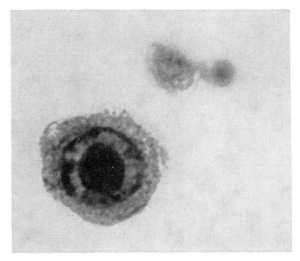

FIG. 35.14. Congenital salivary gland virus disease of childhood, cytomegalic inclusion disease, renal epithelial cell in urine. The large, dark intranuclear inclusion body with smudged chromatin on its surface, has a cleared parachromatin "halo" about it. This is surrounded by the rest of the degenerated chromatin which has marginated onto the nuclear membrane leaving radially arranged strands behind bridging the cleared gap, or "halo." There are no recognizable cytoplasmic inclusions present in this cell, but the cytoplasm is dark and heavily textured. A leukocyte is in the *upper corner* of the field (Papanicolaou stain, ×1200).

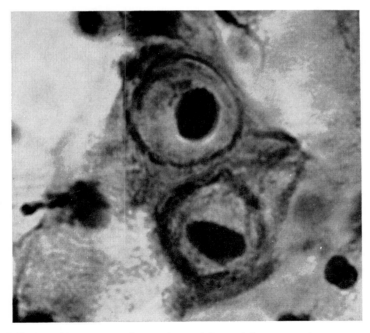

FIG. 35.15. Cells in a Fast smear of a patient with condyloma acuminata. These two huge bizarre cells each have a large intranuclear inclusion body, surrounded by a "halo" of clear parachromatin. The degenerated chromatin is very bland and smudged, and marginates against the nuclear membrane. The cytoplasm is poorly defined. A neutorphil nucleus is evident in the *lower right corner* (Papanicolaou stain, ×1100). (Courtesy of Z. M. Naib.)

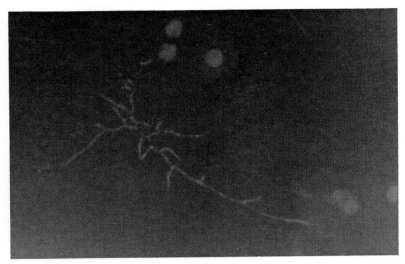

FIG. 35.16. Candida; acridine orange stain viewed with ultraviolet light. The hyphae and yeast buds show brilliantly against the black background, giving a rapid identification under low power (×480).

a Papanicolaou stained cellular spread, the proper method for accurate identification is culture and Gram's stain in the diagnostic microbiology laboratory.

Mycotic Infection. The usual fungus of vulvovaginitis, *Candida albicans*, is best diagnosed by a NaOH crush preparation of a "cotton patch." Its discovery in routine vaginal smears prepared for cancer detection is laborious, fortuitous, and unpredictable. When found it is tentatively identifiable if it consists of both forms: "long" and "round" bodies. The former are septate hyphae, whereas the latter are elongate or budding yeast forms. An excellent method for rapid detection of fungi is the use of acridine orange stain viewed with proper filters in low visible or high ultraviolet light (Fig. 35.16), where a few scattered bodies stand out brilliantly under low power. Other fungi of both the superficial mycoses (dermatophytes) and deep systemic mycoses (actinomycoses, coccidioides, aspergillus, mucor, blastomyces) are found rarely in routine smear, and can be tentatively classified morphologically. Positive identification of all fungi should be made by cultural characteristics. Many contaminating pollens and plant cells closely mimic mycotic morphology.

Mycotic infection becomes more severe during pregnancy.

Protozoal Infections. *Trichomonas vaginalis* produces a true infection involving the tissues in some women, while in others it appears to be merely a superficial symbiote. Its pathogenicity varies according to strain of the organism; it varies between different hosts (patients); and it varies in a given individual according to her state of reaction or of resistance. Its pathogenicity is much more severe in pregnancy and during the late secretory and menstrual phase. The organism can be found in virtually any vaginal pH, but is more florid around 6 or 7. When the vaginal pH changes or other factors become hostile to the organism, it retreats to the endocervix, the urethra, and the glands. Host factors undoubtedly play a great part in its varying degrees of tissue involvement and damage, but the pathogenicity of the organism itself differs greatly among strains.

Its clinical manifestations are found in two major phases, the *florid* vaginitis and the *latent* endocervicitis and urethritis.

During the *florid* vaginitis the patient is troubled and symptomatic. In both the hanging drop and routine vaginal smear, the organisms can usually be identified.

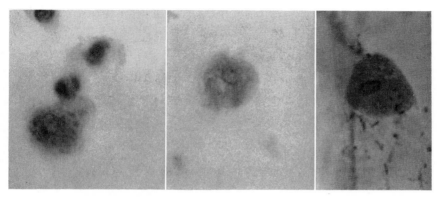

FIG. 35.17. *Trichomonas vaginalis* on a routine Fast smear (single slide, vaginocervical) with Papanicolaou stain. Positive diagnostic identification is to be made only on well preserved organisms with all of the following critical criteria. There is a small, pale but definite, eccentric nucleus; their rounded bodies take a cytoplasmic stain (neither a bare nucleus or mucus) (see Plate XXXV. II B); and they range in size from a neutrophil up to a small parabasal cell (neutrophils in *upper part of left picture*). When a florid vaginitis is not present, they are best found in endocervical material (×700).

Routine vaginal smears reveal an acute, obscuring infection with cellular degeneration, debris and, often, old and new blood. The multinucleated giant cell histiocyte is frequent. The trichomonads are numerous and of a fairly large size but, paradoxically, they may be hard to find and extremely difficult to identify positively in this fixed preparation because of great disruption. For positive identification one must be careful to rule out a bare epithelial cell nucleus, neutrophil, histiocyte, or parabasal cell with a small pyknotic nucleus; each of these can closely mimic a trichomonad in certain circumstances. Flagella, undulating membrane, axostyle, and internal cytoplasmic structures are rarely identified in the routine cytological smear. There are three positive morphological characteristics, however, which are present and are most important for a diagnostic identification (Fig. 35.17): a small pale nucleus must be present which is not pyknotic; the rest of the organism must be definitely cytoplasmic, not vague mucus or a bare epithelial nucleus (Plate XXXV.III *B*). The over-all size falls between that of a neutrophil and a parabasal cell.

During the *latent* phase of infection with *Trichomonas vaginalis* the patient is usually asymptomatic in marked contrast to the symptoms of the florid vaginitis. Mild dysuria may accompany urethral involvement, or a slight discharge may result from a chronic endocervicitis; however, most of these latent infections go unnoticed by both patient and examining physician. The routine Fast smear (single slide, combined vaginocervical, Fig. 35.27) will contain the organism where it can usually be diagnostically identified (Fig. 35.17). In this latent phase, it can also be cultured from endocervical and urethral material. The hanging drop is usually negative, unless adequate endocervical or urethral material is examined. How much of the role of the Trichomonas is saprophytic and how much pathogenic has not been clearly ascertained; furthermore, there is likewise controversy as to the quantity and quality of direct etiologic influence which the organism has in producing dyskaryotic cellular changes and dysplastic tissue alterations. Suffice it to say that while the most frequent cellular change associated with *Trichomonas vaginalis* is that of degeneration, there is an extremely high association of this organism with those bizarre epithelial cell changes within the endocervix which are nondegenerative in nature.

At times cancer is hidden in this obscuring, cell-degenerating infection. The presence of alarming cells bears the same indications for biopsy when Trichomonas is present as it does in the absence of the organism. If in the presence of a severe dysplasia no cancer is found on apparently adequate tissue examination, one must not be content here; by directing intensive therapy at this endocervical infection, a clearer interpretation of the basic cellular change is possible, with identification of the malignant or benign character of any missed remaining lesions. Flagyl is most valuable for such therapy, as its systemic administration is effective in endocervical infections without distorting the picture by such techniques as cauterization. A severe infection with cellular degeneration causes malignant cellular changes to be modified and

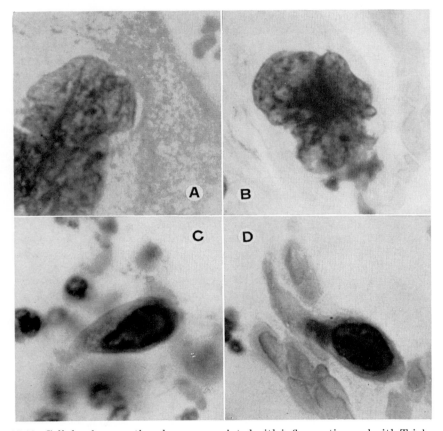

FIG. 35.18. Cellular degenerative changes associated with inflammation and with Trichomonas, causing benign cells (A and C) to take on some neoplastic characteristics and malignant cells (B and D) to lose many diagnostic criteria. A, nuclear size increase and hyperchromasia in a benign cell with degenerative early chromatin smudging, perinuclear "halo," and abundant cytoplasm. The bizarre changes approach those of B. B, a malignant cell with degenerative chromatin smudging in its nucleus. The diagnostic value of the nuclear irregularities, abnormally cleared areas, gigantism, and hyperchromasia is greatly diminished by the loss of sharp detail from degenerative chromatin smudging. C, intense nuclear hyperchromasia from chromatin degeneration in a benign cell with scant cytoplasm. The extreme peripheral smudging and central laking of chromatin bespeak degenerative changes (compare with D). D, degenerative smudging in the nucleus of a malignant tadpole cell from squamous cell carcinoma. The malignant chromatin clumps are so smudged by degeneration that their criteria are inconclusive and are mimicked by the degenerative processes in the benign cell (C).

rendered nondiagnostic; conversely, it produces serious cytological degenerative alterations in benign cells, which can be sufficiently bizarre as to be confusing with cancer (Fig. 35.18).

Helminthic Infestation. At times pinworm and other ova are found in the vaginal vault or picked up on the specimen from the labia. They must not be confused with some pollens or plant cells which might contaminate and which appear morphologically similar. Schistosomes in the bladder and urine have been found in the vaginal pool.

Mixed and Nonspecific Infections. Most infections are mixed. One agent might initiate the process or develop into the major cause of the inflammation, but many are involved in any given case. In spite of some apparently efficacious "shot-gun" therapy now available, it is advantageous to identify certain agents or states in order to direct specific therapy which otherwise might not be included in a general broad spectrum approach. Such is the case for Trichomonas and Candida. Furthermore, recognition of teleatrophy of the aged or the child, so prone to mixed or nonspecific infections, may allow for the production of a lush and resistant epithelium by vaginal estrogens with subsequent disappearance of infection and associated disturbing epithelial reactions. It is important also to recognize the predilection to infection in the pregnant and diabetic states so that appropriate vaginal and cervical therapy may be instituted.

RADIATION CHANGES

General Changes

Ionizing irradiation causes both tissue *damage* of general nature, and tissue *response* of a peculiar host significance. The former, tissue *radiation damage*, ranges from mild and reversible to severe and irreversible leading to death of tissues. It evokes a general inflammatory reaction with leukocytic and fluid outpouring, reflected in the vaginal pool cellular spread as a nonspecific acute inflammation. On the other hand, tissue *radiation response*

reflects the host's response peculiar to such energy and, more specifically, heralds its pattern of reaction to the neoplasm it harbors.

Cellular Response Patterns

Radiation Response. Striking changes occur in cells of benign and malignant tissue *following* irradiation. In therapy for carcinoma of the cervix, the changes which occur in the *nonmalignant* squamous cells (Fig. 35.19) were first shown by Graham to have considerable prognostic correlation. Of greatest significance are these findings when evaluated 10 to 14 days after radium application, and on the 5 days around the last day of external therapy. With these 10-day specimens prepared from the vaginal pool material, the percentage of cells showing the specific radiation response (RR) changes is determined. When good RR (over 70%) is found in patients treated for Stage II carcinoma of the cervix, approximately 80% are alive and well after 5 years. When poor RR is found in the same Stage II group of patients, about 80% are dead within 5 years. The highest degree of RR correlation with salvage is found in Stage II. Many workers (Kjellgren, Nielsen, Merrill and Wood) have corroborated these findings, and they appear to be well established.

Sensitization Response. *Prior* to irradiation for cervical carcinoma, morphological changes may be discerned in normal parabasal cells. Graham named this "sensitivity to radiation" (SR) and found a high correlation with both the host response to subsequent irradiation (RR) and the prognosis of host ability to overcome its tumor (survival).

Since the initial work, many investigators have repeated various studies of radiation response. Very careful and meticulous cytological observation and correlation with follow-up has clearly established certain relationships—others remain obscure. The significance of the SR, in the Grahams' hands, is high; others' results are disappointing and probably represent subjective differences in cellular evaluation. On the other hand,

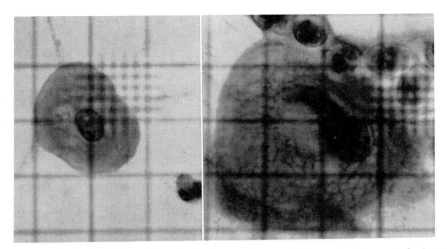

FIG. 35.19. Cellular response to irradiation in carcinoma of the cervix. Many of the important features of radiation response (RR) are present in these two nonmalignant parabasal cells from a vaginal pool smear, Papanicolaou stained. *Left*, an untreated parabasal cell and neutrophil taken on first day of therapy. *Right*, parabasal cell and neutrophils following external irradiation therapy. The cytoplasm has swollen and is vacuolated. The nucleus has also swollen, is folded and distorted. Neutrophils have swollen (×1100).

results of RR when carefully done appear to be consistently corroborative.

Buccal Irradiation. Jones *et al.* have demonstrated that cellular changes on a buccal smear, following single dose irradiation of the buccal mucosa at the start of cervical irradiation, closely correlate with survival in carcinoma of the cervix. By using this method, some disadvantages of vaginal smears are overcome; but of perhaps greater importance, this clearly indicates a basic host factor complex taking place in the patients overcoming cancer with the help of irradiation. Normal epithelial cells of the buccal mucosa react in manners which herald the ability of this host to handle its carcinoma in the pelvis—a "body" away.

Endocrine-Radiation Host Response Relationships

The cytohormonal patterns, both *before* radiation therapy and during the months *following* therapy, have high correlation with patient survival. Graham found that patients with an M.I. shift to the left, with increased parabasal cell exfoliation *before* radiation therapy, had a good cellular RR during therapy and a high survival rate. When not normally

present, this M.I. shift to the left and an increase in SR were accomplished by administration of androgens and vitamin E before radiation therapy. This was also followed by good RR after therapy and increased survival.

After radiation therapy to the cervix, the M.I. usually shifts to the left toward teleatrophy (100/0/0). If this were due merely to ovarian irradiation with functional oophorectomy, the M.I. shift would be to the midzone producing estratrophy (0/100/0). That it progresses toward teleatrophy is, at least in part, due to direct radiation injury to the vaginal epithelium. It is significant to note that this pattern of teleatrophy is usually present in those patients whose tumor is conquered, while a persistent M.I. shift to the right is found in patients harboring residual cancer. Wachtel and others find a high correlation between this persistence of the M.I. to the right following full therapy, and tumor recurrence.

NEOPLASIAS AND RELATED LESIONS

In the detection, diagnosis, and study of the biological behavior of neoplastic lesions of the genital tract, exfoliative cytology offers many unique advantages and opportunities.

First, a properly taken cellular sample provides surface biopsy material from a *wide* area of epithelium, rather than the restricted limits of a small excised bit of tissue. This makes possible the detection of early, small, or hidden lesions.

Second, when proper cellular material is available which is adequate, well preserved, and evaluated by qualified individuals, definitive diagnoses can be made which are as reliable as those based upon proper tissue biopsy, and frequently more comprehensive in biological information. Therapy is to be based upon tissue biopsy study of the disease whenever possible, however, to determine its exact anatomical *location* and to assure complete evaluation as to the *nature* and *extent* of the most serious lesion.

Third, as the lesion is not altered from biopsy interference, it can be left intact to continue its normal growth during the study of exfoliated elements. In this way, biological behavior can be closely observed and followed without fear of biopsy disturbance or even removal of essential parts of the lesion. As knowledge and experience with the exfoliated elements from lesions grow, our correlation of cellular pattern with existing tissue pattern becomes definite and closer to absolute.

For study of tissue, either cellular or surgical, one must carefully choose the biopsy material as to site, adequacy of amount, and quality of preservation. A cellular specimen for routine use must be adequate, containing material from both the vaginal pool (for endocrine, endometrial, and ovarian determinations) and endocervical-external os-exocervical scrapings (for cervical lesions). For routine gynecological work the Fast smear (single slide, combined vagino-cervical, see p. 710) has been very satisfactory. It provides more material for examination than most multiple slide techniques, with less time expended by the clinician, cytotechnologist, and pathologist.

Immediate fixation is necessary for the fine nuclear detail of adequate, satisfactory specimens. *Ethyl* alcohol, 95%, has been found to be most satisfactory. It can be disastrous to dry *before* fixation, even for fractions of a second, as there is no satisfactory method for reconstitution without sacrificing quality. One needs all the assistance possible to extract every bit of evidence from the cells, and should not be handicapped with material degenerated by drying or improper fixation. On the other hand, *after* immediate and proper fixation, the specimens can then be air-dried for transportation without sacrifice in quality.

Cervix Uteri

Anatomical Considerations. The junction of the noncornified, stratified squamous epithelium with the columnar epithelium is present *near* the external os. At times columnar epithelium presents itself on the pars vaginalis (ectropion, etc.) bringing portions of the squamocolumnar junction into view. In the presence of persistent and chronic cervicitis, areas of columnar epithelium in the endocervical canal may become tongues and islands of stratified squamous epithelium through the process of *metaplasia*. Also the squamous epithelium of the exocervix may extend up the canal, through the process of *epidermidization*. Thus by both processes, squamocolumnar junctions may exist high up in the canal, even centimeters above the external os. Most are confined to the distal 2 cm., but still remain hidden from even the experienced and careful examiner's view. This area is also hidden from careful colposcopic examination.

Early carcinomas and *severe dysplasias* are found here, in these important areas of squamocolumnar junction (Johnson *et al.*, Marsh; Carson and Gall; Fennell; Przybora and Plutowa; Pund and Auerbach; Gusberg and Moore; Fluhmann), hidden from the clinician's view but easily accessible to proper cellular examination.

For cervical disease, therefore, a satisfactory cellular sample must contain adequate material from this *endo*cervical area as *high* up the canal as the cervical instrument will allow (Figs. 35.27 and 35.28). Lesions on the exocervix of the portio vaginalis are visible for biopsy; but it is the first 1 or 2 cm. of the *endo-cervical* canal *proximal* to the external os which must be carefully examined cytologically for lesions.

DYSPLASIA, CARCINOMA IN SITU, AND INVASIVE CARCINOMA. Dysplasia, used in the broad sense of the International Committee (Wied 1958), includes such "shades-of-gray" lesions as regenerative, defensive, and neoplastic epithelial reactions. Morphologically they include epidermidization and squamous metaplasia with varying degrees of atypia, transitional metaplasia, atypical regeneration, atypical hyperplasia, prosoplasia, dysplasia, pseudoepitheliomatous hyperplasia squamous cell hyperactivity, basal cell hyperactivity, reserve cell hyperplasia, and subcylindrical cell anaplasia.

While this "shades-of-gray" spectrum morphologically runs imperceptibly into carcinoma in situ, their separation must be attempted morphologically, and correlated on the biological basis of reversibility *versus* irreversibility.

As this is true with the histopathologic study of surgically removed tissues, so it is true with the cytopathologic study of cellular specimens.

One of the most valuable features which is well correlated with biologic behavior in the critical zone between severe dysplasia and carcinoma in situ, is the ability for cells to *mature* in *orderly* fashion throughout *all* layers of the epithelium. Thus carcinoma in situ tissue sections have extremely scanty cytoplasm in all layers with extreme crowding, loss of stratification, and loss of polarity. In exfoliated material this phenomenon of loss of orderly maturation is reflected in the loss of cytoplasmic maturation with extremely scant cytoplasm, high nucleo-cytoplasmic (N/C) ratio, and loss of squamification or columnarization in individual cells (Figs. 35.20 and 35.21).

Cells of this "shades-of-gray" spectrum and carcinoma in situ have a peculliar type of nucleus, forms of which have

been described variously by Papanicolaou as a dyskaryotic cell, Graham as a "third type" cell, and Reagan as an "impending prophase." Cells shed from an invasive squamous cell carcinoma have a characteristically different nucleus (Fig. 35.22 and Plate XXXV.III, *B* and *C*).

Only rarely are epithelial changes in a cervix of purely one type, but usually represent mixtures of the "shades-of-gray" lesions, at times including carcinoma in situ and, less often, invasive carcinoma. This has been well shown by Hertig *et al.*, McKay *et al.*, Galvin *et al.* and others who have serially sectioned cervices and plotted the anatomical distribution of these lesion variants. This mixture of epithelial lesions is directly reflected in the cellular spread.

It is important to realize that the presence of *only* dysplastic cells in a patient's smear does *not* rule out carcinoma, as exfoliated material from carcinoma in situ also contains dysplastic cells and a small area can easily be missed in obtaining the cellular sample with loss of representation in the cell population available for examination. Likewise, if cells from dysplasia and from carcinoma in situ are present, they indicate the presence of carcinoma in situ but do *not* rule out invasive cancer. However, experience has shown that, with adequate cellular samples, both of these situations have around 95% correlation with the highest lesion represented on the cell spread to be the highest lesion histologically demonstrable. Accuracy of this correlation is directly proportional to *adequacy* of cellular sample *and* interpretation. The clinical preparation of an adequate and satisfactory specimen is thus of fundamental importance. With proper material and interpretation, detection of these early endocervical lesions is over 97% (see "Clinical Preparation of Specimens").

Adenocarcinoma of the cervix at times has a fairly characteristic cell type. Its cytological pick-up is good, especially with adequately high endocervical specimens. Mixed, or mucoepidermoid, car-

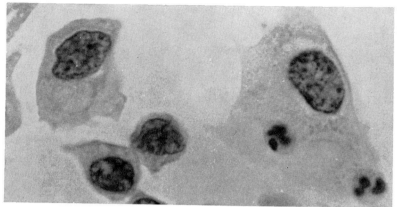

FIG. 35.20. Dyskaryotic cells shed from a "shades-of-gray" lesion (severe dysplasia) of the cervix. Many malignant criteria are present in these dyskaryotic nuclei, such as coarse granularity of the chromatin, increase in nuclear size, nuclear membrane irregularities, and hyperchromasia; but each whole cell does not admit to a diagnosis of malignancy. The cell on the *right* has mature squamous cytoplasm, a mature squamous dyskaryotic cell; the cell in the *upper left* has moderately mature cytoplasm, a moderately mature dyskaryotic cell; the two cells in the lower left have scanty immature cytoplasm, immature dyskaryotic cells (×1200).

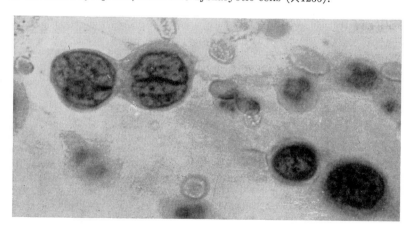

FIG. 35.21. Diagnostic cells shed from a carcinoma in situ of the cervix. Essentially the same malignant criteria are present in these nuclei as are present in the "shades-of-gray" lesions (see Fig. 35.21); but cytoplasm is completely immature with a nucleocytoplasmic ratio high enough for the whole cell to admit to a diagnosis of malignancy. Note the extremely scanty cytoplasm of the cell in the *lower right* (×1200).

cinomas enjoy the same high degree of cellular detection (Howdon *et al.*)

For greater detail regarding diagnostic cytomorphology, consult specific texts (Papanicolaou, 1954; Koss, 1961; Frost, 1961, 1962; Graham, 1963).

Pregnancy Considerations. The visit which is *earliest* in the pregnancy is the best time to obtain a cytological specimen.

Cervical infections increase as pregnancy progresses, with resulting obscuring and degeneration of cellular samples. An early cellular examination obviates much of this cellular distortion. It also gives more opportunity to clear inflammation, if necessary, or to carry out any therapeutic or diagnostic procedures indicated.

The incidence of cervical carcinoma is

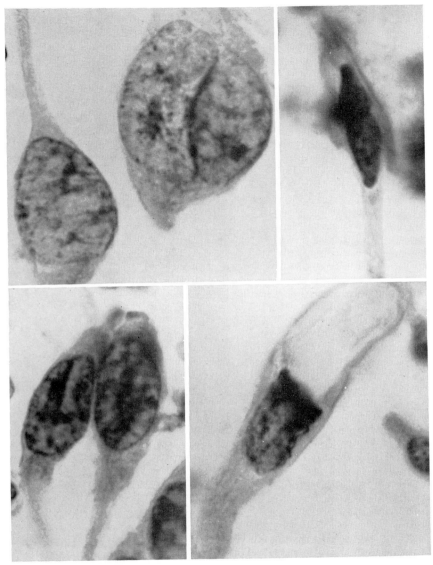

FIG. 35.22. Cells shed from invasive squamous cell carcinoma. The nuclei are of bizarre shapes, have angular and distorted membranes of varying thickness, contain huge and irregular chromatin aggregates and nucleoli, and have abnormally cleared areas of parachromatin. Nuclei in cells shown in *upper right* and *lower right* photomicrographs are becoming pyknotic. The cytoplasm is asymmetrical, with bizarre and uncontrolled squamous cell maturation of thinning and keratinization with, in the *lower right*, ectoendoplasm and beginning formation of a fibullar apparatus of the tail extending downward (×1200).

appreciable even though pregnant patients are of a young age group. Spjut *et al.* found 7 carcinomas in situ among 3,000 pregnant women, 2.3 per 1,000. Schmitz, Isaacs, and Fetherston found 12 invasive and 13 in situ carcinomas among 10,369 obstetrical patients, 2.4. per 1,000. Among 2,828 consecutive private and clinic patients at the Johns Hopkins Hospital, 10 were found by a routine Fast smear to have carcinoma of the cervix, 3.5 per 1,000; on tissue examination, 6 of these were in situ, 2 were in situ with questionable invasion, and 2 were frankly invasive. At the University Hospital in Baltimore carcinoma of the cervix was cytologically detected in a 16-year-old pregnant patient who, in spite of prompt and full therapy, died 2 years later of recurrent disease.

Dysplasias, while they are no different than in the nonpregnant patient, seem to progress in atypicality during pregnancy and then may regress in the postpartum months. This regression usually is not complete and with each subsequent pregnancy the cervical dysplasia may begin at a more atypical level.

There appears to be *no* innocuous atypical cellular change which is specific for, characteristic of, or caused by pregnancy. A careful cytological and histological evaluation is as indicated in patients with severe atypicalities during pregnancy, as in those of the nonpregnant state. Present knowledge of these sinister lesions is far too meager for dogmatism.

Recurrence of Carcinoma Following therapy. Carcinoma of the cervix recurring *within* the lumen of the genital tract is cytologically detected to a high degree, provided sufficient and proper cellular specimens are examined—frequently before gross evidence is present. Extraluminal recurrences are, of course, not detected vaginally.

Usually, the recurrences are of the original histological variety; frequently they can recur as an extremely small and undifferentiated type, which may be difficult to distinguish from reactive histiocytes. Koss has pointed out that occasionally an invasive carcinoma recurs as an in situ lesion. The question of a recurrence *versus* a second primary always arises. Because of persisting radiation cellular changes, interpretation of postradiation specimens may be most difficult and the unwary may overcall reaction. On the other hand, however, the small undifferentiated carcinoma cells may be missed or mistaken for histio-

cytes. It is a very frequent cell type, unfortunately, in recurring or residual carcinoma. When carefully done, however, the accuracy rate is similar to that of initial detection.

Vagina and Labia

Dermatoses, dysplasias, carcinoma in situ, and invasive carcinoma are usually easily detected and diagnosed by biopsy in these areas. Depending upon the site of the lesion, either a vaginal pool smear or a direct scraping yields good cytological diagnosis. A direct scraping of a leukoplakic or condylomatous lesion may be necessary to insure cellular representation of the entire lesion; such a specimen, taken in conjunction with tissue examination of the lesion, augments and tends to compensate for the patchy nature of biopsies. Use of normal saline, to moisten growing margins of a labial lesion before scraping and to remove keratotic and necrotic debris, is suggested for obtaining satisfactory cells. A cotton swab dipped in egg albumen or serum, or a wooden or plastic spatula, are good instruments for preparing these specimens.

Endometrium

Related Findings other than Specific Cells. Atypical hyperplasia and adenocarcinoma are not associated with teleatrophy, even in the very aged. At times the associated *cytohormonal pattern* is bizarre enough for the M.I. to fall to the right of normal limits. When one is aware of the significance, this finding can account for an additional 15 to 20% detection (see "Endocrine Evaluation" and "Clinical Preparations").

The finding of *endometrial-type cells* at a time in the cycle other than during menses is abnormal. Degenerated endometrial cells may be found 3 or 4 days after bleeding stops. In the luteal phase, however, their presence is distinctly abnormal. The cytological distinction between these degenerating endometrial cells shed at the end of menses, poorly preserved cells from endometrial hyperplasia, and degenerating adenocarcinoma can be very difficult at times. This may reflect a poor state of preservation resulting from long travel down the canal, a difficult histological differentiation in the given case, or both.

The term "*endometrial-type cell*" is useful to connote a cell-type (including: atypical endocervicals, atypical endometrials, bizarre histiocytes) whose exact identity is not obvious, but one cannot definitally rule out endometrial disease. When found in the cell spread, further identification is necessary.

Bleeding is a frequent occurrence with endometrial lesions. It is important, thus, that cellular specimens be taken at any time the patient is seen, menstruating or not; however, as a bloody smear may be less than satisfactory and may have to be repeated later, the patient should be alerted for the possible necessity of repeating the specimen to allay anxiety if that should become necessary.

To take a smear when bleeding is present is well worth the possibility of an occasional unsatisfactory specimen. Many times the bloody smear is the only one to contain diagnostic cells.

Clinical Specimen Preparations of Choice for Endometrial Carcinoma. As opposed to cervical carcinoma, cervical scrapings yield a poor detection of endometrial carcinoma; vaginal pool specimens are better, and endometrial specimens are optimal.

As a *routine* procedure in the study of *endometrial* disease, *vaginal pool* material, with its clinical simplicity, is the best suited either as a separate smear or as a combined Fast smear. As a special procedure, however, endometrial aspiration or endometrial brush techniques give superb cellular samples. For a routine detection and cellular study, the vaginal pool contains identifiable cells in 75% of the cases (Fig. 35.23) and, with the added evaluation for abnormal cytohormonal pattern (above), it detects over 90% of endometrial adenocarcinomas.

Endometrial specimens obtained directly from the cavity (*via* aspiration, brush, irrigation techniques) yield superb cellular samples. They are, how-ever, sufficiently more difficult and time-consuming that they do not lend themselves well as a *routine* screening procedure of all asymptomatic women. Furthermore, they should *never* replace a dilatation and curettage, when that procedure is indicated. They are very valuable in detecting over 97% of endometrial carcinomas, and should be in everyone's armamentarium. Before their use, of course, intrauterine pregnancy must be excluded.

A well prepared Fast combined vagino-cervical smear is thus well suited as a routine examination specimen as it contains not only a cellular scraping of the endocervical canal and external os for cervical disease, but also an adequate vaginal pool sample.

Placenta

During the first trimester, trophoblast cells are not infrequent in vaginal pool specimens. Their presence may indicate a low lying placenta or a threatened abortion, but they are also present in some pregnancies which continue as apparently perfectly normal. They have been found in hydatidiform moles, but cytology has been of very little assistance in predicting the grade of mole or the presence of a choriocarcinoma. The presence of decidual cells is of little significance.

Miscellaneous Uterine Lesions

Myomas and endometriosis at times are found to be associated with a peculiar cytohormonal pattern, with the M.I. shifted to the right. Most of the cases fall within normal limits. Leiomyosarcomas, mixed mesodermal sarcomas, and carcinosarcomas may shed diagnostic cells into the vaginal pool. Usually there is quite a bit of necrosis with cellular breakdown, so that cytological pick-up of sarcomas is discouraging unless the cervix or vault is involved to allow a viable surface scraping.

Sarcomas usually shed cells which are undifferentiated. On occasion the exfoliated cells do manifest differentiating

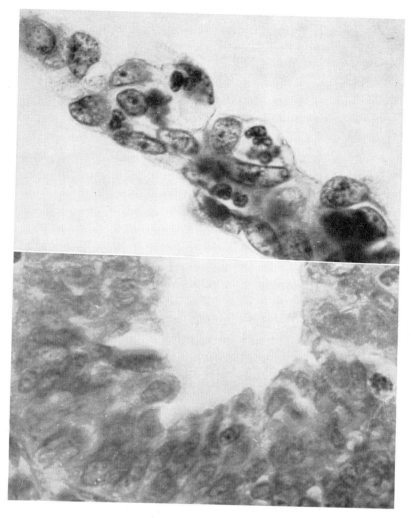

FIG. 35.23. Adenocarcinoma of the endometrium, in an 80-year-old patient. The cytohormonal pattern was distinctly abnormal with a maturation index of $\overrightarrow{0/77/23}$ shifted toward the right. *Upper*, cells present on a Fast smear. Nuclear malignant criteria marked. Hyperdistended secretory vacuoles contain neutrophils which are phagocytosing the mucus in the intact secretory cell. *Lower*, tissue obtained at dilatation and curettage, showing malignant gland lined by cells having many malignant criteria. The whole cells are not available, as in the cellular spread, so that malignant criteria are less pronounced. Note mitosis on *right* and hyperdistended secretory cell at lumen on *left* (×1200).

characteristics such as fat, myofibrils, cross striations, etc., sufficient to suspect, or even diagnose, tumor-type. The finding of a *biphasic* cellular pattern with both sarcomal cells and adenocarcinoma cells, should make one consider a mixed mesodermal tumor (Howdon *et al.*).

Fallopian Tubes

Adenocarcinoma of the oviducts at times will shed diagnostic cells into the vaginal pool. It is usually associated with a watery discharge. The vaginal cytohormonal pattern may be that of an abnormal M.I. shift to the right. Unexplained adenocarcinoma cells or an abnormal cytohormonal pattern in a vaginal specimen should provoke consideration of a lesion of the Fallopian tube.

Ovaries

Tumors of the ovary which produce hormones, express their presence by a cytohormonal pattern characteristic for the endocrine substances being secreted. Granulosa cell tumors shift the M.I. to the right (toward $\overrightarrow{0/0/100}$) depending upon the amount of circulating estrogens, their biologic activity, and the age of the patient. Luteinized mesenchymal tumors shift the M.I. toward the midzone (toward $\overrightarrow{0/100/0}$) if progesterone alone is

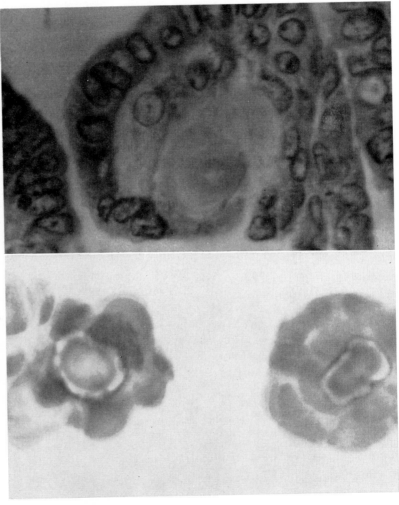

FIG. 35.24. Psammoma bodies present in peritoneal fluid of a patient with a serous cystadenocarcinoma of the ovary. *Upper*, a papillary frond in tissue section with one psammoma body. *Lower*, two psammoma bodies and associated cellular groups which exfoliated into the peritoneal cavity. The peritoneal fluid was extremely bloody and, as this was the first paracentesis, the cells had sat in this degenerating fluid for a period of time sufficient to lose their fine nuclear detail. Their general nuclear outline is evident enough, however, to demonstrate severe molding and size variation (×1200).

being produced, or give a mixed pattern if estrogens are also secreted. Hilar cell tumors and arrhenoblastomas may show the M.I. "spread" pattern of androgen (toward $\overleftrightarrow{33/34/33}$) or the shift to the left (toward $\overleftarrow{100/0/0}$). These hormone-producing tumors of the ovary do not shed diagnostic cells into the vaginal pool, the abnormal cytohormonal pattern being all that is present; however, abnormal columnar cells frequently do appear in the vaginal specimen, shed from the endometrial hyperplasia which is frequently associated with the abnormal endocrine milieu, and may be noted as "endometrial-type cells".

Tumors of the ovary *without known hormone* production, paradoxically, are also frequently found in an abnormal cytohormonal M.I. shift to the right. These not only include the solid and cystic adenomas and adenocarcinomas, but tumors metastatic to the ovary and other lesions. There is evidence that the ovarian stroma may be stimulated into increased steroid production by the presence of such lesions. Furthermore, when the tissues of Müllerian origin of an individual have increased sensitivity to estrogens, an otherwise normal endocrine milieu produces an abnormal response of these structures. This can result in a shift to the right of the M.I. and hyperplastic lesions of the endometrium, tubes, and ovaries.

About one-half of the time the M.I. is sufficiently shifted to the right to be abnormal (Fig. 35.11). Cells exfoliate from these tumors into the peritoneal cavity, where they can be detected in culdocentesis, or travel down the tubes to appear in the vaginal pool. The serous cystadenocarcinomas may shed psammoma bodies with their cellular groups (Fig. 35.24).

About one-third of the patients with ovarian cancer shed recognizably abnormal cells into the vaginal pool specimen, while an additional third have an abnormal M.I. only. By observing *both* abnormal cells and abnormal cytohormonal pattern, over 60% of the ovarian lesions are detectable by using specimens with vaginal pool component (Rubin and Frost).

Abnormal Patterns Associated with Malignancies. CYTOHORMONAL PATTERNS. Even in the absence of cells exfoliated from a tumor surface, there may be an abnormal *cytohormonal pattern* which should arouse suspicion. In addition to the ovarian, tubal, and endometrial lesions noted above, one must also be alerted for adrenal, hypophysial, and mammary tumors (see "Endocrine Evaluation by Cytohormonal Studies").

SEROUS, BLOODY, DEGENERATING, AND OBSCURING PATTERNS. These nonspecific patterns frequently accompany neoplasms without diagnostic cells being present. Paradoxically, some of the largest and most invasive tumors present in this fashion, with necrotic cellular debris and serosanguineous fluid the only material from the lesion. These patterns are *serious warnings* which mandate repeat cellular examinations attempts to clear the condition sufficiently to identify cellular elements, and/or adequate biopsy or dilatation and curettage, depending upon the nature of the case.

Microscopic Aspects. Because of limited space and the clinical nature of this text, more detailed microscopic aspects (Fig. 35.25) will not be dealt with here but can be found elsewhere (Papanicoulaou, 1954 and supplements; Koss, 1961; Frost, 1961 and 1962; Graham, 1963).

CLINICAL PREPARATION OF SPECIMENS

When to Take Specimens for Routine Detection and Diagnosis

Contraindications. A carefully taken gynecological specimen may be obtained at virtually *any* time. It should be taken when the opportunity first arises, rather than being postponed for minor reasons. Certain conditions such as recent douche or active menstrual flow do yield a higher percentage of unsatisfactory specimens, so that at times they are referred to as

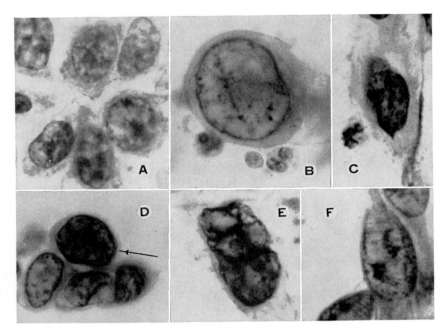

FIG. 35.25. General criteria of malignancy. *A*, undifferentiated cells with scant cytoplasm and indistinct borders. There is a moderate nuclear size variation. Note irregular chromatin patterns with large cleared areas and chromatin clumps with sharp points and angles. Nuclear rims vary abruptly in thickness. *B*, nucleocytoplasmic ratio high in a large cell. Although the nuclear pattern is bland, the total chromatin is increased and there are large, abnormally cleared areas and chromatin spindles. *C*, the nuclear outline is irregular with a sharp, pointed angle protruding. *D*, prominent chromatin clumping with abnormally cleared areas; sharp, angled nucleolus to the right of the largest nucleus; very scant cytoplasm with poor borders; crowding. *E*, marked hyperchromasia with chromatin clumping and sharply delineated parachromatin. Two nucleoli are large and prominent. They are perfectly round, however, and offer no diagnostic assistance. *F*, well preserved sharp, pointed nucleoli and chromatin clumps with abnormal clearing. Marked cytoplasmic attenuation over nuclear sides (×1200).

contraindications; however, in such situations one should take a specimen, with full understanding that it may have to be repeated, and arrange with the patient for a repeat cellular examination at the proper time and with proper preparation.

Bleeding is thus *not* a contraindication, although sometimes a repeat cellular sample may be necessary for a satisfactory examination. Although it is theoretically ideal to avoid menstruation, some cancers shed diagnostic cells *only* during the time of bleeding. Harsh scraping to produce excessive hemorrhage or trauma to the tissues is to be avoided, of course. Bleeding, rather than being a contraindication to cell examination, is itself a strong indication for the consultation.

Douching also is *not* a contraindication. Whereas for certain things it is preferable that the patient refrain from douching for about 24 hours, cell spreads should be prepared even if it is determined that she had just douched. Remarks should be made on the consultation request to that effect, and the patient should be advised that another specimen will have to be obtained after an interval of 24 hours without a douche. Very little change is usually made in the endocervical scraping specimen, but the vaginal pool is frequently useless for cytohormonal evaluation, endometrial lesions, and ovarian disease in an immediate postdouche specimen.

Pregnancy. The *first visit* of a patient *during* her pregnancy is the best time for a cell examination. It should include a *high* endocervical scraping component, unless specifically contraindicated by an obstetrical difficulty, as many early lesions of pregnancy lie within the canal. While the cervix everts, cervical infections tend to increase in severity as the pregnancy progresses, causing increased difficulty of interpretation and obscuring

of diagnostic material. Examination early in pregnancy will allow adequate time to clear any obscuring conditions, determine underlying lesions, and institute proper therapy. After delivery, cervical lacerations and infections take many weeks or even months to heal sufficiently to provide a satisfactory cellular examination of cervical lesions. At the 6-week visit a repeat cellular examination should be performed, regardless of previous findings.

Frequency of Repeat Examination.

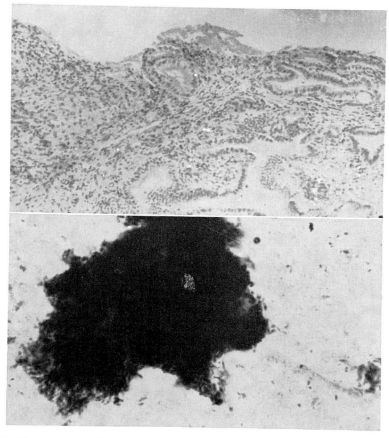

Fig. 35.26. *Upper, unsatisfactory* endocervical biopsy following antiseptic (alcohol) cotton pledget "gently" placed in canal to reduce bacterial contamination before procedure. Lumen, *above;* stroma, *below.* The lumenal epithelium, for which the biopsy was obtained, is entirely missing; the endocervical glands and stroma, only, are intact. *Lower,* same patient; the cotton pledget was rinsed in saline, which was then passed through a Millipore-SM cellulose membrane filter. A large sheet of basal cell hyperactivity epithelium, (a "shades-of-gray" or dysplastic lesion) and numerous endocervical cells are present, which should have been intact on the biopsy (*upper*), for a satisfactory epithelial diagnosis (×30).

Following completely negative cellular examinations, the frequency with which routine cytopathology consultation should be requested must be individualized. The interval to be considered for any one *asymptomatic* patient following *negative* cellular examination usually falls between 6 months and 2 years. The chosen interval mainly depends upon age, but also upon various other factors such as parity, previous or present disease, dependability of revisit, etc. The availability of cytopathological consultation should *not* have to be a factor at this time for the clinician to consider.

Biopsy, Conization, Dilatation, and Curettage

Cytopathology and histopathology are complementary, not competitive, so that tissue confirmation of cytological findings should be sought at all times for determination of extent, degree of invasiveness, and localization of the lesion. As the early endocervical lesions (dysplasias and in situ) are extremely friable and easily rub off on even gentle manipulation, endocervical biopsies or conization should be obtained *before any* instrumentation or dilitation of the canal. The vaginal epithelium and the pars vaginalis of the cervix should be well cleansed; but the external os and the endocervical canal should *not* be touched by anything for cleansing (Fig. 35.26), for dilatation, or for curettage before obtaining the cervical biopsy.

Minimal clean-up and trauma of any kind should therefore be the rule in obtaining cytological and pathological specimens. Indications and technique for biopsy, conization, and curettage have been discussed in preceding chapters.

Technique for Proper Cellular Specimen

So many methods have been devised and advocated for preparation of specimens for cellular examination that it at first appears confusing. Before deciding upon the form of gynecological cell specimen to prepare, one must have clearly in mind what type of information he wishes to obtain.

Routine and Specific Information. An ideal procedure should encompass all realms of desired information adequately, and yet be sufficiently simple to be used in a general gynecological examination for *routine* all-inclusive gynecological cellular examination. The *Fast smear* (Fig. 35.27) with its two specimens (vaginal pool material and endocervical scraping sample) mixed on one slide, is most convenient and valuable in this regard. The *upper* portion of the cell spread, along the edge of the slide away from the endocervical mixture, is pure *vaginal pool* material. This gives an accurate hormonal evaluation, adjudgment of radiation response, determination of sex, detection of endometrial hyperplasia and cancer (90%), and detection of salpingeal and ovarian lesions (60%). The lower portion of the cell spread contains a rich and well preserved endocervical component, giving high detection of carcinoma of the cervix (97%) and associated lesions.

Special Indications. A few techniques have proved themselves to be of outstanding value in well chosen instances: cervical neoplasia (endocervical scraping, swab, aspiration), endometrial neoplasia (vaginal pool; endometrial aspiration, irrigation; brush), salpingeal and ovarian neoplasia (vaginal pool culdocentesis), localization of inflammatory site and determination of etiological agents (V-C-E, differential direct swab), endocrine evaluation (vaginal pool, lateral vaginal wall), daily cytohormonal evaluation (serial vaginal pool aspirations by patient), evaluation of tissue capacity for response to irradiation (vaginal pool, buccal scraping), determination of chromosomal sex (vaginal pool, buccal scraping), population surveys (irrigation smear).

Specific Clinical Cyto-Preparatory Techniques

Fast Smear (Single Slide, Combined Vaginocervical, Routine). This

£ 12800   17/11/06 $ 16
            22075